MASTER TECHNIQUES IN ORTHOPAEDIC SURGERY

■

THE SHOULDER

Second Edition

MASTER TECHNIQUES IN ORTHOPAEDIC SURGERY

Series Editor
Roby C. Thompson, Jr., M.D.

THE FOOT AND ANKLE
Second Edition: Harold B. Kitaoka, M.D.
First Edition: Kenneth A. Johnson, M.D.

RECONSTRUCTIVE KNEE SURGERY
Douglas W. Jackson, M.D.

KNEE ARTHROPLASTY
Second Edition: Paul A. Lotke, M.D. and Jess H. Lonner, M.D.
First Edition: Paul A. Lotke, M.D.

THE HIP
Clement B. Sledge, M.D.

THE SPINE
Second Edition: David S. Bradford, M.D. and Thomas A. Zdeblick, M.D.
First Edition: David S. Bradford, M.D.

THE SHOULDER
Edward V. Craig, M.D.

THE ELBOW
Bernard F. Morrey, M.D.

THE WRIST
Richard H. Gelberman, M.D.

THE HAND
Second Edition: James W. Strickland, M.D. and Thomas J. Graham, M.D.
First Edition: James W. Strickland, M.D.

FRACTURES
Donald A. Wiss, M.D.

THE SHOULDER

Second Edition

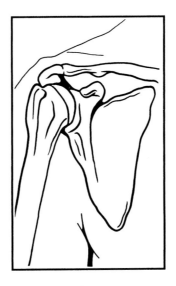

Editor

EDWARD V. CRAIG, M.D.
Professor of Clinical Surgery
Department of Orthopaedics
Weill Medical College of Cornell University
Attending Surgeon
Hospital for Special Surgery
New York, New York

Illustrators

Elizabeth Dempsey
Joel Herring
Robert W. Williams

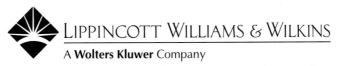

LIPPINCOTT WILLIAMS & WILKINS
A **Wolters Kluwer** Company
Philadelphia · Baltimore · New York · London
Buenos Aires · Hong Kong · Sydney · Tokyo

Acquisitions Editor: James Merritt
Developmental Editor: Grace Caputo
Production Editor: Elaine Verriest McClusky
Manufacturing Manager: Ben Rivera
Cover Designer: Karen Quigley
Compositor: Maryland Composition
Printer: Walsworth Publishing Co.

© 2004 by LIPPINCOTT WILLIAMS & WILKINS
530 Walnut Street
Philadelphia, PA 19106 USA
LWW.com

Printed and bound in the United States of America

Library of Congress Cataloging-in-Publication Data

The shoulder / editor, Edward V. Craig; illustrators, Elizabeth Dempsey, Joel Herring,
    Robert W. Williams.—2nd ed.
        p. ; cm.—(Master techniques in orthopaedic surgery)
    Includes bibliographical references and index.
    ISBN 0-7817-3590-4
        1. Shoulder—Surgery. I. Craig, Edward V. II. Master techniques in orthopaedic surgery
    (2nd ed.)
        [DNLM: 1. Shoulder—surgery. 2. Orthopedics—methods. WE 810 S558611 2003]
    RD557.5.S49 2003
    617.5′72059—dc21

                                                                                        2003050634

Care has been taken to confirm the accuracy of the information presented and to describe generally accepted practices. However, the authors, editor, and publisher are not responsible for errors or omissions or for any consequences from application of the information in this book and make no warranty, expressed or implied, with respect to the currency, completeness, or accuracy of the contents of the publication. Application of this information in a particular situation remains the professional responsibility of the practitioner.

The authors, editor, and publisher have exerted every effort to ensure that drug selection and dosage set forth in this text are in accordance with current recommendations and practice at the time of publication. However, in view of ongoing research, changes in government regulations, and the constant flow of information relating to drug therapy and drug reactions, the reader is urged to check the package insert for each drug for any change in indications and dosage and for added warnings and precautions. This is particularly important when the recommended agent is a new or infrequently employed drug.

Some drugs and medical devices presented in this publication have Food and Drug Administration (FDA) clearance for limited use in restricted research settings. It is the responsibility of the health care provider to ascertain the FDA status of each drug or device planned for use in their clinical practice.

10 9 8 7 6 5 4 3 2 1

Second editions mark time's passage. Some things change. Shoulder surgery certainly has. Fortunately, some things don't change. This book remains dedicated to the people who have been my "constants." To my wife Kathryn, partner and friend to me; mother and role model to our daughters. To Mackenzie, Kelsey, and Taylor, who have grown from "my trifecta of little girls" to delightful preteens and teenagers. Thank you for what you have given me and for helping me to keep my work in perspective.

■

CONTENTS

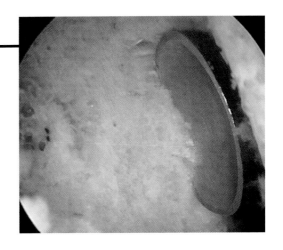

PART I   ARTHROSCOPY

CONTRIBUTORS

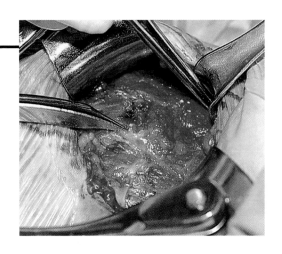

David Altchek, M.D.
Associate Attending Surgeon and Assistant Attending Surgeon, Department of Orthopaedics, Hospital for Special Surgery, New York, New York

Robert H. Bell, M.D.
Associate Professor, Department of Orthopaedics, Northeast Ohio Universities College of Medicine; and Chief, Shoulder Service, Crystal Clinic and Summa Health System, Akron, Ohio

Louis U. Bigliani, M.D.
Professor and Chairman, Department of Orthopaedic Surgery, Columbia University Center for Shoulder, Elbow and Sports Medicine; and Director, Orthopaedic Surgery Service, Columbia-Presbyterian Medical Center, New York, New York

Pascal Boileau, M.D.
Professor, Department of Orthopaedic Surgery, University of Nice-Sophia Antipolis; and Head, Department of Orthopaedic Surgery and Sports Traumatology, Archet 2 Hospital, Nice, France

John J. Brems, M.D.
Head, Section of Shoulder Surgery, Department of Orthopaedic Surgery, Cleveland Clinic Foundation, Cleveland, Ohio

Stephen S. Burkhart, M.D.
Clinical Associate Professor, Department of Orthopaedic Surgery, The University of Texas Health Science Center at San Antonio; and Director of Medical Education, The Orthopaedic Institute, San Antonio, Texas

Wayne Z. Burkhead, Jr., M.D.
Clinical Associate Professor, Department of Orthopaedics, University of Texas Southwestern Medical School, W. B. Carrell Memorial Clinic; and Attending, Department of Orthopaedics, Baylor University Medical Center, Dallas, Texas

Robert H. Cofield, M.D.
Professor, Department of Orthopedics, Mayo Medical School; and Chairman, Department of Orthopedic Surgery, Mayo Clinic, Rochester, Minnesota

Stephen Copeland, M.D., F.R.C.S.
Consultant Orthopaedic Surgeon, Shoulder Surgery Unit, Berkshire Independent Hospital, Coley Park, Reading-Berkshire, Reading, United Kingdom

Charles N. Cornell, M.D.
Associate Professor, Department of Surgery (Orthopaedics), Weill College of Medicine of Cornell University; and Associate Attending Physician, Department of Orthopaedic Surgery, Hospital for Special Surgery, New York, New York

Edward V. Craig, M.D.
Professor of Clinical Surgery, Department of Orthopaedics, Weill Medical College of Cornell University; and Attending Surgeon, Hospital for Special Surgery, New York, New York

Norman Espinosa, M.D.
Resident, Department of Orthopaedic Surgery, University of Zurich, Balgrist University Hospital, Zurich, Switzerland

Larry D. Field, M.D.
Clinical Instructor, Department of Orthopaedic Surgery, University of Mississippi School of Medicine; and Co-Director, Upper Extremity Service, Mississippi Sports Medicine and Orthopaedic Center, Jackson, Mississippi

Evan L. Flatow, M.D.
Lasker Professor of Orthopaedics, Department of Orthopaedics, Mount Sinai School of Medicine; and Chief of Shoulder Surgery, Department of Orthopaedics, Mount Sinai Hospital, New York, New York

Christian Gerber, M.D.
Professor, Department of Orthopaedics, University of Zurich; and Chairman, Department of Orthopaedics, Balgrist University Hospital, Zurich, Switzerland

Thomas P. Goss, M.D.
Professor of Orthopaedic Surgery, Department of Orthopedics, University of Massachusetts Medical School; and Attending Orthopaedic Surgeon, Department of Orthopedics, University of Massachusetts Memorial Health Care, Worcester, Massachusetts

Stephen B. Gunther, M.D.
Department of Orthopaedics, California Pacific Medical Center, San Francisco, California

Peter Habermeyer, M.D., PH.D.
Chief, Department of Shoulder and Elbow Surgery, ATOS Klinik, Heidelberg, Germany

Richard J. Hawkins, M.D.
Clinical Professor, Department of Orthopaedics, University of Colorado, Denver; and Orthopaedic Consultant, Steadman Hawkins Clinic, Vail, Colorado

David L. Helfet, M.D.
Professor, Department of Orthopaedic Surgery, Weill Medical College of Cornell University; and Director, Orthopaedic Trauma Service, Hospital for Special Surgery, New York, New York

Thomas F. Holovacs, M.D.
Instructor, Department of Orthopaedic Surgery, Harvard University Medical School; and Harvard Shoulder Service, Massachusetts General Hospital, Boston, Massachusetts

Chunyan Jiang, M.D., PH.D.
Attending Surgeon, Shoulder Service, Department of Orthopedic Trauma, School of Medicine, Peking University; and Beijing Ji Shui Tan Hospital, Beijing, People's Republic of China

Frank W. Jobe, M.D.
Clinical Professor, Department of Orthopaedic Surgery, University of Southern California Keck School of Medicine; Associate, Kerlan-Jobe Orthopaedic Clinic, Los Angeles, California; and Orthopaedic Consultant, Los Angeles Dodgers, PGA Tour, and Senior PGA Tour

Timothy S. Johnson, M.D.
Instructor, Department of Orthopaedic Surgery, Johns Hopkins School of Medicine; and Attending, Department of Orthopaedic Surgery, Good Samaritan Hospital, Baltimore, Maryland

Steven P. Kalandiak, M.D.
Assistant Professor of Clinical Orthopaedics, Department of Orthopaedics and Rehabilitation, University of Miami School of Medicine; and Jackson Memorial Hospital, Miami, Florida

Earl J. Kilbride, M.D.
Sports Medicine Fellow, Department of Orthopaedics, Southern California Orthopaedic Institute, Van Nuys, California

Steven Klepps, M.D.
Orthopedic Associates, Yellowstone Medical Center, Billings, Montana

Peter Kloen, M.D., PH.D.
Director, Division of Orthopaedic Trauma, Department of Orthopaedic Surgery, Academic Medical Center, Amsterdam, The Netherlands

Sumant G. Krishnan, M.D.
Assistant Clinical Professor, Department of Orthopaedic Surgery, The University of Texas Southwestern Medical Center; and Attending Physician, Shoulder Service, W. B. Carrell Memorial Clinic, Dallas, Texas

Gregory N. Lervick, M.D.
Staff Physician, Department of Orthopaedics, Park Nicollet Clinic/Methodist Hospital, St. Louis Park, Minnesota

Sven Lichtenberg, M.D.
Chief, Department of Shoulder and Elbow Surgery, ATOS Klinik, Heidelberg, Germany

Ian K. Y. Lo, M.D., F.R.C.S.C.
Orthopaedic Fellow, The San Antonio Orthopaedic Group, San Antonio, Texas

David S. Morrison, M.D.
Director of Shoulder and Elbow Surgery, Southern California Center for Sports Medicine; and Department of Orthopaedic Surgery, Memorial Hospital of Long Beach, Long Beach, California

Tom R. Norris, M.D.
Assistant Clinical Professor, Department of Orthopaedics, University of California, San Francisco; and Attending Physician, Department of Orthopaedic Surgery, California Pacific Medical Center, San Francisco, California

Robert J. Nowinski, D.O.
Assistant Professor of Orthopaedic Surgery, Ohio University College of Osteopathic Medicine, Athens; and Private Practice, Orthopaedic Specialists & Sports Medicine, Inc., Newark, Ohio

James D. O'Holleran, M.D.
Resident, Department of Orthopaedics, Harvard Combined Orthopaedic Surgery, Massachusetts General Hospital, Boston, Massachusetts

J. Randall Ramsey, M.D.
Upper Extremity Service, Mississippi Sports Medicine and Orthopaedic Center, Jackson, Mississippi

Robin R. Richards, M.D., F.R.C.S.C.
Professor, Department of Surgery, University of Toronto; and Surgeon-in-Chief, Department of Surgery, Sunnybrook and Women's College Health Sciences Centre, Toronto, Ontario, Canada

Charles A. Rockwood, Jr., M.D.
Professor and Chairman Emeritus, Department of Orthopaedics, The University of Texas Health Science Center at San Antonio, San Antonio, Texas

Felix H. Savoie III, M.D.

Clinical Associate Professor, Department of Orthopaedic Surgery, University of Mississippi School of Medicine; and Co-Director, Upper Extremity Service, Mississippi Sports Medicine and Orthopaedic Center, Jackson, Mississippi

Theodore F. Schlegel, M.D.

Englewood, Colorado

Stephen J. Snyder, M.D.

Medical Director, Center for Learning Arthroscopic Skills, Southern California Orthopedic Institute; and Staff Physician, Southern California Orthopedic Research and Education; and Center for Orthopedic Surgery, Inc., Van Nuys, California

Larry R. Stayner, M.D.

Sports Medicine Fellow, Kerlan-Jobe Orthopaedic Clinic, Los Angeles, California; and Staff Orthopedic Surgeon, Department of Orthopedic Surgery, Missoula Community Medical Center, Missoula, Montana

Sabrina Strickland, M.D.

Assistant Attending, Department of Orthopaedics, Beth Israel Medical Center, Singer Division, New York, New York; and Department of Orthopaedic Surgery, Albert Einstein College of Medicine, Montefiore Medical Center, Bronx, New York

R. Stacy Tapscott, M.D.

Shoulder/Sports Medicine, Decatur Orthopaedic Clinic, Decatur, Alabama

James E. Tibone, M.D.

Clinical Professor, Department of Orthopaedics, University of Southern California Keck School of Medicine; and Associate, Kerlan-Jobe Orthopaedic Clinic, Los Angeles, California

Gilles Walch, M.D.

Orthopaedic Surgeon, Department of Shoulder Surgery, Clinic St. Anne Lumiere, Lyon, France

Jon J. P. Warner, M.D.

Associate Professor, Department of Orthopaedic Surgery; and Chief, Harvard Shoulder Service, Massachusetts General Hospital and Brigham and Women's Hospital, Boston, Massachusetts

Russell F. Warren, M.D.

Hospital for Special Surgery, New York, New York

Raymond R. White, M.D.

Associate Professor, Department of Orthopaedics, University of Vermont, Burlington, Vermont; and Chairman, Orthopaedic Trauma Division, Maine Medical Center, Portland, Maine

Riley J. Williams III, M.D.

Assistant Professor, Department of Orthopaedic Surgery, Weill Medical College of Cornell University; and Attending Surgeon, Sports Medicine and Shoulder Service, Hospital for Special Surgery, New York, New York

Michael A. Wirth, M.D.

Professor, Department of Orthopaedics, The University of Texas Health Science Center at San Antonio, San Antonio, Texas

Paul H. Woodworth, M.D.

Sports Medicine Fellow, Shoulder and Elbow Surgery, Southern California Center for Sports Medicine; and Surgeon, Department of Orthopaedic Surgery, Long Beach Memorial Medical Center, Long Beach, California

Bertram Zarins, M.D.

Associate Clinical Professor, Department of Orthopaedic Surgery, Harvard Medical School; and Chief, Sports Medicine Service, Massachusetts General Hospital, Boston, Massachusetts

Joseph D. Zuckerman, M.D.

Professor, Department of Orthopaedic Surgery, New York University School of Medicine; and Chairman, Department of Orthopaedic Surgery, NYU-Hospital for Joint Diseases, New York, New York

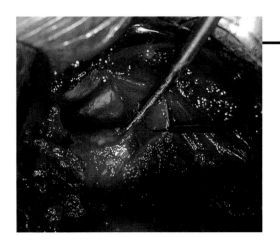

ACKNOWLEDGMENTS

Many people are responsible for the completion of this project. My thanks, admiration, and appreciation go to each of the contributing authors for the time and effort that went into preparing their manuscripts and ensuring that the illustrative material was of the necessary quality to teach their techniques. I thank them for their intellect, honesty, teaching ability, and willingness to share surgical "rough spots" so others' cases go smoothly. I recognize and respect the planning involved in trying to bring these techniques to life and make them reproducible.

Second, I appreciate the encouragement, support, and, when necessary, poke in the ribs from the staff at Lippincott Williams & Wilkins, particularly Jim Merritt and Grace Caputo, without whose persistence this project would have stalled many times.

Finally, I acknowledge the role played by the series editor, Roby C. Thompson, Jr.—mentor, colleague, and friend—one of the very few orthopedists with the clarity of thought, breadth of knowledge, wealth of experience, and scope of vision to lead a project such as the *Master Techniques in Orthopaedic Surgery* series.

SERIES PREFACE

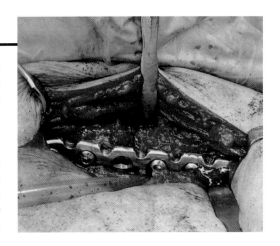

The first volume of the series *Master Techniques in Orthopaedic Surgery* was published in 1994. Our goal in assembling the series was to create easy-to-follow descriptions of operative techniques that would help orthopaedists through the challenges of daily practice. The books were intended to be more than just technical manuals, they were designed to impart the personal experience of the "master orthopaedic surgeons."

Master Techniques in Orthopaedic Surgery has become precisely what we hoped for—books that are used again and again, and are found at home and in the offices of practicing orthopaedists and residents in training. Most importantly, they are recommended by orthopaedists who look to them for practical advice and suggestions concerning the difficult but common problems they encounter.

The series is now in its second edition phase. You will again find recognized leaders as volume editors, known for their contributions to research, education, and the advancement of the surgical state of the art. Chapter authors have been selected for their experience, operative skills, and recognized expertise with a particular technique. The classic procedures are still included; some techniques have changed as new technology has been incorporated; and new procedures that have been popularized during the last several years have been added.

We are maintaining the same user-friendly format that was so well-received when the series was first introduced—a standardized presentation of information replete with tips and pearls gained through years of experience, with abundant color photographs and drawings to guide you step-by-step through the procedures.

With these new editions, we again invite you into the operating room to peer over the shoulder of the surgeon at work. It is our goal to offer the orthopaedic surgeon seeking an improved proficiency in practice access to the maximum confidence in selecting and executing the appropriate surgery for the individual patient.

Roby C. Thompson, Jr., M.D.
Series Editor

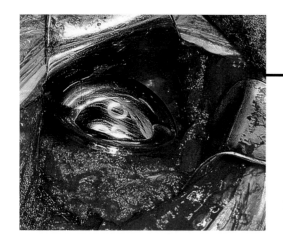

PREFACE TO THE FIRST EDITION

The Shoulder is part textbook, part road map, part atlas. Is is also part diary, part reflection, and part personal experience. Is it exhaustive? No. Are these operations the only way? No. But each one is an approach you can use, safely and effectively, for a broad range of common surgical problems of the shoulder.

Each of the authors has been asked to describe a technique as if dictating an operative report: patient position, position of retractors, surgical approach, pitfalls, and what to do when. The guiding principle was, if we could not be by their side, then they were to come to us. These surgeons were chosen both for what they have to teach and for whom they are. Each is a proven, effective communicator. I know them. I know their operations. Each procedure is a good solution to the problem. Each author was asked to include expectations (not only of the surgeon but also of the patient), the time course, and what milestones could be expected along the way.

Buy any "how to" is little more than a cookbook unless accompanied by personal indications, contraindications, assessment and evaluation of the patient, hints to make the procedures reproducible, the treatment, and strategy for avoiding complications.

There are many ways to use this book. Read it when deciding how to treat an individual problem, or as an instructional manual before performing a procedure for the first time, or after routine as well as difficult surgery. Read it for how the authors handled or avoided the inevitable rough spots, for how you can do it better next time. Peruse the diagrams and photographs before, during, or between cases. This book is designed to be flexible, useful, appreciated, and friendly.

This volume is part of the *Master Techniques in Orthopaedic Surgery* series. The word *master* is an adjective. It means skilled or proficient. It is also a noun. It means a worker qualified to teach others; an artist of considerable skill. However the word is defined, these "masters" indeed have much to teach. Learn from them. Take advantage of them. And enjoy the process.

Edward V. Craig, M.D.

PREFACE

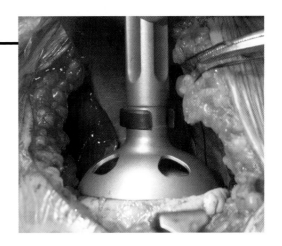

Since the first edition of *The Shoulder* was published, the dramatic technologic advances that have improved and changed our approach to diagnosis and treatment of all musculoskeletal conditions have inevitably altered and modified operative management of many shoulder conditions. An increased spectrum of treatment alternatives now exists which is reflected in the changes, modifications, additions, and updates in the second edition of *The Shoulder*. Despite this, the fundamental mission of the book—to take the clinician inside the operating room of the "master" surgeon—is unchanged. Thus, the preface to the first edition is included because it continues to reflect this book's purpose.

The contents of the book have been expanded from 24 to 33 chapters. Directly reflecting technical advances in arthroscopic techniques, new chapters have been added on arthroscopic approaches to the rotator cuff, shoulder instability, biceps pathology, frozen shoulder, calcific tendinitis, and glenohumeral arthritis. The section on open management of rotator cuff tears has been expanded to include tendon transfers. Fracture management has been updated and augmented with new chapters on percutaneous fixation of humeral fractures and operative treatment of glenoid fractures. The section on surgical approaches for glenohumeral arthritis has been expanded to reflect additional options for shoulder arthroplasty—including resurfacing arthroplasty, revision arthroplasty, and arthroplasty in the face of soft tissue deficiency. In every instance in which a chapter from the first edition has been retained, it has been reviewed and updated to reflect current approaches or modification where appropriate.

With the expansion accompanying this second edition, my intent is that you will continue to find this volume useful, valuable, practical, easy to navigate, and enjoyable.

Edward V. Craig, M.D.

PART I

Arthroscopy

1

Arthroscopic Subacromial Decompression and Rotator Cuff Débridement

Timothy S. Johnson and Russell F. Warren

INDICATIONS/CONTRAINDICATIONS

Impingement syndrome is a common cause of shoulder pain and dysfunction. Table 1-1 shows the etiology of subacromial pathology. Traditionally, these causes have been grouped into structural factors and dynamic factors. Structural factors lead to mechanical obstruction and decreased space for clearance of the rotator cuff within the supraspinatus outlet. The obstruction abrades the rotator cuff, producing tears and degeneration. When structural factors are the primary cause of subacromial pain, alleviation of the obstruction is curative. Alternatively, dynamic factors cause subacromial impingement secondarily due to superior migration of the humeral head during arm elevation (3). Abnormal superior migration leads to abutment of the greater tuberosity against the coracoacromial (CA) arch and thus, tendon injury. Rotator cuff dysfunction and fatigue cause most dynamic imbalance. These patients respond well to rehabilitation of the shoulder musculature, which centers the humeral head within the glenoid fossa during arm elevation. Successful treatment of dynamic impingement due to glenohumeral instability may require operative stabilization to achieve centering (9).

Arthroscopic subacromial decompression (ASD) has become a mainstay of treatment for patients with impingement syndrome that has failed conservative management. Since its introduction in 1985, ASD has reliably produced clinical success comparable to that of open anterior acromioplasty with better cosmesis, low morbidity, and early return of function (1,12). The most important indications for ASD are as follows: (a) primary mechanical impingement, (b) partial-thickness rotator cuff tears, (c) massive irreparable rotator cuff tears (where limited decompression combined with tuberoplasty may be helpful), and (d) mal-

T. S. Johnson, M.D.: Department of Orthopaedic Surgery, Johns Hopkins School of Medicine; and Good Samaritan Hospital, Baltimore, Maryland.

R. F. Warren, M.D.: Hospital for Special Surgery, New York, New York.

Table 1-1. *Causes of subacromial pathology*

Structural	Dynamic
Abnormal acromial morphology	Scapular dysfunction
Calcific tendonitis (thickening of the rotator cuff)	Primary tendon overload
	Glenohumeral instability
Osteophytes of the acromioclavicular joint	Repetitive microtrauma
Hypertrophy of the coracoacromial ligament	Imbalance of shoulder musculature
Os acromiale	
Inflammatory bursitis	
Malunion of the greater tuberosity, distal clavicle, or acromion	
Partial tear of the rotator cuff	
Full-thickness tear of the rotator cuff	

unions of the greater tuberosity with superior displacement of less than 1 cm. (Malunion of the greater tuberosity with displacement of more than 1 cm is best treated with osteotomy and repositioning of the tuberosity.)

Diagnostic arthroscopy of the glenohumeral joint at the time of ASD is extremely useful. The indications are as follows:

1. *When subacromial decompression is being considered for impingement in patients under 40 years old.* Instability is present with impingement and cuff pathology in a significant percentage of these younger patients, especially in those who are overhead athletes (1,9). Often this instability is subtle, difficult to demonstrate on routine physical examination, and evident only at the time of examination under anesthesia. Arthroscopic examination of the capsuloligamentous complex is valuable in making the diagnosis.
2. *When there is a suspicion of a cuff contusion or partial-thickness tearing of the rotator cuff.* Arthroscopic débridement of the cuff is simple and often beneficial in this setting (4).
3. *When there is a suspicion of a full-thickness cuff tear amenable to repair.* Arthroscopic inspection and probing are instrumental in assessing the ability to achieve a successful repair. Furthermore, recent advances in arthroscopic instrumentation have rendered many tears easy to repair arthroscopically. As discussed later, when a massive irreparable tear is encountered, débridement of the torn tissue is advantageous and easily performed arthroscopically.
4. *When the preoperative diagnosis is uncertain.* Abnormalities such as labral tears, biceps tendon pathology, synovitis, and adhesive capsulitis may be missed when the glenohumeral joint is not inspected arthroscopically. If left untreated, these problems can lead to residual pain after decompression.

It is worth noting that impingement syndrome may be confused with other causes of shoulder pain, such as osteoarthritis. Table 1-2 lists other causes of shoulder pain. Isolated

Table 1-2. *Other causes included in the differential diagnosis for impingement syndrome*

Acromioclavicular joint arthrosis
Adhesive capsulitis
Bicep tendonitis
Brachial plexopathy
Cervical radiculitis
Glenohumeral arthrosis and neoplasm of the shoulder girdle
Pancoast tumors
Thoracic outlet syndrome
Visceral problems (e.g., coronary disease, cholecystitis)

subacromial decompression in these patients may not be curative. However, mechanical impingement may occur concurrently with these disorders. Subacromial decompression may provide some pain relief in this setting but successful long-term treatment depends on management of the primary pathology. Hence, careful preoperative assessment cannot be overemphasized.

PREOPERATIVE PLANNING

The preoperative evaluation of a patient with rotator cuff pathology includes consideration of the history, physical examination, and imaging studies. The history should include the patient's age, activity level, occupation, and goals. The onset, duration, and severity of symptoms are equally as important. Note the effect of prior treatments such as medications, injections, physical therapy, or surgical procedures. Although most patients with full-thickness cuff tears are over 40 years old, we see a significant number of younger contact and throwing athletes with cuff tears requiring operative treatment. Manual laborers and recreational athletes are also susceptible to cuff injury. Patients with partial-thickness or small full-thickness tears will often complain of pain without weakness. Those with larger full-thickness tears are disabled by weakness as well as pain. The pain associated with rotator cuff disease is often worse at night and keeps the patient awake. Patients with long-standing pain associated with overhead activity are more likely to have a degenerative cuff tear than are patients in whom an acute, traumatic event initiated their symptoms.

Examination

We routinely perform a thorough physical examination of the cervical spine and upper extremity in the patient with shoulder pain. We assess atrophy of the shoulder girdle, active and passive range of motion, strength, neurovascular status, and impingement signs. Proximal rupture of the tendon of the long head of the biceps is often associated with chronic cuff tendonitis and degeneration. Patients with symptomatic cuff tears have difficulty initiating abduction and present with altered scapulothoracic rhythm. More specifically, a "shrug sign" is present during arm elevation, demonstrated by increased scapulothoracic motion and decreased glenohumeral motion. With the forearm fully pronated, weakness of shoulder elevation indicates a tear in the supraspinatus. Weakness of the external rotators indicates involvement of the infraspinatus. Although patients with a massive tear may exhibit full active elevation, strength testing frequently reveals marked weakness. We use the lift-off test and or the belly press test to assess subscapularis function (6,7). Again, glenohumeral instability can be the cause of the impingement and cuff tendonitis in young overhead athletes (9). A careful examination for anterior, posterior, and multidirectional instabilities should be performed.

Diagnostic Imaging

In patients over 40 years old, we obtain routine radiographs of the affected shoulder to assess the glenohumeral joint, acromion, and acromioclavicular (AC) joint. These include anteroposterior (AP) views in internal and external rotation, an axillary view, and a supraspinatus outlet view. A high-riding humeral head with a narrowed subacromial space suggests a large or massive rotator cuff tear. Calcific tendonitis may be readily apparent on the AP view (Fig.1-1A). A curved or beaked anterior acromion, as seen on the outlet view, is often associated with impingement (Fig. 1-1B and C). An axillary view may show os acromiale. Osteophytes secondary to arthritis of the AC joint can contribute to impingement and cuff tendonitis. In patients under 40 years old, obtain AP, West Point axillary, and Stryker notch views to better visualize the glenoid rim and to detect Hill-Sachs lesions associated with instability.

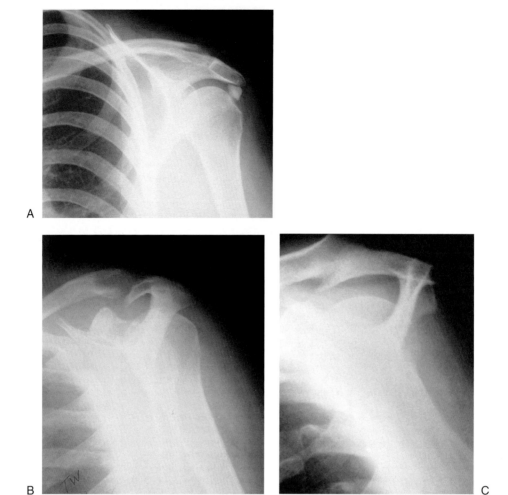

Figure 1-1. A: Anteroposterior view of left shoulder showing calcific tendonitis. **B:** Outlet view demonstrating a "curved" type II acromion. **C:** "Beaked" type III acromion.

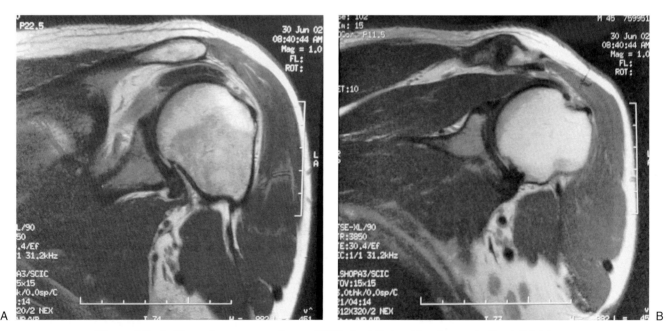

Figure 1-2. A: Magnetic resonance image (MRI) of a left shoulder demonstrating full-thickness tear of the rotator cuff tendon with separation of the infraspinatus from its insertion onto the greater tuberosity. **B:** MRI demonstrating separation of the supraspinatus from its insertion onto the greater tuberosity.

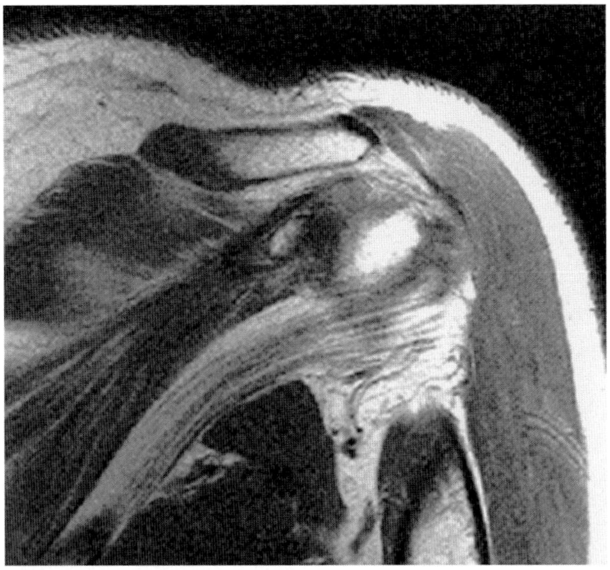

Figure 1-3. Chronic full-thickness rotator cuff tear with fatty infiltration of the teres minor and infraspinatus muscles and retraction of the tendon edge medially.

When a rotator cuff tear is suspected, a variety of imaging studies may be performed to confirm the diagnosis. If only full-thickness tears must be ruled out, arthrography is an acceptable imaging modality. It has the drawback of being invasive and does not detect partial tears on the bursal side of the cuff. It is also difficult to define the size of the tear and the quality of the remaining tissue with arthrography. Alternatively, ultrasonography may be used. However, the utility of ultrasound depends heavily on the experience of the radiologist. At our institution, magnetic resonance imaging (MRI) is the preferred imaging modality. MRI combines accuracy in detecting full-thickness rotator cuff tears with comprehensive imaging of the shoulder joint (Fig. 1-2). Furthermore, the MRI scan has the distinct advantage of being able to reveal the size of the tear, the extent of retraction, and the quality of the remaining tissue. Fatty infiltration of the cuff musculature with retraction on MRI examination indicates a poor prognosis (Fig. 1-3). Knowing this preoperatively is important as it may alter the operative plan.

SURGERY

Instrumentation

In addition to basic arthroscopic instruments, we use an inflow pump for shoulder arthroscopy (Arthrotek, Biomet, Warsaw, IN or Oratec, Oratec Interventions Inc., Menlo Park, CA). We typically use a 5.5-mm full-radius resector for subacromial decompression. An arthroscopic burr is useful when removing hard bone. We prefer using a tissue ablator (Arthrocare Corp., Sunnyvale, CA) for soft-tissue removal and coagulation. If a rotator cuff repair is anticipated, we prepare instruments designed for suturing the cuff back to bone. A variety of tacks, staples, and suture anchors are available for this purpose, but we prefer using a suture repair.

Positioning

Regional anesthesia for shoulder procedures is advantageous because it provides excellent postoperative analgesia without the use of intravenous narcotics. Most patients will require only oral analgesics postoperatively and can be discharged from the hospital on the day of

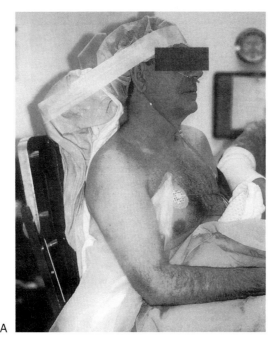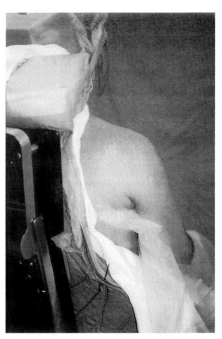

A   B

Figure 1-4. A, B: Beach-chair position for shoulder arthroscopy. The patient is positioned on a full-length beanbag mattress or a beach-chair table attachment so that the torso is 70 to 80 degrees upright and rotated 20 degrees away from the affected side.

surgery. We prefer to place patients in the beach-chair position. It avoids the potential neural complications that may occur when a patient is in the lateral decubitus position with the arm in traction. It also facilitates freedom to manipulate the humerus during intraarticular examination. Furthermore, we find it easier to convert the arthroscopic procedure to a miniarthrotomy from this position if necessary.

To achieve beach-chair positioning, lower the foot of the table and flex it 20 degrees at the waist after inducing anesthesia. Raise the back of the table so that the patient's torso is positioned 70 degrees from the horizontal plane. Rotate the upper body roughly 20 degrees so that the operative shoulder is lifted away from the table. Recess the beanbag beneath the operative shoulder so that there is access to the medial aspect of the scapula. After deflating the beanbag, move the patient and beanbag toward the operative edge of the table (Fig. 1-4). Alternatively, a shoulder-specific table with a removable back component may be used to enhance visualization.

Before prepping and draping the surgical field, examine the range of motion and stability of the affected shoulder. If passive range of motion is restricted, manipulate the shoulder at this point.

Diagnostic Arthroscopy

After preparing the sterile surgical field, palpate the osseous landmarks (acromion, coracoid process, and distal end of the clavicle). With a skin marker, outline these landmarks to establish reference points for the arthroscopic portals (Fig. 1-5). Mark the portal sites for diagnostic arthroscopy (posterior and anterior). The posterior portal is located 2 cm inferior and 2 cm medial to the posterolateral margin of the acromion. With interscalene anesthesia, the skin in this region may not be anesthetized. Infiltrate the skin with 3 mL of 1% lidocaine hydrochloride solution. The anterior portal is located 2 cm medial and 1 cm inferior to the anterolateral border of the acromion, just lateral to the coracoid process. At both portal sites, inject 3 mL of a 1:3,000,000 epinephrine solution subcutaneously to reduce potential bleeding.

Make a 5-mm posterior portal incision through the skin only. Assemble the blunt trocar and cannula for the arthroscope. Insert this assembly into the glenohumeral joint through this incision. Direct the trocar toward the coracoid process to reliably enter the joint. With the cannula remaining in the joint, exchange the trocar for the arthroscope. After visual ver-

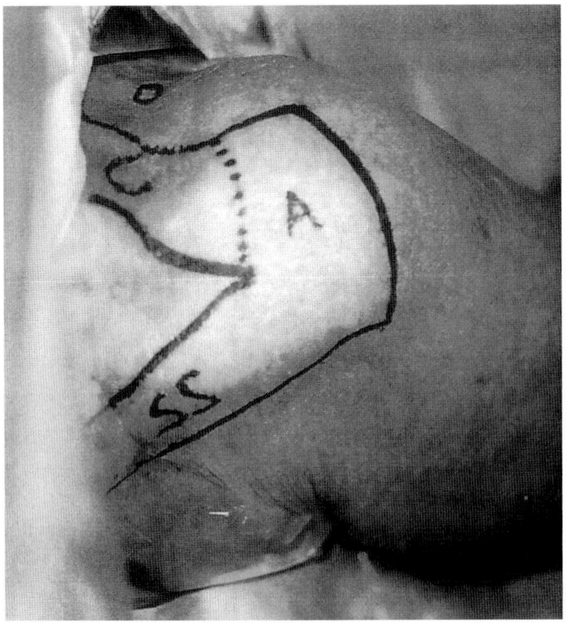

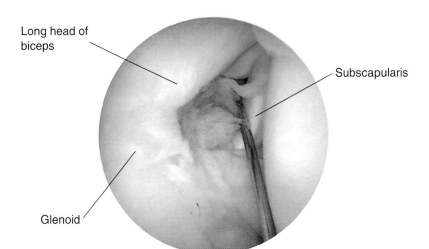

Figure 1-5. Osseous landmarks marked with a surgical marker on a right shoulder. *A*, acromion; *C*, clavicle; and *SS*, scapular spine. A circle marks the coracoid process anteriorly.

ification of an intraarticular location, distend the joint with fluid to a pressure of 40 mm Hg using the pump. The intraarticular location of the anterior portal is the triangular area outlined by the margin of the glenoid medially, the tendon of the long head of the biceps superiorly, and the tendon of the subscapularis inferiorly. Under arthroscopic guidance, localize this point with a spinal needle. Starting on the skin just lateral to the coracoid process, direct the needle into this triangular area (Fig. 1-6). Once properly positioned, make a 5-mm portal incision and exchange the needle for a 4.5-mm cannula with a diaphragm and a side port. The side port is used for outflow. Through the anterior cannula, introduce into the joint a probe with a 3-mm tip.

Perform a diagnostic arthroscopy of the glenohumeral joint, using the probe for palpation. Inspect the biceps tendon and superior labral complex for pathology. Make an effort to observe the synovium above the biceps origin. Synovitis and a pannuslike reaction superior to the labrum are common in shoulders with cuff pathology (Fig. 1-7). Conversely, synovitis inferiorly is usually not present with cuff disease; it is more consistent with ad-

Long head of biceps

Subscapularis

Glenoid

Figure 1-6. The intraarticular site for the anterior portal is located with a spinal needle. The space is defined by the long head of the biceps superiorly, the glenoid medially, and the subscapularis tendon inferiorly. (Patient is in the beach-chair position.)

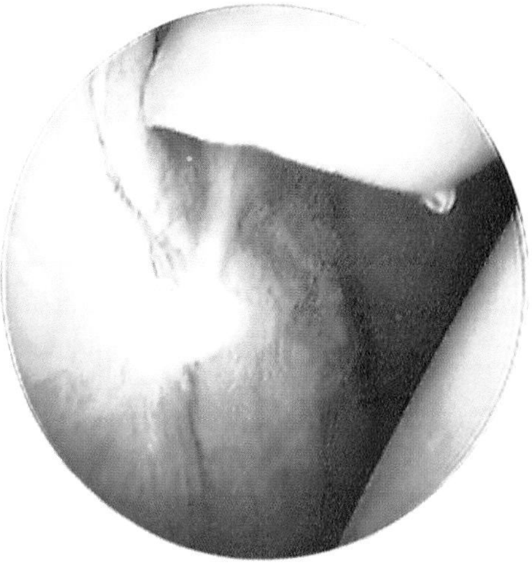

Figure 1-7. Synovitis superior to the biceps insertion into the labrum is often seen in shoulders with rotator cuff pathology. Here, the synovium extends anteriorly and inferiorly over the anterior labrum.

hesive capsulitis. Examine the anterior labrum, posterior labrum, and glenohumeral ligaments for detachment, tears, and laxity. These findings suggest instability and may require operative treatment. Be sure to visualize the axillary recess and the rest of the labrum, followed by the articular surface of the glenoid and humerus.

Begin examining the rotator cuff by following the biceps tendon distally to the point at which it exits from the joint. Subluxation or dislocation of the bicep tendon from the bicipital groove indicates either a partial or a complete tear of the subscapularis. Look for a curved arch of tendon on the undersurface of the cuff, just medial to the insertion of the supraspinatus and infraspinatus into the greater tuberosity. The arch is oriented in an anterior to posterior direction. Supraspinatus tears are usually found just lateral to this area. Visualization of the subacromial space from this intraarticular location is consistent with a full-thickness tear (Fig. 1-8). If present, make note of the location, size, and character of the tear. Assess the amount of cuff retraction and the quality of the torn tissue.

Partial tears present as fraying of the cuff without complete disruption of the tendon (Figs. 1-9 and 1-10). Recall that the supraspinatus tendon inserts less than 1 mm from the articular margin of the humerus, along the anterior 2 cm of the greater tuberosity. Normal tendon thickness at this location averages 14 mm (5). Thus, the degree of partial tearing can be estimated fairly accurately. When an articular sided partial tear is present, mark its location with a suture. Do this by passing a spinal needle through the tear, followed by a polydioxanone synthetic (PDS) suture (Ethicon Inc., Somerville, NJ) through the spinal needle (11). The location of the partial tear is now tagged for subsequent inspection from the subacromial space (11).

In throwers with internal impingement, partial-thickness tears will be located more posteriorly involving the infraspinatus tendon. These tears contact the posterosuperior labrum with the arm in the 90-degree/90 degree position where degeneration and/or a superior labrum anterior and posterior (SLAP) lesion may be present.

We use a classification system for cuff tears (Table 1-3) that is a modification of that described by Snyder et al. (11). Tears are classified on the basis of type, size, mobility, and tissue quality. Partial-thickness tears on the articular side are classified as "A." Those on the bursal side are classified as "B." Full-thickness or complete tears are classified as "C." We measure tear size in two dimensions. Cuff retraction is classified as (a) none, (b) minimal, (c) moderate, and (d) severe. We characterize the quality of the cuff tissue as good, fair, or poor. As shown in Table 1-3, we assign numeric values to tears on the basis of their size, level of retraction, and quality of tissue. Thus, a full-thickness, massive, fixed tear with poor-quality tissue is described as a C-10 tear. A partial articular surface tear measuring less than 2 cm^2, without retraction and with good quality tissue, is an A-2 tear.

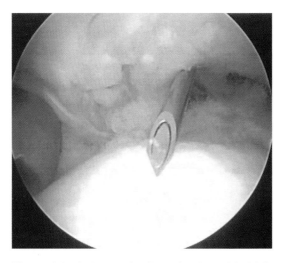

Figure 1-8. Arthroscopic view of a right-sided full-thickness rotator cuff tear with fraying of undersurface of supraspinatus.

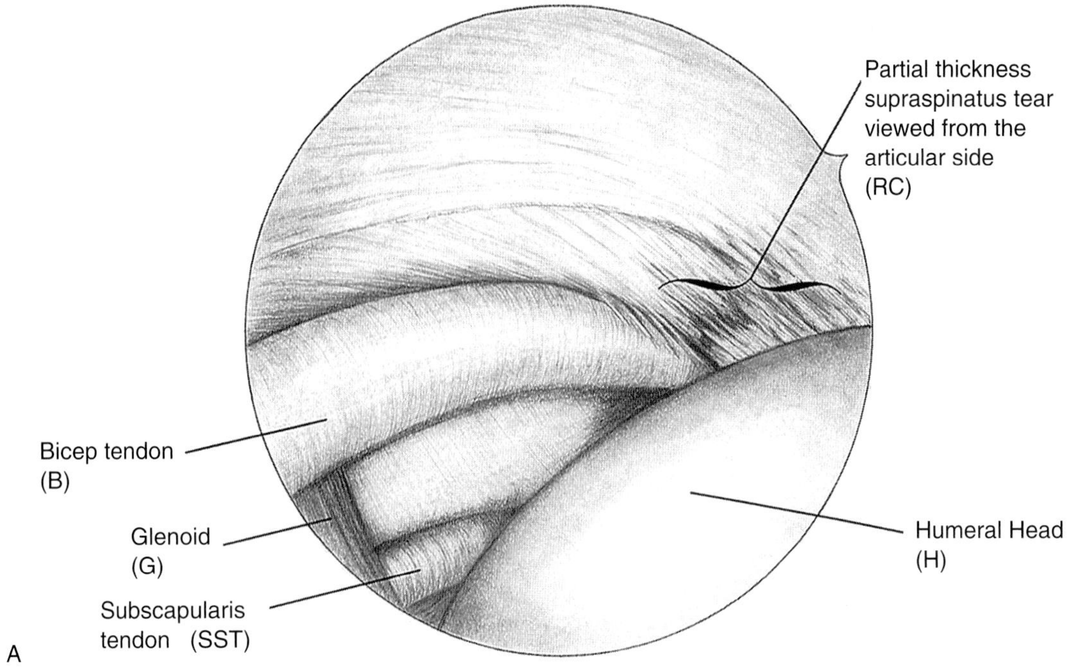

Partial thickness
supraspinatus tear
viewed from the
articular side
(RC)

Bicep tendon
(B)

Glenoid
(G)

Subscapularis
tendon   (SST)

Humeral Head
(H)

A

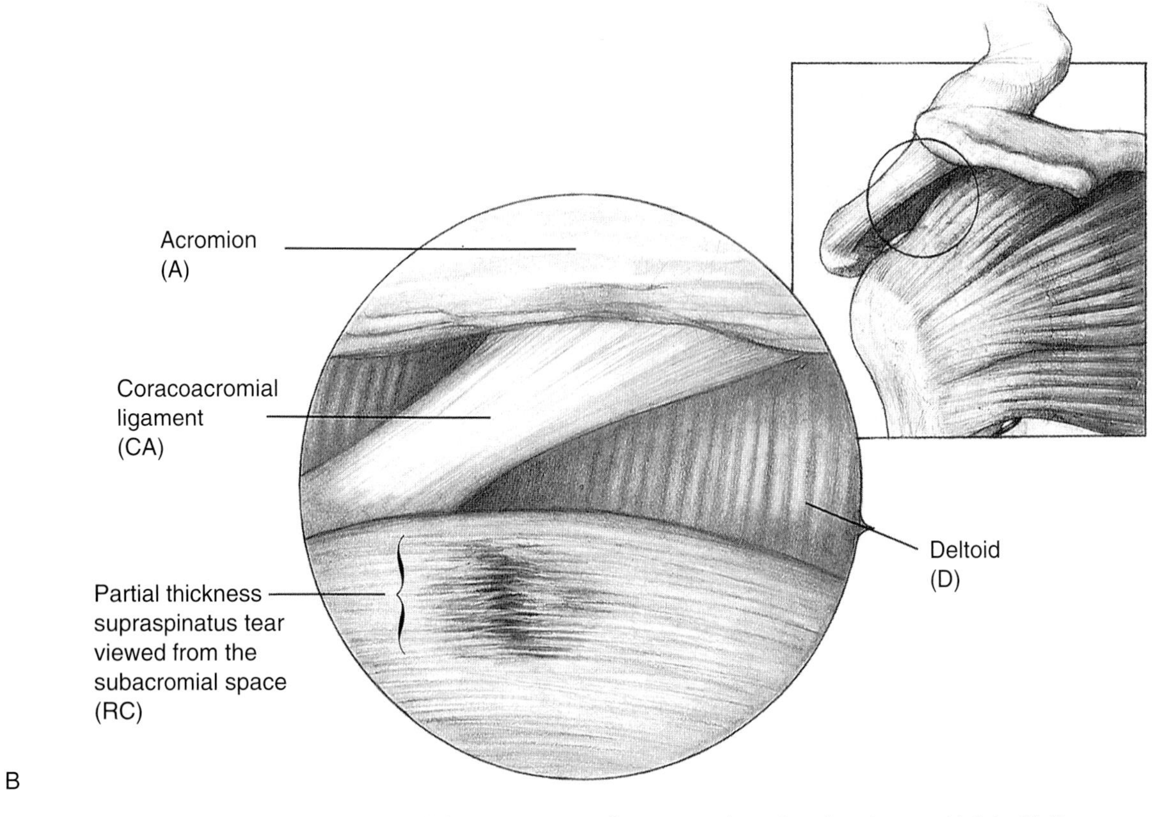

Acromion
(A)

Coracoacromial
ligament
(CA)

Deltoid
(D)

Partial thickness
supraspinatus tear
viewed from the
subacromial space
(RC)

B

Figure 1-9. A: A partial-thickness rotator cuff tear seen from the glenohumeral joint with the arthroscope in the posterior portal. *B*, biceps tendon; *G*, glenoid; *H*, humeral head; *RC*, rotator cuff; *SST*, supraspinatus tendon. **B:** A partial-thickness rotator cuff tear of the bursal surface as seen from a posterior arthroscopic portal. *A*, acromion; *CA*, coracoacromial ligament; *D*, deltoid; *RC*, rotator cuff.

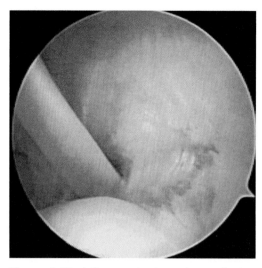

Figure 1-10. Arthroscopic view of an articular-sided partial-thickness tear in a right shoulder.

Acromioplasty

Examine the subacromial space next. Do this by removing the arthroscope from the posterior cannula and reinserting the trocar. Withdraw from the joint and redirect the trocar/cannula assembly into the subacromial space. Advance in an anterolateral direction beneath the acromion to enter the bursa, which is most prominent on the anterolateral edge of the acromion. The trocar must pass anterior to the midpoint of the acromion in order to pierce the veil of the bursa at this point (Fig. 1-11). If the trocar is inserted posterior to the bursa, the subacromial space will not be visualized when the arthroscope is inserted. Once in position, sweep the trocar in a medial to lateral direction to break up any adhesions in the bursa.

Table 1-3. *Hospital for Special Surgery rotator cuff tear classification system*

	Points
Tear type	
A Partial thickness, articular surface	
B Partial thickness, bursal surface	
C Full thickness, complete	
Size (cm^2)	
No tear	0
Small ($<$2)	1
Medium ($<$6)	2
Large ($<$15)	3
Massive ($\geq$15)	4
Retraction/mobility	
No retraction	0
Extracapsular release required[a]	1
Extra- and intracapsular release required[a]	2
Unable to reapproximate tear to insertion site	3
Tissue quality	
Normal (normal cuff tissue surrounding the tear)	0
Good (vascular, elastic, slightly thinned, or frayed)	1
Fair (thin, frayed, vascular, holds structure well)	2
Poor (thin, shredded, avascular, and brittle)	3
Surgeon's subjective assessment of repair	
Excellent	
Good	
Fair	
Poor	

[a]Releases required to reapproximate cuff tear to anatomic insertion site.

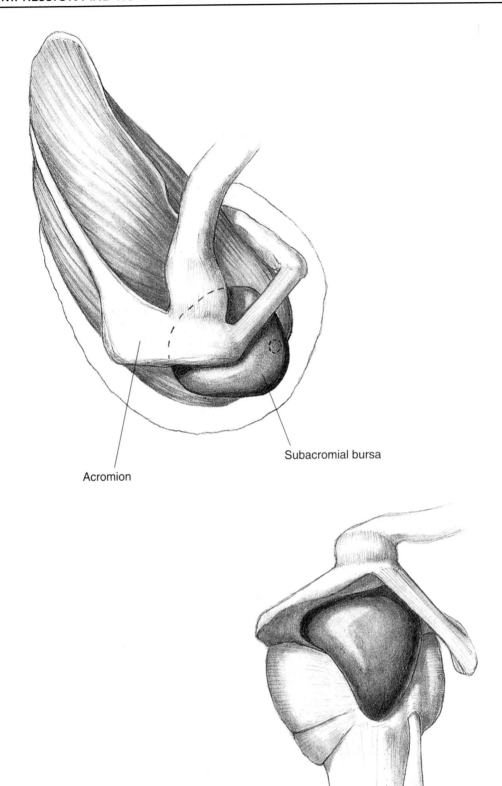

Acromion

Subacromial bursa

Figure 1-11. Subacromial bursa. The posterior aspect of this bursa acts as a veil of tissue that must be pierced by the arthroscope in order to visualize the anterior acromion. Note the anterolateral position of the bursa.

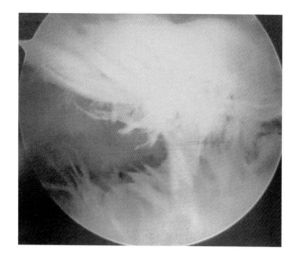

Figure 1-12. Fraying and degeneration of the coracoacromial ligament at the acromial insertion consistent with impingement.

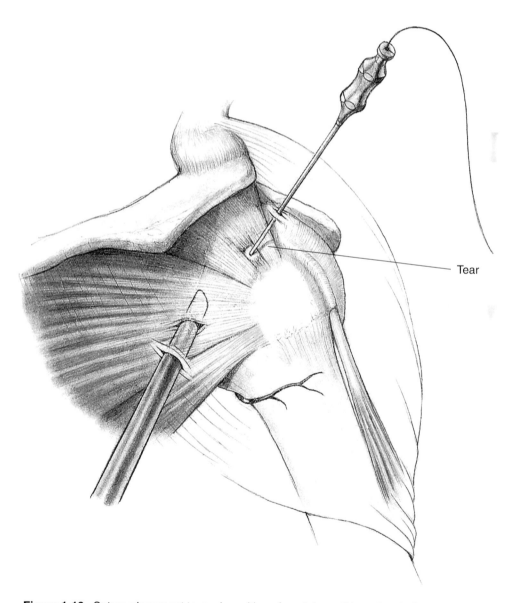

Tear

Figure 1-13. Suture placement to mark position of a rotator cuff tear. A polydioxanone synthetic (PDS) suture (Ethicon Inc., Somerville, NJ) may be placed through a spinal needle introduced laterally to mark the location of a rotator cuff tear viewed from the glenohumeral joint. A grasper is used to bring the suture out the anterior portal. The spinal needle is removed, and the two ends of the suture are clamped with a hemostat.

Next, withdraw the trocar and insert the arthroscope through the cannula. If there is inflammation of the bursal tissue, it may be difficult to see all parts of the subacromial space. However, skillful placement of the arthroscope will generally allow visualization of the anterior acromion, CA ligament, and rotator cuff. For impingement to be diagnosed, one should clearly see degeneration of the CA ligament at the acromial insertion (Fig. 1-12).

Establish a lateral portal 2 cm distal to the lateral border of the acromion. If no tear is present, we make this portal in line with the posterior border of the clavicle. If a tear is present, the AP position of this portal varies between the midpoint and the anterior margin of the acromion, depending on the location of the cuff tear. Similar to the technique used to mark partial-thickness tears, tag full-thickness tears with a PDS suture as described by Snyder et al. (11) (Fig. 1-13). Use this suture to identify the AP position of the lateral portal incision. The suture may also be used for traction during subsequent cuff repair.

Place a 5.5-mm cannula through the lateral portal into the subacromial space. Obtain visualization by removing all inflamed bursae with a 5.5-mm full-radius shaver and a tissue ablator. Unresected bursae will compromise the surgical result by impairing visualization, particularly if a rotator cuff repair will be performed. Retained bursae may also continue to impinge on the subacromial space leading to persistent pain after surgery. After the bursectomy, identify the anterior and lateral margins of the acromion. Establish the position of the AC joint. Identify the CA ligament. Remember, patients with impingement will have fraying of the CA ligament (Fig. 1-12). Remove the bursa from the cuff gently with a shaver. Test the integrity of the rotator cuff by palpating it with a probe. Reassess the depth, size, thickness, and quality of the tissue as discussed previously.

Begin the subacromial decompression by removing the CA ligament with a tissue ablator and cautery. Assess the acromion and the AC joint for overhang and spurs. Be sure to identify the most anterolateral aspect of the acromion. Failure to do this may lead to an inadequate decompression. Perform the acromioplasty starting from the lateral portal using the 5.5-mm resector or a burr. The goal is to remove enough of the undersurface and anterior border of the acromion to ensure a flat inferior surface. Define the plane of resection laterally first. Then progressively work in a medial direction toward the AC joint. Resect the spur with a sweeping motion from the anterior acromial edge to the midportion of the acromion. Take care to leave the deep fascia of the deltoid intact. Aim to achieve a wedge-shaped resection, removing more bone anteriorly than posteriorly. Be sure to remove adequate bone from the anterolateral corner, because pressures are maximal at this location (10). Avoid leaving a ridge between the resected and unresected bone at the midportion of the acromion. Do this by progressively "feathering" the resection posteriorly so that bone is no longer being removed when the resector reaches the midportion of the acromion. At the completion of the resection, the leading edge of the acromion should lie even with the anterior edge of the clavicle (Figs. 1-14 and 1-15). If a subclavicular spur is present, remove it in a similar fashion, coplanar to the acromioplasty. Take care to avoid the plexus of small vessels around the clavicle. We have not encountered subsequent problems with AC joint pain when coplaning was performed.

Rotator Cuff Débridement

Partial-thickness tears with loose flaps of torn rotator cuff tissue can be a source of impingement. Débride the torn tissue to alleviate this potential source of residual pain. Repair is often unnecessary if sufficient tendon remains attached to the greater tuberosity (see Results). Massive tears with severe retraction and poor tissue quality are not repairable. In this situation, débridement is also helpful. Approach these tears by removing the torn tissue with a full-radius resector. Perform a synovectomy and smooth the acromion as needed. In an effort to avoid future anterosuperior instability, do not remove the CA ligament. If the greater tuberosity is enlarged, remove the bony prominence to decrease impingement and subsequent pain. Débridement provides pain relief in this setting; however, restored rotator cuff function is unlikely. Be sure to discuss these limited goals with the patient.

(text continues on page 18)

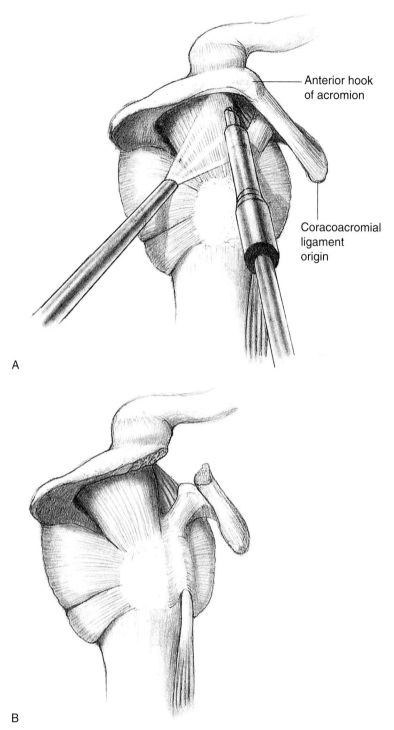

Anterior hook
of acromion

Coracoacromial
ligament
origin

A

B

Figure 1-14. Acromioplasty. The anterior hook of the acromion is resected along with the origin of the coracoacromial ligament, leaving a flat acromial undersurface. **A:** Prior to resection. **B:** After arthroscopic acromioplasty.

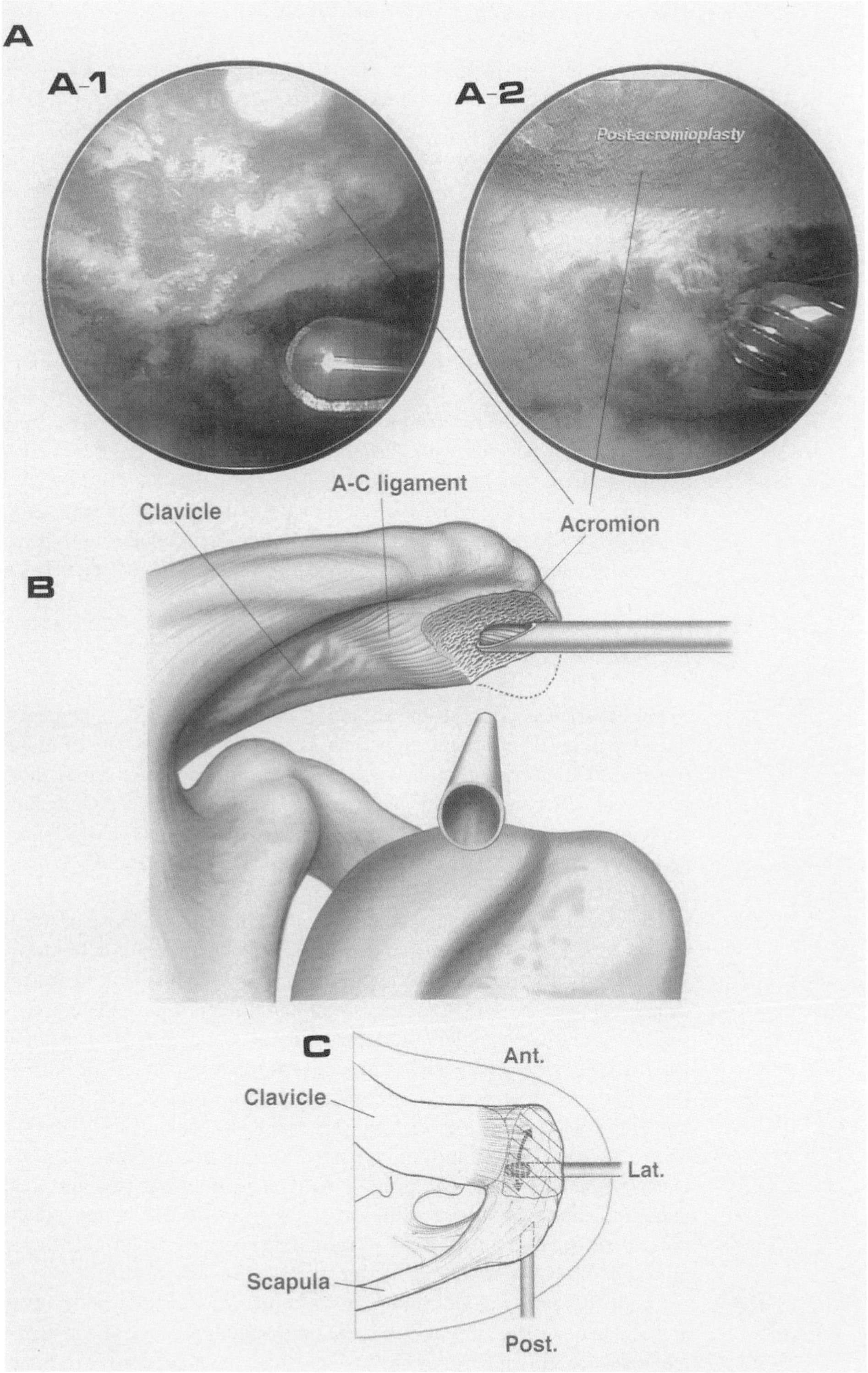

Figure 1-15. A: Acromioplasty. The anterior hook of the acromion is resected along with the origin of the coracoacromial ligament, leaving a flat acromial undersurface. **A1,** Prior to resection; **A2,** after arthroscopic acromioplasty. **B, C:** Schematic representation.

POSTOPERATIVE MANAGEMENT

Start rehabilitation by giving a sling to patients immediately after the operative decompression. Begin Codman/pendulum exercises on the first postoperative day and remove the sling by the third postoperative day. Initiate passive and active-assisted range-of-motion exercises during the first week. In the second postoperative week, commence light resistive exercises for the rotator cuff using elastic tubing. We aim for full range of active motion by the third or fourth week after surgery. Continue progressive strengthening of the rotator cuff and deltoid with the arm at the patient's side for 2 to 3 months.

Following acromioplasty, most patients can return to nonstrenuous work in a week. Full return to sports and heavy labor usually requires 2 to 3 months. The amount of rehabilitation after acromioplasty varies based on the amount of rotator cuff disease. The muscle-tendon unit must be returned to function that is more normal by stretching and strengthening exercises. This slow process will require several months. If an adequate acromioplasty has been performed, the compromised cuff can be rehabilitated to restore its function. Treat patients with partial-thickness tears that are débrided and decompressed similar to those who have been simply decompressed. As noted, return of full active motion and strength may be delayed in this group due to the higher degree of tendon injury. Exercises to strengthen the anterior deltoid and periscapular muscles are particularly important for patients with massive irreparable tears that have been débrided.

RESULTS

In our experience, arthroscopic acromioplasty for chronic impingement syndrome has produced high levels of long-term patient satisfaction. In a review of more than 80 consecutive cases at our institution, more than 80% of patients were satisfied with the result at up to 10 years after surgery (12). However, as many as one of three competitive athletes involved in overhead sports may have difficulty returning to heavy throwing activities after surgery. Failures can be divided into three distinct categories: diagnostic error, surgical error, and rotator cuff pathology.

The most common diagnostic error is the failure to diagnose occult instability. As discussed earlier, a comprehensive preoperative evaluation and a high level of suspicion in younger patients are critical to avoiding this error. Subsequent treatment of the instability usually relieves the symptoms of secondary impingement in these patients.

Failure to diagnose glenohumeral arthrosis can also lead to residual pain after ASD. Radiographically severe glenohumeral arthropathy coincident with impingement syndrome is not uncommon. A preoperative 5-lb–weighted AP radiograph of the glenohumeral joint is helpful in making this diagnosis. The efficacy of shoulder arthroscopy with subacromial decompression in patients with full-thickness loss of articular cartilage is not predictable. However, mild to moderate concurrent glenohumeral arthrosis is not a contraindication to subacromial decompression. In our hands, ASD for resistant impingement syndrome can improve shoulder function and provide durable results despite mild to moderate glenohumeral degenerative joint disease (8).

Surgical errors include removing too much or too little bone from the subacromial arch. Inadequate decompression is the more common of these two errors. There are a few methods to avoid this oversight. First, evaluate the preoperative radiographs and estimate the amount of resection to be performed. Second, verify the adequacy of decompression intraoperatively by moving the arm through a full range of motion while observing the subacromial space with the arthroscope. Finally, place the resector in the posterior portal while viewing laterally to obtain an alternative perspective on the amount of bone resected.

Primary failure to treat rotator cuff pathology leads to poor outcome after ASD. Débridement and decompression of a full-thickness cuff tear without repair is not advised in patients with good soft tissue and a repairable cuff lesion. Young active patients are typically good rehabilitation candidates and are therefore likely to regain function when the cuff is repaired. Furthermore, early surgical repair affords the best opportunity for maximal recovery of shoulder function when compared to late repair (2). Elderly patients with painful massive rotator cuff tears are good candidates for arthroscopic débridement and decompression. Retraction and fatty infiltration of the cuff musculature consistent with tissue atrophy are often evident on preoperative MRI of these patients (Fig. 1-3). These fragile tissues are difficult to mobilize and do not tolerate fixation well. In our experience, simply débriding the cuff provides pain relief in this setting. Restored rotator cuff function is less predictable.

Débridement and decompression may successfully treat partial-thickness and minimal full-thickness cuff tears. In our experience, patients with articular-sided partial tears comprising less than 50% of the tendon thickness have done well with arthroscopic acromioplasty and cuff débridement. The clinical outcome in these patients is not significantly different when compared with arthroscopic acromioplasty in patients without rotator cuff pathology. This is in contrast to patients with bursal-sided partial-thickness tears ($< 50\%$). Bursal-sided pathology may be better served with primary repair (4).

COMPLICATIONS

Intraoperative Bleeding

Intraoperative bleeding impairs visualization making it difficult to perform adequate subacromial decompression. There are several easy steps to avoid this complication. Instruct patients to discontinue the use of nonsteroidal medication 1 week before surgery. Meticulously and expeditiously coagulate bleeding vessels as they are encountered. When bleeding impairs visualization, use rapid intermittent suction to clear the surgical field so that the "bleeder" may be identified. Alternatively, raise the pump pressure temporarily. Be sure to lower the pump pressure after hemostasis is obtained to avoid fluid extravasation into the soft tissues. The anesthesiologist can also decrease bleeding by lowering the patient's blood pressure. Injection of the subacromial space with 20 mL of 1:300,000 epinephrine/saline solution at the beginning of the procedure may help control bleeding. However, we do not favor this technique as it distorts the bursa making visualization of the subacromial space difficult.

Residual Pain

In addition to the causes discussed above, residual pain after acromioplasty may stem from the failure to address all the pathology. Some examples include the failure to identify and treat concurrent adhesive capsulitis, AC joint arthrosis, or fatigue from permanently weakened muscles. Avoid these complications by carefully selecting and assessing patients preoperatively. Intraoperative examination under anesthesia is equally as important. Pay careful attention to the postoperative rehabilitation as well. Before surgery, discuss with patients the limited goals of débriding irreparable tears and the role of ASD in the shoulder with concurrent degenerative joint disease.

Postoperative Stiffness

If the patient is adequately decompressed, the rotator cuff repaired, and careful attention paid to early institution of postoperative range-of-motion exercises, this avoidable complication is unlikely to occur.

RECOMMENDED READING

1. Altchek, D.W., Warren, R.F., Wickiewicz, T.L., et al.: Arthroscopic acromioplasty: technique and results. *J Bone Joint Surg Am* 72(8): 1198–1207, 1990.
2. Bassett, R.W., Cofield, R.H.: Acute tears of the rotator cuff: the timing of surgical repair. *Clin Orthop* 175: 18–24, 1983.
3. Chen, S.K., Simonian, P.T., Wickiewicz, T.L., et al.: Radiographic evaluation of glenohumeral kinematics: a muscle fatigue model. *J Shoulder Elbow Surg* 8(1): 49–52, 1999.
4. Cordasco, F.A., Backer, M., Craig, E.V., et al.: The partial-thickness rotator cuff tear: is acromioplasty without repair sufficient? *Am J Sports Med* 30(2): 257–260, 2002.
5. Dugas, J.R., Campbell, D.A., Warren, R.F., et al.: Anatomy and dimensions of the rotator cuff insertions. *J Shoulder Elbow Surg* 11(5):498, 2002.
6. Gerber, C., Hersche, O., Farron, A.: Isolated rupture of the subscapularis tendon. *J Bone Joint Surg Am* 78(7): 1015–1023, 1996.
7. Gerber, C., Krushell, R.J.: Isolated rupture of the tendon of the subscapularis muscle: clinical features in 16 cases. *J Bone Joint Surg Br* 73(3): 389–394, 1991.
8. Guyette, T.M., Bae, H., Warren, R.F., et al.: Results of arthroscopic subacromial decompression in patients with subacromial impingement and glenohumeral degenerative joint disease. *J Shoulder Elbow Surg* 11(4): 299–304, 2002.
9. Jobe, F.W., Kvitne, R.S., Giangarra, C.E.: Shoulder pain in the overhand or throwing athlete: the relationship of anterior instability and rotator cuff impingement. *Orthop Rev* 18(9): 963–975, 1989.
10. Payne, L.Z., Deng, X.H., Craig, E.V., et al.: The combined dynamic and static contributions to subacromial impingement: a biomechanical analysis. *Am J Sports Med* 25(6): 801–808, 1997.
11. Snyder, S.J., Pachelli, A.F., Del Pizzo, W., et al.: Partial thickness rotator cuff tears: results of arthroscopic treatment. *Arthroscopy* 7(1): 1–7, 1991.
12. Stephens, S.R., Warren, R.F., Payne, L.Z., et al.: Arthroscopic acromioplasty: a 6- to 10-year follow-up. *Arthroscopy* 14(4): 382–388, 1998.

2

Arthroscopic Distal Clavicle Excision

David S. Morrison and Paul H. Woodworth

INDICATIONS/CONTRAINDICATIONS

Intraarticular pathology of the acromioclavicular (AC) joint is seen frequently in an active and athletic population, where it is usually secondary to a traumatic episode. It is also frequently seen in the elderly, where the primary pathology is advancing degenerative arthritis. In either case, the treatment is usually conservative, consisting of nonsteroidal antiinflammatory agents and an occasional steroid injection in an attempt to control the inflammation and subsequent pain. In cases where conservative management is not successful, intraarticular surgery may be indicated. The choice of surgery depends on the pathology present. In patients in whom the AC pain is secondary to instability of the joint, a reconstruction of the coracoclavicular ligaments, with or without an excisional arthroplasty of the distal clavicle, is the treatment of choice. In patients in whom the primary pathology is an intraarticular meniscus lesion similar to that seen in the knee, the technique used is a simple microsurgical procedure for removal of the offending cartilage. The latter disorder is rare and is seen mainly in young athletes such as gymnasts or swimmers. In those cases in which the intraarticular pathology has progressed to the point where there are also degenerative changes of the clavicular or acromial articulation, the treatment of choice is an excisional arthroplasty of the AC joint.

Arthroscopic excisional arthroplasty of the AC joint is not performed on all patients with AC arthritis, but rather on those selected according to strict criteria. Patients with a very productive osteoarthritis of the joint or a hypermobile distal clavicle are often better treated by open excisional arthroplasty or open excisional arthroplasty with clavicular stabiliza-

D. S. Morrison, M.D.: Southern California Center for Sports Medicine; and Department of Orthopaedic Surgery, Memorial Hospital of Long Beach, Long Beach, California.

P. H. Woodworth, M.D.: Shoulder and Elbow Surgery, Southern California Center for Sports Medicine; and Department of Orthopaedic Surgery, Long Beach Memorial Medical Center, Long Beach, California.

tion. In the case of hypertrophic osteoarthritis, the diameter of the distal clavicle can measure up to 4 cm. An AC joint of this size takes quite a long time to treat arthroscopically, and the amount of damage done to the surrounding ligaments and muscle attachments closely approximates that caused by an open surgical procedure. In these patients, we prefer to perform an open excisional arthroplasty so the deltoid–trapezius aponeurosis can be repaired after excising the large distal clavicle fragment.

A relative contraindication for an arthroscopic excisional arthroplasty of the AC joint is a patient's pending worker's compensation claim. In our clinic, we have found that the arthroscopic technique is successful in 90% of private patients, whereas it is satisfactory in only 70% of worker's compensation cases. Therefore, it may be better to do the "definitive" procedure with open techniques in this patient population.

The ideal patient for the arthroscopic procedure has isolated AC joint arthritis without massive hypertrophic spur formation and who has a stable distal clavicle. Unfortunately, the incidence of concomitant rotator cuff tendinitis and subacromial impingement syndrome in patients with symptomatic AC arthritis is as high as 38.5%. Therefore, a large percentage of patients will require not only the excision of the AC joint but also an arthroscopic subacromial decompression with or without rotator cuff repair to completely alleviate the symptoms in their shoulder.

PREOPERATIVE PLANNING

The patient who has degenerative disease that is isolated to the AC joint or disease in this joint in conjunction with subacromial impingement syndrome is a candidate for arthroscopic distal clavicle excision. The patient with isolated AC joint problems has pain well localized to the superior aspect of the shoulder in the area of the AC joint. The patient's pain is usually aggravated by use of the arm above shoulder level or by reaching behind the back or across the chest to the contralateral shoulder. However, while each of these motions may be painful, it is the localization of the pain precisely to the AC joint that identifies this joint as the pathologic site. There may be a history of an athletic injury, a repetitive stress to this joint as in gymnastics or weightlifting, or a job requiring repeated use of the arm above shoulder level. Physical examination may reveal an increased bony prominence at the AC joint. The AC joint is typically tender and boggy, although it is useful to compare the painful AC joint with the contralateral AC joint to see if the local tenderness is asymmetric.

Clinically significant pain in the AC joint can also be elicited by provocative tests. Having the patient hold his or her arm straight in front and at shoulder level is the first and most specific test. The patient is instructed to resist any motion as the examiner applies a force attempting to move the arm into horizontal abduction first and then into horizontal adduction. Reproduction of pain at the AC joint with either maneuver is considered a positive provocative test for the AC joint, although the former is usually more telling. Another more sensitive but less specific test is performed by horizontally adducting the internally rotated arm across the patient's chest. It is positive if it reproduces pain. This provocative test is sensitive for AC joint pathology, but not specific because it can also be positive with rotator cuff problems.

Posterior clavicular instability occurs in about 20% of patients with AC arthritis. To test for it, the patient holds the arm in 90 degrees of elevation in the frontal plane. The examiner places the index finger of one hand on the posterior cortex of the distal clavicle right behind the AC joint and pushes down hard on the patient's arm with the other hand. The distal clavicle will normally shift posteriorly about 2 mm. In patients with posterior clavicular instability, however, the clavicle will displace 5 to 8 mm posteriorly. In some cases, it will slide so far back that it pinches the spine of the scapula at the base of the acromion and reproduces a component of the patient's pain. Minimal posterior instability can be addressed at surgery by rounding off the back of the clavicle, whereas gross instability requires open treatment at the time of the excisional arthroplasty.

Range of motion is typically unaffected by AC joint pathology unless the pain has been of such long duration that a secondary frozen shoulder is present. If this has occurred, there will be painful limitation of the arm's range of motion in forward elevation, external rotation, and internal rotation. This can make it difficult to differentiate AC joint pain from capsular or cuff pain. The strength of the shoulder girdle is typically normal in these patients except for protective weakness due to pain.

Useful radiographic studies are anteroposterior (AP), lateral, and axillary views, which may show spurring, sclerosis, or narrowing of the AC joint. To best visualize the AC joint, obtain a 20-degree cephalic-tilt AP view of the clavicle. This view shows the AC joint without any bony overlap and is the most useful view for identifying subtle changes within the AC joint. If there is neither a history of a specific traumatic episode nor clinical suspicion of an AC joint separation, weighted views are not necessary. There is little need for more sophisticated imaging studies in isolated AC joint disease because the joint is readily palpable on physical examination and plain radiographs show the pathology well.

SURGERY

The technique is essentially the same whether or not arthroscopic subacromial decompression is performed in the same operation. The exposure and orientation are somewhat more difficult in the absence of subacromial decompression, but the length of the procedure and the quality of the resection are not significantly altered. Our preferred technique uses virtually the same portals and instrumentation that are normally used for routine arthroscopic surgery of the shoulder. Once the patient is anesthetized, the subacromial space is injected with 20 mL of 1% lidocaine hydrochloride with epinephrine for preemptive analgesia. The patient is then placed in the lateral decubitus position, our standard position for glenohumeral arthroscopy. The beach-chair position can also be used; however, it has the disadvantage that the irrigation fluid leaking from the posterior portal tends to track down the arthroscope and onto the operator's hand and arm. In a dry-camera situation, this frequently results in irrigation fluid leaking through the drape material and fogging the optics of the arthroscope. In the lateral position, this does not happen, and although the anterior portal is somewhat awkward for instrumentation in this position, we still prefer it for the majority of our arthroscopies. Sufficient traction is used to counterbalance the weight of the arm, to stabilize it, and to displace the humeral head from the field (usually 5 kg). A position of 10 to 15 degrees of abduction and 15 to 20 degrees of forward flexion is ideal (Fig. 2-1).

The procedure is performed through two portals: a posterior portal used for glenohumeral and subacromial visualization and the standard anterior operative portal in the area of the rotator interval (Fig. 2-2). The posterior portal lies in such a location that with a 30-degree arthroscope, it is possible to look down the length of the AC joint from posterior to anterior and to look directly up into the AC joint to visualize its superior aspect and the superior AC ligaments. The skin location of the standard anterior glenohumeral operative portal through the rotator interval will lie approximately 5 cm anterior and inferior to the AC joint. An instrument placed through this portal into the subacromial space will come to lie inferior and parallel to the AC joint, in an excellent position to perform the removal of the distal clavicle (Fig. 2-3).

The posterior portal is developed primarily 2 to 3 cm posterior and 2 to 3 cm medial to the posterolateral corner of the acromion (see portal A, Fig. 2-2). This portal is 1 cm more medial than a standard posterior glenohumeral portal to allow better visualization of the AC joint; however, a standard arthroscopic glenohumeral examination is still easily performed via this portal. A changing rod is then used to enter the subacromial space, followed by the arthroscope cannula over the changing rod. The cannula is swept from medial to lateral in the subacromial space to break up any adhesions and to facilitate visualization. We use a high-flow arthroscope that obviates the need for a second irrigation portal, but if this is not available, the standard anterolateral operative portal used for arthroscopic subacromial decompression can be used as an inflow portal. It is placed approximately 1 cm posterior and 3 cm distal to the anterolateral corner of the acromion (see portal B, Fig. 2-2). For good visualization, a minimum inflow of 1 L per minute is required. We are able to obtain this vol-

(text continues on page 26)

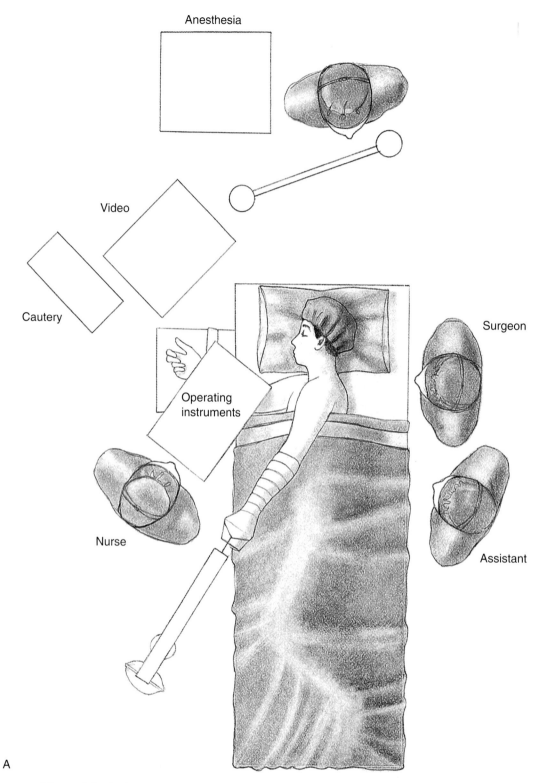

Figure 2-1. A: Arrangement of the operating room: The patient is in the lateral decubitus position with the nurse, video equipment, and anesthesia off to the opposite side of the table. This arrangement allows the surgeon easy access to both sides of the shoulder and places an assistant on each side of the operating room table. *(continued)*

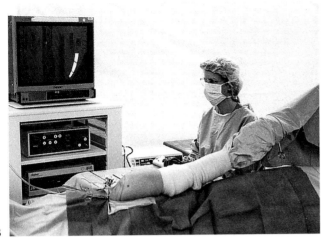

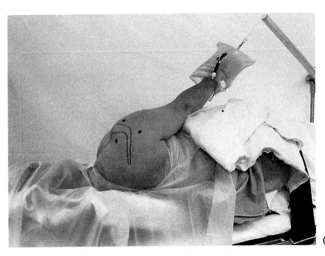

B   C

Figure 2-1. *Continued.* **B:** Patient positioning: We prefer the lateral decubitus position with minimal abduction and forward flexion. **C:** Five kilograms of traction is used for stabilization of the arm and slight traction.

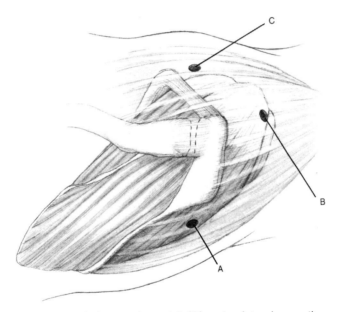

Figure 2-2. Arthroscopic portal *(A)*, anterolateral operative portal *(B)*, and anterior rotator interval portal *(C)* for intraarticular instrumentation of the glenohumeral joint and the acromioclavicular joint.

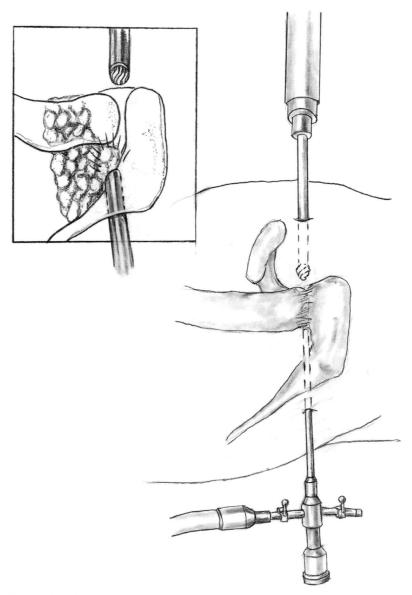

Figure 2-3. Instrument placement for acromioclavicular (AC) arthroplasty. The arthroscopic burr is parallel to the AC joint. The 30-degree arthroscope in the posterior portal allows easy visualization of the entire AC joint. A hypervascular fat pad, found beneath the distal clavicle and the posteromedial acromion, should be avoided or bleeding may be brisk.

ume using gravity inflow and a high-flow cannula but others advocate the use of an arthroscopic pump. We have found that a pump is rarely necessary if the patient's blood pressure is controlled. The rotator interval portal just lateral and approximately 1 cm superior to the tip of the coracoid is then established, and a full-radius power resector is advanced into the subacromial space (see portal C, Fig. 2-2). A partial subacromial bursectomy is carried out until visualization of the undersurface of the clavicle is sufficient. If there is difficulty in orientation, a needle can be placed through the AC joint into the subacromial space to act as a marker for this débridement. At this point in the procedure, extreme care must be taken to not resect the subacromial and subacromioclavicular joint fat pad, which is normally found posteromedial to the AC joint and is remarkably hypervascular (Fig. 2-3). If the resector is placed in this area and débridement is performed indiscriminately, the result will be massive bleeding that will be very difficult to control through any means, even electrocautery. Therefore, débridement should take place along the anteromedial acromion and under the anterior surface of the AC joint to avoid this hypervascular fat pad. The periosteum of the distal clavicle is quite vascular and electrocautery is essential during this procedure. We routinely do a subperiosteal cauterization of the distal 8 mm of the clavicle (anterior, inferior, and posterior cortices) at the beginning of the procedure before the removal of the periosteum (Fig. 2-4). This decreases bleeding significantly throughout the remainder of the case. Once the periosteum is removed from the undersurface of the anterior portion of the acromial and clavicular articulation of the AC joint, the subperiosteal débridement is carried posteriorly until the entire undersurface of the AC joint is exposed down to bone. The periosteal resection and bursectomy are then carried medially under the distal clavicle for about 8 mm, exposing the undersurface of the clavicle. Again, care is taken not to drift posterior to the clavicle into the fat pad.

Once the AC joint has been identified and the inferior capsule released, a 5-mm full-radius resector is used to round off the inferior edge of the acromial articulation to allow better visualization into the AC joint. This is a very important part of the surgical procedure because rounding off this edge will make it much easier to look up into the area of the AC resection later in the case. The full-radius resector is removed and a 5.5-mm high-speed burr is introduced into the same portal. The axis of the burr lies directly along the axis of the AC joint, making resection a simple task of superior and inferior movement of the burr over the distal end of the clavicle (Figs. 2-5 and 2-6). The full diameter of the burr is buried into the most anteroinferior portion of the distal clavicle. This divot in the clavicle is used as a reference point for the amount of bone to be removed from the clavicle and will yield a resection of about 6 mm of clavicular bone. The resection of the distal clavicle is carried posteriorly at the same depth using a superior and inferior sweeping motion. The most difficult portion of the resection is the posterior cortex of the clavicle. This is mainly because once the resection is carried posteriorly, blood vessels are frequently encountered not only in the subclavicular fat pad, but also in the posterior joint capsule and the AC ligaments. It is important to remove the same amount of bone from the posterior portion of the clavicle as from the anterior portion so that a consistent excision width is obtained across the entire

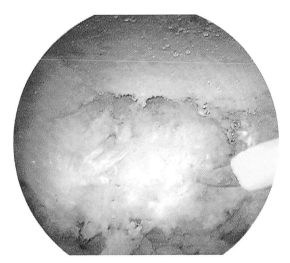

Figure 2-4. The periosteum of the distal clavicle is quite hypervascular and electrocautery is essential during acromioclavicular (AC) arthroplasty. In this intraoperative photograph, the acromion (after acromioplasty) is on top, the rotator cuff is on the bottom, and the electrocautery is introduced from the right, pointing at the distal clavicle. The AC joint space is at the upper middle portion of the picture, oriented left to right.

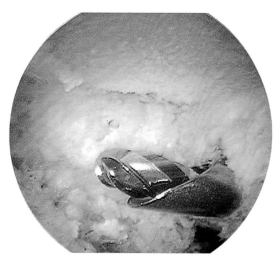

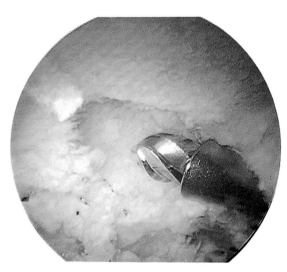

Figure 2-5. The burr is introduced through the anterior portal before beginning the resection of the distal clavicle. The axis of the burr lies directly along the axis of the acromioclavicular joint.

Figure 2-6. Resection consists of superior and inferior movements of the burr over the distal end of the clavicle. Here a partial resection of the distal clavicle is shown.

AC joint (Fig. 2-7). We try to remove approximately 6 to 7 mm from the distal clavicle and 2 mm from the acromial articulation of the AC joint. In this way, all cartilage is removed from the acromial side and 6 mm of bone is removed from the clavicular side. Including the 1 to 2 mm of original AC joint space, this yields a total resection of 8 to 10 mm as seen in the postoperative radiographs (Figs. 2-8 and 2-9).

Occasionally, degenerative cysts are encountered while resecting the distal clavicle. It is important to fully excise these cysts, because they can be a source of postoperative pain. If the cyst is very deep and would require too much of the distal clavicle to be resected, the remainder of the cyst can be removed with a small angulated curette (Fig. 2-10).

The second most difficult portion of the procedure is the resection of the superior cortex of the clavicle without disrupting the superior AC ligaments. Preservation of these liga-

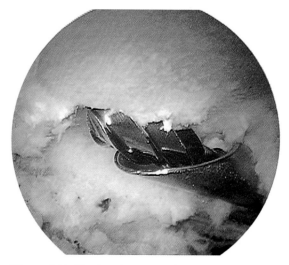

Figure 2-7. The burr is seen on its way superiorly up into the acromioclavicular joint. A portion of the acromial facet may be removed at this time. It is important that the same amount of bone be removed from the posterior clavicle as from the anterior clavicle so that a consistent width of excision is obtained.

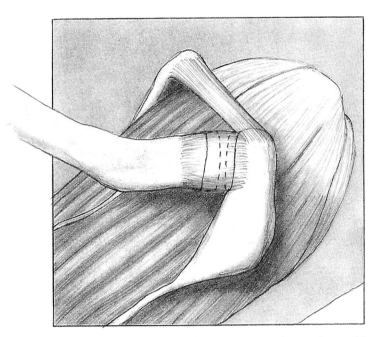

Figure 2-8. Acromioclavicular resection: 1 to 2 mm of acromion and 5 to 7 mm of distal clavicle are excised. The same amount of bone is removed from the anterior as from the posterior clavicle.

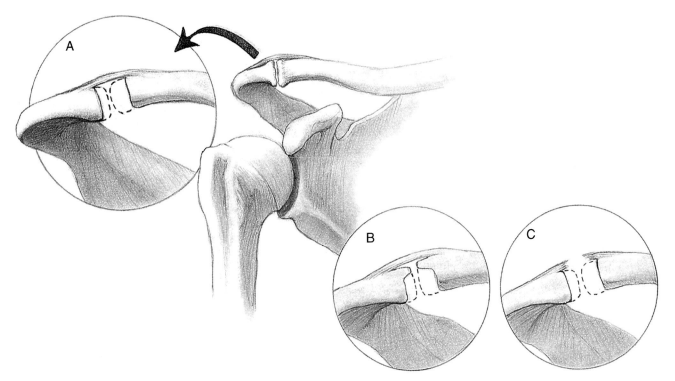

Figure 2-9. A: Satisfactory completion of an acromioclavicular (AC) arthroplasty with the posterior and superior AC ligaments intact. **B:** Incomplete resection superiorly will lead to continued symptoms postoperatively and failure. **C:** Satisfactory bone resection with disruption of the AC ligaments can result in postoperative instability and skin puckering with continued pain.

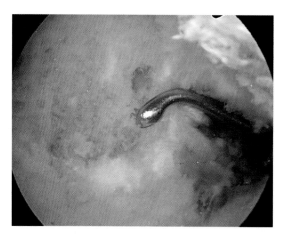

Figure 2-10. Degenerative cyst in the subchondral bone of the distal clavicle after partial resection of the distal clavicle. A small, angulated curette has been used to remove soft tissue from the cyst. An attempt should be made to remove these cysts during the resection. If they are too deep in the cancellous bone then they can be curetted as shown here.

ments prevents postoperative instability of the distal clavicle, it also eliminates the problem of the dent or puckering of the skin that may occur in the area of an AC arthroplasty, which can cause so much trouble with women's clothing, particularly bra straps. To accomplish this, the arthroscope is placed directly posterior to the AC joint and rotated so that it is looking straight up into the joint. This gives an excellent view of the superior aspect of the joint and allows complete visualization while the superior resection is performed. When it is apparent that the resection is completed satisfactorily, a probe is placed through the anterior operative portal, and the ligament is probed posteriorly, superiorly, and anteriorly for fragments of retained bone (Figs. 2-11 and 2-12). During the resection, it is often possible to shell out and thin the cortical bone so that it appears to be a portion of ligament, but with probing it will become apparent that there are some bone fragments retained within the ligamentous structures. It is imperative that these fragments be removed before the completion of the procedure or they may act as a nidus for heterotopic ossification postoperatively. A curette introduced through the anterior portal is often helpful for shelling out the remaining bone and leaving the superior AC ligament intact (Fig. 2-13).

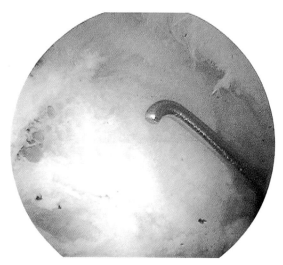

Figure 2-11. A probe is placed through the anterior portal, and the ligament is probed posteriorly, superiorly, and anteriorly for fragments of retained bone. In this photograph, the probe is seen in the acromioclavicular (AC) joint. At the 12-o'clock position is the edge of the acromion; the superior AC ligaments are just inferior to this, and the resected clavicle (appearing *yellow*) is in the center of the picture. With this 5-mm probe, approximately 7 mm has been resected between the clavicle and the acromion.

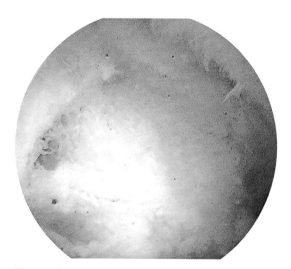

Figure 2-12. The completed distal clavicle excision.

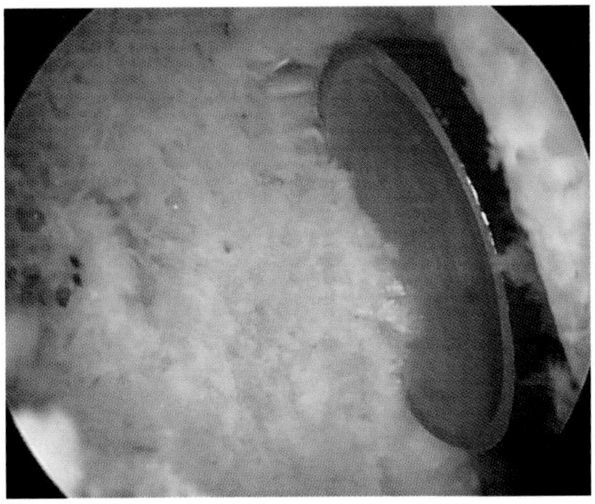

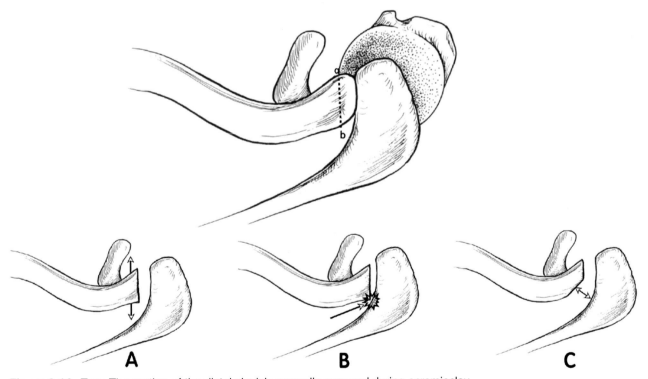

Figure 2-13. A medium curette is helpful for removing thin pieces of the superior cortex of the distal clavicle, which may be left behind by the burr. This manual method leaves the superior acromioclavicular ligament intact.

If overaggressive resection results in disruption of the superior AC ligament and an unstable clavicle, it is important to resect more bone from the posterior aspect of the distal clavicle. This is because the unstable clavicle has a tendency to impinge on the spine of the scapula at the base of the acromion. The rounding of the posterior clavicle will decrease the incidence of this painful impingement (Fig. 2-14). However, the best way to prevent this

A   **B**   **C**

Figure 2-14. Top: The portion of the distal clavicle normally removed during acromioclavicular (AC) arthroplasty. **A:** The edges of the distal clavicle have not been rounded off, the sharp points anteriorly and posteriorly can be a source of pressure sensitivity after surgery. In addition, if the AC ligaments have been damaged during the surgery, there can be anteroposterior instability of the distal clavicle. **B:** The posterior aspect of an unstable distal clavicle can impinge on the spine of the scapula at the base of the acromion. This causes pain with resisted forward elevation of the arm or overhead lifting. **C:** Rounding off or beveling of the posterior aspect of the distal clavicle decreases the incidence of this painful impingement.

problem is to avoid damaging the ligaments in the first place. If, however, mild to moderate AP clavicular instability is part of a patient's presenting pathology, then this same technique can be used to eliminate scapuloclavicular impingement postoperatively.

The subacromial space and AC joint are then copiously irrigated to remove fragments of bone, periosteum, and bursa, and inflow pressure is decreased to visualize and control bleeding prior to wound closure. Probably the most important factor in controlling bleeding during shoulder arthroscopy is the control of the patient's blood pressure. In a recent study, we found that a pressure differential of 50 mm Hg between the systolic blood pressure and the subacromial space irrigation pressure was necessary to prevent capillary bleeding. Subacromial surgery is a painful procedure and if uncontrolled, blood pressure will frequently elevate to 150 to 170 mm Hg intraoperatively. This would require a subacromial space irrigation pressure of over 100 mm Hg to control bleeding. Not only is this almost impossible to obtain, but the massive extravasation of fluid caused by such pressure is detrimental to good surgical technique and the welfare of the patient. Keeping the systolic blood pressure at about 95 mm Hg, whenever medically feasible, will allow excellent visualization with simple gravity inflow and a high-flow arthroscope.

We then instill the subacromial space with 20 mL of 0.5% Marcaine with epinephrine in an effort to control postoperative pain and to decrease postoperative bleeding. The wound is closed in the standard fashion and the arm is placed in a sling.

In patients in whom concomitant subacromial decompression is required, the AC arthroplasty is easier to perform because it is facilitated by that procedure. During the midportion of the subacromial decompression, the AC joint is almost always identified and at times it may be accidentally entered.

We do not believe in "coplaning" of the asymptomatic AC joint. This is the practice of removing osteophytes from the undersurface of the acromial and clavicular articulations of the AC joint. In our experience, entering an arthritic but asymptomatic AC joint in this fashion causes symptomatic postoperative AC joint pain in about 17% of patients. True impingement from these osteophytes is extremely rare and only in these rare cases would we recommend their removal at the time of subacromial decompression.

When we perform an arthroscopic subacromial decompression and an AC arthroplasty, we carry the acromial resection medially under the AC joint. The acromial articulation of the AC joint is then rounded off to expose the entire distal clavicle. Marker needles are not needed in this case because the AC joint is readily identified. At this point, the distal 8 mm of clavicle is cauterized along the anterior, inferior, and posterior surfaces, and then the procedure as described above is accomplished.

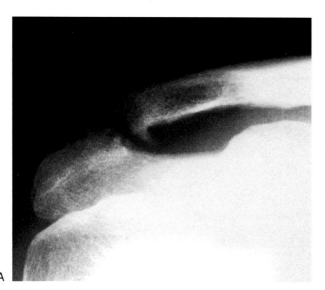

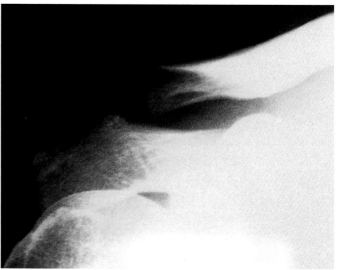

A   B

Figure 2-15. Preoperative **(A)** and postoperative **(B)** radiographs of a successful arthroscopic acromioclavicular arthroplasty.

If for some reason, visualization of the AC joint from the standard posterior portal is difficult or incomplete, then the arthroscope can be moved to the anterior operative portal, and the entire AC joint is easily visualized. If any retained bone is found, then the high-speed burr or a curette is reintroduced to complete the AC arthroplasty (Fig. 2-15).

POSTOPERATIVE MANAGEMENT

The arm is placed in a sling in the operating room and the patient is sent home from the hospital the same day. We recommend that the patient rest the arm for 1 day postoperatively, but within 48 hours the patient is encouraged to take the arm out of the sling, use it for all normal activities at the side, and then discard the sling. Two days postoperatively, the patient begins progressive passive assistive range-of-motion exercises for the shoulder to avoid adhesive capsulitis. We have the physical therapist and patient concentrate on internal and external rotation exercises and avoid any range-of-motion exercises in shoulder flexion or abduction. Overhead passive range-of-motion exercises are often very painful for the patient and may affect the maturation of scar tissue within the resected AC joint leading to long-term pain and hypermobility of joint. If a patient has full external rotation at the side and internal rotation behind the back, he or she will have obligate forward elevation within 10 degrees of his or her normal range. (Unfortunately, full forward elevation does not carry with it obligate full internal or external rotation.) Thus, these overhead restrictions will not result in loss of elevation due to adhesive capsulitis. These limitations are for formal exercises only and the patient may perform overhead activities in the course of usual activities of daily living, but not on a repetitive basis.

We work on range of motion only for the first 4 to 6 weeks. Then, if the patient has normal range of motion, strengthening exercises are begun as pain allows. Because the postoperative immobilization and restrictions are minimal, an extensive strengthening program is not usually necessary because very little atrophy has taken place in the perioperative period. Once the patient has regained normal strength and range of motion, full normal activities may be resumed using pain as a guide. Competition in contact athletics or overhead or throwing sports is delayed for 8 to 12 weeks to allow healing and maturation of scar tissue.

Because this procedure is done arthroscopically without interfering with the deltoid origin, return of range of motion is usually rapid. Within 2 to 4 weeks from the time of surgery, motion in all planes is usually full and strength is near normal. The patient, however, may continue to experience pain with arm movement, although frequently the pain is clearly different from that which was present preoperatively. Pain is typically present with range-of-motion exercises, but it is unusual to have pain at rest. By 3 months after surgery, the pain in this area is usually gone except for weather ache and fatigue ache when the arm is used repetitively above shoulder level. By 6 months after surgery, the patients have usually returned to their normal activities with a shoulder that has normal strength, normal motion, and normal function. If the diagnosis was correctly isolated to the AC joint and the arthroscopic AC joint resection was well performed, virtually all patients should experience significant relief of pain and return to normal activities.

RESULTS

We have found the arthroscopic technique successful in 90% of our private patients. As stated previously, this decreases to 70% satisfaction in the patients with worker's compensation claims. Of the failed arthroscopic procedures, revision distal clavicle excision via open technique yields excellent results in only 20% of patients; 50% of patients noting a significant decrease, but not complete elimination of their pain; 25% experiencing no change in their symptoms; and 5% claiming to be worse after revision open surgery. It is therefore best to perform a good operation the first time and obviate the need for further treatment.

COMPLICATIONS

The most common complication is incomplete resection of the AC joint and persistent pain localized to this area. Careful surgical technique to ensure complete AC joint excision, as described above, should help minimize this complication. Arthroscopic surgical success can also be optimized by careful patient selection and choosing an open procedure for a patient with a very thick, mobile, or hypertrophic degenerative AC joint.

A second complication not infrequently seen is that of residual bone fragments in the area of clavicle excision. This bone debris may serve as a nidus for heterotopic ossification in the area of the joint and may be an important reason for failure of some arthroscopic resections. Making certain that there is adequate visualization, all fragments of bone are removed from the capsule, and the joint is vigorously irrigated to remove loose bone before skin closure may minimize this complication.

Although it is more common to err on the side of the underresection of bone, an excessive amount of bone may be resected and the stability of the clavicle threatened. The preoperative radiograph should be evaluated to determine the amount of bone that needs to be resected and to keep the distal clavicle resection well lateral to the insertion of the coracoclavicular ligaments.

Finally, persistent pain due to an untreated additional diagnosis is not uncommon. AC joint disease frequently accompanies subacromial impingement syndrome. Addressing the pathology in the AC joint without addressing the concomitant pathology in the subacromial space may lead to residual pain from subacromial impingement. A thorough preoperative evaluation to accurately identify the exact source(s) of the patient's pain will minimize the occurrence of this complication. In addition, posterior clavicular instability needs to be diagnosed preoperatively and a decision made as to whether rounding off the posterior clavicle during arthroscopy can adequately treat it or whether it requires open stabilization at the time of AC joint resection.

RECOMMENDED READING

1. Gartsman, G.M., Combs, A.H., Davis, P.E., et al.: Arthroscopic AC joint resection: an anatomical study. *Am J Sports Med* 19: 2–5, 1991.
2. Johnson, L.L.: *Arthroscopic surgery: principles and practice.* St. Louis: Mosby–Year Book, 1986.
3. Johnson, L.L.: *Diagnostic and surgical arthroscopy of the shoulder.* St. Louis: Mosby–Year Book, 1993.
4. Morrison, D.S., Schaefer, R.K., Friedman, R.L.: The relationship between subacromial space pressure, blood pressure, and visual clarity during arthroscopic subacromial decompression. *Arthroscopy* 11: 557–560, 1995.
5. Myers, J.F.: Arthroscopic debridement of the AC joint and distal clavicle resection. In: McGinty, J.B., Caspari, R.B., Jackson, R.W., et al. eds.: *Operative arthroscopy.* New York: Raven Press, 557–560, 1991.
6. Synder, S.J.: Arthroscopic AC joint debridement and distal clavicle resection. *Tech Orthop* 3: 41–45, 1988.

3

Arthroscopic Repair of the Rotator Cuff

Robert H. Bell

INDICATIONS/CONTRAINDICATIONS

Tears of the rotator cuff mechanism remain one of the more common problems we as orthopaedists need to treat. Because this is a disease with a broad continuum, these patients can present with various levels of pathology. Tears may be partial-thickness lesions or full-thickness lesions ranging from 1 cm small tears to massive, irreparable tears. Often, these patients will have associated disease of the acromioclavicular (AC) joint, biceps tendon, and labrum. While impingement from the overlying acromion is a part of this disease entity, many tears may have an intrinsic pathology unrelated to the impingement process or an extrinsic process such as instability. As such, the surgeon must be careful in his or her assessment of these patients and understand the origin of the pathology in order to best treat the disease.

The principal indication for rotator cuff surgery is pain. Lack of mobility and diminished strength, while often of concern to patients, are secondary to that of pain relief in these patients. The patients should understand that the intent of the surgery is to remove the offending acromial prominence and repair the damaged tendons. It is important that they realize the results of such surgery are dependent on many factors, including tear size, retraction, tissue quality, preoperative mobility, and a patient's overall health. Furthermore, they should understand their role in the postoperative rehabilitation and the length of time required for recovery.

Relative and absolute contraindications to this surgery are rare but include active infection or a recent history of such, significant medical problems, advanced degenerative joint disease requiring arthroplasty, and advanced cuff arthropathy. Patients with fixed superior migration of the humeral head on anteroposterior (AP) films, an absent acromiohumeral interval, fatty infiltrates, atrophy, and marked retraction of tendon edges on magnetic reso-

R. H. Bell, M.D.: Department of Orthopaedics, Northeast Ohio Universities College of Medicine; and Shoulder Service, Crystal Clinic and Summa Health System, Akron, Ohio.

nance imaging (MRI) are not candidates for an arthroscopic rotator cuff repair much less an open one and should be recognized preoperatively.

PREOPERATIVE PLANNING

Patients with impingement and associated rotator cuff pathology can and will present with a constellation of physical findings, however, in most cases, the history these patients provide is remarkably similar regardless of the size of the tear. Nearly all of these patients will describe pain with routine overhead activities such as reaching to the top shelf in the kitchen or closet, trouble putting on a coat and reaching behind their back to hook a bra, an inability to participate in their normal level of recreational activities such as tennis or golf and most significantly, trouble with sleep. Pain at rest is common in this group of patients owing to the edema of the cuff tendons and secondary inflammation encountered when they become dependent lying in bed. This night pain classically improves after they get up in the morning and once again assume an upright posture. Those patients with large and massive tears may describe a more significant functional limitation than those with smaller tears given that they have lost much of their ability to externally rotate the arm and position it for daily activities. Nevertheless, even patients with smaller lesions may have trouble with many activities of daily living due to pain and occasionally a secondary adhesive capsulitis.

The physical examination may provide some subtle evidence of rotator cuff problems even on the inspection. Not uncommonly, patients with only moderately advanced cuff disease will have a torn long head of the biceps tendon with the classic "Popeye" muscle appearance. The AC joint, if arthritic, will be more prominent and may even have an associated ganglion making it that much more noticeable to a patient. This is glenohumeral joint fluid that has leaked out into the subacromial space and through the absent inferior capsule of the AC joint. This ganglion enlarges superiorly to present as a prominence on the dorsal surface of the AC joint. If the cuff tear is long-standing and advanced, there will often be an empty fossa due to atrophy of the supra- and infraspinatus muscles and a relative prominence of the scapular spine. Palpation will elicit some tenderness if the AC joint is inflamed, however, for the most part, patients with rotator cuff disease will be most symptomatic with motion testing, not palpation. Motion should be assessed as both passive and active and recorded as such. These patients will, depending on the size of their tears, demonstrate varying losses of both types of motion. Patients with small tears typically will have preservation of active and passive motion with limitation only due to pain on extremes. As the tear enlarges, the supraspinatus and ultimately the infraspinatus and teres minor become involved and not only will a patient begin to lose forward elevation but also external rotation. If there is little capsular adhesion, passive motion will be preserved and active motion decreased proportionally. Strength in these planes will decrease as well and may be most noticeable on resisted external rotation. To test this I use a maneuver called the drift sign in which I help the patient position the arm in slight external rotation and ask him or her to hold the arm in that position after I let go. An inability to maintain this position of external rotation is indicative of a larger tear. Similarly, the lift off test, belly push, or Napoleon sign allows the surgeon to test for the integrity of the subscapularis.

The classic Neer impingement sign will often be positive, as will the Hawkins test and the painful arc. All these confirm the presence of subacromial impingement and likely cuff pathology but do not necessarily help to quantitate the size of tear. However, in concert with the test for motion, they do provide enough information to make one suspect larger tears. If the AC joint is pathologic due to painful arthritic changes or an inflammatory arthropathy without radiographic changes, the cross-arm abduction test will help to elicit pain well localized to the joint.

Diagnostic Tests

There are a number of diagnostic studies that can aid the surgeon in not only defining the existence of a full-thickness rotator cuff tear, partial-thickness rotator cuff tear or other associated pathology, but also help to better define those lesions that may be amenable to an arthroscopic repair given their level of technical ability. Arthroscopic rotator cuff surgery requires an understanding of basic shoulder arthroscopy, arthroscopic subacromial decompressions, arthroscopic excisions of the distal clavicle, repair of superior labrum anterior and posterior (SLAP) lesions, biceps pathology, and capsulolabral disruptions.

Routine imaging begins with radiographic studies of the shoulder, including but not limited to a true AP to the glenohumeral joint, lateral, and outlet views. These three views will give the surgeon an appreciation for associated glenohumeral degenerative disease, loose bodies, and the relative acromiohumeral interval. Furthermore, the outlet view will show relative acromial morphology (types I –III), inferior clavicular osteophytes that compromise the outlet, and the relative prominence of the greater tuberosity, if there were prior trauma. Additional views such as the Zanca view will better demonstrate the status of the AC articulation, degenerative changes within this joint, and cystic changes consistent with idiopathic osteolysis and its inclination, which may be important in operative planning. Axillary views can also help to demonstrate associated glenohumeral narrowing consistent with early degenerative arthritis, posterior subluxation, and posterior glenoid osteophytes, often seen in throwing athletes.

Arthrography, once the gold standard in defining rotator cuff pathology, is used less often because of the advent of MRI. Although arthrography is a reliable tool for determining the presence of a full-thickness rotator cuff tear, it is limited in its ability to determine the size of full-thickness rotator cuff tears or the existence of partial-thickness rotator cuff tears.

MRI, on the other hand, clearly has overshadowed other diagnostic modalities in the area of shoulder problems. Its sensitivity and specificity are unmatched by other conventional means and afford the surgeon the ability to know preoperatively the size and character of a rotator cuff lesion. A combination of sagittal, tangential, and coronal oblique images may allow the surgeon to determine AP and mediolateral dimensions of a tear as well as coexistent atrophic changes and fatty infiltrates within the muscle bodies of the supraspinatus and infraspinatus thereby better defining the age of a rotator cuff tear. In addition, the existence of such changes coexistent with fixed superior migration of the humeral head on routine AP films of the shoulder should lead one to suspect an irreparable lesion and give consideration to other options.

Rotator cuff surgery, in order to be most successful, requires not only a skillful surgeon but also a well-informed patient. I use a number of teaching aids to facilitate this process of learning for the patient including written materials and a self-made teaching video. While a number of teaching tapes exist for open rotator cuff surgery, few are commercially available for arthroscopic repair. A personalized tape showing his or her surgeon allows the patient a greater comfort level in the preoperative discussion. A simple 5-minute video of the doctor discussing the mechanics of the surgery, the postoperative course, and potential outcomes and complications will allay many concerns and make for a ready partner in the recovery process. In these preoperative teachings, I touch on a number of different issues, including the following:

1. The success rate for the arthroscopic approach has been proven comparable to that of open repairs.
2. The morbidity following the surgery will be less than that of an open repair but will still encompass pain requiring analgesics for the first few weeks.
3. The tendon repair while painful at first will rapidly become less painful over the first month but the actual healing of the tendon to the bone will take as long as 6 months to reach a strength comparable to a normal shoulder. This requires that they protect their repair carefully especially for the first 2 to 3 months, before any strengthening begins.
4. I typically discharge most patients after their third or fourth visit at the 5- to 6-month mark, but inform them that additional gains in motion and strength may take a year.
5. Many patients ask if they really need to fix the tendon. I tell them that likely half of all tears enlarge over time and become more painful and functionally debilitating but that we cannot predict which will do this but that if they have noted a progression of their

symptoms that this often indicates a tear that is enlarging and, thus, should be addressed.

6. I warn them that if their tear does enlarge, it may become irreparable due to size and retraction and may, in rare cases, go on to develop cuff arthropathy.

7. Patients always want percentages for a procedure and I state a 85% to 90% chance for success, meaning improvement in pain, not necessarily in motion; 10% chance of no improvement; and less than 1% chance of being made worse. Arthroscopic repairs, because they preserve the deltoid, lessen the risk of serious deltoid problems postoperatively but patients need to be aware of this possibility.

8. The intent of rotator cuff surgery is pain relief and the patients must understand that the goal of their surgery will be primarily to help relieve their pain and any secondary improvement in motion and function, while anticipated, will be a bonus.

9. Finally, I let all patients know that repairs can fail, early and late, and that the larger the tear, the greater the likelihood of such an occurrence. I ask them to keep me apprised of their status during the recovery even after discharge. I do explain that it is common to notice periods of pain during their recovery and that should they be significant we will investigate accordingly.

SURGERY

Operating Room Setup

I do all rotator cuff surgery with the patient in the lateral decubitus position. This allows ready access to the posterior, anterior, and superior aspects of the shoulder while holding the arm in an appropriate position of slight abduction thereby facilitating approximation of the free tendon edge to the region of the greater tuberosity. In this position, the arm may be rotated as necessary to facilitate anchor placement and reduce tension during suture tying. In the vast majority of patients, 10 lb of traction at approximately 30 to 40 degrees of abduction is more than adequate to provide appropriate positioning (Fig. 3-1A). I make certain that anesthesia is moved out of the immediate operative field so that I have access to the entire shoulder region, front and back. This allows me to work on the decompression and anchor placement from the posterior aspect and then move to the top of the table to tie knots (Fig. 3-1C).

The traction apparatus that we use is a very simple device that uses a pulley system: an inflatable hand holder that negates any risk of potential nerve injury or skin problems (Fig. 3-1B). Because this device is attached at a single centered hole, we are able to readily rotate the arm in internal and external rotation. As in all orthopaedic procedures, instruments can make or break any operation. This is no different with arthroscopic rotator cuff repairs. I use a basic set of instruments that are necessary for every case and they include a simple knot pusher, a ring grabber or crab claw device for retrieving individual sutures, a set of pigtail suture passers, a cannula for fluid management, and one of a number of different suture retrievers.

Portals

All arthroscopic repairs require three principal portals and an additional ancillary anterior portal (Fig. 3-2). The viewing portal is located 1 cm medial and 2 cm inferior to the posterolateral corner of the acromion. The working portal is located immediately anterior to the "finish line"—a line drawn perpendicular to the lateral margin of the acromion beginning at the posterior extent of the AC joint. The working portal is then located anterior to this line 2 to 3 cm inferior to the lateral margin of the acromion. The anchor portal is determined by subacromial viewing with the arthroscope and using needle localization technique and is typically at the anterolateral corner of the acromion. An additional fourth portal may be made anterior to the acromion and is called the "waiting room" portal. We use this in large tears in which three or more anchors and six or more sutures are used. This portal allows us to position sutures that are not being worked with anteriorly to free up the viewing area while posterior sutures are tied. This aids greatly in suture management.

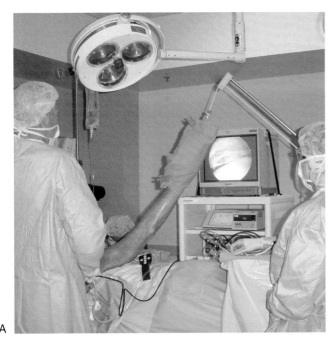

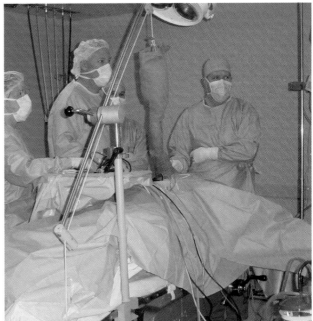

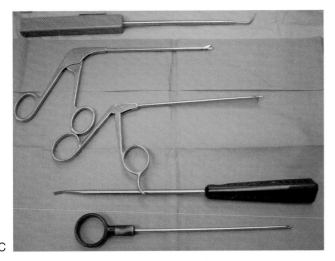

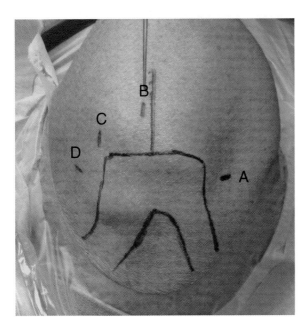

Figure 3-1. A: The patient is placed in the lateral decubitus position held by a beanbag device and the arm is abducted 40 degrees. **B:** An inflatable hand holder is used to hold the arm during suspension. Anesthesia is moved remote from the immediate area so the surgeon has nearly unrestricted access to the posterior aspect of the shoulder for the decompression and anchor placement and the lateral and anterior portals for knot tying and suture passing. **C:** Basic instruments for cuff repairs including (from **top** to **bottom**) suture snare or retriever, arthroscopic scissors, ring grabber, liberator for mobilizing, and knot pusher.

Figure 3-2. Right shoulder. The viewing portal *(A)* is 1 cm medial and 2 cm inferior to the posterolateral corner of the acromion. The working portal *(B)* is 1 cm anterior to the finish line and 3 cm lateral to the lateral acromion. The anchor portal *(C)* is just off the anterolateral corner of the acromion. The waiting room portal *(D)* is 1 cm anterior to the anterior border of the acromion.

Glenohumeral Inspection

All rotator cuff repairs begin with a thorough inspection of the glenohumeral joint to identify and treat other associated pathology such as SLAP lesions, capsulolabral disruptions, biceps tears, and loose bodies. Additionally, partial-thickness tears of the rotator cuff can be assessed, localization sutures placed, and if a high-grade lesion is encountered, a formal débridement of the lesion with conversion to a full-thickness tear may be accomplished during glenohumeral inspection (Fig. 3-3).

Acromioplasty

All chronic full-thickness rotator cuff tears and most acute full-thickness rotator cuff tears undergo a concomitant arthroscopic subacromial decompression using standard technique. Viewing from the posterior portal, initial subacromial débridement is performed consisting of a bursectomy to provide visualization of the inferior surface of the acromion. If a large rotator cuff tear has been identified, an extensive bursectomy is necessary with attention directed toward the lateral and posterior bursal tissue. This ensures that visualization will be optimal during the repair. With the bursectomy complete, a radiofrequency device is used to remove

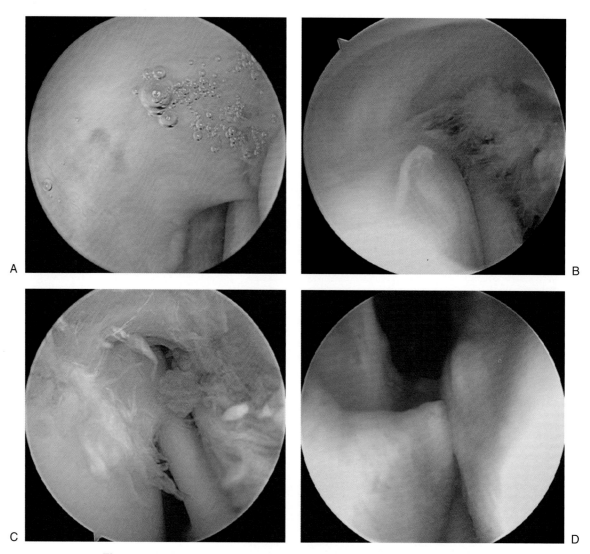

Figure 3-3. A: Normal-appearing articular side of supraspinatus. **B:** Low-grade partial thickness rotator cuff tear (RCT). **C:** High-grade partial-thickness RCT seen from articular side. **D:** Full-thickness RCT seen from within the glenohumeral joint on the articular side.

all residual soft tissue from the undersurface of the acromion and to release the coracoacromial ligament from the inferior and anterior aspects of the acromion (Fig. 3-4). The burr is then introduced from the lateral working portal and the decompression is begun at the anterolateral corner of the acromion, working both medial and posterior. The completion of the decompression is noted when the acromioplasty is tapered and terminates at or about the finish line drawn at the time of initial portal placement. The surgeon's shaver or burr should be aligned parallel to the finish line at this transition point to ensure appropriate resection. I confirm and complete the decompression using a "cutting block" technique. This is accomplished by moving the scope to the lateral portal, bringing our burr in posteriorly from the initial viewing portal, and smoothing the undersurface of the acromion to convert to a type I acromion.

Mobilization

As in open repairs, mobilization of the rotator cuff tendons may be necessary to facilitate a tension-free repair. This is accomplished in a technique similar to that used during open procedures. Traction sutures may be applied to the tendon edges and using either a shaver or a small periosteal elevator introduced through the lateral working portal, viewing from the posterior portal; the subacromial adhesions are gently released. If intraarticular adhesions are present, they may be released during the glenohumeral inspection by applying traction to the rotator cuff tendons and carefully releasing the capsulolabral junction. Care

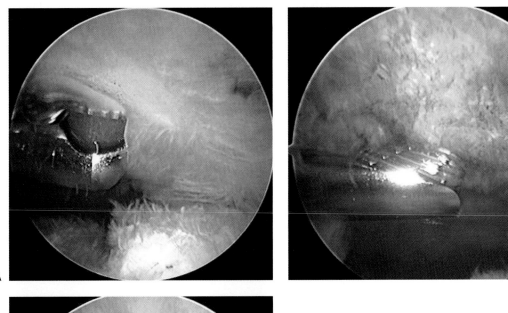

A   B

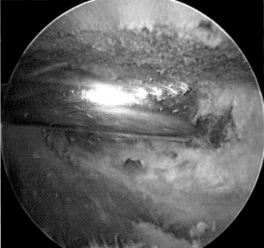

C

Figure 3-4. Left shoulder. A radiofrequency device is used to clean the inferior surface of the acromion. **A:** After this, the coracoacromial ligament (shown) is resected. **B:** Beginning at the anterolateral corner of the acromion, the decompression progresses medially and posteriorly. **C:** The completed acromioplasty.

should be taken to preserve the biceps insertion and to avoid posterior excursion of sharp instruments because of the location of the suprascapular nerve. This is also the time at which the surgeon should anticipate and plan the repair. It may be necessary to first consider a convergence repair, side to side, of the medial extent of a rotator cuff tear before placing anchors and performing the tendon-to-bone repair.

Anchor Placement

With the acromioplasty complete, the tendon edges mobilized, and the repair planned, anchors should be placed in a position that affords minimal tension on the tendon margin at the time of repair. In most cases, this will be immediately medial to the greater tuberosity, in the sulcus between that structure and the articular surface. In small and medium tears requiring no more than one or two anchors and two to four sutures, all anchors will be placed before suture passing. Anchor choice is dependent on the surgeon's preferences, however, most anchors are double-loaded with a no. 2 nonabsorbable suture material, which provides adequate suture strength and repair capability. My preference in anchors has been metallic devices, double-loaded with no. 2 nonabsorbable suture. I have avoided absorbable anchors

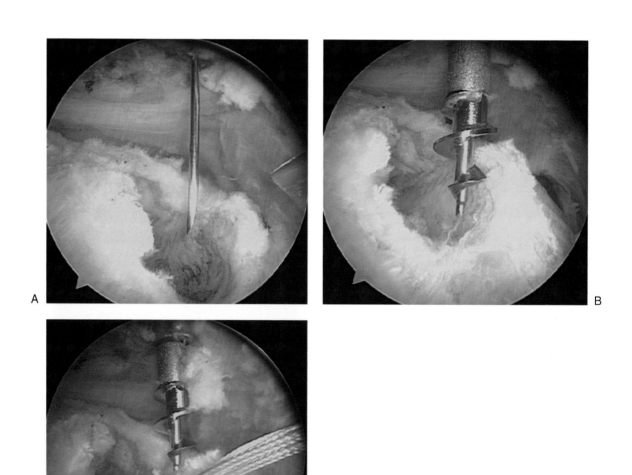

Figure 3-5. A: A needle is introduced just off the anterolateral corner of the acromion and directed toward the anticipated site of anchor placement to locate the proper anchor portal. **B:** Anchor placement begins posterior, just medial to the greater tuberosity. **C:** Each subsequent anchor is placed 1 cm anterior to the last.

simply because I have not had any evidence of anchor pullout and the metallic anchors obviate the risk of inflammatory reaction sometimes seen with absorbable ones. Anchor placement begins posterior (Fig. 3-5). A spinal needle is introduced from the anchor portal to ensure an appropriate angle for anchor insertion. The first anchor is placed beginning at the posterior aspect of the tear, and each additional anchor is placed 1 cm anterior to the last.

Suture Passing

A number of different techniques are available to facilitate suture passing through the rotator cuff tendon before tying. These include direct placement of the anchor through the substance of the tendon, retrograde passing of the suture through the tendon using a suture retrieval device, and the use of pulling stitches or suture shuttles to draw the anchor suture through the tendon. Tear morphology often determines the use of these various techniques, and the surgeon should be comfortable with a number of different methods.

Retrieval Technique for Suture Passing

In this technique, the scope is moved to the lateral working portal so that the surgeon has a direct view of the rotator cuff tear from above (Fig. 3-6). The anchors have been placed, and the retrieval device is introduced from the posterior portal, the waiting room portal, or through an additional anteromedial portal determined by need. Most retrieval devices or snares allow the surgeon to introduce the device through the tendon edge, 1 cm back from its margin. Once through the tendon, the snare is opened and an individual suture limb is grasped. The snare is closed only enough to contain the suture but not so as to impede its motion through the snare eyelet. The retriever is then pulled out bringing the suture limb along creating a simple stitch ready for tying. This process would then be repeated for each subsequent double-loaded anchor.

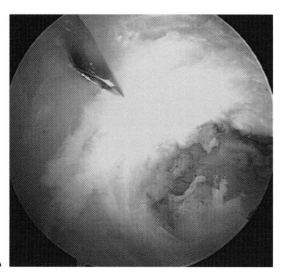
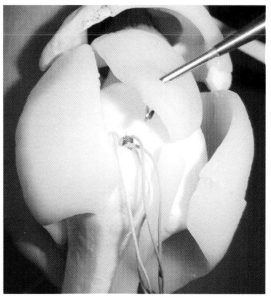

A   B

Figure 3-6. Viewing from the lateral working portal **(A)**, looking directly down on a right shoulder cuff tear, the snare-type retriever is introduced from either the anterior **(B,C,E,F,H)** or posterior **(D,G,I)** portals and passed through the tendon 1 cm from its margin **(B–D)**. *(continued)*

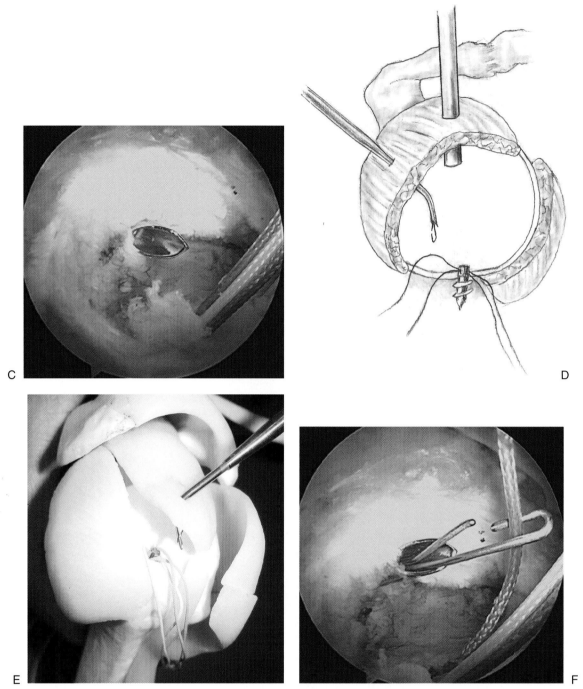

Figure 3-6. *Continued.* **E–G:** The snare is opened and one limb of one of the two sutures on that anchor is captured. *(continued)*

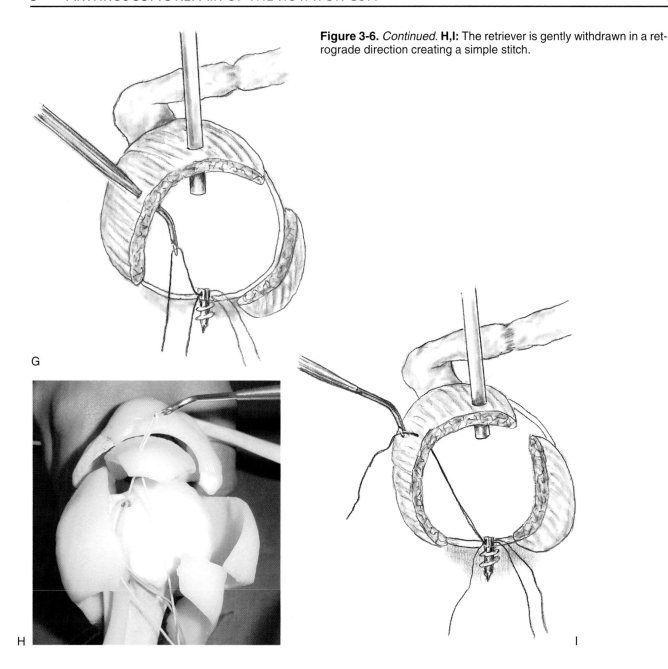

Figure 3-6. *Continued.* **H,I:** The retriever is gently withdrawn in a retrograde direction creating a simple stitch.

Pulling Stitches or Suture Shuttles

Alternatively, anchor sutures may be passed using a pulling suture technique (Fig. 3-7). The pulling suture is a monofilament suture such as O-PDS (Ethicon Inc., Somerville, NJ), which is passed using any of a number of different cannulated devices such as a pigtail or Caspari punch. With a monofilament suture passed, this is then tied to one limb of one of the anchor sutures, and used to pull that suture through the substance of the tendon margin. This process is repeated for each subsequent anchor suture. Alternatively, a loop is created of 2-0 PDS through which the free end of one of the anchor sutures is placed allowing the suture to be drawn through the tendon margin in a fashion similar to the previous description (Fig. 3-8).

When the tear is very small or most of a repair has been completed and an additional suture needs to be passed, a pigtail can be used (Fig. 3-9). Its low profile allows it to be passed beneath the tendon edge and rotated up and through the tendon. The pulling suture is tied to the anchor suture completing the simple stitch.

(text continues on page 50)

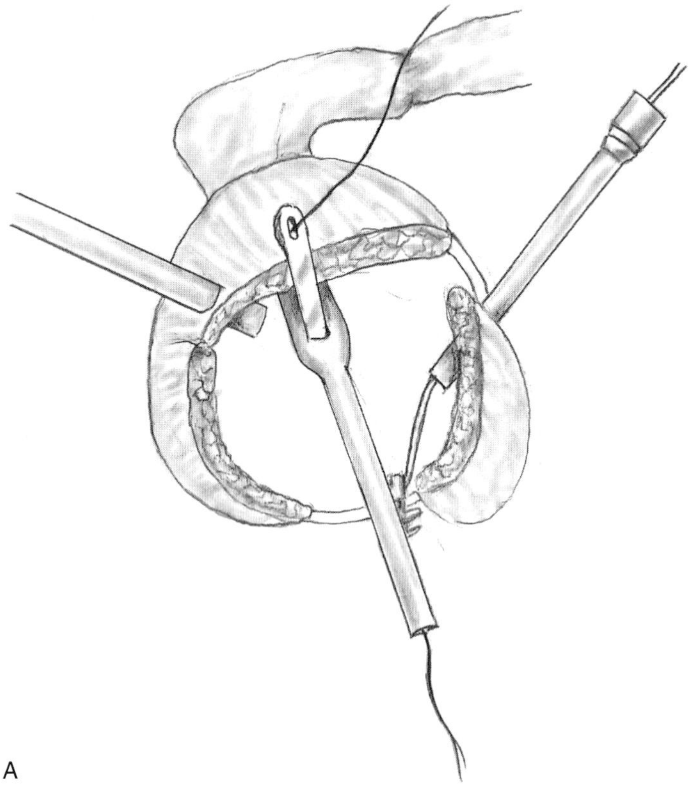

A

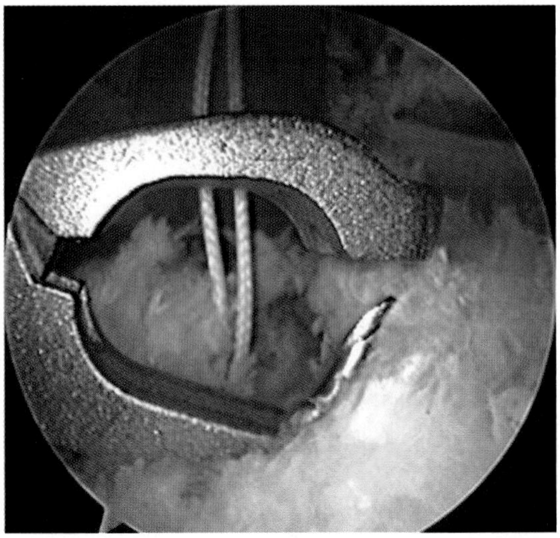

B

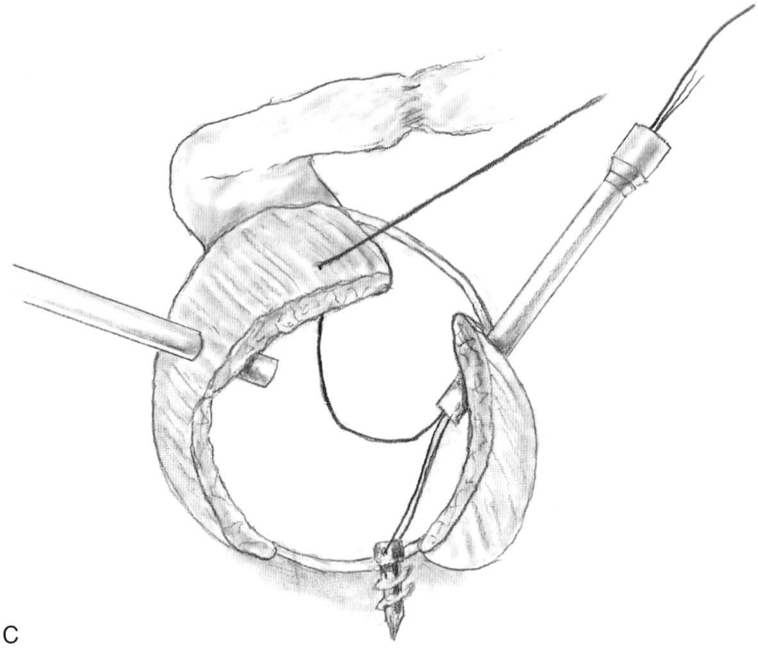

C

Figure 3-7. A: Caspari suture punch is used to capture the tendon edge. **B,C:** A monofilament suture is passed through the tendon and retrieved. One limb of the anchor suture is retrieved. *(continued)*

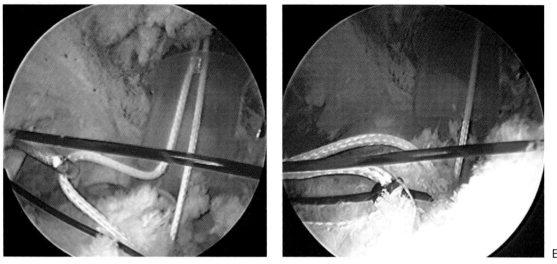

Figure 3-7. *Continued.* **D,E:** The anchor suture, tied to the monofilament suture, is pulled back through the tendon to create a simple stitch.

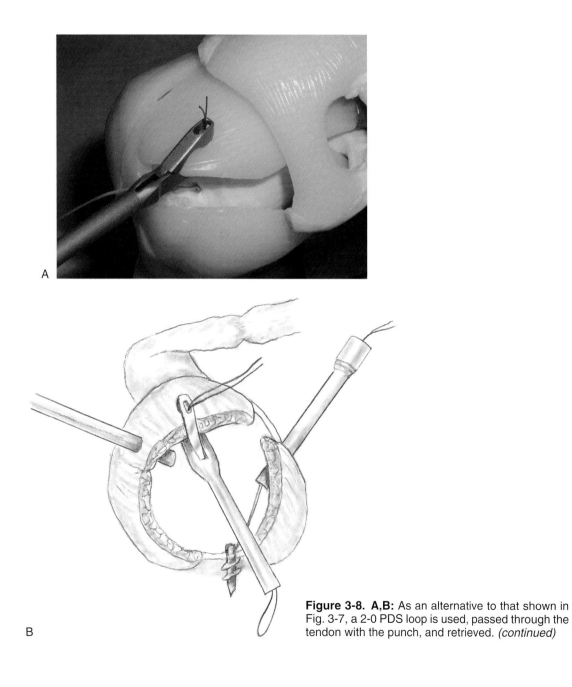

Figure 3-8. A,B: As an alternative to that shown in Fig. 3-7, a 2-0 PDS loop is used, passed through the tendon with the punch, and retrieved. *(continued)*

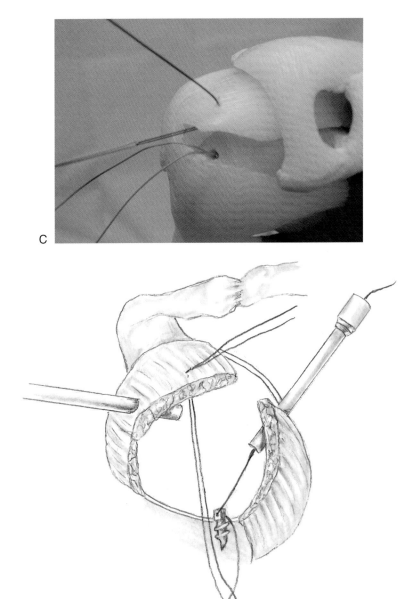

Figure 3-8. *Continued.* **C,D:** One limb of the anchor suture is placed in the loop of PDS and drawn back through the tendon edge.

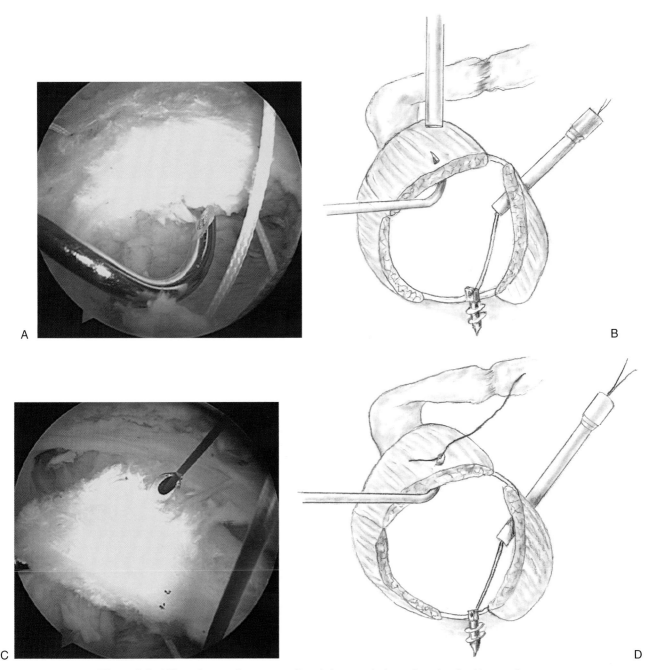

Figure 3-9. When the tear is very small and size precludes using standard types of passers or if most of a repair is complete and most of the tendon is already affixed to the bone **(A,B),** a pigtail can be used. **C–F:** The passed PAS is retrieved. *(continued)*

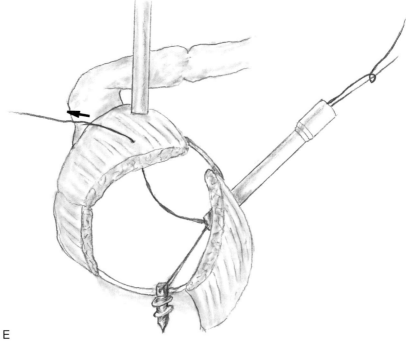

E

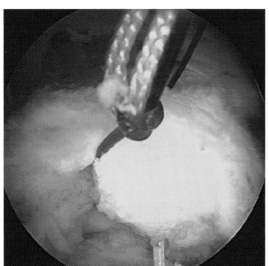

F

Figure 3-9. *Continued.* Using a ring grabber, the portion of the PAS entering the deep surface of the tendon is grouped along with one limb of the anchor suture. Both of these are brought out the anterior cannula and tied together, and the other end of the PAS is pulled, drawing the anchor suture through the tendon.

Side-to-side and Convergence Repairs

Large tears often have an interval component to their defect and it is necessary to close this defect before advancing the lateral portion of the tear to the area of the tuberosity for anchor placement and repair. As in open repair, these defects require simple or figure-eight, side-to-side sutures. My preference is to place multiple simple stitches beginning medially working my way out laterally to close down the AP dimension of the tear (Fig. 3-10). This technique uses an 18-gauge spinal needle introduced from the front of the shoulder, just beneath the acromial edge to perforate the anterior tissue, typically the upper border of the subscapularis. A monofilament suture is passed through the needle and a retriever, brought in from the posterior portal through the posterior tendon, grasps the suture and brings it out the posterior portal. I then use this monofilament suture as a pulling suture to pull a no. 2 nonabsorbable suture back across the tear. I typically pass

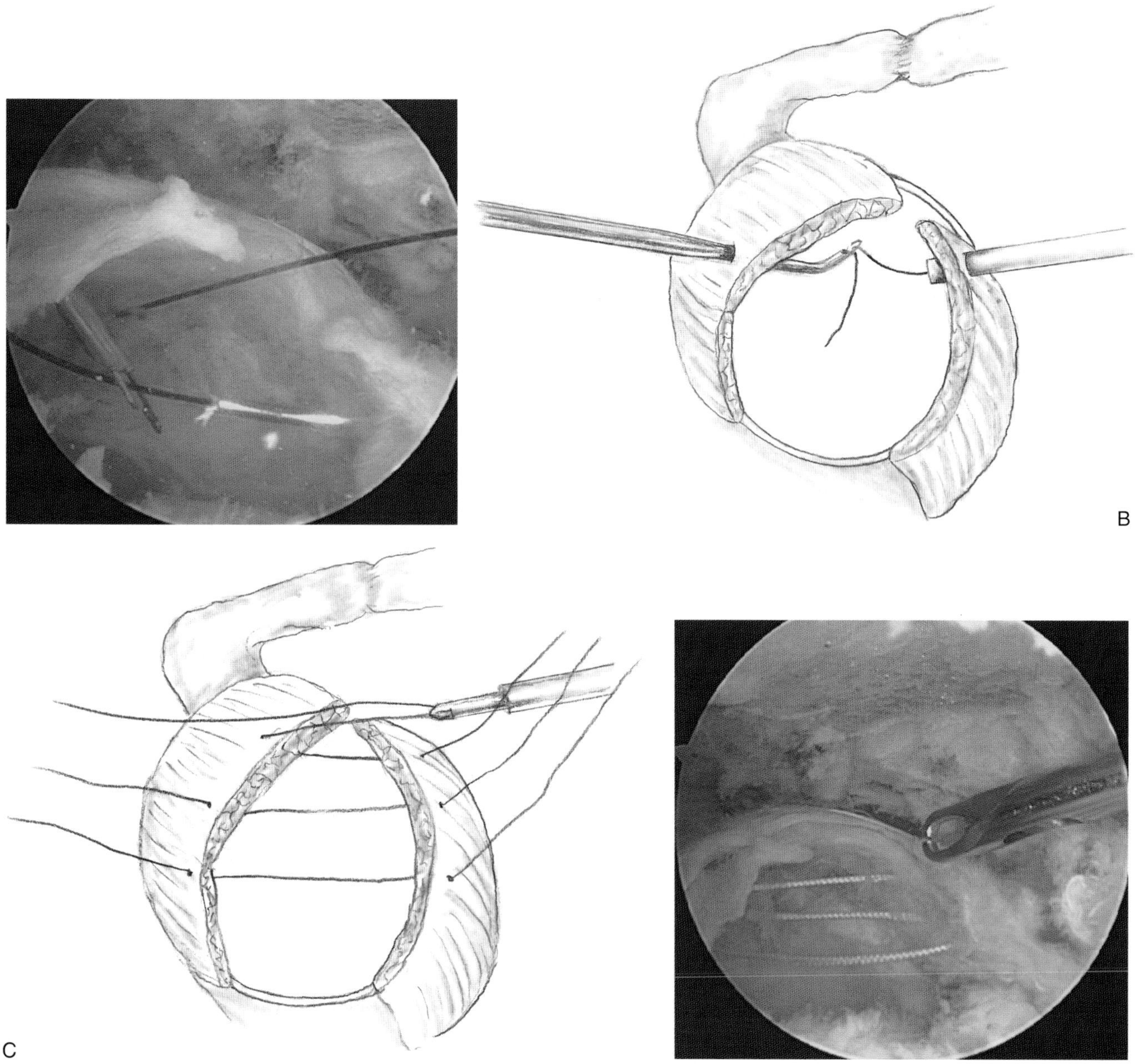

A

B

C

D

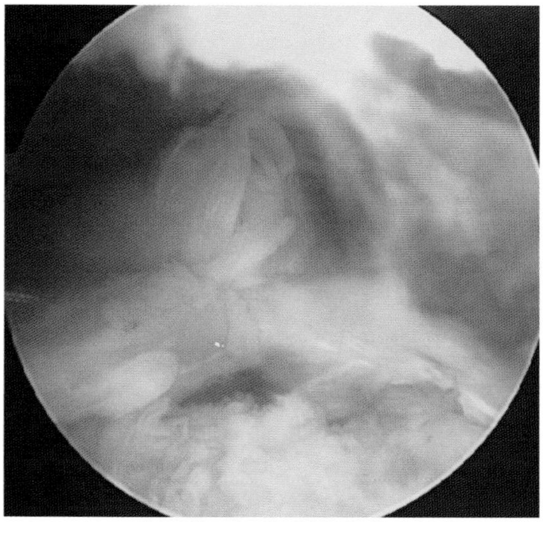

E

Figure 3-10. A,B: Spinal needle is passed through the anterior portion of the tear and polydioxanone synthetic (PDS) suture (Ethicon Inc., Somerville, NJ) is passed and retrieved by the snare. The PDS is tied to the no.-2 nonabsorbable suture and pulled back through creating a simple stitch. **C,D:** Multiple sutures have been passed. **E:** Side-to-side stitches are tied beginning medially and working out laterally to close the defect and bring the tendon margins closer to the tuberosity. *(continued)*

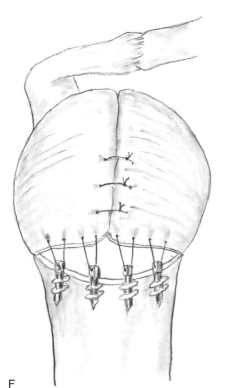

F

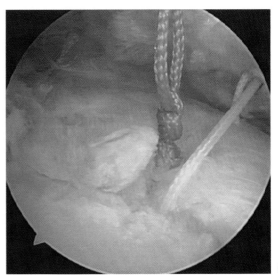

G

Figure 3-10. *Continued.* **F,G:** Anchor placement near the tuberosity completes the repair.

all these sutures first and then tie. If another stitch is needed, it can readily be placed in similar fashion. Once the apex of the tear is closed down, this complex tear becomes a simple tear, which can be repaired directly to the region of the tuberosity as described previously.

Some tears will be simple avulsions of the supraspinatus in which there remains a sizable tag or residual cuff material. In these cases, a side-to-side repair is readily accomplished without the need for anchors.

Knot Tying

A number of different arthroscopic knots have been described and each has its applicability and proponents. The surgeon should become familiar and comfortable with one knot and proficient in its use. I use the Tennessee slider knot, which has excellent sliding and locking characteristics. Furthermore, it is a simple knot to tie and to teach and is very reproducible from surgeon to surgeon and resident to resident (Fig. 3-11). The first step in knot tying is identification of the initial post, which should be the suture end that passes through the rotator cuff tendon. It is on this post that the sliding knot will be tied and introduced into the subacromial space. I shorten the first post and hold it in my left hand. This will accommodate for the length gained when the knot is pulled into the shoulder and keep the two suture limbs even. The knot is made by bringing the right-hand, long limb around the index finger, under the left-hand post limb, back over both suture limbs and then up and through the D-shaped space created. The slack is taken out of the knot but it is not tightened. The knot pusher is then placed over our first post, pushing the sliding knot down into the subacromial space to the tendon. Gentle traction simultaneously on our initial left-hand post while pushing the knot against the tendon will tighten the knot and it is then set and locked in place by pulling on the opposite right-hand post. Step 2 involves switching my knot pusher to the other post and placing five alternating half hitches. The suture is then cut and its stability confirmed. This process is repeated for each subsequent suture.

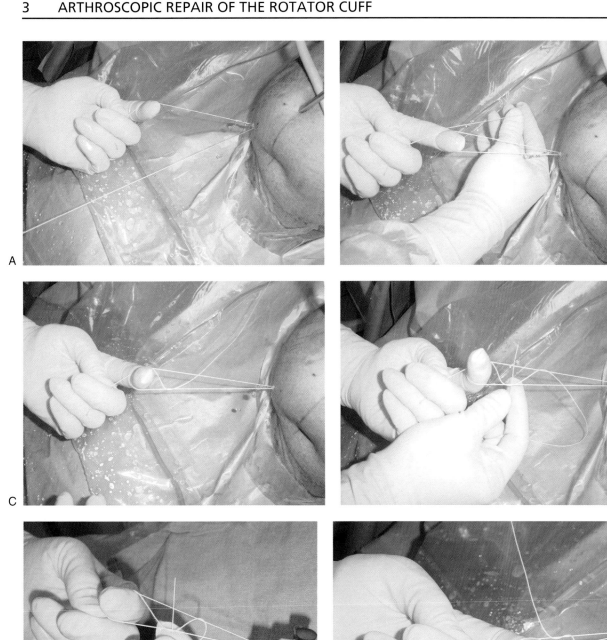

Figure 3-11. A–F: I shorten the first post and hold it in my left hand. This will accommodate for the length gained when the knot is pulled into the shoulder and keep the two suture limbs even. The knot is made by bringing the right-hand, long limb around the index finger, under the left-hand post limb, back over both suture limbs, and then up and through the D-shaped space created. The slack is taken out of the knot but it is not tightened. *(continued)*

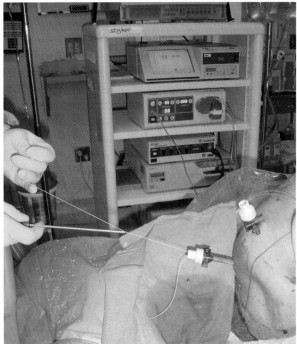

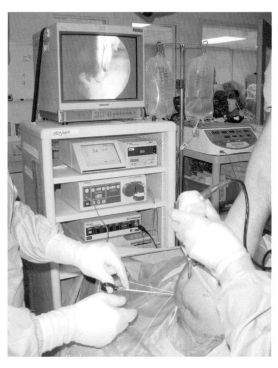

G
H

Figure 3-11. *Continued.* **G:** The knot pusher is then placed over our first post, pushing the sliding knot down into the subacromial space to the tendon. **H:** Gentle traction simultaneously on our initial left-hand post while pushing the knot against the tendon will tighten the knot. It is then set and locked in place by pulling on the opposite right-hand post. Note the monitor view showing the pusher against the knot.

RESULTS

I have done more than 700 arthroscopic rotator cuff repairs, yet during my first year of attempting repairs, I did only 40 and all with tacks, not anchors and sutures. Although I was able to achieve a repair in many small tears, the larger tears and my inability to do arthroscopically what I had become accustomed to in an open repair frustrated me. I made a commitment then to acquire the necessary skills to move forward. Over the following years, my confidence and skill grew, and I have come to the point where I do all cuff repairs via the arthroscope, save the rare chronic subscapularis lesion. As my technique has improved, so have the results. Of the past 300 repairs, more than 90% showed good and excellent results with only 8 known retears. Reoperation took place in 12 patients, 6 for retears, 2 underwent manipulations for adhesive capsulitis, and 4 patients developed painful AC joints requiring arthroscopic excision. Two patients with retears became asymptomatic after a period of rest and declined revision surgery. The most significant finding in this group has been uniformly less postoperative pain and more rapid return of motion and function. Clearly, a procedure that is less invasive does not necessarily mean it will be better for the patient, however, the literature supports this concept and patients are more and more going to be asking for an arthroscopic approach over the traditional open repair for rotator cuff repair.

POSTOPERATIVE MANAGEMENT

The postoperative management of patients who have undergone arthroscopic rotator cuff repair must be individualized, much as we do with open rotator cuff repairs. The most significant difference between those individuals with an arthroscopic repair and those with the traditional open repair is the substantial decrease in postoperative morbidity and the tendency to accelerate their rehabilitation. Very often, the surgeon will find that these patients return 1 week after surgery with very little discomfort in comparison to the more traditional open repair and the ability to do much more than is desired in terms of motion with the repaired shoulder. With that in mind, we follow the following rehabilitation protocol for most arthroscopic rotator cuff repairs.

Postoperative Days 1 to 7

During the first 24 hours after surgery, we ask the patient to perform gentle elbow and wrist range-of-motion exercises actively or passively to decrease joint stiffness and the risk of venous stasis and deep venous thrombosis. The patient is allowed to shower at the 36-hour mark and allows the arm to rest comfortably at the side with the elbow in an adducted position. For the first week, the patient is encouraged to perform gentle pendulum exercises that had been taught earlier in the outpatient ambulatory facility recovery room. The patient also continues active range-of-motion exercises for the elbow and wrist. The patient is further instructed to wear his or her sling, ultra-sling immobilization, or abduction pillow at all times while out in public and in bed. The patient may take the sling and ultra-sling off to dress, placing all garments over the involved arm first, and the normal contralateral side second. Abduction pillows are not to be removed.

Weeks 2 to 4

This constitutes phase I of the exercise program and is passive in nature. In those individuals with small or medium tears, in whom compliance is felt to be strong, I teach a passive range-of-motion program for forward elevation and external rotation in a supine position. If there is any question about the patient's ability to participate in this program, he or she is sent to a physical therapist close to home. During the first few weeks, I avoid extension and internal rotation and the use of pulleys. No resistive exercises are performed at this time; however, I do add scapular rotation exercises.

Weeks 5 to 10

Phase II consists of active-assisted and active range-of-motion exercises for the involved shoulder beginning in a supine position and then progressing to the seated or standing position. I have the patient use either their contralateral normal arm to assist or a cane to first perform active-assisted motion. All planes of motion are incorporated, including forward elevation, abduction, external rotation, and gentle internal rotation. One must be cautious when adding internal rotation because it places the greatest strain on the repair. During this time, the patient will gradually note an improvement in the ability to actively forward elevate comfortably. The surgeon must be cautious about how rapidly the patient is allowed to progress in this exercise program and if any pain is encountered during the addition of active exercises, I recommend that the patient drop back to a passive range of motion until symptoms improve.

Week 10

At this point, phase III, the progressive-resistance, strengthening program is instituted. This is only to be incorporated when a comfortable range of active motion has been achieved. Terminal stretching is also continued during the strengthening program. This begins with the addition of different levels of resistance bands and progresses on to the use of light free weights and closely monitored isokinetic strengthening machines. It is imperative that a patient not be placed into a strengthening program prematurely. I have found that both the patient and the therapist will often ask to start strengthening too early because the patient is more comfortable early on than a patient with open repairs. When strengthening exercises are added, it is not uncommon for the patient to note an increase in his or her level of discomfort. The patient should be reassured and monitored accordingly. I tell the patient that mild aching during exercises is normal but should improve between sessions. If pain persists, the rehabilitation program should be adjusted.

The time for a return to athletic endeavors and/or manual labor will differ from patient to patient depending on the size of the tear as well as rehabilitation potential and individual motivation. Most patients are told that discharge should be anticipated at the 4- to 6-month mark but that ultimate return to athletic endeavors and/or heavy manual work may take 6 to 9 months. Furthermore, they are instructed that full maturation of their repair and ultimate return of strength can take more than 12 months and that they should not be frustrated by some residual discrepancy in strength relative to their normal contralateral shoulder. In addition, these patients will note some achy discomfort, weather-related symptoms, and problems after repetitive overhead use even after discharge. Instruct these patients to use antiinflammatories judiciously and to contact the surgeon for reevaluation if they have persistent symptoms.

COMPLICATIONS

Persistent Pain

The etiology of residual or persistent pain following an arthroscopic rotator cuff repair is no different from that seen after an open repair and may be due to any one of a number of sources. An inadequate decompression must be considered in those patients in whom motion and strength seem to be improved from the preoperative status, yet pain relief has been only partial. The diagnosis of a failed decompression is made using selective injections of the potential offending structures such as the subacromial space, the AC joint, and the biceps. Failed decompressions are frequently due to inadequate decompression of the anterolateral corner of the acromion. This is best noted on an AP view, whereas inadequate anterior decompression alone is best seen on the outlet view.

Occasionally the AC joint may be painful after a repair. Clearly, careful preoperative planning and treatment of symptomatic AC problems during the initial surgery should help avoid later trouble, however, occasionally a patient will develop pain after a repair and this can represent a source of frustration for both patient and surgeon. If the AC joint is painful postoperatively, injections may provide adequate relief to avoid further surgery. If not, an arthroscopic resection will be needed.

A painful biceps tendon can be seen during the early phase of strengthening exercises, and will usually pass. However, additional modalities such as phonophoresis and/or injections may be helpful. Once again, preoperative recognition of a painful biceps may warrant it being addressed at the time of the initial procedure with either a tenodesis or tenotomy.

Retear

Retear following an arthroscopic repair is uncommon but may be seen more commonly in patients with larger tears and those with poor-quality tissue and or significant retraction. Patients with suspected retears will often note an improvement in their postoperative pain to the point where nothing further is needed. In those individuals with confirmed retears and ongoing symptoms, repair is warranted if the tissue quality at the time of the initial repair was adequate.

Stiffness

Every patient undergoing rotator cuff surgery will note a different rate of recovery in terms of pain relief and return of motion. A hallmark of arthroscopic rotator cuff repairs is the uniformly more comfortable rehabilitation. Occasionally, these patients, as do patients with open repairs, develop postoperative adhesive capsulitis. More often than not I see this in those patients with preoperative stiffness and in patients with acute tears repaired in the first few weeks following their injury. In response, I have begun to delay the repair in those patients for 3 weeks to allow them to regain full passive motion and to allow resolution of the postinjury inflammatory component. This delay has not been a problem in terms of reparability of even large tears and their postoperative stiffness has been less. If stiffness and pain are significant enough to warrant treatment, the addition of nonsteroidal antiinflammatory drugs and judicious use of an injection may be helpful. An alteration in the therapy routine may be needed, especially if one suspects a patient has advanced too rapidly thus creating an inflammatory response.

RECOMMENDED READING

1. Burkhart, S.S.: A stepwise approach to arthroscopic rotator cuff repair based on biomechanical principles. *Arthroscopy* 6: 82–90, 2000.
2. Burkhart, S.S., Danaceau, S.M., Pearce, C.E. Jr.: Arthroscopic rotator cuff repair: analysis of results by tear size and by repair technique-margin convergence versus direct tendon-to-bone repair. *Arthroscopy* 17: 905–912, 2001.
3. Gartsman, G.M.: Arthroscopic rotator cuff repair. *Clin Orthop* 390: 95–106, 2001.
4. Murray, T.F. Jr., Lajtai, G., Mileski, R.M., et al.: Arthroscopic repair of medium to large full-thickness rotator cuff tears: outcome at 2- to 6-year follow-up. *J Shoulder Elbow Surg* 11: 19–24, 2002.
5. Snyder, S.: Technique of arthroscopic rotator cuff repair using implantable 4-mm Revo suture anchors, suture shuttle relays, and no. 2 nonabsorbable mattress sutures. *Orthop Clin N Am* 28: 267–275, 1997.
6. Stollsteimer, G.T., Savoie, F.H. III: Arthroscopic rotator cuff repair: current indications, limitations, techniques, and results. *Instr Course Lect* 47: 59–65, 1998.
7. Weber, S.C., Abrams, J.S., Nottage, W.M.: Complications associated with arthroscopic shoulder surgery. *Arthroscopy* 18[Suppl 1]: 88–95, 2002.
8. Wilson, F., Hinov, V., Adams, G.: Arthroscopic repair of full-thickness tears of the rotator cuff: 2- to 14-year follow-up. *Arthroscopy* 18: 136–144, 2002.

4

Arthroscopic Partial Repair of the Rotator Cuff

Ian K. Y. Lo and Stephen S. Burkhart

INDICATIONS/CONTRAINDICATIONS

The advent of arthroscopy and arthroscopic repair techniques has opened new frontiers in the treatment of shoulder disorders including rotator cuff disease. While the vast majority of rotator cuff tears can be completely repaired using either open or arthroscopic techniques, there exists a subset of patients whose rotator cuff tears are considered "irreparable." In the past, such patients were often treated with acromioplasty and débridement alone (2). Although this treatment frequently resulted in pain relief, functional improvement was unpredictable and sometimes unsatisfactory.

The concept of partial rotator cuff repair evolved from the observation of patients who had normal function despite large rotator cuff tears (2). Such tears, termed "functional rotator cuff tears," have normal function by satisfying five biomechanical criteria:

1. Force couples must be balanced in the coronal and transverse planes.
2. A stable fulcrum kinematic pattern must exist.
3. The shoulder's "suspension bridge" must be intact (Fig. 4-1).
4. The tear must occur through a minimal surface area.
5. The tear must possess edge stability.

Thus, in a patient whose massive, dysfunctional rotator cuff tear is not completely repairable, the goal of partial rotator cuff repair is to effect enough of a repair to regain overhead function. This is primarily achieved by balancing the force couple between the anterior and posterior portions of the shoulder and requires an intact subscapularis tendon anteriorly and an intact inferior half of the infraspinatus tendon posteriorly. Anatomically,

I. K. Y. Lo, M.D., F.R.C.S.C.: The San Antonio Orthopaedic Group, San Antonio, Texas.

S. S. Burkhart, M.D.: Department of Orthopaedic Surgery, The University of Texas Health Science Center at San Antonio; and The Orthopaedic Institute, San Antonio, Texas.

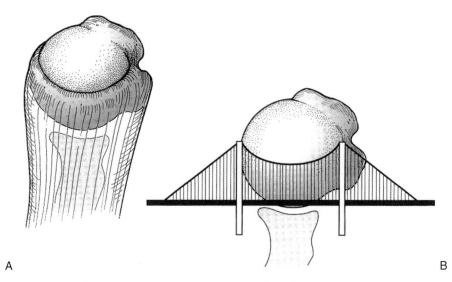

A   B

Figure 4-1. A rotator cuff tear **(A)** can be modeled after a suspension bridge. **B:**
The free margin corresponds to the cable, and the anterior and posterior attachments of the tear correspond to the supports at each end of the cable's span.

this corresponds to the anterior and posterior attachments of the rotator cable (Fig. 4-2).
Partial rotator cuff repair is preferable to tendon transfer because the former respects and
preserves the normal mechanics of the rotator cuff, whereas tendon transfers adversely affect shoulder mechanics.

The indications for partial rotator cuff repair comprise persistent pain and dysfunction
due to any rotator cuff tear that is not completely repairable. Obviously, a complete rotator
cuff repair is the primary goal of surgery. However, this can only be determined intraoperatively, and thus the indications for partial rotator cuff repair are similar to those for any rotator cuff tear. Partial repairs are recommended whenever complete closure of the defect is
not possible.

There are few contraindications for partial rotator cuff repair. In low-demand patients
with preoperative functional rotator cuff tears, who require pain relief only and who do not

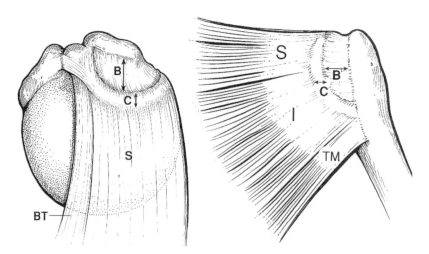

Figure 4-2. Superior and posterior projections of the rotator cable and crescent.
The rotator cable extends from the biceps to the inferior margin of infraspinatus,
spanning the supraspinatus and infraspinatus insertions. *C,* width of rotator cable; *B,* mediolateral diameter of rotator crescent; *S,* supraspinatus; *I,* infraspinatus; *TM,* teres minor; *BT,* biceps tendon.

wish to participate in a long rehabilitation program, the surgeon may consider a subacromial decompression and débridement alone. Patients with advanced cuff tear arthropathy are relative contraindications to arthroscopic partial rotator cuff repair and may require a more extensive combined procedure (hemiarthroplasty with or without partial rotator cuff repair). In addition, arthroscopic partial rotator cuff repair is contraindicated in patients with significant permanent neurologic deficits or medical conditions precluding surgery.

PREOPERATIVE PLANNING

The clinical presentation of patients with rotator cuff tears that are only partially repairable is similar to those for whom complete rotator cuff repair is possible. However, patients are usually older (approximately 60 years old) with a prolonged history of pain in the anterolateral aspect of the shoulder. Pain is typically aggravated by repetitive use of the arm overhead and in chronic cases, pain can be constant with a significant component of night pain. In patients whose tears are only partially repairable, symptoms are usually prolonged, severe, and functionally disabling.

Physical examination in these massive tears demonstrates atrophy of the supraspinatus and infraspinatus muscles, tenderness over the anterolateral humerus, and palpable subacromial crepitus. Impingement signs are usually positive. Although passive range of motion is generally full, active range of motion is typically significantly limited, with many patients demonstrating only a shoulder "shrug." Strength is also severely limited, particularly in external rotation, flexion, and abduction. In patients with concomitant subscapularis tendon insufficiency, the lift-off test or Napoleon test results may be positive. Acromioclavicular (AC) joint derangement is a common associated condition and therefore patients may have tenderness over the AC joint and pain with cross-body adduction.

We routinely obtain five views of the shoulder [anteroposterior (AP) views in internal and external rotation, axillary view, outlet view, 30 degrees caudal-tilt view] preoperatively in all shoulder patients. The AP view commonly shows sclerosis of the undersurface of the acromion and sclerosis and cystic changes in the region of the greater tuberosity. AC joint arthritis may be variably present. In massive tears, patients may demonstrate chronic proximal migration of the humerus. We do not consider chronic proximal migration of the humerus a contraindication for partial rotator cuff repair. In some cases, the proximal migration may be reversed following repair.

The axillary view is carefully evaluated for early glenohumeral arthritis or an os acromionale. The outlet view is evaluated and the acromial morphology classified. Patients with massive tears commonly have type III acromia, with ossification of a portion of the coracoacromial ligament. In addition, the 30-degree caudal-tilt radiograph provides another view of the anterior acromial spur, particularly, the portion anterior to the clavicle.

We routinely obtain a magnetic resonance imaging (MRI) scan on all preoperative shoulder patients. The MRI can provide information on tear size, tear configuration, and tendon involvement and findings to suggest whether a massive rotator cuff tear is potentially repairable. Careful evaluation of the axial views is necessary to identify subscapularis tendon involvement, which significantly increases the complexity of repair. (This chapter however will focus exclusively on posterosuperior rotator cuff tears.) An MRI may also demonstrate a spinoglenoid ganglion cyst, which can cause symptoms that mimic a rotator cuff tear.

We do not believe that long-standing tears with their associated fatty degeneration are a contraindication to surgical repair. Although we agree with Gerber et al. (8) that rotator cuff repairs should be performed as soon as possible, in our experience, patients have shown marked improvement even when undergoing repair of chronic tears more than 10 years after initial injury (6).

Because we now understand how to repair massive rotator cuff tears using techniques such as margin convergence (see below), we never perform open repairs. Arthroscopic techniques, in our hands, accomplish rotator cuff repair that is as secure as open repair with less operative morbidity (6).

SURGERY

The indications for arthroscopic partial rotator cuff repair are persistent pain and dysfunction due to any rotator cuff tear that is not completely repairable. Thus, the principles and techniques used for arthroscopic partial rotator cuff repair are the same as those used when the rotator cuff tear is completely repairable. Although technically demanding, the essential elements of any arthroscopic rotator cuff repair are the following:

1. Visualization
2. Angle of approach
3. Tear-pattern recognition

Visualization

During arthroscopic shoulder surgery, nothing is more frustrating than poor visualization. Particularly in the subacromial space, bleeding can obscure visualization and frustrate attempts to obtain an effective rotator cuff repair. To maximize visualization, we use several techniques. First, the patient's systolic blood pressure is maintained at below 100 mm Hg (preferably less than 90 mm Hg) if not medically contraindicated. This will require close cooperation between the surgeon and anesthesiologist. Second, we routinely maintain the subacromial pressure at 60 mm Hg using an arthroscopic pump (Arthrex, Inc., Naples, FL). If bleeding occurs, the pressure may be temporarily increased up to 90 mm Hg to tamponade bleeding or to enhance visualization until bleeding is controlled. However, the duration of high subacromial pump pressures is restricted to minimize subcutaneous swelling. Electrocautery [3.5 mm × 90-degree, right-angle Arthrowand (Arthrocare, Sunnyvale, CA)] may be used to cauterize bleeding, although this can sometimes be difficult and time-consuming.

Most important, careful attention must be paid to fluid leakage from noncannulated portals. Fluid flow from these portals creates a suction effect by virtue of the Bernoulli principle and draws blood into the subacromial space. Simply blocking these portals using digital pressure will facilitate a clear view by controlling turbulence within this closed system.

Angle of Approach

The proper angle of approach is essential in repairing rotator cuff tears arthroscopically. This is achieved using a combination of proper portal placement and proper instrument configuration. Although the most commonly used portals for arthroscopic repair are the anterior, posterior, and lateral subacromial portals, one should not hesitate to establish accessory portals for anchor placement or suture passage if the current portals (combined with manipulation of the arm) do not afford a proper angle of approach.

Tear-pattern Recognition

Arthroscopy has vastly improved the surgeon's ability to evaluate rotator cuff tears from several different perspectives. Unlike traditional open surgery, which exposes the rotator cuff through an anterolateral incision, arthroscopy is not restricted by spatial constraints. Rotator cuff tears may now be approached and assessed from several different angles with minimal disruption to the overlying deltoid. In the senior author's (S.S.B.) experience, most massive rotator cuff tears can be classified into two major categories (1,3):

1. Crescent-shaped tears (Fig. 4-3A), which reduce easily with minimal tension to the bone bed;
2. U-shaped tears (Fig. 4-4A), which are massive tears that extend medially, with the apex of the tear at the level of the glenoid.

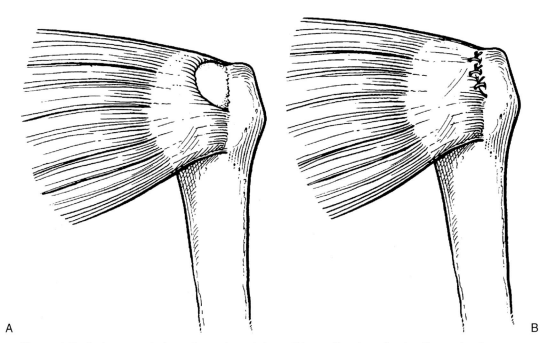

Figure 4-3. A: A crescent-shaped massive rotator cuff tear without much retraction and sufficient medial to lateral mobility can be repaired directly to bone with minimal tension. **B:** Posterior view of repair of crescent-shaped rotator cuff tear.

Crescent-shaped tears comprise approximately 25% to 30% of massive tears and although massive, do not typically retract medially. These tears demonstrate excellent mobility from a medial-to-lateral direction and may be repaired directly to bone with minimal tension (Fig. 4-3B).

U-shaped rotator cuff tears comprise approximately 70% to 75% of massive tears and extend much farther medially than crescent-shaped tears, with the apex of the tear at or medial to the glenoid rim (Fig. 4-4A). In these seemingly irreparable tears, it is important to recognize that the apex of the tear is not a result of medial retraction but represents the shape an L-shaped tear assumes when placed under physiologic load from its muscle tendon components. It is essential to recognize such tears because attempting to medially mobilize and repair the apex of the tear to a lateral bone bed will result in overwhelming tensile stresses in the middle of the repaired rotator cuff margin and subsequent failure. These tears demonstrate significant mobility from an anterior-to-posterior direction and should be initially repaired in a side-to-side fashion using the biomechanical principle of margin convergence.

In such cases, sequential side-to-side suturing, from medial to lateral, of the anterior and posterior leaves of the tear causes the free margin of the rotator cuff to converge toward the bone bed on the humerus (Fig. 4-4B). The free margin of the rotator cuff can then be easily repaired to the bone bed in a tension free manner (Fig. 4-4C). The technique of "margin convergence" not only allows repair of seemingly irreparable tears but also minimizes strain at the repair site. This theoretically decreases the risk of rerupture and subsequent failure of the rotator cuff repair.

Operating Room Setup

Place the patient in the center of the operating room with the audiovisual equipment, power equipment, and electrocautery unit on the side facing the front of the patient. Position the audiovisual and power equipment toward the head of the patient and the arthroscopy pump and electrocautery unit toward the foot of the patient.

Ensure that there is enough room between the patient and the above equipment for a

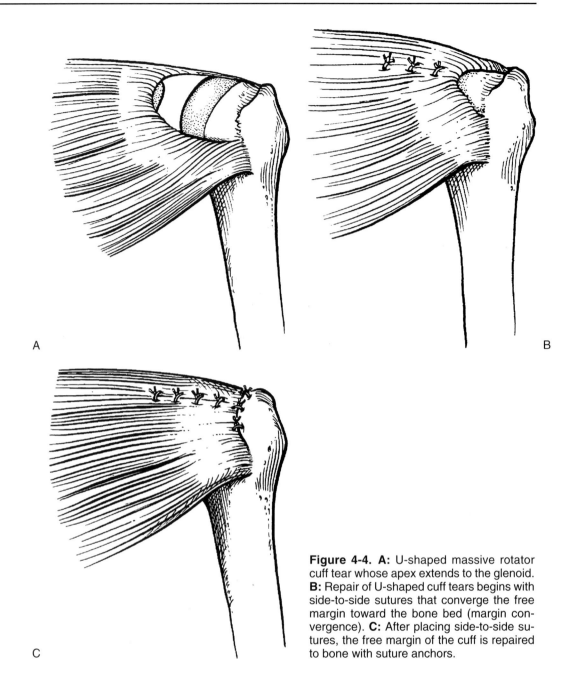

Figure 4-4. A: U-shaped massive rotator cuff tear whose apex extends to the glenoid. **B:** Repair of U-shaped cuff tears begins with side-to-side sutures that converge the free margin toward the bone bed (margin convergence). **C:** After placing side-to-side sutures, the free margin of the cuff is repaired to bone with suture anchors.

Mayo stand and an assistant. Use the Mayo stand to hold the arthroscope, electrocautery instruments, and motorized shaver/burr. The assistant on this side can vary the position of the arm intraoperatively to maximize visualization.

The surgeon and second assistant are behind the patient. Use an instrument table to hold all arthroscopic instruments, anchors, and sutures. The second assistant passes instruments to the surgeon and assists in positioning.

Patient Induction, Positioning, and Draping

All shoulder arthroscopies are performed under general endotracheal anesthesia. Position the anesthesiologist at the head of the bed, allowing easy access to the patient's airway. Following induction, place the patient in the lateral decubitus position. Secure the patient using a beanbag around the thorax and abdomen. Position the nonoperative arm in 90 degrees of forward flexion and place a roll in the axilla to protect the brachial plexus. Flex the patient's legs and place pillows between and beneath the patient's legs. Recheck all bony prominences and soft tissues to ensure there are no pressure points. Secure the patient's thorax and legs to the operating room table using tape. Apply a warming blanket to the patient to help maintain core body temperature, particularly for longer, more complex procedures. Isolate the upper extremity using an adhesive U-drape in the axilla with tails directed toward the patient's head and a 1010 Steri-Drape (3M Worldwide, St. Paul, MN) across the superior aspect of the shoulder. Ensure there is adequate exposure of the entire shoulder, particularly anteriorly and posteriorly.

Prepare the skin using an iodine cleansing and topical solution encompassing the entire shoulder to the distal fingertips and sterilely isolate and drape the shoulder. Place the arm in a Buck traction sleeve and connect the sleeve to a Star Sleeve Traction system (Arthrex, Inc.). Use balanced suspension of 5 to 10 lb to maintain the arm in 30 degrees abduction and 20 degrees forward flexion. By varying the amount of abduction and rotation, the assistant can maximize exposure and visualization.

Portals

Three standard portals are used during arthroscopic rotator cuff repair (anterior, lateral subacromial, posterior) (Fig. 4-5).

Posterior Portal. By palpating the posterior soft spot of the glenohumeral joint, establish a standard posterior portal approximately 4 cm inferior and 4 cm medial to the posterolateral corner of the acromion. Use this portal for initial glenohumeral arthroscopy. The same skin puncture can be used as a posterior viewing portal and instrument portal during subacromial bursoscopy and rotator cuff repair.

Anterior Portal. Establish a standard anterior glenohumeral portal using an outside-in technique just superior to the lateral half of the subscapularis tendon for diagnostic glenohumeral arthroscopy. Use an 18-gauge needle as a guide to ensure accurate placement of the anterior portal. This same skin puncture can be used as an anterior working portal and inflow subacromial portal and can be used during distal clavicle resection if indicated.

Lateral Subacromial Portal. Create this portal approximately 3 cm lateral to the lateral aspect of the acromion, in line with the posterior border of the clavicle. Ensure the portal is parallel to the undersurface of the acromion. This portal serves as a viewing and working portal in the subacromial space.

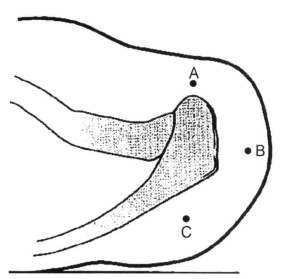

Figure 4-5. Standard portals used during arthroscopic rotator cuff repair: *A,* anterior portal; *B,* lateral subacromial portal; *C,* posterior portal.

Initial Diagnostic Glenohumeral Arthroscopy

Perform a diagnostic arthroscopy using a posterior viewing portal and an anterior instrument portal. Switch viewing and instrument portals to ensure a complete evaluation of the posterior glenohumeral joint. Treat all associated intraarticular pathologies [e.g., superior labrum anterior and posterior (SLAP) lesions, chondromalacia]. Diagnostic glenohumeral arthroscopy will confirm a massive rotator cuff tear with the subacromial space visible through the defect in the rotator cuff (Fig. 4-6). From the glenohumeral joint, make an initial assessment of the size and extent of tearing.

Initial Subacromial Bursoscopy and Tear-pattern Recognition

After arthroscopic inspection and treatment of the glenohumeral joint, place the arthroscope into the subacromial space through the posterior portal. Establish a lateral subacromial working and viewing portal as described above. Create an anterior portal as described above, which may function as a working and inflow portal.

Before assessing and classifying the rotator cuff tear, all bursal and fibrofatty tissue must be débrided from the margins of the rotator cuff. Start the débridement with the arthroscope posterior and the shaver lateral (5.0-mm resector), débriding the anterior, medial, and posterior margins of the tear. Débride the posterior margin of the rotator cuff tear by viewing through the lateral portal and introducing the shaver through the posterior portal (Fig. 4-7). A judicious bursectomy/débridement is essential since adventitial swelling during arthroscopic repair can obscure visualization. Furthermore, the true margin of the tear may be obscured by a synovialized "leader" of thickened bursal tissue. Such tissue margins should be followed laterally, and if they are found to insert into deltoid fascia rather than bone, they are not tendons and must be débrided until the tendon insertion into bone is clearly visualized.

The tear pattern can now be assessed by determining the mobility of the tear margins in the mediolateral and AP directions. To determine the mediolateral mobility of the rotator cuff tear, introduce an atraumatic tendon grasper, through the lateral portal while viewing posteriorly. Grasp the medial margin of the tear and pull this laterally toward the bone bed

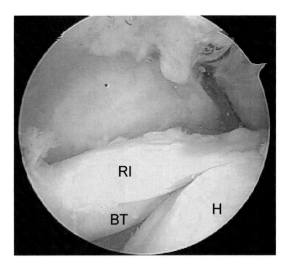

Figure 4-6. Arthroscopic view through a posterior glenohumeral portal of a massive recurrent rotator cuff tear in a right shoulder. Note how the subacromial space is visible through the tear. (All arthroscopic views are of right shoulders oriented in the beach-chair position with the patient's head toward the top of the figure.) *BT,* biceps tendon; *H,* humeral head; *RI,* rotator interval; *,* acromion.

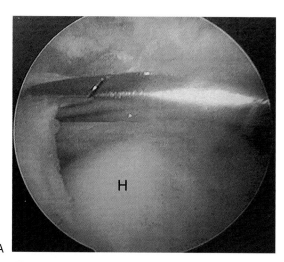

Figure 4-7. Arthroscopic débridement of the posterior margin of a rotator cuff tear through the posterior portal while viewing through the lateral portal. The overlying bursa *(B)* is débrided until the margins of the rotator cuff *(RC)* are exposed. *G,* glenoid; *H,* humeral head.

(Fig. 4-8). If the tear can be easily brought to the bone bed with minimal tension, the tear is classified as crescent-shaped and may be directly repaired to bone with suture anchors (Fig. 4-3).

If the tear cannot be brought easily to the lateral bone bed, the surgeon must determine if the tear is a mobile U-shaped tear and therefore amenable to repair by margin convergence. Place the arthroscope in the lateral portal and determine where the apex of the tear is located. If the apex is at or medial to the glenoid margin, the tear likely represents a U-shaped tear (Fig. 4-9). Next, assess the AP mobility of the tear margin. Using an atraumatic tendon grasper, through the posterior portal grasp the anterior leaf of the tear and test its mobility in the posterior direction (Fig. 4-10A). Then introduce the grasper through the anterior portal, grasp the posterior leaf, and test its mobility in the anterior direction (Fig. 4-10B). If sufficient mobility is present to allow contact of the anterior and posterior leaves

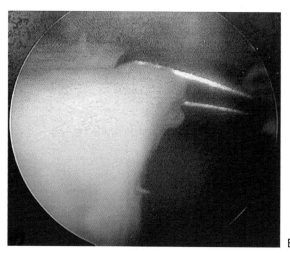

A   B

Figure 4-8. Assessing medial-to-lateral mobility. With the arthroscope in the posterior portal, a tendon grasper is introduced through the lateral portal grasping the margins of the rotator cuff tear **(A)** and pulling it laterally toward the bone bed **(B).** *H,* humeral head.

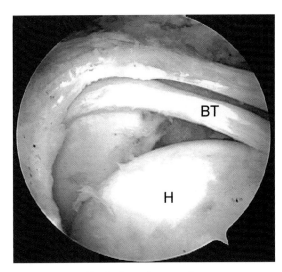

Figure 4-9. Typical arthroscopic appearance, through the lateral portal, of a U-shaped massive rotator cuff tear with the apex above the level of the glenoid. *BT,* biceps tendon; *H,* humeral head.

to each other, then the tear is a U-shaped tear and may be initially sutured with side-to-side sutures using the principle of margin convergence.

Those tears without significant mediolateral or AP mobility represent massive, fixed, severely contracted rotator cuff tears. These tears represent less than 10% of massive tears and may be candidates for mobilization techniques such as an interval slide (2).

Cuff Mobilization and Subacromial Decompression

Significant rotator cuff mobilization along the glenoid margin is rarely required during arthroscopic rotator cuff repair. However, in patients who have previously undergone surgery, ad-

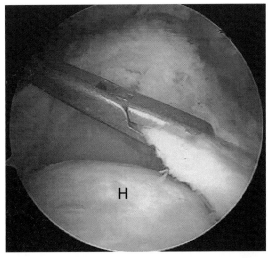
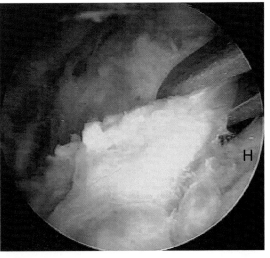

Figure 4-10. Assessing mobility in a U-shaped massive rotator cuff tear. Arthroscopic view through a lateral portal in a recurrent massive rotator cuff tear. The lateral mobility of the medial margin of the massive rotator cuff tear demonstrates minimal to no mobility. The anteroposterior mobility is then assessed. **A:** The posterior mobility of the anterior leaf is assessed by introducing a grasper through the posterior portal and pulling the anterior leaf posteriorly. **B:** The anterior mobility of the posterior leaf is assessed by introducing a grasper through the anterior portal and pulling the posterior leaf anteriorly. *H,* humeral head.

hesions between the rotator cuff and deltoid and between the rotator cuff and acromion may occur. These adhesions must be lysed or excised for sufficient cuff mobility.

To locate the proper plane of dissection, begin the dissection medially at the apex of the tear, beneath the medial acromion, and locate the fibrofatty layer above the rotator cuff (Fig. 4-11A). Follow this layer posteriorly and dissect the posterior leaf of the rotator cuff tear off the deltoid using a shaver (Fig. 4-11B). Even in chronic adhesed tears, this fibrofatty layer separates the deltoid from the rotator cuff and thus may be used as a guide to separate the peripheral tear margins from the deltoid. Continue to excise these adhesions between the deltoid and rotator cuff using a shaver or electrocautery until the tear is fully defined.

For massive rotator cuff tears, particularly those in which only partial repair may be feasible, do not perform a formal arthroscopic acromioplasty. Alternatively, perform a subacromial "smoothing." Decompress the subacromial space by débriding the soft tissues on the undersurface of the acromion and resecting any small osseous irregularities. Be sure to preserve the coracoacromial ligament because it is an essential restraint to anterosuperior migration of the humeral head if the rotator cuff repair fails or is nonfunctional.

Bone Bed Preparation

The bone bed on the humeral neck and greater tuberosity is prepared next. While viewing through the posterior portal, introduce a shaver through the lateral portal and débride the soft-tissue remnants from the residual rotator cuff footprint. Next, introduce a burr through the lateral portal to lightly "dust" a shallow bone bed (i.e., not a bone trough) to bleeding bone. Do not decorticate the bone bed. This maximizes the bone's resistance to suture anchor pullout. Furthermore, *in vivo* animal studies have demonstrated that tendon healing to a bleeding surface of cortical bone is as strong as tendon healing to cancellous bone. The bone bed may be medialized by 5 mm, if necessary, to maximize tendon-to-bone contact and to minimize resting muscle tension, a common cause of failure of rotator cuff repair.

Margin Convergence (Side-to-side) Suturing

Following preparation of the lateral bone bed, the rotator cuff tear can be initially closed by side-to-side suturing of the anterior and posterior leaves of the tear. Place the arthroscope

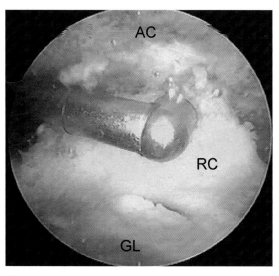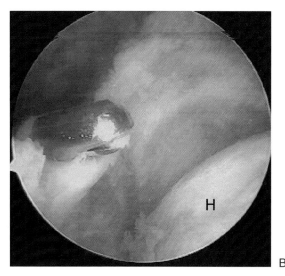

A   B

Figure 4-11. Arthroscopic views through a lateral portal during rotator cuff mobilization in adhesed rotator cuff tears. **A:** The rotator cuff is initially dissected beneath the medial acromion and the fibrofatty layer is identified above the rotator cuff. *AC*, acromion; *GL*, glenoid; *RC*, rotator cuff. **B:** The same layer is then followed posteriorly to identify the posterior margin of the tear. *H*, humeral head.

through the lateral portal and observe the rotator cuff defect. This view provides an excellent "Grand Canyon" view of the massive tear, which is necessary for side-to-side suturing (Fig. 4-9). Depending on the angle of approach and the availability of assistants, two methods are commonly used for passage of side-to-side sutures.

Hand-off Technique. This technique requires two sutures passers. We prefer to use either BirdBeak suture passers (Arthrex, Inc.) or Penetrator suture passers (Arthrex, Inc.). In this technique, load one of the suture passers with no. 2 Ethibond (Ethicon; Somerville, NJ). Through the posterior portal, introduce the "loaded" suture passer and penetrate the posterior leaf of the rotator cuff tear near the apex of the tear medially (Fig. 4-12A). Next, introduce a second, empty suture passer through the anterior portal and penetrate the anterior leaf of the rotator cuff tear. Finally, "hand-off" the suture from the posterior to the anterior suture passer (Fig. 4-12B) and withdraw the anterior suture passer. This draws the suture through the anterior leaf and out the anterior portal, effectively creating a side-to-side suture.

Continue placing side-to-side sutures in a similar fashion progressing from medial to lateral. Space the sutures at 5- to 10-mm intervals alternating the color of suture to facilitate suture management. Ordinarily, four to five side-to-side sutures are required for massive U-shaped tears, with the most lateral suture abutting against the medial portion of the bone bed. Place all side-to-side sutures before knot tying to allow unobscured suture passage through the rotator cuff.

Viper Technique. In this technique, an anterograde suture passing instrument such as the Viper suture passer (Arthrex, Inc.) is required (see below for a detailed description of anterograde suture passing using the Viper suture passer). In this technique, load the Viper suture passer with no. 2 Ethibond and introduce the instrument through a posterior portal (Fig. 4-13A). Pass the suture in an anterograde fashion through the anterior leaf (Fig. 4-13B) and place successive sutures along the anterior leaf margin, alternating the color of suture (Fig. 4-13C). Next, introduce a Penetrator suture passer through the posterior portal, penetrate the posterior rotator cuff medially, and grasp the suture limb on the undersurface of the rotator cuff of the medial suture (Fig. 4-13D). Withdrawing the Penetrator suture passer passes the suture limb through the posterior cuff, completing a side-to-side suture (Fig. 4-13E). Repeat this procedure, grasping each of the undersurface suture limbs in sequence while moving laterally with each successive suture.

Following placement of side-to-side sutures, the sutures are then tied in a sequential

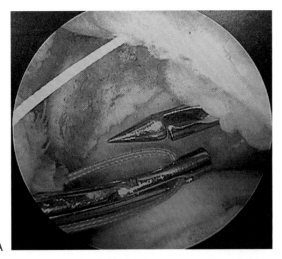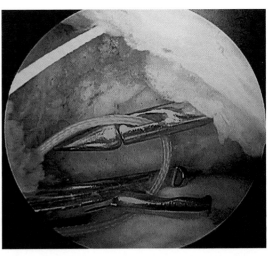

A   B

Figure 4-12. Side-to-side suturing using a hand-off technique. Arthroscopic views through the lateral portal. **A:** A loaded suture passer (Penetrator, Arthrex, Inc., Naples, FL) is introduced through the posterior portal and penetrates the posterior leaf of the rotator cuff tear. A second empty suture passer (Penetrator) is introduced through the anterior portal and penetrates the anterior leaf of the rotator cuff tear. **B:** The posterior suture passer "hands-off" the suture to the anterior suture passer, which is withdrawn, passing the suture through the anterior leaf.

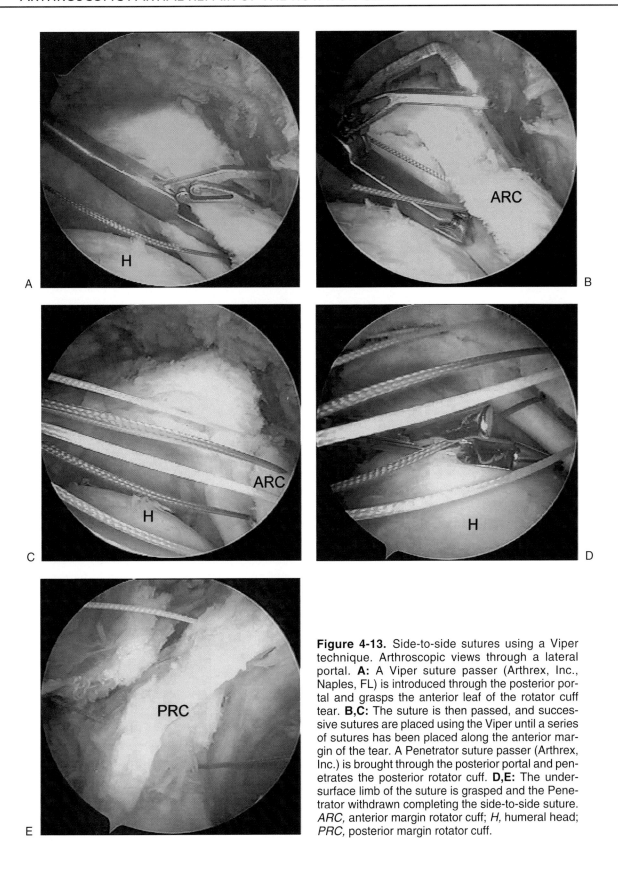

Figure 4-13. Side-to-side sutures using a Viper technique. Arthroscopic views through a lateral portal. **A:** A Viper suture passer (Arthrex, Inc., Naples, FL) is introduced through the posterior portal and grasps the anterior leaf of the rotator cuff tear. **B,C:** The suture is then passed, and successive sutures are placed using the Viper until a series of sutures has been placed along the anterior margin of the tear. A Penetrator suture passer (Arthrex, Inc.) is brought through the posterior portal and penetrates the posterior rotator cuff. **D,E:** The undersurface limb of the suture is grasped and the Penetrator withdrawn completing the side-to-side suture. *ARC,* anterior margin rotator cuff; *H,* humeral head; *PRC,* posterior margin rotator cuff.

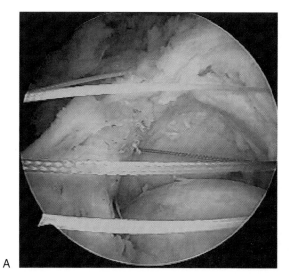
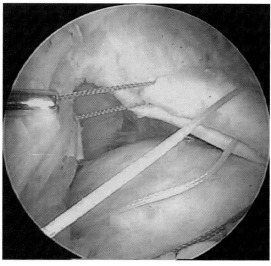

A

B

Figure 4-14. Tying of side-to-side sutures. Lateral arthroscopic view demonstrating side-to-side suture tying. **A:** Side-to-side sutures have been placed at 5- to 10-mm intervals. The apical suture is retrieved through the posterior portal, and sutures are tied over the posterior leaf of the tear. **B:** Sutures are sequentially retrieved through the posterior portal and tied, effecting a margin convergence of the rotator cuff tear.

fashion from medial to lateral to effect a margin convergence of the rotator cuff tear (Fig. 4-14). Tie side-to-side sutures through a cannulated posterior portal starting with the apical stitch (Fig. 4-14A). Retrieve all the other sutures though the anterior cannula to avoid suture "fouling." Tie the knots over the posterior leaf of the tear to avoid the theoretic problem of knot impingement on the undersurface of the anterior acromion. (See later for a complete description of arthroscopic knot tying.)

As the sutures are tied in a sequential fashion from medial-to-lateral, the free margin of the rotator cuff will converge laterally toward the bone bed (Fig. 4-14B). If the rotator cuff converges completely over the lateral bone bed, a complete rotator cuff repair is achievable (Fig. 4-15). However, in some cases, the margin of the rotator cuff will not converge sufficiently to completely cover the articular surface (Fig. 4-16). In these cases, only partial rotator cuff repair is possible, and a defect must be left in the superior portion of the rotator cuff. In these cases, side-to-side suturing is continued as far laterally as possible and then

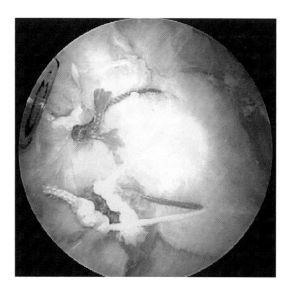

Figure 4-15. Arthroscopic views from a lateral portal following placement of side-to-side sutures and after knot tying with convergence of the rotator cuff margin to the lateral bone bed. A complete repair is possible.

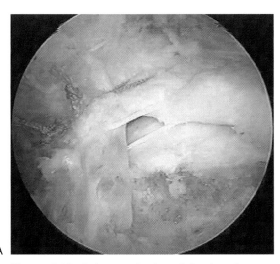
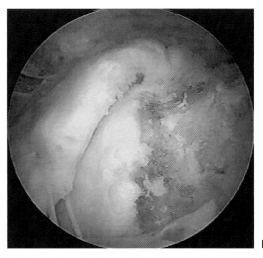

A   B

Figure 4-16. Arthroscopic views following placement and knot tying of side-to-side sutures. The margin of the rotator cuff tear converges to the lateral bone bed but not completely. Only partial repair is feasible. **A:** Lateral view. **B:** Posterior view.

each leaf is repaired to bone with suture anchors. This effectively mobilizes and shifts the rotator cuff superiorly, restoring the posterior moment and balancing the transverse plane force couple.

Special consideration must be given to the deficient rotator interval. In these cases, there is no anterior leaf to effect a margin convergence type repair. In this situation, we have used the biceps tendon as a temporary stent to assist in converging the posterior rotator cuff superiorly and laterally (4). This is accomplished by advancing the posterior leaf to the intraarticular biceps tendon and securing the posterior cuff to the biceps with side-to-side sutures (Fig. 4-17). The posterior cuff is then secured to bone as described below.

Tendon Fixation to Bone

Anchor Insertion. After effecting as much of a margin convergence as possible, each leaf of the rotator cuff must be fixed securely to the lateral bone bed. For partial rotator cuff repairs, use one suture anchor for each leaf. We prefer biodegradable corkscrew suture

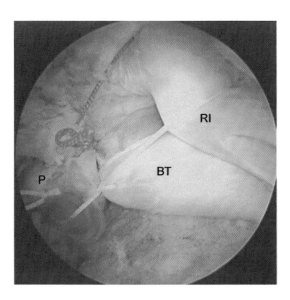

Figure 4-17. Arthroscopic view from a lateral portal demonstrating side-to-side suturing of a massive U-shaped rotator cuff tear with a partially deficient rotator interval. The biceps tendon has been incorporated into the repair. *BT,* biceps tendon; *P,* posterior cuff; *RI,* rotator interval.

anchors (BioCorkscrew; Athrex, Inc.) double loaded with no. 2 Ethibond or no. 2 Fiberwire (Arthrex, Inc.) for secure tendon fixation to bone.

This anchor is designed with an eyelet consisting of a flexible loop of no. 5 polyester suture that is insert-molded into the body of the anchor. Unlike metallic anchors where the eyelet must be directed toward the rotator cuff margin, the flexibility of the BioCorkscrew eyelet allows the suture to slide easily through it without regard to orientation. This minimizes suture "fouling" due to tangling and friction in the eyelet. When using corkscrew anchors, the suture must be passed through the tendon after the anchor has been placed in the bone.

While viewing through a posterior portal, the suture anchors can be inserted through 3-mm percutaneous skin punctures immediately adjacent to the lateral acromion. Use a spinal needle to locate the optimal position for each anchor and to ensure placement of anchors at a "dead man's" angle of 45 degrees. Placing anchors at this angle increases the pullout strength of the anchor and minimizes tension in the suture, thus minimizing suture breakage.

Incise the skin, and create a bone socket for the anchor in the lateral bone bed using a pointed bone punch (Fig. 4-18A). Anchors are generally placed 1 cm from the anterior and posterior leaves to shift the leaves to the anchors as the knots are tied. This maneuver

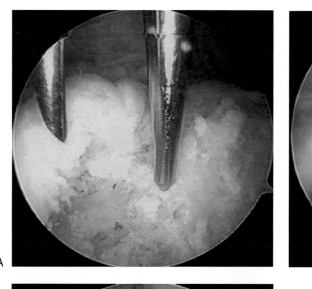

A

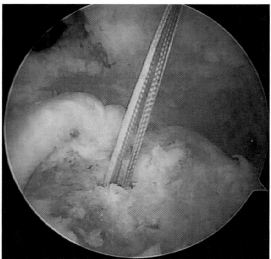

B

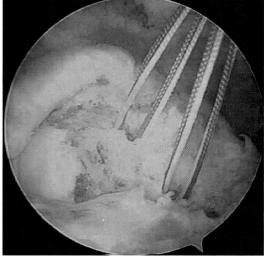

C

Figure 4-18. Suture anchor insertion. Arthroscopic views through a posterior portal. An 18-gauge needle is initially used as a guide to ensure the proper angle of approach for insertion of anchors at a "dead man's" angle of 45 degrees. **A:** A pointed bone punch is introduced parallel to the 18-gauge needle through a percutaneous skin puncture and impacted into bone. The anchor (5.0-mm BioCorkscrew; Arthrex, Inc., Naples, FL) is then inserted, replicating the direction of the bone punch until seated. **B:** The insertion device is removed, leaving the sutures protruding from the bone. **C:** A minimum of two anchors is inserted, one for each leaf.

maximizes the moment of the posterior rotator cuff in the transverse and coronal planes to effectively balance the force couples.

In most cases, tapping the bone socket is not necessary. However, in particularly hard bone, a conical threaded socket may be created using a tap. The anchor is then inserted into the bone socket until seated completely into bone. Confirm the anchor fixation in bone by pulling on the sutures (Fig. 4-18B). Usually a minimum of two suture anchors is inserted, one for the anterior leaf and one for the posterior leaf (Fig. 4-18C).

Suture Passage. Following anchor placement, the sutures must be passed through each leaf of the tear. We prefer simple sutures through the rotator cuff passed in an antegrade or retrograde fashion.

Retrograde Passage.

1. *Posterior Cuff:* To pass sutures through the posterior rotator cuff, place the arthroscope in the lateral portal and a suture-passing instrument through the posterior portal. The Penetrator suture passer provides an excellent angle of approach for the posterior leaf. Next, withdraw the arthroscope so that the suture passer and suture anchor are both within the view. Then "line-up the putt" (Fig. 4-19A) and pass the Penetrator suture passer through the posterior leaf toward the suture anchor (Fig. 4-19B). Use the Penetrator suture passer to grasp one suture limb from the anchor (Fig. 4-19C) and withdraw it through the posterior leaf.

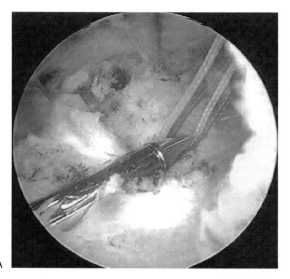

A

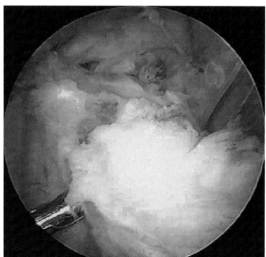

B

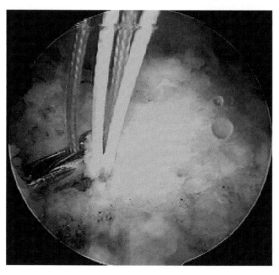

C

Figure 4-19. Posterior rotator cuff: retrograde passage. Arthroscopic views through a lateral portal. **A:** A 15-degree Penetrator suture passer (Arthrex, Inc., Naples, FL) is introduced through the posterior portal and "lines up the putt." **B:** The Penetrator is withdrawn slightly and penetrates the posterior cuff in a direction toward the suture anchor. **C:** One limb of the suture from the anchor is grasped, and the Penetrator is withdrawn. The suture limb is then drawn through the posterior cuff in a retrograde fashion.

2. *Anterior Cuff:* To pass sutures through the anterior leaf of the rotator cuff, the same sequence is repeated. However, the 45-degree BirdBeak suture passer provides a better angle of approach to the anterior leaf than does the Penetrator (Fig. 4-20).

3. *Central Cuff:* To pass sutures retrograde through the central portion of the rotator cuff, a modified Nevaiser portal is utilized. This portal is created approximately 2 to 3 cm posteromedial to the AC joint, in the "soft spot" bordered by the posterior clavicle, medial acromion, and the scapular spine (Fig. 4-21A). While viewing from a lateral portal, use a spinal needle as a guide to determine the proper position of the portal to allow an adequate angle to the central cuff (Fig. 4-21B). Because no cannula is necessary, only a small 3-mm skin puncture is required to accommodate suture-passing instruments. Using the needle as a guide, "walk" a Penetrator suture passer down the needle and visualize its entry into the subacromial space. As described above, penetrate the central cuff, retrieve one limb of the suture, and withdraw the suture through the rotator cuff (Fig. 4-21C).

Anterograde Suture Passage. Anterograde suture passage is particularly useful for the central rotator cuff. Anterograde suture passage requires a special instrument such as the Viper suture passer. This invaluable instrument allows the surgeon to grasp the tissue, deliver the suture, and retrieve the suture in a single step. In addition, the tissue may be grasped and pulled toward the bone bed before stitch delivery to ensure that the proposed suture location is satisfactory.

This instrument is designed with a lower jaw, which is used to hold the suture to be passed, and an upper hooked jaw, which is used to penetrate the tissue and retrieve the suture from the lower jaw. The lower jaw is constructed so that the suture may be held in an anterior or a posterior position, which is controlled by a separate trigger on the handle of the instrument. In the posterior suture position, the suture is stowed safely out of reach of the upper hook (Fig. 4-22A). In the anterior position, the suture may be grasped by the upper jaw (Fig. 4-22B).

For suture passage, place the arthroscope through the posterior portal. Place a larger 8.25-mm twist-in instrument cannula through the lateral portal and retrieve one suture limb from the suture anchor (Fig. 4-23A). Place this suture into the lower jaw of the Viper suture passer extracorporeally and load it into the posterior position. Introduce the Viper through the lateral portal and grasp a portion of the rotator cuff (Fig. 4-23B). The rotator cuff can then be tensioned or pulled laterally to ensure that suture placement is satisfactory. Then, move the suture into its anterior position using the separate trigger, open the jaws of the Viper instrument (Fig. 4-23C), and pull the suture out the lateral portal (Fig. 4-23D).

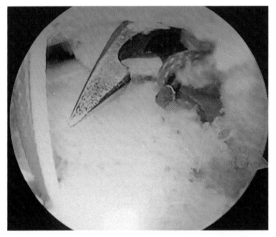

Figure 4-20. Anterior rotator cuff: retrograde passage after a 45-degree BirdBeak (Arthrex, Inc., Naples, FL) is introduced through the anterior portal to "line up the putt." The BirdBeak is used to penetrate the anterior cuff, grasp one limb of the suture, and draw it through the rotator cuff in a retrograde fashion.

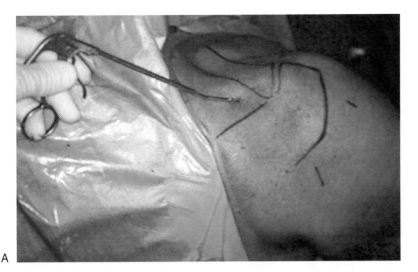

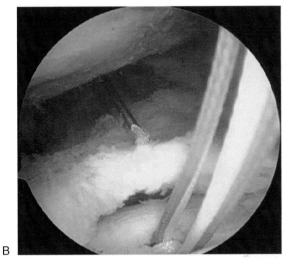

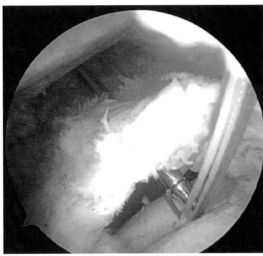

Figure 4-21. Central rotator cuff: retrograde passage **(A)**. The modified Nevaiser portal is created in the soft spot bordered by the posterior clavicle, medial acromion, and scapular spine. **B:** An 18-gauge spinal needle is used as a guide to determine the proper position of the portal to allow an adequate angle to the central rotator cuff. Using the needle as a guide, a Penetrator (Arthrex, Inc., Naples, FL) is "walked" down the spinal needle. **C:** The rotator cuff is penetrated and the suture grasped and passed in a retrograde fashion. Arthroscopic views from a lateral portal.

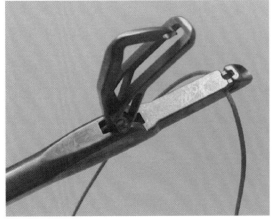

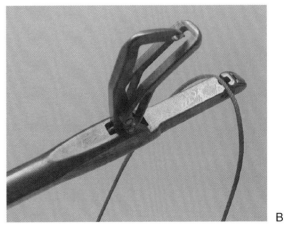

Figure 4-22. The Viper suture passer (Arthrex, Inc., Naples, FL). **A:** The posterior suture position stows the suture safely away from the upper hook. **B:** The anterior suture position allows the suture to be engaged by the hook from the upper jaw.

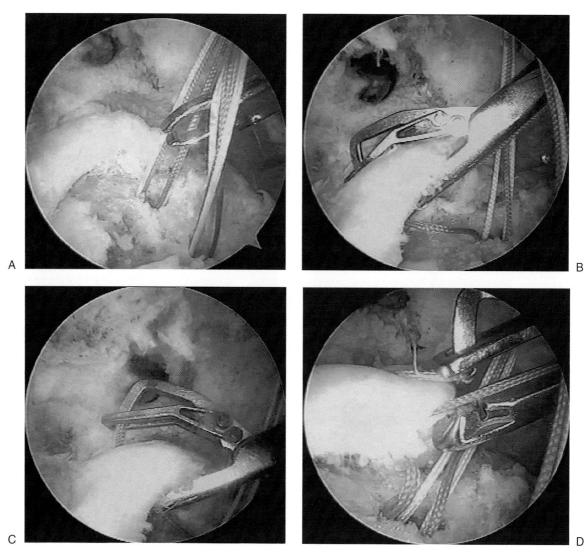

Figure 4-23. Anterograde suture passage using the Viper suture passer (Arthrex, Inc., Naples, FL). Arthroscopic views through a posterior portal. **A:** An 8.25-mm twist-in instrument cannula has been placed through the lateral portal and one limb of the suture from the anchor is retrieved through this cannula. The Viper has been loaded with the suture limb in the posterior position and introduced through the lateral cannula. **B:** A portion of the rotator cuff is then grasped and the proposed suture placement is assessed. **C:** The suture is moved into the anterior position using the separate trigger and engages the hook from the upper jaw. The jaws are then opened passing the suture through tendon. **D:** The suture is then pulled out the lateral portal.

Following passage of all sutures, simple sutures are tied in a sequential fashion. By passing all sutures before tying, it is easier to manipulate the suture retriever under the rotator cuff margin, because the cuff is not bound down by sutures that have already been tied. Arthroscopic knot tying for fixation of tendon to bone is usually performed through a lateral portal with all other sutures retrieved through a holding portal (usually anterior). Tie the knots over the rotator cuff.

Knot Tying

For knot tying, use a 7.0-mm translucent "fish-bowl" instrument cannula, which allows better visualization of knot tying. When there is significant deltoid or adventitial swelling, knots may be tied entirely within the cannula. While some authors prefer the use of sliding knots, this can potentially damage the tendon as it slides through the rotator cuff or abrade and weaken the suture as it slides against the eyelet of the anchor (especially metal anchors).

To ensure both loop security (maintenance of a tight suture loop around the enclosed soft tissue) and knot security (resistance of the knot to failure by slippage or breakage), stacked half-hitches are tied with a double-diameter knot pusher. By using the Surgeon's Sixth Finger (Arthrex, Inc.) knot pusher, the tissue to be secured can be manipulated into place using the end of the Sixth Finger, and most important, continuous tension can be maintained on the post limb as knots are tied to prevent loosening of the soft-tissue loop between throws (i.e., loop security). Although several combinations of knots are possible, we prefer to initially stack three half-hitches (base knot) followed by three consecutive half-hitches on alternating posts.

To tie knots, retrieve both limbs out a separate cannula and hold all other sutures in temporary holding portals. Thread one limb of the suture (the post limb is threaded through the inner metallic tube using the suture threader and is usually the limb that penetrates the soft tissue) through the lumen of the knot pusher and run the inner metallic tube of the knot pusher through the cannula down to the tissue. While maintaining tension on the post limb, tie a base knot consisting of three stacked half-hitches in the same direction. When pushing half-hitches down the inner metallic sleeve, unravel any twists in the suture by turning the outer plastic sleeve followed by past-pointing to tighten each throw (Fig. 4-24). In this way, knot security is maximized by minimizing slack between throws. This initial base knot is followed by three additional half-hitches in which the post is reversed for each throw.

Switching posts can be easily performed without rethreading by flipping the half-hitch through differential tensioning of the suture limbs. Since the post limb is always the limb under the most tension, the wrapping limb can be converted to the post limb by tensioning it to a greater degree than the original post limb, thereby "flipping" the post (Fig. 4-25). This is not only easy but it also optimizes the strength of any knot. Tissue indentation by the suture is a final indicator of good loop security (Fig. 4-26). In partial rotator cuff tears, a defect will persist in the superior portion of the rotator cuff (Fig. 4-27).

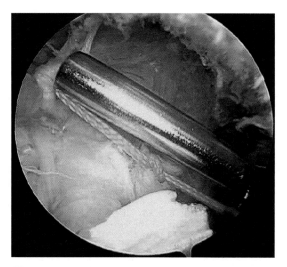

Figure 4-24. Past-pointing tightens each throw maximizing knot security.

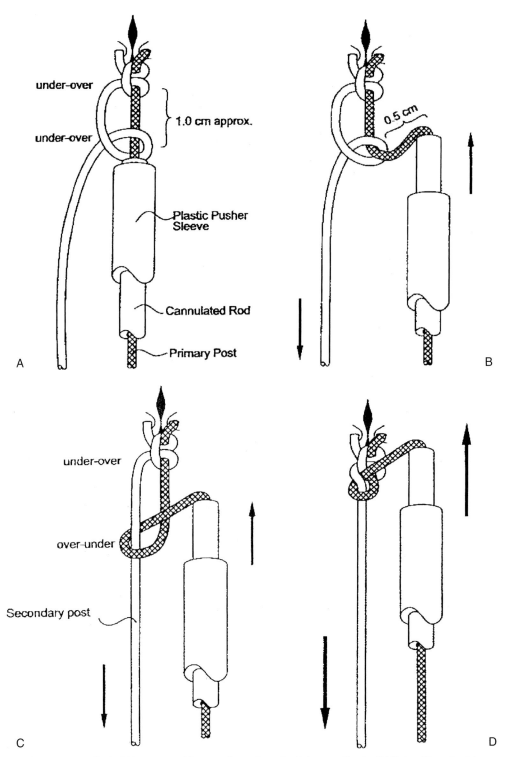

Figure 4-25. Switching posts without rethreading. **A:** Advance the half-hitch with a double-diameter knot tier. **B:** Back off the knot tier by approximately 0.5 cm and then advance the knot tier. **C:** While advancing the knot tier, pull on the secondary-post limb. **D:** Past point to tighten the knot.

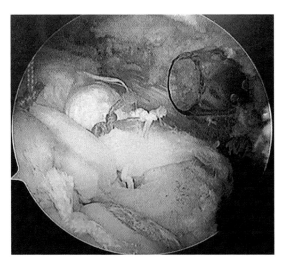

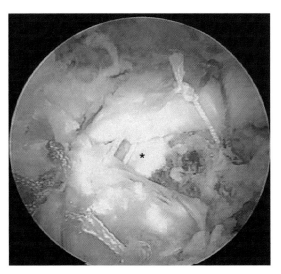

Figure 4-26. Arthroscopic view through a posterior portal demonstrating tissue indentation by suture loops, a good indicator of loop security.

Figure 4-27. Completed arthroscopic partial rotator cuff repair. Arthroscopic views through a lateral portal demonstrating a partial rotator cuff repair with a small residual defect in the superior portion of the rotator cuff exposing the articular cartilage of the humeral head (*).

POSTOPERATIVE MANAGEMENT

All arthroscopic rotator cuff repairs are performed on an outpatient basis. Patients leave the surgical center approximately 90 minutes after surgery. Following the procedure, place the operated arm at the side in a sling with a small pillow. The sling is worn continuously for 6 weeks except during bathing and exercises.

Encourage active elbow flexion and extension avoiding terminal extension if a biceps tenodesis was also performed. Patients may perform passive external rotation exercises immediately. However, overhead stretching is avoided until 6 weeks postoperatively to avoid stressing the repair. Stresses on the cuff can be significant even with passive overhead stretching.

At 6 weeks, the sling is discontinued and overhead stretches with a rope and pulley and internal rotation stretches are commenced. Isotonic strengthening is not begun until 10 to 12 weeks after surgery at which point we begin rehabilitation of the rotator cuff, deltoid, and scapular stabilizers. Progressive activities are incorporated as strength allows and unrestricted activities are usually resumed from 6 to 12 months after surgery.

RESULTS

Although the results of partial rotator cuff repair are not as good or as consistent as complete rotator cuff repair, they are superior to débridement and decompression alone. It is important to remember that these patients represent a small subgroup of patients with massive tears and are usually significantly disabled. Our previous review of patients who underwent partial rotator cuff repair demonstrated significant improvements in pain, range of motion, and overall joint function (7).

A recent review of 12 patients indicated that at a mean follow-up of 35.2 months after arthroscopic partial rotator cuff repair, the mean University of California Los Angeles (UCLA) score improved from 8.9 to 31.7 (9). Good to excellent results were obtained in 83% of patients. The mean forward elevation increased to 160 degrees, with most patients obtaining overhead function. Seventeen percent of patients had fair or poor results. However, because of their poor preoperative status, even those with fair results demonstrated significant improvements in pain and function. Interestingly, three patients had durable reversal of proximal humeral migration.

COMPLICATIONS

No major intraoperative complications have been noted during arthroscopic partial rotator cuff repair. During prolonged procedures, however, the shoulder and particularly the deltoid can become quite swollen, thus impairing visualization and making repair more difficult. Although compartment syndrome of the deltoid has not been reported in the published literature, we are aware of one case of deltoid necrosis presumably secondary to extravasation of fluid into the deltoid during a prolonged arthroscopic procedure. For this reason, we recommend that if visualization is impaired or the surgeon cannot easily complete the entire case within 2 ½ hours, conversion to an open repair should be strongly considered.

Anchor pullout is a theoretic possibility, particularly in osteoporotic bone. However, inserting a corkscrew anchor at a "dead man's angle" of 45 degrees or less maximizes pullout. We have not noted any fixation problems when anchors are appropriately inserted.

RECOMMENDED READING

1. Burkhart, S.S.: Arthroscopic repair of massive rotator cuff tears: concept of margin convergence. *Tech Shoulder Elbow Surg* 1: 232–239, 2000.
2. Burkhart, S.S.: Arthroscopic treatment of massive rotator cuff tears. *Clin Orthop* 390: 107–118, 2001.
3. Burkhart, S.S.: A stepwise approach to arthroscopic rotator cuff repair based on biomechanical principles. *Arthroscopy* 16: 82–90, 2000.
4. Burkhart, S.S.: Partial repair of massive rotator cuff tears: the evolution of a concept. *Orthop Clin N Am* 28: 125–132, 1997.
5. Burkhart, S.S.: Reconciling the paradox of rotator cuff repair versus débridement: A unified biomechanical rationale for the treatment of rotator cuff tears. *Arthroscopy* 10: 4–19, 1994.
6. Burkhart, S.S., Danaceau, S.M., Pearce, C.E.: Arthroscopic rotator cuff repair: analysis of results by tear size and by repair technique—margin convergence versus direct tendon-to-bone repair. *Arthroscopy* 17: 905–912, 2001.
7. Burkhart, S.S., Nottage, W.M., Ogilvie-Harris, D.J., et al.: Partial repair of irreparable rotator cuff tears. *Arthroscopy* 10: 363–370, 1994.
8. Gerber, C., Fuchs, B., Hodler, J.: The results of repair of massive tears of the rotator cuff. *J Bone Joint Surg Am* 82: 505–515, 2000.
9. Tehrany, A.M., Burkhart, S.S.: Massive rotator cuff tears: results of arthroscopic partial repair. Presented at: The 21st Annual meeting of the Arthroscopy Association of North America, Washington, DC, April, 2002.

5

Arthroscopic Repair of Anterior Instability

Peter Habermeyer and Sven Lichtenberg

Shoulder dislocation occurs in 2% to 8% of the population and represents one third of all emergency cases around the shoulder. Recurrence is age-related and may be as high as 95% in patients under 20 years old (6). Recurrence rates drop with age and will be less than 50% in patients over 25 years old (7).

The gold standard for anterior instability will always be the open Bankart procedure for anatomic reconstruction of the shoulder. In the early 1980s, the former author of this chapter, Richard Caspari, and Craig Morgan developed an arthroscopic suture technique of reconstruction to decrease perioperative morbidity. In the beginning of arthroscopic surgery, enthusiasm in these new techniques led to their uncritical use and therefore to high failure and recurrence rates of up to 49%.

In the late 1990s, there was a tendency to reevaluate the indications/contraindications for arthroscopic stabilization. Analyses of mistakes and pitfalls, better understanding of the pathoanatomy, and improved instruments (e.g., suture anchors, suture passing devices) have led to a more careful treatment of unstable shoulder in regard to arthroscopic procedures (4).

INDICATIONS/CONTRAINDICATIONS

First-time Traumatic Dislocations

The ideal patient for arthroscopic treatment after first-time traumatic dislocation is the young athlete with instability after an adequate trauma. These patients usually present with

P. Habermeyer, M.D., PH.D. and S. Lichtenberg, M.D: Department of Shoulder and Elbow Surgery, ATOS Klinik, Heidelberg, Germany.

a labral tear off the glenoid rim and no capsular redundancy. A Hill-Sachs lesion is obligate and proves the traumatic onset. Reduction must be performed by a physician, sometimes under anesthesia. It was shown that in young cadets after conservative treatment of first-time traumatic dislocation the recurrence rate was 80%. McLaughlin and McLellan (7) report a recurrence rate of 95% in patients younger than 20 years, thus in these patients, primary surgery is favorable.

Chronic Posttraumatic Instability

Recurrent posttraumatic instability without hyperlaxity [type II according to Gerber (4); see Table 5-1] is characterized by an adequate trauma that destroys the passive stabilizing mechanisms [inferior glenohumeral ligament (IGHL), labrum], a Hill-Sachs lesion is obligate in these patients. Habermeyer et al. (5) proved that with an increasing number of dislocations, pathologic changes will also increase. The labrum, capsule, and ligaments will undergo plastic deformation and recurrences will occur more atraumatically, sometimes at night. The presence of a robust inferior glenohumeral ligament is a key selection criterion. This leads to the recommendation that a patient should not have more than five dislocations before arthroscopic surgery. Some authors report a higher recurrence rate after arthroscopic stabilization in patients who have experienced more than five dislocations before surgery (11).

Traumatic instability with hyperlaxity [type III according to Gerber (4)] first becomes apparent by a trauma to the shoulder in external rotation and abduction. Under examination of the contralateral shoulder, the hyperlaxity becomes obvious. These patients tend to have an earlier onset of recurrences without adequate trauma and are able to reduce the shoulder themselves.

Multidirectional Instability

Real multidirectional instability with anteroinferior and posterior dislocations is a very rare entity. More often the term is wrongly used for instability with hyperlaxity as mentioned above. In our experience, real multidirectional instability is an indication for open surgery. You even have to consider a combined surgical approach from anterior and posterior.

In those cases with an anterior dislocation and hyperlaxity [type III according to Gerber (4)], the posterior laxity must be controlled by a capsular plication; this will be described later.

Anterior Subluxation

This uncomfortable entity is seen in patients who are involved in overhead sports and who experience repetitive microtrauma to the shoulder from throwing or pitching. Most of these patients also demonstrate capsular laxity.

Table 5-1. *Classification of instability according to Gerber*

Type I	Locked dislocation
Type II	Unidirectional instability without hyperlaxity
Type III	Unidirectional instability with hyperlaxity
Type IV	Multidirectional instability without hyperlaxity
Type V	Multidirectional instability with hyperlaxity
Type VI	Voluntary instability

From Gerber, C.: Observations on the classification of instability. In: Warner, J. J. P., Ianotti, C., Gerber, C., eds. *Complex and revision problems in shoulder surgery.* Philadelphia: Lippincott–Raven Publishers, 1997: 9–18.

There have been reports on arthroscopic posterior instability repairs. At this point we recommend these techniques only to the experienced arthroscopic surgeon.

On the basis of a review of the literature and our own experience, we recommend arthroscopic stabilization for patients with the following:

1. First-time traumatic dislocation in young and athletic patients

- Hills-Sachs lesion
- Bankart/Perthes lesion
- No hyperlaxity

2. Recurrent posttraumatic dislocation with or without hyperlaxity and no more than five dislocations

- Good quality and competence of IGHL and middle glenohumeral ligament (MGHL)
- No osteochondral lesion (lack of concavity compression)
- Symptomatic subluxation

Contraindications

Contraindications include the following:

1. Bony Bankart lesion
2. Hypoplasia or lack of labrum
3. Severe damage to IGHL or MGHL
4. Humeral avulsion of glenohumeral ligament (HAGL)
5. Concomitant rotator cuff lesion
6. Voluntary instability (type VI Gerber) and multidirectional instability (type IV + type V)
7. Suspicion of posterior instability
8. Nondisplaced fracture of the greater tuberosity (recurrence rate, 3%)

PREOPERATIVE PLANNING

History

Important information can be obtained from the patient's history. The mechanism of injury and whether the trauma was a high-speed injury or a minor trauma are of interest to judge if there will be concomitant hyperlaxity or not. The patient is asked if the reduction was performed by him- or herself or by a physician with or without anesthesia or if the shoulder reduced spontaneously. The number of dislocations will lead to a critical review of the pathology and the chosen procedure.

Examination

After testing range of motion, which is usually normal, isometric strength tests follow to exclude rotator cuff tears. In patients with chronic instability, external rotation can be limited. Typical signs for instability are positive results in the apprehension sign, relocation test, and fulcrum test. In cases of susceptible hyperlaxity, the anterior and posterior drawer laxity test must be carried out: The test will show a ++ translation, allowing the humeral head to subluxate as far as to the glenoid rim in an anteroposterior (AP) direction.

The sulcus sign is positive when the rotator interval is too wide. By pulling the arm caudally, a sulcus appears between the lateral border of the acromion and the humeral head.

The hyperabduction test is performed by passively abducting the arm with one hand while fixing the scapula with the other hand. The test is positive if the arm can be abducted more than 100 degrees without moving the scapula.

Radiography

Routinely, the following radiographs should be obtained:

1. True AP: This view can show a concomitant bony lesion of the glenoid.
2. Y-view: It is important to rule out a posterior dislocation.
3. Axillary view: With this view, glenoid fractures can be ruled out.
4. Bernageau view: This view shows a good profile of the glenoid and helps to rule out bony lesions.
5. Stryker-notch view: This view reveals the Hill-Sachs lesion.

Magnetic Resonance Imaging

Preoperatively, a magnetic resonance arthrography with intraarticularly applied gadolinium contrast medium can be performed to view the type of Bankart lesion and the size of the capsular structure; this will also provide a clue of capsular redundancy. Rotator cuff lesions are to be ruled out.

Diagnostic Arthroscopy

During diagnostic arthroscopy, the type and size of the labral lesion and the glenoid rim are to be defined (Fig. 5-1).

Glenoid Labrum. Pathologic findings are a disruption of the labrum off the glenoid rim with or without disruption of the glenohumeral ligaments (Bankart lesion). A periosteal avulsion of the labrum together with the glenohumeral ligaments off the scapular neck is referred to as a Perthes lesion. The labrum tends to ectopically scar beneath the glenoid rim to the scapular neck, diminishing the glenoid cavity [anterior labrum periosteal sleeve avulsion (ALPSA lesion)].

In traumatic cases, the force leading to the labral tear continues either caudally–posteriorly or cranially–posteriorly, thus creating a capsulolabral tear beyond the 6-o'clock position at the inferior glenoid or a superior labral tear from anterior to posterior (SLAP lesion). These lesions are crucial because they increase instability and therefore also require repair.

Glenohumeral Ligaments and Capsule. Pay attention to the capsular insertion at the labrum. Check the insertion site of the IGHL and MGHL, whether they are still attached to the labrum, whether they are disrupted from the labrum, and whether they are scarred in a dislocated position beneath the glenoid rim. With a probe, ensure that the quality of the capsule and its ligaments is normal or thinned. Evaluate the humeral insertion site to assess

Figure 5-1. Different lesions in anteroinferior shoulder instability. **A:** Normal anatomy of a right shoulder in the sagittal plane, smooth-confluence articular cartilage, labrum, inferior glenohumeral ligament (IGHL), and axillary recess. **B:** Bankart line. A classic Bankart lesion involves disruption of the glenoid labrum off the glenoid rim without periosteal avulsion. A double labral lesion involves labral disruption off the glenoid rim and the IGHL. In a bony Bankart lesion, a small bony fragment is avulsed from the glenoid. **C:** Perthes line. In a classic Perthes lesion, there is complete disruption of the labrum and the IGHL together off the scapular neck. In an anterior labrum periosteal sleeve avulsion (ALPSA) lesion, labrum and IGHL are avulsed off the scapular neck and scarred below the plane of the glenoid. A triple labral lesion involves a lesion of the labrum off the glenoid rim and off the IGHL and disruption of the IGHL off the scapular neck. An extralabral ligament lesion involves the IGHL of the glenoid rim and scapular neck but leaves the labrum intact. **D:** Capsular line. In a non-Bankart lesion, the IGHL is not confluent with the labrum but inserts more medially on the scapular neck. This is often seen in atraumatic instability. In a substance defect of IGHL, intraligamentous defects, elongation, or plastic deformation leads to capsular redundancy. A quatro lesion involves disruption and attenuation of the labrum–ligament complex. A humeral avulsion of glenohumeral ligament lesion is defined by an avulsion of the IGHL off its humeral insertion. **E:** In a glenoid labrum articular disruption (GLAD) lesion, there is a chondral defect in the transition zone toward the labrum without disruption of the labrum. This is often caused by direct trauma and causes pain but no instability.

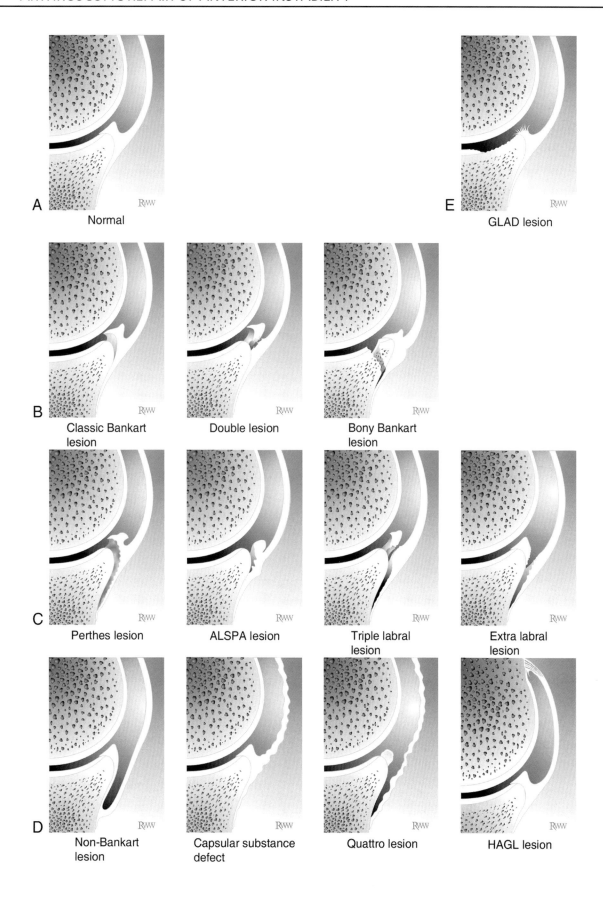

A — Normal
B — Classic Bankart lesion, Double lesion, Bony Bankart lesion
C — Perthes lesion, ALSPA lesion, Triple labral lesion, Extra labral lesion
D — Non-Bankart lesion, Capsular substance defect, Quattro lesion, HAGL lesion
E — GLAD lesion

for humeral avulsion (HAGL lesion). In cases of a HAGL lesion or a substantial defect of the capsule–ligament complex, open surgery is advisable.

Hyperlaxity or elongation is obvious in the presence of the following:

- Drive-through sign (you can easily drive with the scope from anterosuperior down into the axillary pouch along the anterior glenoid without damaging the humeral head)
- Non-Bankart defect
- Open or elongated rotator interval

Glenoid. Rule out chondral defects of the glenoid rim [GLAD (glenoid labrum articular disruption)] lesions or bony lesions like a bony Bankart fracture.

Humeral Head. Visualizing the whole humeral head is only possible by rotating the arm in all directions. At the posterosuperior aspect, an impression fracture (Hill-Sachs lesion) emphasizes the traumatic onset. According to Calandra (2), there are three grades of defects: (a) chondral, (b) osteochondral, and (c) osseous.

The typical Hill-Sachs lesion is not a contraindication for arthroscopic repair. A Hill-Sachs lesion of more than 30% of the humeral sphere or a posterocentral lesion has to be considered for rotational osteotomy.

SURGERY

Patient Positioning

After induction of general anesthesia, the patient is placed in the lateral decubitus position with the scapula dorsally rotated by 30 degrees to have the glenoid parallel to the ground. The arm is placed in a double-arm holder with horizontal traction weight of 5 kg and a vertical traction weight of 3 kg. Place the arm in about 30 to 45 degrees of abduction and neutral rotation. Prepare the arm from the mandible to the lower ribs, from sternum to the spinous process and down to the wrist (Fig. 5-2). Mark the bony landmarks.

Make sure that the anesthesiologist and anesthesia machines are moved to the contralateral side and ask the anesthesiologist to use long hoses, so you can stand freely cranial of the patient's head.

Portals

Enter the joint through a standard *posterior* portal, which is located 2 cm distally and medially of the posterolateral corner of the acromion. First use a sharp obturator to go gently

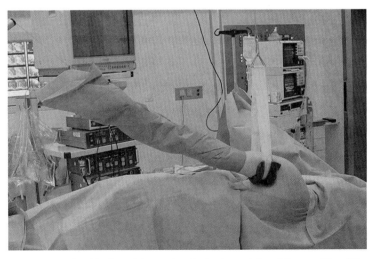

Figure 5-2. Positioning of the patient in the lateral decubitus position. The arm (right shoulder) is extended by 5 kg horizontally and 3.5 kg vertically.

through the deltoid fascia, then switch to a blunt obturator to penetrate the capsule. Ride along the humeral head to feel the joint space between head and glenoid and fall into it. Then with gentle force, penetrate the capsule. A first "dry" look follows. Then infuse the fluid, irrigate the joint, and inspect it thoroughly. Use a continuous-flow pump to have a steady intraarticular pressure of 60 mm Hg with high flow rate. Try to avoid higher fluid pressure to minimize fluid extravasation.

An *anteroinferior* portal is established in outside-in technique. Locate the portal with a needle in the rotator interval just superior to the subscapularis tendon and make sure you can reach the glenoid rim from the 12- to the 6-o'clock positions easily. Always stay lateral of the coracoid process. We use an 8.25-mm translucent twist-in cannula so the instruments and sutures are visible. Now introduce a probe and perform an inspection of the joint. Pay attention to all possible pathologies as mentioned above under Diagnostic Arthroscopy.

After deciding that arthroscopic surgery is adequate, a third *anterosuperior* portal is placed. Introduce a needle anterior to the acromioclavicular joint so it will penetrate the capsule posterior of the biceps anchor. Then incise the skin and introduce a changing rod. Take the arthroscope out of the shaft and place another changing rod through the posterior portal. Next, take the shaft of the arthroscope and insert it into the joint over the rod in the anterosuperior portal. Using the rod in the posterior portal another 8.25-mm translucent twist-in-cannula is inserted. Now two cannulas are located anterior and posterior, while the scope is superior (Fig. 5-3).

Surgical Technique

The following steps are crucial for a sufficient capsulolabral repair:

1. Release and mobilization of the ectopically scarred tissue
2. Decortication of scapular neck
3. Correct placement of suture anchors
4. Labral fixation
5. Sufficient ligament shift
6. Handling of sutures and knot management
7. Stable knot tying

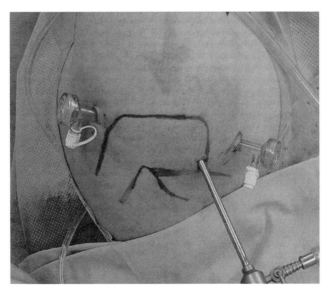

Figure 5-3. Portals on a right shoulder: The anterosuperior portal in front of the acromioclavicular joint is used for the scope. The posterior and anteroinferior portals are working portals with an 8.25-mm translucent cannula.

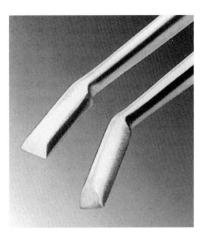

Figure 5-4. Tissue elevator.

Release and Mobilization of the Ectopically Scarred Tissue. Good stabilization depends on this surgical step. Only an extensive release enables you to perform a ligament shift to reduce joint volume.

Use a meniscal punch to release the labrum–ligament complex (LLC) off the glenoid rim. At the beginning, you may find it difficult to find a starting point because the tissue is tightly scarred to the scapular neck. In this case, take a tissue elevator (Fig. 5-4) to sharply dissect the tissue off the bone for a short distance. From this point, use the punch. Continue the dissection all the way down to the 6-o'clock position. Because you view the glenoid rim from superior, you have easy access to the scapular neck. Release all tissue off the neck to reach good mobilization of the LLC. If you cannot reach down inferior enough, use a glenoid rasp (Fig. 5-5) to get all tissue off the bone. Once a good release is achieved, the tissue will float up to the glenoid level. The release is finished when you can see the subscapularis muscle (Fig. 5-6).Sometimes it will bleed from there, but it is not worrisome.

If the joint is tight or small, ask your assistant to pull the arm more lateral so you can reach more inferior. Always stay close to the bone while releasing the tissue to stay away from the axillary nerve safely.

A holding or pulling stitch can be applied if you need more resistance while passing through the tissue later on. This step is not mandatory but can help in suture passing. Load a suture hook (Linvatec Corp., Largo, FL) with a no. 1 polydioxanone synthetic (PDS) suture (Ethicon Inc., Somerville, NJ) and from anterior, perforate the LLC at the anterior band of the IGHL. Advance the suture into the joint and redraw the suture hook out of the

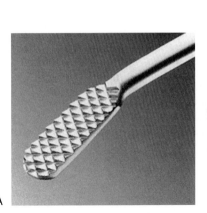

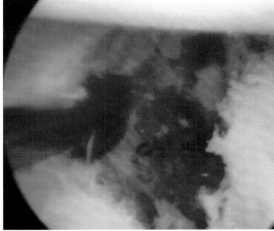

A   B

Figure 5-5. A: Glenoid rasp. **B:** Tissue mobilization on the scapular neck with a rasp.

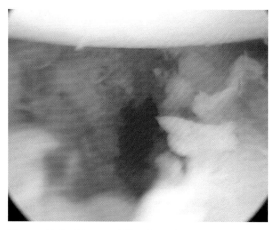

Figure 5-6. After mobilization, the tissue floats up to the glenoid level. In the background the subscapularis muscle belly becomes visible.

joint. With a suture retriever, pull the suture out anteriorly. Secure the PDS suture with a clamp. This holding stitch can be pulled on to reach inferior enough when you pass the sutures for definite refixation.

In patients with atraumatic instability, the capsular release must be continued beyond the 6-o'clock position (12). Dissect the capsule from the 6-o'clock position into the axillary pouch straight down. You receive a triangle-shaped tissue complex that can be shifted similar to a V-Y-plasty. This way an additional shift can be achieved (Fig. 5-7).

Decortication of Scapular Neck. Now decortication of the scapular neck is performed, using the rasp to create bleeding. You can also use a motorized burr (Fig. 5-8) to do so. Bleeding is imperative for fibroblastic healing of the tissue to bone. Creation of a bony trough is not necessary. With a slotted whisker shaver, débride the chondral rim (Fig. 5-9).

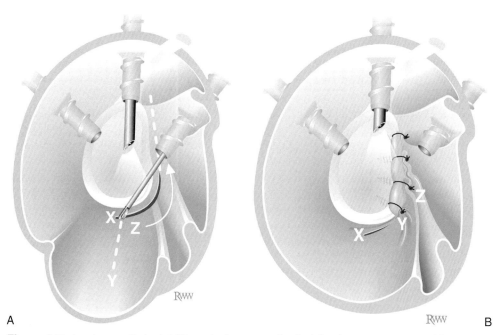

A   B

Figure 5-7. In atraumatic instability, a further capsular incision is necessary to achieve a sufficient capsular shift. **A:** The axillary recess is incised to point Y. **B:** The capsular triangle is then shifted superiorly and the axillary recess is removed.

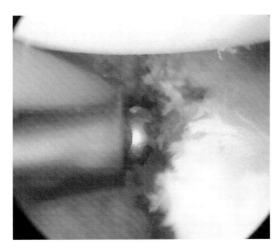 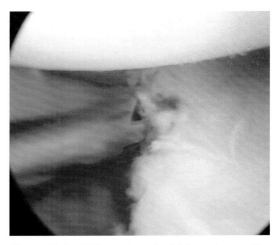

Figure 5-8. A motorized burr is used to create bleeding on the scapular neck, which is mandatory for fibroblastic healing.

Figure 5-9. With a slotted whisker shaver, the transition zone is débrided.

Placement of Suture Anchors. The use of suture anchors (e.g., Bio-FASTak, Arthrex Inc., Naples, FL; Panalok anchor, Mitek Worldwide, Norwood, MA) is now widely accepted as the standard in arthroscopic instability surgery. According to Barber et al. (1), the pullout strength of all available suture anchors is more than what is needed in their applications.

After using metal anchors, we now only use bioabsorbable anchors because of the danger of implant dislocation or misplacement with implant-induced arthritic changes. The anchor is preloaded with a no. 2 braided suture and has a soft suture eyelet. This diminishes the aberration of the suture in the eyelet compared to that of metal anchors, minimizes the risk of suture breakage, and facilitates the sliding of the suture.

The anchor is placed using a guiding instrument, the so-called spear (Arthrex Inc.). Introduce the spear with a sharp-tipped trocar through the anterior portal and place it at the 5- to 5:30-o'clock position (Fig. 5-10A). With the central trocar, penetrate the cortical bone at the glenoid rim to create a pilot hole. Remove the trocar, allowing the fish-mouth design of the spear to sit on the glenoid rim. Attach the tap to the ratcheting screwdriver handle and advance it through the spear to the pilot hole. Advance the tap into the bone until the distal laser mark is flush with the bone surface (Fig. 5-10B). The mark can be seen through the holes at the distal end of the spear as well as on the tap itself. This way a threaded hole is established.

Take out the taper and insert the anchor. When the laser mark on the inserter equals the bone level, the anchor is fully inserted (Fig. 5-10C). With a short and fast pull the inserter is then removed from the anchor. Control the anchor by looking into its hole. It should be fully covered by bone (Fig. 5-10D).

The anchor must not be placed too superficially in order not to create chondral damages on the humeral head. If it is inserted too deep into the bone, the sutures could be abraded by the bone. You would rather place the anchor 2 to 3 mm more toward the articular cartilage than placing it too medial on the scapular neck. If the anchor is too medial, reconstruction of glenoid concavity is not possible.

It is imperative to introduce the anchor not too shallow (tangential), because this again will cause chondral damage ("anchor arthritis"). Be absolutely sure about your anchor, if you are not, take it out, and do it again.

After perfect positioning of the anchor, retrieve the suture strand that faces away from the glenoid rim (outer strand) through the posterior portal. This maneuver will avoid intermingling of the sutures while passing them through the tissue. If the sutures run criss-cross through the eyelet, they might get caught by themselves and will lock to early. They will not slide through the eyelet and a sliding knot is not applicable.

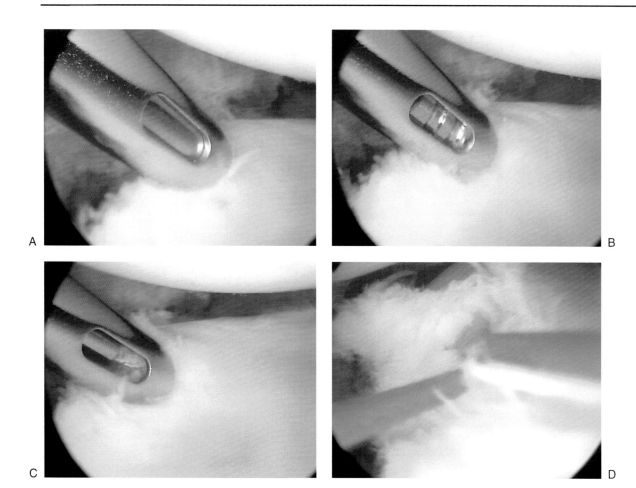

Figure 5-10. The spear cannula with the sharp trocar is placed on the glenoid rim creating a pilot hole **(A)**, the tap, which is connected to the ratcheting screwdriver creates a threaded hole for the uptake of the anchor **(B)**. **C:** A bioabsorbable Bio-FASTak (Arthrex, Inc., Naples, FL) is inserted through the spear cannula. The anchor's position has to be controlled and it must be fully inserted into bone **(D)**.

Labral Fixation and Ligament Shift. Aiming at a good labral fixation and ligament shift, it is necessary to place the sutures through the released tissue at the correct site.

Use a suture hook with a shuttle relay device (Linvatec Corp.) or a Suture Lasso (Arthrex, Inc.) and penetrate the IGHL and labrum at the most inferior position even more caudad of the holding stitch (Fig. 5-11). Take a good bite of the tissue about 1 cm lateral of the glenoid rim to accomplish a good capsular shift. Single labral repair, which leaves the

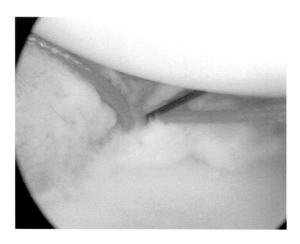

Figure 5-11. A suture hook (not visible in the arthroscopic view) loaded with a shuttle relay is inserted to perforate the inferior glenohumeral ligament–labrum complex at an inferior position and 1 cm lateral of the glenoid to achieve a good capsular shift.

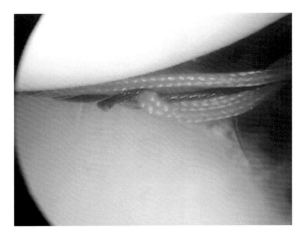

Figure 5-12. The shuttle relay has been loaded with one of the anchor's suture strands outside of the posterior cannula. It is now pulled from anterior and the suture is located in the shuttle relay's metal eyelet.

capsular redundancy untouched, will not reduce extensive joint volume, leading to early recurrence.

If you have trouble perforating the tissue and it moves away from your needle, pull on the holding stitch to have more resistance. Perforating the LLC can be done with various instruments, but we have found it the easiest to use a suture hook for the first one or two stitches because you can grasp more inferiorly. Moving more superior, we prefer to use a tissue penetrator or BirdBeak (Arthrex Inc., Naples, FL). These instruments allow fast and precise tissue penetration and suture passing.

From the posterior portal, pull out the shuttle relay and insert the suture strand that was moved there before into the small metal eyelet of the shuttle relay. It is pulled back through the anterior portal (Fig. 5-12). Now the outer strand is located in the tissue and the inner strand runs free. If the sutures are intermingled, use a probe or a suture retriever to straighten out the sutures. Do not loose patience when the sutures are mixed up. There is always a way out.

Suture Handling and Knot Tying. Only secure knot tying ensures good results. Two different techniques are possible: sliding or nonsliding knots. For the use of a sliding knot, make sure that the suture slides freely through both the tissue and the eyelet of the anchor.

Different knots have been described. For further details, review the recommended reading of Nottage and Lieurance (10). We prefer the Duncan loop sliding knot and a single nonsliding knot with alternating half-hitches. After advancing the loop down onto the tis-

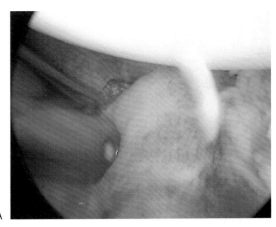

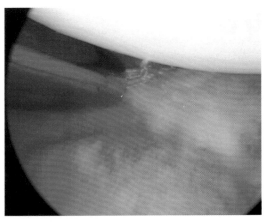

A   B

Figure 5-13. A: The suture is tied with a sliding knot. **B:** The knot pusher helps to correctly place the knot. The suture is cut with a suture cutter and the final knot is located on the scapular neck.

sue, use a knot pusher to direct the knot. The knot should not impinge on the articular surface but should be placed beneath the tissue to push it upwards to enhance concavity (Fig. 5-13).

Depending on the size of the lesion, three to four anchors are used. Take enough tissue to reduce capsular redundancy. The ligament shift has to be performed in inferosuperior (south–north) *and* lateromedial (east–west) direction. The quality of repair depends on the number of anchors and security of knots.

As a variation of this technique you can pass not only one but both of the suture strands of one anchor through the LLC. You might increase the shift by this procedure, but might face the risk that in weak tissue the sutures cut through the tissue and you will end up with an "air knot" not fixing the LLC back to the glenoid (8). When you pass both strands through the tissue, it is mandatory to place the anchor exactly on the rim. Otherwise the sutures will not pull the tissue onto the glenoid rim but will leave it below (medial) the rim not creating glenoid cavity.

A concomitant SLAP-lesion must be repaired.

Additional Techniques

In patients with traumatic instability with hyperlaxity (type III), you often find a posterior capsular redundancy and an insufficient rotator interval. The interval is a stabilizer in inferior direction and in these patients, you see a positive sulcus sign and a positive drive-through sign at arthroscopy.

As mentioned earlier, the force tearing the labrum off the glenoid rim can extend superior–posterior creating a SLAP lesion or inferoposterior, creating a posterior Bankart lesion. The technique of posterior Bankart repair is the same as that for the anterior one, but you work from the posterior portal, park your sutures in the anterior portal, and still view from the anterosuperior portal.

Posterior Capsular Plication. Posterior plication (Fig. 5-14) is advisable when during diagnostic arthroscopy you see a huge posterior capsular pouch. In these cases it is possible to look at the posterior glenoid rim and labrum from the posterior portal and even see the capsular insertion more medial on the scapular without gliding out of the joint with the scope. Examination under anesthesia shows increased posterior translation.

The scope is in the superior portal. Abrade and débride the posterior capsule with a slotted whisker shaver to create some bleeding in the capsule. This is needed for healing of the plicated capsule. With a suture hook loaded with a no. 1 PDS suture enter the joint, perforate the capsule far inferior about 1 to 1.5 cm lateral of the glenoid. Guide the instrument from intra- to extraarticular and then back to intracapsular. A good portion of the capsule is on your hook. Again guide it toward extraarticular and then bring it back into the joint by aiming between labrum and glenoid. Advance the suture out of the suture hook. Take a suture grasper and pull the suture out of the posterior portal. Tie the knot using a sliding knot. For a good and sufficient plication, at least three sutures must be used (13).

In posterior plication, you may find it easier to locate your posterior portal a bit more lateral toward the humeral head and more inferior to achieve a good plication. If you feel that posterior plication might be suitable because examination under anesthesia showed abnormal posterior translation, start the procedure with a modified posterior portal and posterior capsular plication before you reconstruct the LLC and before closing the rotator interval.

SLAP Repair. Change your scope to the posterior portal. Similar to the anterior Bankart repair the SLAP complex has to be mobilized (Fig. 5-15). From anterior you use a special SLAP rasp to débride the bone of the superior glenoid to create bleeding. If the rasp does not give enough decortication take a motorized burr to do so.

Then enter, in a right shoulder, an anchor at the 10:30- to 11:00-o'clock position (1:30 to 2:00 o'clock in the left shoulder) from the anterosuperior portal. Introduce a suture hook with a shuttle relay from anterior and perforate the SLAP complex from superior to inferior pointing the tip of the suture hook toward the glenoid. Forward the shuttle relay and take it out from superior. Put one suture strand into the eyelet of the shuttle relay and re-

(text continues on page 98)

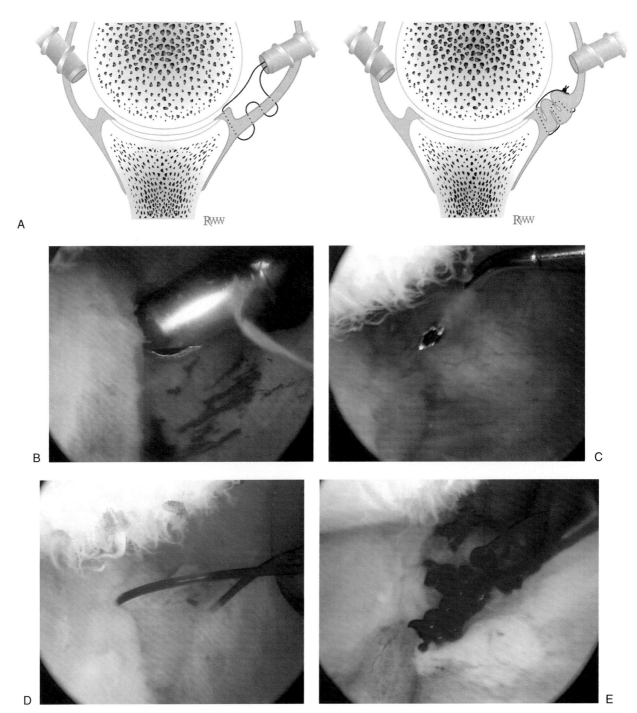

Figure 5-14. Posterior capsular plication. **A:** Schematic drawing. The suture is first passed from interior to exterior and then interior again. Then it is again passed extracapsular and located between the labrum and the glenoid. **B:** After the suture is tied, the posterior capsule is plicated on itself. During arthroscopy, the capsule is first débrided to create bleeding. **C:** Then a suture hook is introduced to perforate the capsule laterally and perforate it again close to the glenoid between the labrum and the cartilage. The suture is tied with a sliding knot. A couple of sutures **(D)** are necessary to perform a sufficient plication **(E)**.

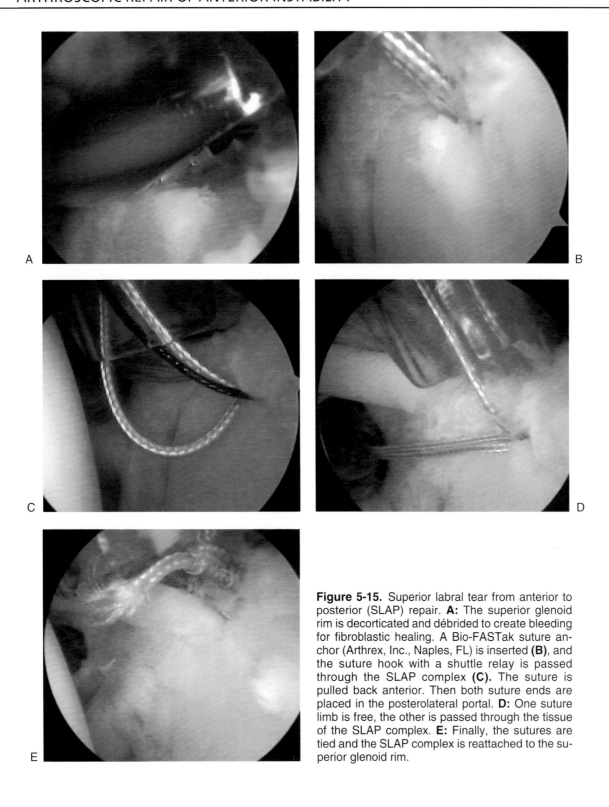

Figure 5-15. Superior labral tear from anterior to posterior (SLAP) repair. **A:** The superior glenoid rim is decorticated and débrided to create bleeding for fibroblastic healing. A Bio-FASTak suture anchor (Arthrex, Inc., Naples, FL) is inserted **(B)**, and the suture hook with a shuttle relay is passed through the SLAP complex **(C).** The suture is pulled back anterior. Then both suture ends are placed in the posterolateral portal. **D:** One suture limb is free, the other is passed through the tissue of the SLAP complex. **E:** Finally, the sutures are tied and the SLAP complex is reattached to the superior glenoid rim.

trieve it from anterior. Now one suture strand is located in the SLAP-complex. Pull this strand out to the superior portal and tie the knot. Then place one or two more anchors at the 12:00- to 12:30-o'clock position and perform the repair. Take care not to squeeze the biceps tendon. If your anchor is directly under the biceps you would rather pass both limbs of the suture through the SLAP complex and tie the knot on top of the complex.

Rotator Interval Closure. Rotator interval closure (Fig. 5-16) is performed at the end of the procedure after reconstruction of the LLC and other additional steps. When performing a rotator interval closure, change the scope into the posterior portal, because it provides a better view of the structures to repair. For this additional procedure use a suture hook with a no. 1 PDS suture and perforate the MGHL just above the superior border of the subscapularis tendon. Advance the suture in the joint and release it from the suture hook. After taking the suture hook out, turn the twist-in cannula back just outside the joint capsule. Then enter with a BirdBeak or another sharp suture passer and penetrate the rotator interval capsule close to the supraspinatus. Advance to the suture and retrieve one end of it out of the joint. With a sliding knot tie the suture thoroughly. You will not see this knot with the arthroscope, because you fix it extraarticular on the interval capsule. You check the knot by

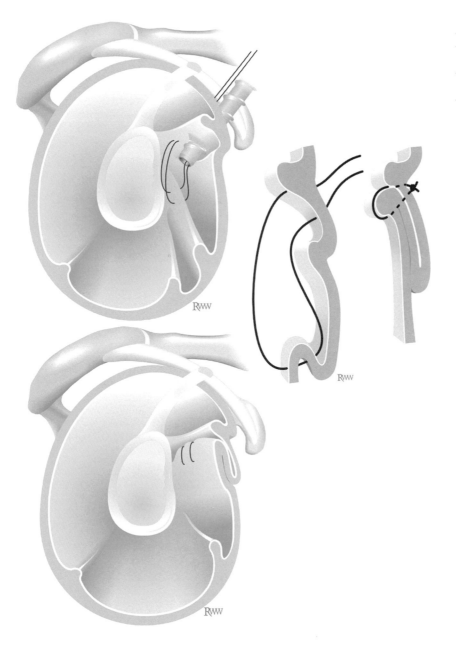

Figure 5-16. Schematic drawing of rotator interval closure. The suture is passed through the middle glenohumeral ligament just superior to the subscapularis tendon into the joint. With a BirdBeak (Arthrex, Inc., Naples, FL), the rotator interval capsule is penetrated superior to retrieve the free end of the suture. The knots are tied extracapsular.

changing your scope to the anterior portal. Repeat this procedure with another one or two sutures. Do not overtie the interval. It can cause additional limitation in external rotation. Therefore, tie the rotator interval with the arm at 30-degrees external rotation minimum.

At the end of all arthroscopic stabilizing procedures, we use a drain to support the vacuum effect of the joint for 24 hours. After skin closure, local anesthetics are instilled. Sterile wound dressing and a sling are applied.

POSTOPERATIVE MANAGEMENT

The arm is fixed in a sling for 48 hours. Immediate ice and antiinflammatory drugs are given. Then an abduction brace (cushion) of 20 degrees of abduction with the forearm in only slight internal rotation is used for 3 weeks. During the first 3 weeks, passive mobilization to 30 degrees of abduction, 30 degrees of flexion, 0 degrees of external rotation, and 60 degrees of internal rotation is allowed. Then range of motion is subsequently increased. Avoid aggressive glides and manipulation. The limits of 90 degrees of abduction and flexion, free internal, and 0 degrees of external rotation are enforced. After week six, range of motion, especially external rotation, increases further and muscle-strengthening exercises can begin. A well-balanced exercise program for the rotator cuff muscles, the deltoid, and the scapula stabilizing muscles (Musculi trapezius, serratus anterior, rhomboidei, and levator scapulae) is initiated. Follow up on the patient in your outpatient clinic after 6 weeks and, if necessary, modify rehabilitation. Rehabilitation should always be pain-free and gentle to avoid frozen shoulder.

Return to contact sports or overhead athletic activities should not commence before 6 months.

RESULTS

The literature includes many reports on arthroscopic stabilization procedures. Recurrence rates vary from as low as 2% to as high as 49%. The worst results have been reported in those series in which patients with all kinds of instability were treated the same way, without discussion of the etiology. Patients with one or two dislocations were arthroscopically operated on as were patients with more than 20 or 30 dislocations prior to surgery. The problem of hyperlaxity was often not addressed. Recently, a few prospective studies with very strict inclusion and exclusion criteria were published. These reports show low recurrence rates in patients selected according to the criteria mentioned above. In these studies, the authors achieved good results with transglenoid (11) or anchor techniques (3,8,12). Failure analysis has been helpful in establishing the recommendations for patient selection that are summarized in this chapter.

In our own experience since 1987, we have gone through the same process of enthusiasm for arthroscopic procedures but had to face high recurrence rates of up to 35%. In our own prospective, not yet published study with strict criteria, we compared the results of 46 patients treated with arthroscopic stabilization. Twenty-three patients were randomly assigned to surgery with a transglenoid technique and 23 with suture anchors. In the transglenoid group, three (13%) patients and one (4.3%) patient in the anchor group experienced recurrence. Furthermore, patients treated with a transglenoid technique suffered from pain in the back because of the suture knots on their infraspinatus fascia. One patient had to undergo revision surgery for this problem. We therefore favor the use of suture anchors.

COMPLICATIONS

The overall complication rate in arthroscopic stabilization is low. Besides the perioperative complications of wound or deep infection, deep vein thrombosis, hematoma, and postoperative frozen shoulder, inform the patient about the following possible complications:

Stiff Shoulder

The causes that can lead to postoperative stiff shoulder include:

- In acute first-time traumatic dislocation, immediate surgery is not advisable. In this case, the increased activity of proteinases causes a higher risk of arthrofibrosis similar to that for the acute treatment of anterior cruciate ligament ruptures. Therefore, a security interval of 2 to 3 weeks should be respected.
- Overtensioning of MGHL and IGHL can lead to loss of external rotation and therefore to stiff shoulder. In particular, it is important to avoid overtension of MGHL and IGHL in chronic cases with preoperatively decreased external rotation.
- Aggressive rehabilitation with pain during or after physiotherapy will cause intermittent adhesive capsulitis.

Recurrence

Besides technical errors, recurrence is influenced by incorrect patient selection (9). As mentioned above, tissue quality, number of preoperative dislocations, compliance, functional demands, and involvement in contact sports must be considered before treating a patient by arthroscopic Bankart repair. Adequate repair is mandatory: Free all tissue off the bone and perform a sufficient capsular shift in order to get satisfactory results.

The most common mistake that causes recurrence is failure to detect a bony Bankart lesion, which compromises glenoid concavity. Rule out the presence of this lesion with radiographs, magnetic resonance imaging, and arthroscopy.

Recurrence with transglenoid techniques in our experience is higher because of the following points:

1. Suture fixation over swollen soft tissue. After the swelling has resolved the sutures may get loose.
2. If you drill the transglenoid hole too medial on the scapular neck you are not able to restore concavity.

The same is true for misplacement of suture anchors, therefore, put them on the rim or even 2 to 3 mm into the articular cartilage.

Patients over 40 years old who experience a first-time traumatic shoulder dislocation have an increased risk of rotator cuff tears. Therefore in those patients an arthroscopic or mini-open rotator cuff repair, instead of a stabilizing procedure is necessary. Take care to rule out rotator cuff lesions in dislocations of these patients.

Nerve Injury

The risk of damaging the suprascapular nerve is abolished with the use of suture anchors. The axillary nerve is at risk when you have to perform a capsular incision in the axillary pouch to achieve a good shift in cases of atraumatic instability. So stay close to the glenoid bone because the nerve is a safe distance from the glenoid in most of the arm positions during surgery.

The axillary nerve and the plexus could get irritated by too much extension weight on the arm holder. Therefore, do not exceed a weight of 5 kg on horizontal and 3.5 kg on vertical traction.

Hardware

"Anchor arthritis" is the most feared complication in arthroscopic stabilization. Put the anchors deep enough into bone. Always check the anchor's position with the scope.

Do not insert the anchor too shallow (tangential) because that also will cause chondral damage. If unsure about its position, do not hesitate to take it out and give it another shot.

We have changed from metal to bioabsorbable anchors. They, of course, also can damage the humeral head if they are not fully inserted but we believe this is of minor gravity.

Because of foreign-body reaction, we do not recommend bioabsorbable tacks, which are implanted intraarticularly or extraarticularly. Furthermore, we see a limitation in retensioning the IGHL properly. The recurrence rate in arthroscopic stabilization with a bioabsorbable tack ranges from 9% to 21%.

RECOMMENDED READING

1. Barber, F.A., Herbert, M.A.: Suture anchor—update 1999. *Arthroscopy* 15: 719–725, 1999.
2. Calandra, J.J., Baker, C.L., Uribe, J.: The incidence of Hill-Sachs-lesions in initial anterior shoulder dislocations. *Arthroscopy* 5: 254–257, 1989.
3. Gartsman, G.M., Roddey, T.S., Hammerman, S.M.: Arthroscopic treatment of anterior-inferior glenohumeral instability: two-to-five-year follow-up. *J Bone Joint Surg Am* 82: 991–1003, 2000.
4. Gerber C. Observations on the classification of instability. In: Warner, J.J.P., Ianotti, J.P., Gerber, C., eds.: *Complex and revision problems in shoulder surgery.* Philadelphia: Lippincott–Raven Publishers, 1997: 9–18.
5. Habermeyer, P., Gleyze, P., Rickert, M.: Evolution of lesions of the labrum-ligament complex in posttraumatic anterior shoulder instability: a prospective study. *J Shoulder Elbow Surg* 8: 66–74, 1999.
6. Hovelius, L.L.: Anterior dislocation of the shoulder in teenagers and young adults: five-year prognosis. *J Bone Joint Surg Am* 69: 393–399, 1987.
7. McLaughlin, H.L., McLellan, D.I.: Recurrent anterior dislocation of the shoulder, II: a comparative study. *J Trauma* 7: 191–201, 1967.
8. Nebelung, W., Ropke, M., Urbach, D., et al.: A new technique of arthroscopic capsular shift in anterior shoulder instability. *Arthroscopy* 17: 286–289, 2001.
9. Nelson, B.J., Arciero, R.A.: Arthroscopic management of glenohumeral instability. *Am J Sports Med* 28: 602–614, 2000.
10. Nottage W.M., Lieurance, R.K.: Arthroscopic knot tying techniques. *Arthroscopy* 15: 515–521, 1999.
11. O'Neill, D.B.: Arthroscopic Bankart repair of anterior detachments of the glenoid labrum. *J Bone Joint Surg Am* 81: 1357–1366, 1999.
12. Tauro, J.C.: Arthroscopic capsular split and advancement for anterior and inferior shoulder instability: technique and results at a 2 to 5 year follow-up. *Arthroscopy* 16: 451–456, 2000.
13. Wolf, E.M., Eakin, C.L.: Arthroscopic capsular plication for posterior shoulder instability. *Arthroscopy* 14: 153–163, 1998.

6

Arthroscopic Repair of Posterior Instability

Sabrina Strickland, Riley J. Williams III, and David Altchek

INDICATIONS/CONTRAINDICATIONS

Recurrent posterior instability of the shoulder is much less common than anterior instability. The incidence of posterior instability is reportedly between 2% and 12% of all shoulder instability (6,11). Excellent clinical results have been reported with surgical intervention in patients with positional instability, in which posterior subluxation of the humeral head occurs when the arm is adducted at 90 degrees of flexion (1). These patients typically present with posterior shoulder pain with or without distinct symptoms of instability. Pain is exacerbated by activities that posteriorly load the shoulder in the adducted position (bench press or push-up exercises) (4,8). Most commonly, trauma to the affected extremity (fall onto outstretched arm, blow to a forward-flexed adducted arm) precedes the onset of symptoms. However, patients rarely report a history of frank posterior dislocation (4,11). The etiology of injury may also be attributed to chronic overuse that leads to microtrauma and the development of laxity of the capsulolabral complex (5). Athletic activities that predispose the individuals to posterior capsulolabral injury include baseball, softball, football, swimming, and volleyball (8).

Biomechanical evaluation of posterior shoulder translation has demonstrated a continuum between subluxation and dislocation. Weber and Caspari (9) assessed cadaver shoulders with the humerus positioned in full internal rotation, 90 degrees' forward flexion, and neutral horizontal adduction. The humerus was then displaced posteriorly until the humeral head was displaced by at least one head diameter. This humeral head translation resulted in

S. Strickland, M.D.: Department of Orthopaedics, Beth Israel Medical Center, Singer Division, New York; and Department of Orthopaedic Surgery, Albert Einstein College of Medicine, Montefiore Medical Center, Bronx, New York.

R. J. Williams III, M.D.: Department of Orthopaedic Surgery, Weill Medical College of Cornell University; and Sports Medicine and Shoulder Service, Hospital for Special Surgery, New York, New York.

D. Altchek, M.D.: Department of Orthopaedics, Hospital for Special Surgery, New York, New York.

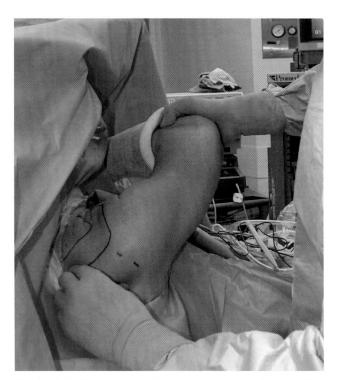

Figure 6-1. Photograph of the examination under anesthesia—specifically the posterior load and shift test.

a posterior Bankart lesion, posterior capsular disruption, or both. Force displacement curves did not show an inflection point to suggest rupture of any single capsular restraint. No injury was noted in the anterior or superior capsule. Although posterior capsular damage was the common denominator for all of the specimens evaluated, labral damage was frequently noted.

Physical examination may reveal posterior joint line tenderness, crepitance with range of motion, posterior subluxation, or dislocation. The posterior load-and-shift maneuver (forward flexion, adduction, and internal rotation) is often positive in this patient group and suggests the presence of a posterior Bankart lesion (Fig. 6-1).

Historically, management of posterior shoulder instability has been complicated by recurrence rates ranging from 7% to 72% with operative management and 16% to 96% with conservative management (3,5,11). Many of the failures with operative treatment have been attributed to unrecognized multidirectional instability (8). Conservative management comprises a formal physical therapy program with emphasis on strengthening of the posterior deltoid, infraspinatus, and teres minor (2). Arthroscopic management of this difficult problem continues to evolve. Several authors have demonstrated successful augmentation of the glenolabral concavity and reduction of capsular laxity (1). In addition, other authors have suggested that traumatic labral lesions of the posterior glenoid may be repaired by arthroscopic means (4).

PREOPERATIVE PLANNING

Patients with suspected posterior shoulder instability upon clinical evaluation should first have plain anteroposterior radiographs in internal and external rotation, to rule out a reverse Hill-Sachs lesion, as well as an axillary view to rule out a posterior bony Bankart lesion and to assess glenoid version. However, magnetic resonance imaging is critical for the assessment of the posterior labrum and to rule out other intraarticular pathology (Figs. 6-2 and 6-3). Ultimately, the surgical procedure chosen is dependent on the findings at examination under anesthesia and diagnostic arthroscopy. Arthroscopy is a reasonable first step for all

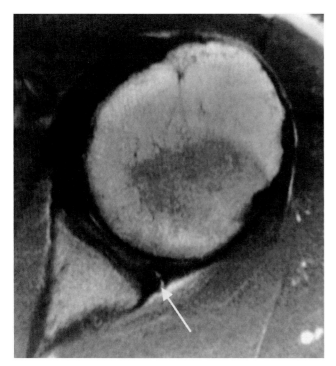

Figure 6-2. Axial magnetic resonance image depicting posterior Bankart lesion (*white arrow*).

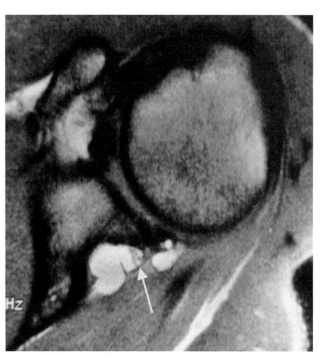

Figure 6-3. Axial magnetic resonance image depicting cyst (*white arrow*) and labral split.

patients under consideration for posterior stabilization. Patients with multidirectional instability or poor tissue quality are better stabilized by an open technique. In addition, voluntary dislocators may be better treated by an open procedure and education to avoid positions of provocation (7).

SURGERY

Typically, a regional interscalene block is performed; general anesthesia is acceptable and allows examination of the contralateral shoulder. The patient should be positioned in the beach-chair configuration using a full-length beanbag on an adjustable operating room table (Fig. 6-4). The bag is carefully molded and positioned on the table to provide access to the medical aspect of the scapula. An examination of the affected shoulder under anesthesia is performed (sulcus sign, anterior and posterior humeral head translation, range of motion) (Fig. 6-1). Grading of joint translation is as follows: grade 1, translation of the humeral head to the glenoid rim; grade 2, translation of the humeral head over the glenoid rim with spontaneous relocation; grade 3, translation of the humeral head over the glenoid rim with locking. Grade 3 humeral head translation implies the presence of glenohumeral capsular laxity and should be surgically addressed (i.e., capsular plication). Bony landmarks are then identified and marked (Fig. 6-4).

A posterior portal is then localized 2 cm medial and 2 cm inferior to the posterolateral border of the acromion. Lidocaine is injected subcutaneously into the intended portal site before the skin incision if regional anesthesia is used. The arthroscope is placed into the shoulder joint. A pump is routinely used to maintain joint distention. An anterior portal is made in the rotator interval. A diagnostic arthroscopy is performed, carefully assessing the glenoid, glenoid labrum, Bankart lesions, humeral Hill-Sachs or reverse Hill-Sachs lesions, rotator cuff, and biceps tendon. The scope should be switched to the anterior portal to fully evaluate the posterior aspect of the glenohumeral joint. The capsule should be carefully inspected for redundancy and evidence of capsular stretch/attenuation.

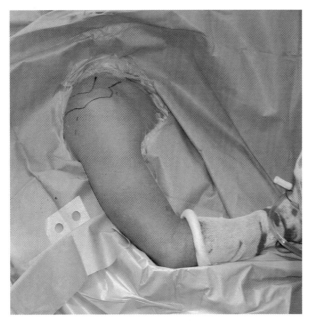

Figure 6-4. Patient in beach-chair position with bony landmarks clearly marked. The standard posterior portal is made 2 cm inferior and 2 cm medial to the lateral border of the posterior acromion. The accessory posterior portal is made 1 cm inferior to the standard posterior portal.

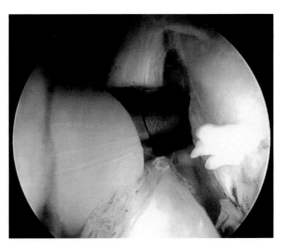

Figure 6-5. Posterior Bankart lesion. The posterior capsule and labrum are elevated from the glenoid with the shaver.

Those cases amenable to arthroscopic posterior shoulder stabilization will demonstrate clear separation of the posterior capsulolabral structures from the posterior glenoid (Fig. 6-5). With the arthroscope in the anterior portal, a second more lateral posterior portal is established to allow access to the glenoid neck (Fig. 6-6). The posterior rim of the glenoid is prepared by using a 4.5 full-radius shaver to débride remaining soft tissue and establish a bleeding, cancellous bony surface immediately adjacent to the rim of articular cartilage (Figs. 6-7 and 6-8). A number of different methods and implants are available for labral repair (Fig. 6-9).

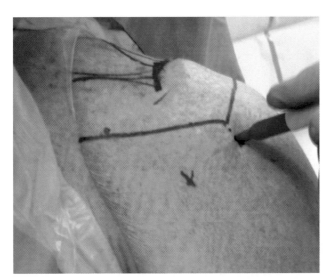

Figure 6-6. An additional lateral portal is made posteriorly to optimize the angle of insertion of the suture anchor; a less oblique angle of insertion may result in anchor penetration of the articular surface. Arthroscope is in the anterior port for viewing.

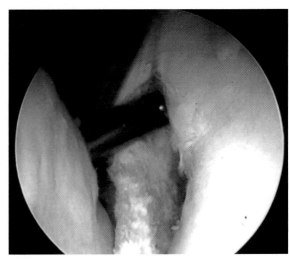

Figure 6-7. A 4.5-mm full-radius shaver is used to débride the posterior glenoid and labrum.

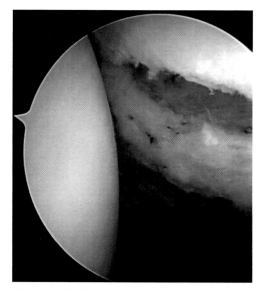

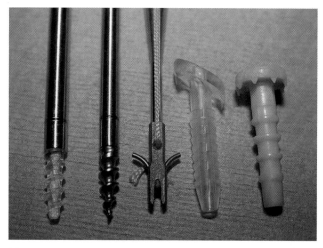

Figure 6-8. When a step-off of articular cartilage is encountered, the shaver can be used to burr down the glenoid bone to the level of the remaining articular surface.

Figure 6-9. Tacks and anchors from right to left: BioFASTak (Arthrex, Naples, FL), FASTak (Arthrex), Knotless Suture Anchor (Mitek, Westwood, MA), Tissuetak (Arthrex), Suretac (Smith and Nephew, Andover, MA).

We currently use a suture-based repair for posterior shoulder stabilization. In this technique, two posterior portals are made and cannulas are placed. The posterior glenoid rim is prepared and capsule is mobilized from the glenoid (Fig. 6-10). The angle of suture anchor insertion should be more oblique to the glenoid surface compared with the angle used for the placement of anterior glenoid anchors. The angle of insertion should be approximately 60 degrees relative to the glenoid surface; a less oblique angle of insertion may result in an-

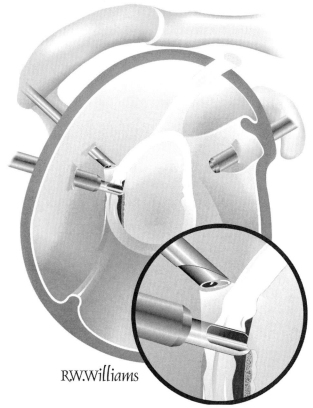

R.W.Williams

Figure 6-10. Débridement of posterior glenoid to bleeding bone with a motorized full-radius shaver.

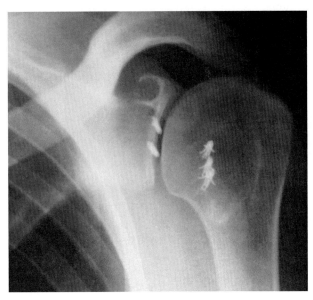

Figure 6-11. Radiograph depicting incorrect anchor placement with violation of the articular surface.

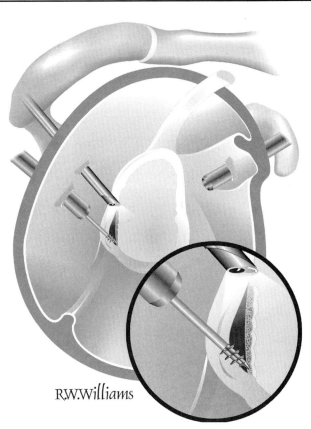

Figure 6-12. Placement of suture anchor at the inferior aspect of the posterior glenoid rim.

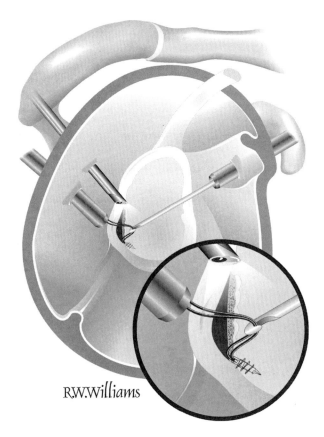

Figure 6-13. Passage of sutures through anterior portal.

chor penetration of the articular surface (Fig. 6-11). An anchor is placed in the desired area of repair, usually at the inferior margin of the capsular detachment (Fig. 6-12). (We prefer to use a 2.8-mm corkscrew-type anchor, metal or bioabsorbable.) Sutures are pulled through the anterior cannula once the anchors are placed and carefully kept separate (Fig. 6-13). Occasionally, it is helpful to place a traction suture inferiorly in the labrum before placing the looped suture; in this case, a single 2.0 Prolene (Ethicon, Inc., Somerville, NJ) is passed and grabbed and pulled through the anterior portal along with the end originating through the posterior portal. A Spectrum (Linvatec Corp., Largo, FL) right-curved suture passer (in a right shoulder) or a straight Arthro-pierce grasper (Orthopaedic Biosystems Ltd., Scottsdale, AZ) is placed through the posteroinferior cannula and used to grab the inferior capsule and labrum; the two free ends of a looped polydioxanone synthetic (PDS) suture (Ethicon, Inc.) is passed through the Spectrum and pulled out the anterior portal (Fig. 6-14). A second PDS suture is shuttled by passing it through this loop (outside the posteroinferior cannula) and the loop is pulled out anteriorly. One end of the Ethibond (Ethicon, Inc.) suture from the inferior suture anchor is then passed through this loop and pulled out the posterior portal (Fig. 6-15). The other end of the Ethibond suture is grabbed intraarticularly and pulled through the posterior cannula (Fig. 6-16). The sutures are then tied using standard arthroscopic knot technique and secured with a knot pusher, alternating direction of the knots and tying six knots in total (Fig. 6-17). A second suture anchor is then placed at the 9-o'clock position (or 3-o'clock in a left shoulder), and the identical technique is used for the more superior anchor(s) (Figs. 6-18 to 6-21).

After the labral repair has been carried out, a probe is used to confirm stability of the anchors and apposition of the labrum to the glenoid edge. Once satisfied with the posterior capsulolabral repair, the scope is placed into the subacromial space and thickened bursa, if present, is débrided with an Arthrocare wand and a 4.5 shaver. Rarely is a formal decompression necessary.

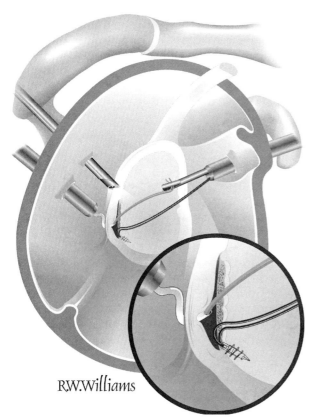

Figure 6-14. Using a corkscrew suture passer, a looped suture is passed through the labrum and posterior capsule, out the anterior portal, and then shuttled back with a second looped suture.

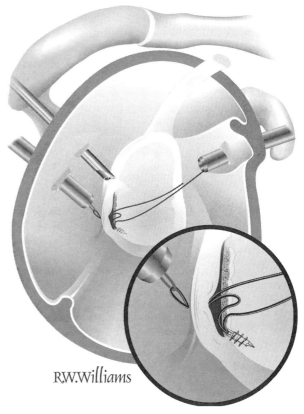

Figure 6-15. One limb of the suture (attached to the anchor) is then passed through the capsulolabral tissue. The remaining suture limb is then brought through the posterior portal and the sutures are tied.

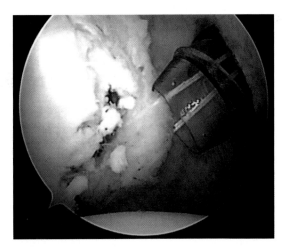

Figure 6-16. After the suture anchor has been placed and sutures have been passed through the labrum but before the labrum has been tied down.

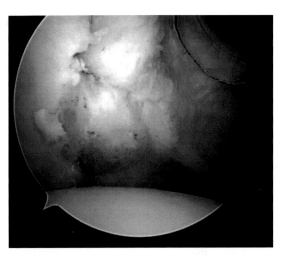

Figure 6-17. Final result after labral repair using suture anchor repair. Note use of different colored sutures in order to facilitate suture management.

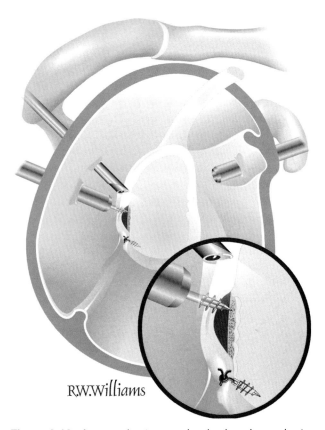

Figure 6-18. A second suture anchor is placed superior to the previously placed anchor.

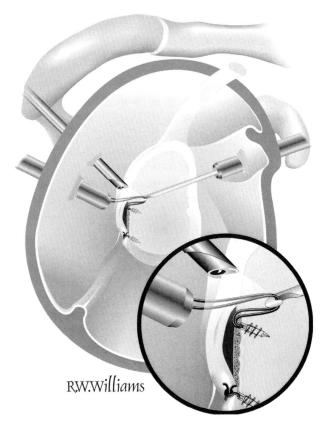

Figure 6-19. The identical technique is used to pass one suture limb through the capsule and labrum.

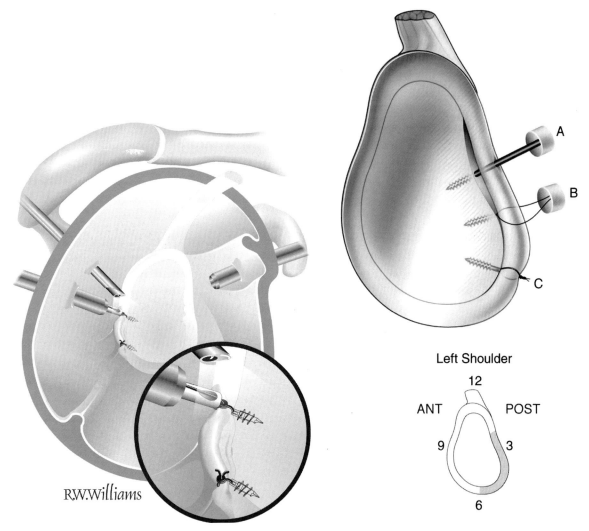

R.W.Williams

Figure 6-20. Arthroscopic knot tying technique is performed and the repair is complete.

Figure 6-21. Drawing depicting placement of suture anchors.

POSTOPERATIVE MANAGEMENT

This procedure should provide the patient with complete resolution of pain and mechanical symptoms (clicking, catching, locking) within the shoulder. The patient can expect to resume activities of daily living within 6 to 8 weeks and return to sports in 5 to 6 months.

Rehabilitation

Postoperatively the affected shoulder is placed in a sling with an abduction pillow. A Cryocuff (Aircast, Summit, NJ) or ice packs are used extensively for the first 72 hours and then intermittently. Shoulder range of motion is restricted for the first 4 weeks, meanwhile, elbow, wrist, and hand range of motion (ROM) are maintained through a home exercise program. Specifically, the patient is instructed to work on deltoid isometrics, grip strengthening, and wrist ROM and strengthening as well as elbow active and active-assisted ROM. At the 4-week mark, patients begin a supervised physical therapy program with an emphasis on ROM and gentle isometrics. The sling is discontinued during the 4- to 6-week period. Passive ROM is instituted with a pulley for flexion along with pendulum exercises. If a pool is available, the patient can work on shoulder active and active-assisted ROM for flexion, extension, horizontal elbow flexion, and extension while avoiding adduction past neutral. The period from 6 to 12 weeks is focused on posterior cuff, latissimus, and scapular muscle strengthening with stress on eccentrics. Therabands are used for resistive exercise and weights are started at 8 to 10 weeks. ROM is continued with active/active assist/passive range of motion with the arm at the side progressing to ROM with the arm in 45 degrees' abduction. During weeks 12 to 16, emphasis is placed on restoration of scapulohumeral rhythm, joint mobilization, and strengthening of scapular stabilizers and progressive resistive exercises. Sports are resumed at approximately 16 to 24 weeks after muscle endurance has been regained and motion and strength have returned to normal.

RESULTS

A retrospective review of patients who underwent arthroscopic repair of a posterior capsulolabral detachment, or posterior Bankart lesion, was performed at our institution (10). Twenty-seven shoulders in 26 patients were included. All 26 patients were male with a mean age of 28.7 years and reported a specific traumatic event that occurred before the onset of symptoms. Overwhelmingly, the most common complaint was pain with athletics and activities of daily living followed by mechanical symptoms ("clicking," "clunking"). Follow-up averaged 5.1 years. In our study, 92% of patients were successfully treated and required no further intervention following arthroscopic stabilization. Moreover, no gross capsular laxity was noted at surgery in our group of patients. There were no perioperative or long-term complications associated with this arthroscopic repair procedure in our study.

Mair et al. (4) described the clinical results of nine patients with symptomatic posterior instability that precluded participation in sport, following athletic trauma. In that study, a posterior labral lesion was repaired using a bioabsorbable tack. At a minimum 2-year follow-up, all patients reported the elimination of pain symptoms and a return to competitive athletics (4).

In summary, our results and those of Mair et al. (4) demonstrate successful arthroscopic treatment of posterior labral lesions. We expect that this procedure will provide appropriately chosen surgical candidates with complete relief of their symptoms.

COMPLICATIONS

Similar complications occur after posterior shoulder stabilization as after any arthroscopic shoulder procedure. Infection is a very small risk and is minimized with the use of prophylactic antibiotics. Axillary nerve injury is possible with incorrect portal placement; an accessory posterior portal that is too low puts the axillary nerve at risk as it exits the quadrilateral space and circles anteriorly approximately 5 cm inferior to the acromion. The last major complication associated with shoulder arthroscopy is brachial plexus traction injury and is usually related to positioning. It is important to avoid excessive traction on the arm and to keep the patient's head aligned with the shoulders. If the patient's head is secured to the table and the operative area is not adequately exposed, the tendency is to pull the patient's shoulder over; this maneuver places excessive traction on the brachial plexus.

RECOMMENDED READING

1. Antoniou, J., Harryman, D.T. II.: Arthroscopic posterior capsular repair. *Clin Sports Med* 19(1): 101–114, vi-vii, 2000.
2. Burkhead, W.Z., Rockwood, C.A.: Treatment of instability of the shoulder with an exercise program. *J Bone Joint Surg Am* 74: 890–896, 1992.
3. Hurley, J.A., Anderson, T.E., Dear, W., et al.: Posterior shoulder instability: surgical versus conservative results with evaluation of glenoid version. *Am J Sports Med* 20(4): 396–400, 1992.
4. Mair, S.D., Zarzour, R.H., Speer, K.P.: Posterior labral injury in contact athletes. *Am J Sports Med* 26(6): 753–758, 1998.
5. McIntyre, L.F., Caspari, R.B., Savoie, F.H. III: The arthroscopic treatment of posterior shoulder instability: two-year results of a multiple suture technique. *Arthroscopy* 13(4): 426–432, 1997.

6. McLaughlin, H.: Posterior dislocation of the shoulder. *J Bone Joint Surg Am* 34: 584–590, 1952.
7. Rowe, C.P., Pierce, D.S., Clark, J.G.: Voluntary dislocation of the shoulder: a preliminary report on a clinical, electromyographic and psychiatric study of twenty-six patients. *J Bone Joint Surg Am* 55: 445, 1973.
8. Tibone, J.E., Bradley, J.P.: The treatment of posterior subluxation in athletes. *Clin Orthop Rel Res* 291: 124–137, 1993.
9. Weber, S.C., Caspari, R.B.: A biomechanical evaluation of the restraints to posterior shoulder dislocation. *Arthroscopy* 5(2): 115–121, 1989.
10. Williams, R.J., Strickland, S.M., Altchek, D.A., et al.: Arthroscopic shoulder stabilization for posterior shoulder instability. *Am J Sports Med* 31(2):203–209, 2003.
11. Wolf, E.M., Eakin, C.L.: Arthroscopic capsular plication for posterior shoulder instability. *Arthroscopy* 14(2): 153–163, 1998.

7

Arthroscopic Treatment of the Arthritic Shoulder

J. Randall Ramsey, Felix H. Savoie III, and Larry D. Field

INDICATIONS/CONTRAINDICATIONS

Advances in arthroscopic technology and training have allowed arthroscopy to become a mainstay in diagnosis and treatment of arthritic joint disorders. Degenerative arthritis of the glenohumeral joint occurs less often than similar arthritis of the weight-bearing joints of the lower extremity. However, it is still relatively common, affecting about 20% of the elderly population. Several authors have reported beneficial effects of arthroscopic treatment of the arthritic shoulder. Recently Weinstein et al. (5) reported their results with arthroscopic débridement for osteoarthritis with significant pain relief postoperatively in all 25 patients. At nearly 34 months of follow-up, 80% were rated as excellent or good.

Glenohumeral arthritis can be thought of as primary or secondary. Primary involvement occurs when no predisposing factor is identified. The structure and function of the shoulder may predispose it to degenerative wear as significant pressure and stresses are placed across the glenohumeral articulation with movement of the upper extremity. As the humeral head serves as a fulcrum to upper limb motion, pressures equal to ten times the weight of the extremity are transmitted across the articular surfaces of the joint. Any additional load or resistance placed on the extremity can only increase this pressure in a similarly exponential fashion. Secondary involvement is more common and occurs as a result of an antecedent event that may include trauma, instability, chronic rotator cuff tear, and previous surgery. While primary arthritis may begin as early as the second decade, it is more common in the elderly. Secondary arthritis on the other hand is more likely to affect

J. R. Ramsey, M.D.: Upper Extremity Service, Mississippi Sports Medicine and Orthopaedic Center, Jackson, Mississippi.

F. H. Savoie III, M.D. and L. D. Field, M.D.: Department of Orthopaedic Surgery, University of Mississippi School of Medicine; and Upper Extremity Service, Mississippi Sports Medicine and Orthopaedic Center, Jackson, Mississippi.

the younger more active patient.

Regardless of the etiology, initial treatment should be directed at resolution of symptoms and improvement of function. Mainstays of nonoperative treatment remain physical therapy, oral nonsteroidal antiinflammatory agents, and the judicious use of corticosteroid injections. Additionally, injection of a synthetic hyluronate (although not yet approved by the Food and Drug Administration) may prove beneficial. For the patient with advanced degenerative changes who has failed nonoperative management, joint replacement arthroplasty may provide satisfactory pain relief and return to function. However, many patients seek other, immediate alternatives and this arthroscopic treatment is an accepted, viable option.

Patients appropriate for arthroscopic débridement include those with stages I to III arthritis who have a functional deficit or intolerable pain despite appropriate nonoperative management. Recently, evidence has shown that those with stage IV arthritis may also have substantial benefit from arthroscopic treatment. It should be emphasized to patients that the goal of treatment is primarily pain relief and that any functional gain is an added benefit. Additionally, many patients with primary osteoarthritis may have additional pathology in the shoulder. Labral tears, partial or complete rotator cuff tears, subacromial spurs, and acromioclavicular (AC) arthritis may exist concomitantly. Arthroscopic management of these additional sources of discomfort may be helpful.

The mechanisms by which arthroscopy alleviates pain in arthritic joints are multifactorial. The benefit of lavage of arthritic joints dates to the first half of the 20th century. While the exact reason for this benefit is poorly understood, it likely results from the removal of degradative enzymes that are produced as part of the inflammatory process. Removal of inflamed synovium is also likely to reduce pain. Removal of mechanical irritants to the joint such as loose bodies and osteophytes is not only pain relieving, it also allows functional improvement. Similarly, débridement of loose chondral flaps serves to reduce potential mechanical irritants. Contouring of articular defects promotes kinematics of the joint that are more normal, thereby reducing inflammation and enhancing function. Addressing coexisting problems such as capsular contracture, instability, a torn rotator cuff, AC pathology, and impingement is also possible and beneficial at the time of arthroscopy.

There are some patients in whom, at the time of arthroscopy for an unrelated surgical problem, full-thickness cartilage loss is identified in the humeral head, glenoid, or both. These may be localized or more widespread chondral defects and may come to the attention of the surgeon unexpectedly. Most frequently, these are associated without clear radiographic findings of glenohumeral arthritis. Arthroscopic débridement, with or without abrasion chondroplasty or microfascia, seems to be a viable way to treat these localized grade 4 lesions. This is similar in concept to abrasion chondroplasty for localized chondral defects in other joints. The long-term effect of abrasion chondroplasty on the shoulder is unknown.

The primary contraindication to arthroscopic management is the posteriorly subluxated shoulder. Walch et al. (4) have reported dissatisfactory results in these patients. Our results have been similar, and we do not routinely recommend arthroscopic débridement for this group.

There are no other specific contraindications to arthroscopic treatment of the arthritic shoulder. However, more advanced glenohumeral arthritis, presence of large osteophytes, deformity of the humeral head, collapse of the humeral head, or significant bone deficits are unlikely to be helped with arthroscopic treatment alone, and more aggressive treatment of the shoulder is usually more predictable. Likewise, if a shoulder exhibits significant joint-space narrowing associated with capsular contracture, not uncommon in end-stage glenohumeral arthritis, the actual establishment of arthroscopic portals may be difficult. In addition, arthritis associated with large deficits in the rotator cuff, arthritis associated with significant rheumatoid arthropathy in soft tissue deficits, and arthritis resulting from fracture and its concomitant deformity are unlikely to be adequately addressed with arthroscopic approaches in soft-tissue releases.

Finally, unrealistic expectations by the patient are probably a relative contraindication to the arthroscopic approach to glenohumeral arthritis. Patients should expect that limited goals of pain relief for a variable period are anticipated with arthroscopic débridement alone for glenohumeral arthritis.

Relative contraindications may include a patient with unrealistic expectations, infection, or postsurgical stiff shoulder with stage IV glenohumeral changes.

PREOPERATIVE PLANNING

The typical patient who is a candidate for arthroscopic treatment of glenohumeral arthritis is a relatively young patient who presents with progressive pain in the shoulder with activity and at rest. The patient has frequently failed the usual nonoperative means, including nonsteroidal antiinflammatory medications, rehabilitation efforts, activity modification, and intraarticular injections. The ideal patient is one in whom intraarticular lidocaine has temporarily relieved the pain, reinforcing for surgeon and patient that the source of pain is intraarticular as opposed to other areas around the shoulder. The pain in glenohumeral arthritis is characteristically located in the top lateral aspect of the arm and radiates down toward the deltoid insertion with any range of motion of the shoulder. Pain may be present with activities and at rest and frequently is described by the patient as a toothache-type of pain. Patients may also note symptoms of clicking, grinding, or catching due to loose cartilage flaps, joint incongruity, and intraarticular loose bodies. Not infrequently, a patient will give a history that the shoulder "goes out." In the presence of glenohumeral arthritis, this is typically not instability, but represents an incongruity in the humeral head sliding over areas of denuded glenoid articular cartilage.

History and Physical

As with all patient interactions, a thorough history and physical examination are the initial steps. Age, activity level, and comorbid illnesses should be reviewed. Those patients who are not candidates for general or regional anesthesia should be excluded. Previous injury and surgical history should be ascertained. Patient expectations should be discussed, and any unrealistic expectations should be discouraged.

Examination should include the observation for asymmetry between affected and unaffected sides. Atrophy, swelling, any surgical incisions, deformity, subdeltoid or subcutaneous cysts, and any other areas of asymmetry are identified. The carrying posture of the extremity should also be noted. Motion should be compared to the opposite extremity as well, although frequently arthropathies are bilateral in nature. The motions typically tested are forward flexion, external rotation with the arm at the side, external rotation in abduction, and internal rotation. In patients with early glenohumeral arthritis, external rotation is the most frequent motion loss. The loss of forward flexion in internal rotation may occur quite late. With the movement of the arm, crepitation, pain, and abnormalities of scapulothoracic rhythm may be noted. Although testing strength and instability is routine, it may be painful for the patient. Strength of internal and external rotation is predominantly determined by inadequacy of the rotator cuff. In many types of arthropathy, such as periosteoarthritis of the shoulder, avascular necrosis, and postcapsulorraphy arthropathy, it is typical to have normal internal and external rotation strength. However, contraction of the rotator cuff may center the humeral head on the glenoid and may be responsible for the deep crepitus, grating, and grinding that frequently occurs in active motion and strength testing in glenohumeral arthritis. Any questions about integrity of neurovascular structures should be investigated further. If there is a discrepancy between passive and active range of motion, this is due to volitional limitation of active motion due to pain, muscle atrophy, neurogenic deficit, or rotator cuff incongruity.

Specific attention should be directed toward eliciting the source of discomfort. Many sources of shoulder pain can mimic the pain from glenohumeral arthritis. These sources include adhesive capsulitis, rotator cuff tearing, subacromial impingement, AC joint disease, synovitis, frozen shoulder syndrome, and even nonshoulder etiologies (cervical spine radiculopathy, Pancoast tumor). The best chance for symptomatic improvement of shoulder pain from glenohumeral arthritis is to specifically identify the glenohumeral joint as the sole source of the shoulder pain. In many instances, differential injection of Xylocaine (AstraZeneca, Wilmington, DE) may aide the surgeon in identifying the precise source of pain, whether subacromial, AC joint, or glenohumeral joint.

Multiple sources of shoulder pain do not preclude successful treatment arthroscopically. For example, early glenohumeral arthritis may coexist with subacromial impingement syndrome or AC joint arthrosis or painful contracture of the shoulder joint. Multiple etiologies of the shoulder pain may be addressed at the time of arthroscopy, such as combining arthroscopic subacromial decompression with débridement for mild glenohumeral joint arthritis. However, it is usually quite helpful to use differential injections to identify the patient's main source of shoulder pain.

Examination should include the observation for asymmetry between the affected and the unaffected sides, including the presence of atrophy, swelling, and surgical incisions. The carrying posture of the extremity should also be noted. Motion should be compared to the opposite extremity as well. While checking motion, crepitus, pain, and abnormality in scapulothoracic rhythm should be noted. Strength and instability testing should be performed and neurologic status verified.

Specific attention should be directed toward eliciting the source of discomfort. Reproduction of symptoms by minimal glenohumeral glide testing signifies the arthritic glenohumeral joint as the source of pain. Loading the humeral head into the glenoid and then shifting it in different directions should produce crepitation and reproduce the patient's pain if glenohumeral arthritis is the main factor producing symptoms. Crepitation or pain at the more extreme load and shift displacement may signify labral pathology in addition to arthritis.

The specific range-of-motion limitation with and without scapulothoracic immobilization should be documented. Although crepitation is common, instability and strength assessment should also be performed.

Palpation for swelling and areas of proximal tenderness is also beneficial. Manual testing for impingement and AC arthritis may elicit those areas as additional sources of pain, signifying potential improvement with arthroscopic management.

Radiographic assessment begins with plain radiographs. Three views are routinely obtained: an anteroposterior view of the glenohumeral joint, a scapular Y view, and an axillary lateral view. These views allow adequate assessment of the glenohumeral joint, including joint-space narrowing, subchondral sclerosis, subluxation, and osteophyte formation. AC degeneration and hypertrophy can be assessed. Acromial morphology can be determined as well. Additional findings may include chondrocalcinosis or signs of associated pathology such as a Hill-Sachs lesion or narrowed subacromial interval.

Nakagawa et al. (3) and Weinstein et al. (5) have proposed staging of glenohumeral arthritis based on radiographic findings. Stage I arthritis has normal-appearing radiographs and is found only at the time of arthroscopy. Stages II through IV are evident radiographically (Fig. 7-1). Stage II is characterized by minimal joint-space narrowing and a concentrically located humeral head in the glenoid. Stage III exhibits moderate joint-space narrowing and inferior osteophyte formation. Stage IV changes include severe loss of joint space, osteophyte formation, and loss of concentricity between the humeral head and glenoid.

Additional studies, including limited computed tomography (CT) scan and magnetic resonance imaging (MRI), may be beneficial. Limited CT through the glenohumeral joint can be used to assess glenoid version and posterior glenoid bone loss and may reveal the presence of osseous loose bodies. MRI scanning can aide in the assessment of associated pathology such as rotator cuff tears, labral pathology, and the presence of osteonecrosis.

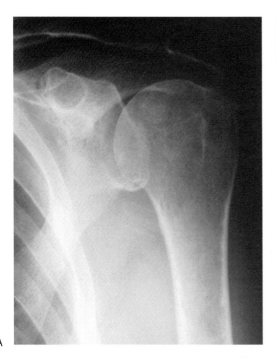

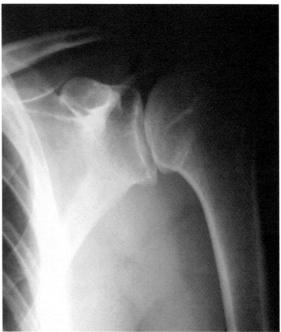

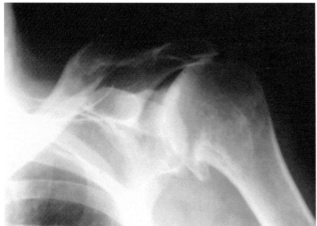

Figure 7-1. Plain anterior-posterior radiographs depicting stages II through IV arthritis. **A:** Grade II changes of minimal joint space narrowing with a concentric glenohumeral articulation. **B:** Grade III changes of moderate space narrowing, a concentric glenohumeral articulation and inferior osteophyte formation of the glenoid and humeral head. **C:** Grade IV changes of severely narrowed joint space, advanced osteophyte formation and superior migration of the humeral head indicative of a large rotator cuff tear.

SURGERY

We prefer a lateral decubitus positioning because it allows easier access to the entire glenohumeral joint. However, beach-chair positioning is an acceptable alternative and allows the arm to be abducted and rotated effectively as well. This procedure can be done with interscalene block, regional anesthesia, or general anesthetic. Gravity inflow or infusion pump and accessory inferior portal may be helpful for the manipulation and arthroscopy débridement of the inferior pouch, particularly if an inferior osteophyte is present. In addition, if the inferior osteophyte is small and contributing to joint incongruity and mechanical symptoms, an accessory inferior portal may aide in specific débridement of the associated inferior osteophyte. A standard posterior portal is then placed. The portal should be located at the equator of the joint in the raphe of the infraspinatus. Locating the posterior portal in this position allows access into even the most severely posteriorly subluxated shoulders without damaging the infraspinatus or remaining articular cartilage. Beginning first with the arthroscope in the posterior portal, a thorough diagnostic glenohumeral joint examination is performed. A diagnostic arthroscopy is then performed. The depth area of cartilage loss on the articular surface of the humerus and glenoid is documented. The degree and location of labral tears, loose bodies, synovitis, and rotator cuff tears are documented.

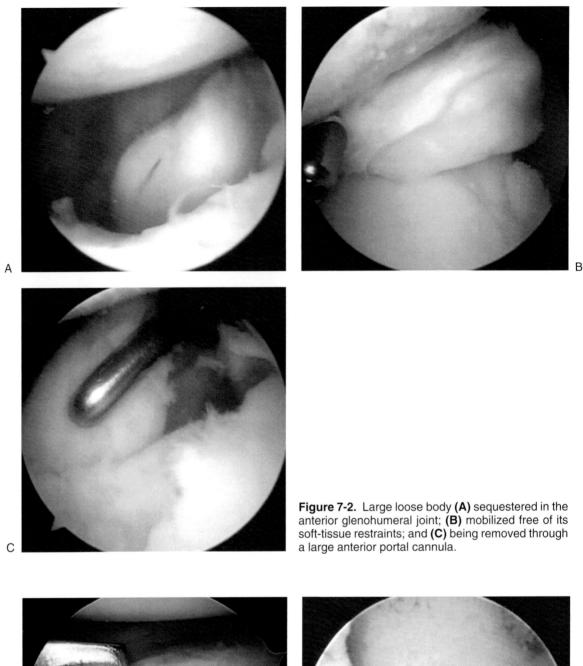

A

B

C

Figure 7-2. Large loose body (A) sequestered in the anterior glenohumeral joint; (B) mobilized free of its soft-tissue restraints; and (C) being removed through a large anterior portal cannula.

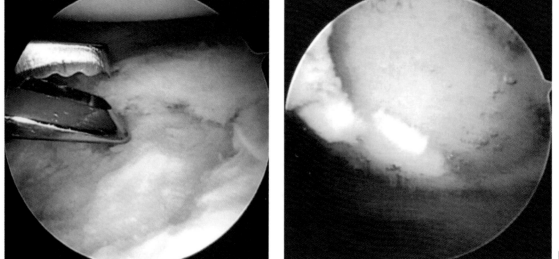

A

B

Figure 7-3. A: Central glenoid wear of primary arthritis. B: Corresponding wear of the humeral head.

An anterior portal is established through the interval from an outside-in technique. The portal is located lateral to the coracoid and is tested by inserting a spinal needle first to ensure adequate access to all pathology. In many cases, a superior Nevaiser portal may be placed to increase fluid flow through the joint and thereby increase the lavage effect of the arthroscopy.

The anterior portal cannula is introduced, which allows probing and manipulation of the arthroscopic instruments. Associated pathology, which is not infrequently seen, may be labral tears, loose bodies, loose cartilage flap, intraarticular scarring, extensive synovitis, and rotator cuff tearing.

Débridement of an arthritic joint should proceed in logical, stepwise fashion. Loose bodies are removed first. These should be readily evident at diagnostic arthroscopy, but sometimes are elusive. The axillary recess and the subscapularis recess are common places to find loose bodies (Fig. 7-2). Labral tears are débrided and a synovectomy performed as needed. Loose articular cartilage is then removed and full-thickness defects on the humerus and glenoid are abraded, drilled, or managed by microfracture. Evaluation of the articular surfaces of the humeral head and glenoid should be done from the anterior and posterior portals. Primary arthritis typically results in central or superior wear of the humeral head and central wear of the glenoid resulting in a "halo"-type pattern on the glenoid (Fig. 7-3). Secondary arthritis results in patterns consistent with the primary pathology (Fig. 7-4). Regardless of the pattern of wear, the edge of the articular cartilage defect should be probed and any loose cartilage systematically débrided. Numerous techniques are available for this purpose, including motorized shavers, arthroscopic punches, and laser (Fig. 7-5). We prefer to use either the motorized shaver or the laser for this purpose. The goal is to remove loose flaps and leave a stable rim of cartilage around the defect. A smooth transition between the cartilage and the base of the defect should be attained. In young active patients, consideration should be given to performing microfracture to the base of the defect allowing fibrocartilage to fill the void. This can be done by drilling with Kirschner wires or using a microfracture awl. Areas requiring repair are then addressed (Fig. 7-6).

Any intraarticular bodies are removed. Labral tears may be débrided and significant synovitis can be removed with the intraarticular shaver or with vaporization techniques. Intraarticular loose bodies are usually readily evident at diagnostic arthroscopy, but may be elusive. Typical locations for intraarticular loose bodies are the axillary recess, the subscapulary recess, and along the bicipital tendon sheath. Manipulation of the bicep sheath and manual manipulation of the subscapular recess can be helpful in bringing these loose bodies into view. If the loose bodies are too large to extract through a cannula and a grabber, the loose bodies can be morsalized and fragmented before removal.

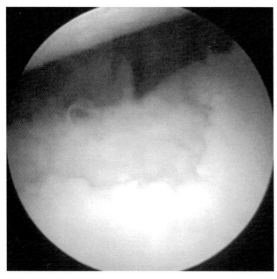
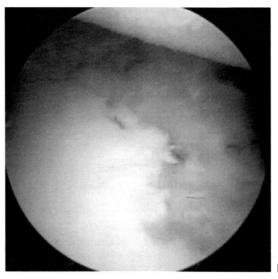

A   B

Figure 7-4. Anteroinferior glenoid arthritis in a patient with a 9-year history of recurrent anteroinferior glenohumeral dislocations. **A:** View from posterior portal. **B:** View from anterior portal.

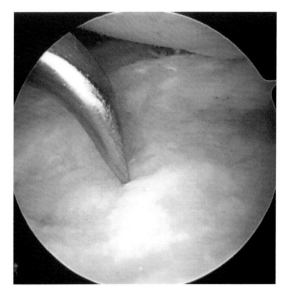

Figure 7-5. Use of a chondral awl to perform microfracture technique on a contained articular defect.

The arthroscope is then placed in the anterior portal and the steps repeated with the instrumentation used through the posterior portal.

Other intraarticular structures are addressed systematically as necessary. The labrum may be frayed or fragmented and can be débrided with a shaver to remove loose tissue (Fig. 7-7). The biceps and rotator cuff tendons may also be degenerative and should be dealt with accordingly (Fig. 7-8). Biceps tenotomy or tenodesis may be performed in patients with significant (greater than 50%) deterioration of that tendon. It is important to pull the tendon into the joint for an adequate inspection. Tears in the bicipital groove area may be a source of discomfort and should be addressed. Any rotator cuff pathology of any significance should be repaired if this has been discussed preoperatively with the patient, because this will alter the postoperative course significantly. Capsular contracture that has been determined preoperatively to limit motion should be released (Fig. 7-9). Synovitis is often a source of pain and can be carefully débrided leaving the underlying capsule intact with a shaver or electrothermal device (Fig. 7-10). Osteophytes, if thought to be a source of

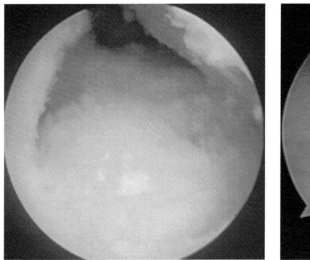
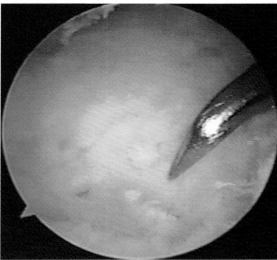

A   B

Figure 7-6. Chondral pick/microfracture technique. **A:** Arthritic area of anterior glenoid. **B:** Microfracture awl in place.

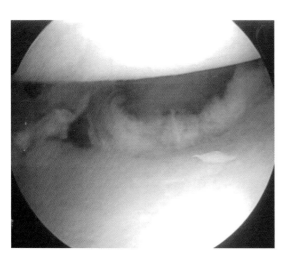

Figure 7-7. Degenerative fraying of the anterior glenoid labrum.

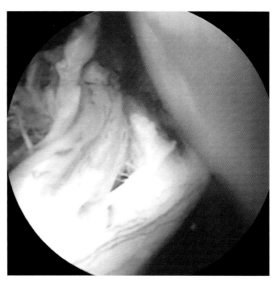

Figure 7-8. Degenerative fraying of the long head of the biceps as it courses through the gleno-humeral joint.

impingement within the glenohumeral joint, can be removed with a burr or bone-cutting shaver. Osteophytes on the inferior aspect of the humeral head are less likely to be troublesome and should be considered for débridement via an accessory posteroinferior portal only if necessary because the axillary nerve may be easily damaged. One must remember the extracapsular position of the axillary nerve during this procedure and maintain the shaver position *within* the joint.

Once work is completed in the glenohumeral joint, the arthroscope is redirected to the subacromial space. A bursectomy is performed and further evaluation of the rotator cuff is carried out. The acromion is converted to a type I morphology through the process of acromioplasty if necessary. The AC joint is assessed and if hypertrophic or degenerative, the distal clavicle is resected (Fig. 7-11). Care is taken to preserve the superior and posterior capsules during this procedure. The biceps sheath may be released and inspected for loose bodies, synovitis, and tendon damage. This is an important part of the management

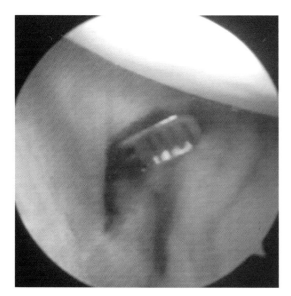

Figure 7-9. Release of the glenohumeral capsule with a suction punch in a patient with a globally decreased motion.

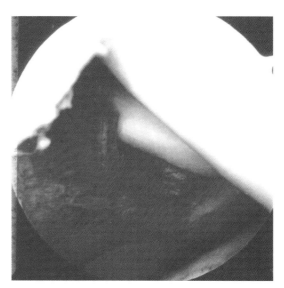

Figure 7-10. Florid hyperemic synovitis in the anterior joint of a patient with secondary arthritis due to recurrent dislocations.

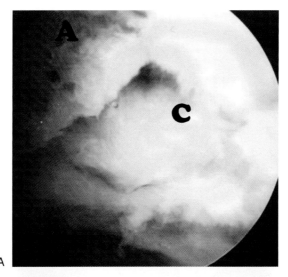

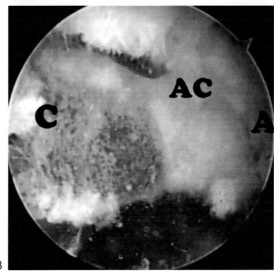

Figure 7-11. Severely degenerative acromioclavicular joint. **A:** Before resection of the distal clavicle. **B:** After resection. *A,* acromion; *C,* clavicle; *AC,* capsule.

of the arthritic shoulder, allowing inspection of the more distal aspect of the biceps tendon while simultaneously removing any constrictions on the tendon from the sheath.

Arthroscopic intraarticular capsule release, particularly involving the anterior capsule, may be able to be combined with arthroscopic rotator interval release to increase external rotation in the patient in whom this is limited with glenohumeral arthritis. Frequently the anterior capsule is thickened and scarred. An arthroscope capsule in rotator interval release can be accomplished with the arthroscope in the posterior portal and in the anterior portal a basket, shaver, or vaporizer used to release these soft tissues. If doing a capsular release to increase range of motion, care must be taken to ensure that the interval between the subscapularis and the capsule is developed so that an intact subscapularis tendon is not interfered with. Because limited range of motion in glenohumeral arthritis is usually from a combination of etiologies, including joint incongruity and encapsulitis, a modest improvement to range of motion is usually expected with soft-tissue releases done arthroscopically.

Synovitis is often a concomitant source of pain accompanying glenohumeral arthritis. Using a combination of alternative anterior and posterior portals, the inflamed synovium can be débrided with a shaver or electrothermal device. Since synovium in an arthritic shoulder is frequently very vascular, it is usually most helpful to do a synovectomy with an electrothermal device rather than a shaver to diminish the amount of intraarticular bleeding. Fragments of scarred synovium after electrothermal vaporization can be removed by an intraarticular shaver. The common areas of significant synovitis are at the biceps tendon, the attachment site, and the superior glenoid posteriorly and anteriorly (Fig. 7-10).

Once the synovium is removed and the biceps and rotator cuff pathology and capsular pathology addressed, a careful examination of the presence, extent, location, and accessibility of the osteophytes can be undertaken. Osteophytes, if thought to be a source of mechanical impingement within the glenohumeral joint, a donor of intraarticular loose bodies, or a source of mechanical symptoms, may be removed with a burr or a bone-cutting shaver. Osteophytes on the inferior aspect of the humeral head are more likely to be troublesome and should be considered for débridement via an accessory plus the inferior portal. The accessory portal is established by direct visualization. The arthroscope is maintained in the posterosuperior portal, and under direct visualization, a needle can be used to establish the site for the accessory inferior portal. Once this is established under direct visualization, a cannula or other instrument to dilate this portal can be added.

Isolated articular defects adjacent to the edge may be covered using adjacent labral tissue. The labrum is freed from its attachment to the glenoid neck and mobilized (Fig. 7-12). The arthritic area is abraded to a bleeding surface. An absorbable suture anchor is then placed adjacent to the normal articular cartilage. The attached sutures are retrieved through the mobilized labrum and as the arthroscopic knot is tied the labrum covers the damaged

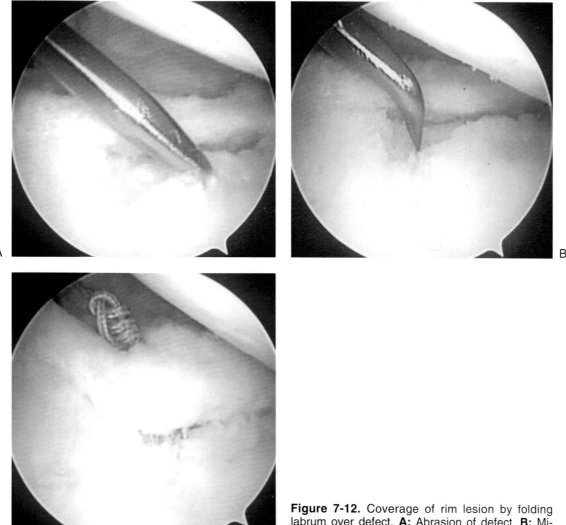

A

B

C

Figure 7-12. Coverage of rim lesion by folding labrum over defect. **A:** Abrasion of defect. **B:** Microfracture. **C:** Labrum repaired over defect.

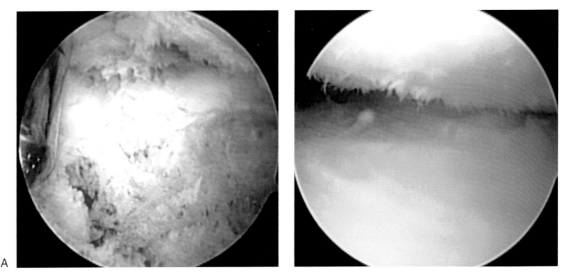

Figure 7-13. Posterior view of the glenoid in an 18-year-old patient with advanced arthritis. **A:** Before resurfacing. **B:** After resurfacing with a porcine small intestine graft.

articular surface. It is extremely important to simply fold down the labrum over the degenerative joint. Any significant superior or medial shift can result in a loss of external rotation, increased articular surface pressure, and more rapid progression of the arthritis.

An additional procedure that is enjoying some early success is interposition arthroplasty. On completion of the débridement as previously described, a piece of autograft, allograft, or xenograft can be inserted through a cannula and sutured arthroscopically to the labrum, using routine labral/capsule repair techniques. The graft is designed to become adherent to the glenoid and hopefully transform to a cartilage substitute, resulting in increased range of motion (Fig. 7-13). This procedure is performed by placing a tagging suture on the graft at the 10-o'clock position. An absorbable anchor is placed at the 1-o'clock position on the glenoid and the sutures are retrieved through the corresponding area of the graft. The tagging stitch is then placed into the joint and retrieved through the corresponding area of the posterior labrum and out posteriorly. As this stitch is pulled, the graft enters the joint through the anterior cannula and is held in position by this suture. The suture or the anchor is then tied, fixing the graft at two points: 10 o'clock and 1 o'clock. A suture hook is then used to attach the graft at the 4- and 7-o'clock positions, covering the previously drilled and abraded glenoid.

POSTOPERATIVE MANAGEMENT

Providing no additional pathology has been addressed, the postoperative course for degenerative arthritis involves restoration of passive motion within the first 2 to 4 weeks. This is followed by initiation of active motion and a functional progression of strengthening exercises. Rehabilitation for instability stabilization or rotator cuff repair should be similar for those patients who do not have associated arthritis. An increase in pain or decrease in motion often is an indication for injection with Depo-Medrol-Man (Pfizer, New York, NY) or hyaluronase.

COMPLICATIONS

The primary complication in arthroscopic management is a failure of the procedure. While arthroscopy may be palliative, it does not correct the primary disease process, resulting in recurrence of symptoms.

The complications of arthroscopic treatment of degenerative arthritis of the shoulder include those seen with other arthroscopic approaches to the shoulder. These include infection, brachial plexus injuries from traction or as an interscalene block effect, stiffness, and incomplete relief of pain. A number of complications may be unique to arthroscopic treatment of glenohumeral arthritis:

1. *If associated capsular releases are performed to regain motion, damage to an anterior subscapularis tendon may be a problem.* The best way to avoid this is to carefully localize the interval between the anterior capsule and subscapularis so that only capsular tissue is released.
2. *Dislocation after capsular release.* While theoretically possible, it is unusual for instability to occur in the presence of glenohumeral arthritis, as shoulder stiffness from joint incongruity is much more common.
3. *Axillary nerve injury.* This may be seen with use of thermal devices adjacent to the inferior capsule in an effort to release the inferior capsule, regaining motion. In addition, the axillary nerve emerges in the quadrilateral space and may be injured during the development of an accessory posterior inferior portal. Care must be taken to establish this accessory inferior portal with a spinal needle to precisely identify the position of the posterior portal. This nerve is also at risk during removal of inferior humeral spurs.
4. *Stiffness.* Patients who have glenohumeral arthritis frequently have some limitation of range of motion. An extensive arthroscopic treatment, which may include AC joint, subacromial space débridement, and intraarticular pathology, can increase the degree of stiffness in the shoulder.
5. *Increased pain.* Occasionally, increasing the range of motion in an arthritic shoulder can bring into contact an area of the humeral head that would ordinarily not be in contact with the glenoid. This may be a new source of pain following apparently successful arthroscopic improvement in range of motion.

Removal of the inferior humeral spur can result in damage to the axillary nerve if the capsule is violated. Removal of the spur contributes very little to the clinical success and should be reserved for those patients whose symptoms can be isolated to that area.

RESULTS

Arthroscopic treatment of glenohumeral arthritis should be considered in terms of limited goals. The successful removal of all loose bodies, articular cartilage, inflamed synovium, and debris would be expected to improve the patient's pain. In approximately three fourths of the patients undergoing arthroscopic débridement, there is a measurable and significant improvement in glenohumeral joint pain. Treatment of any associated impingement syndrome or AC joint arthritis contributing to the pain also increases the degree of pain relief. Approximately one fourth of patients find no improvement in pain in the glenohumeral joint. Degree of improvement of pain relief is in all probability related to the stage of arthrosis for which the arthroscopic treatment is performed. Earlier and more minor degrees of glenohumeral arthritis have a greater ability to have a more predictable response of pain relief than late stages of arthritis, such as grade 4 changes with joint incongruity.

The removal of intraarticular loose bodies, the removal of osteophyte, and capsular and rotator interval releases frequently will result in an increased range of motion for the patient, particularly in external rotation. While these range-of-motion improvements are frequently measurable, it is not uncommon for the patient to have little effective functional improvement in the use of the arm. Whether this is due to failure to completely restore range of motion or is due to ongoing and residual pain from the arthrosis is difficult to ascertain.

In our series of 24 patients, the average visual analog score (VAS) pain scale decreased from 7 to 3. Flexion improved from 100 to 150, and external rotation from 5 to 15. Overall, the patient satisfaction rate was 83%.

RECOMMENDED READING

1. Crawford, D., Safran, M.R., Wolde-Tsaddik, G.: Prospective outcome study of arthroscopic debridement for grade IV glenohumeral arthritis. Presented at AANA Annual Meeting, Washington, D.C., April 26, 2002.
2. Matsen, F.A. III, Ziegler, D.W., DeBartolo, S.E.: Patient self-assessment of health status and function in glenohumeral degenerative joint disease. *J Shoulder Elbow Surg* 4(5): 345–351, 1995.
3. Nakagawa, Y., Hyakuna, K., Otari, S., et al.: Epidemiologic study of glenohumeral osteoarthritis with plain radiography. *J Shoulder Elbow Surg* 8(6): 580–584, 1999.
4. Walch, G., Ascani, C., Boulahia, A., et al.: Static posterior subluxation of the humeral head: an unrecognized entity responsible for glenohumeral osteoarthritis in the young adult. *J Shoulder Elbow Surg* 11(4): 309–314, 2002.
5. Weinstein, D.M., Bucchieri, J.S., Pollock, R.G., et al.: Arthroscopic debridement of the shoulder for osteoarthritis. *Arthroscopy* 16(5): 471–476, 2000.

8

Arthroscopic Biceps Tenodesis and Release

Pascal Boileau, Sumant G. Krishnan, and Gilles Walch

INDICATIONS/CONTRAINDICATIONS

The long head of the biceps is a well-known cause of shoulder pain, due to the multiple possible pathologies of the biceps tendon and its pulley system (4), such as tenosynovitis, prerupture, subluxation, or dislocation of the tendon. The surgical treatment for these disorders is limited to removal of the intraarticular portion of the tendon, by either tenotomy or tenodesis (4,6). Biceps tenodesis, with or without a rotator cuff repair, is a common and well-accepted open surgical procedure (1,4,6). In 1988, we reported for the first time the results of arthroscopic biceps tenotomy for patients with chronic and significant shoulder pain, due to a pathologic biceps tendon, in the presence of a massive irreparable rotator cuff tear (8).

Because we were familiar with the technique of interference screw fixation for hamstring anterior cruciate ligament reconstruction, we developed a personal technique for biceps tenodesis using bioabsorbable interference screws. This technique has been used routinely in open surgery since 1996, and since 1997 has been used under arthroscopic control (2,3). This technique is different from previous techniques described using either isolated sutures or sutures with anchors (5,7,9).

The indications for tenodesis or release of the biceps tendon are multiple (1,4,6). Performing this procedure under arthroscopic control may be beneficial for the patient, in case of pathologic biceps tendon [tenosynovitis, prerupture, subluxation or dislocation, non-reparable SLAP (superior labrum anterior and posterior) lesion], whether or not the rotator cuff is torn. Basically, this procedure can be performed in three different clinical situations:

P. Boileau, M.D.: Department of Orthopaedic Surgery, University of Nice-Sophia Antipolis; and Department of Orthopaedic Surgery and Sports Traumatology, Archet 2 Hospital, Nice, France.

S. G. Krishnan, M.D.: Department of Orthopaedic Surgery, The University of Texas Southwestern Medical Center; and Shoulder Service, W. B. Carrell Memorial Clinic, Dallas, Texas.

G. Walch, M.D.: Department of Shoulder Surgery, Clinic St. Anne Lumiere, Lyon, France.

(a) in association with arthroscopic rotator cuff repairs; (b) in cases of isolated pathology of the biceps tendon with an intact cuff, especially in young athletes; and (c) in cases of massive, degenerative, and irreparable cuff tears with a pathologic biceps tendon, responsible for a painful shoulder. In this last situation, tenodesis of the biceps is performed as an alternative to a simple tenotomy. A tenodesis is preferred to a simple tenotomy, especially in elderly but active and muscular patients. This avoids the distal retraction and bulging of the muscle at the elbow level (which may be a source of pain during work) and the possible slight decrease in supination strength, at least for the first year after surgery.

Contraindications include a thin, fragile, almost-ruptured biceps tendon, which is the technical limit of arthroscopic biceps tenodesis. We do not pretend that arthroscopic biceps tenodesis is superior to a simple tenotomy; it is just another technical option available for the arthroscopic shoulder surgeon. A very old and fragile patient will be a preferable candidate for a biceps tenotomy rather than a tenodesis.

PREOPERATIVE PLANNING

The patient who is a candidate for biceps tenodesis complains of chronic shoulder pain. The dominant side is involved in 80% of the cases. The patient can be elderly and retired, over 65, with or without a history of massive and irreparable cuff tear. The patient can also be younger, around 30 or 40, with a history of an "overused shoulder" because of his or her profession (mason, painter, gardener) or sports activity (throwing athlete). Onset is progressive in half of the cases; the other half has a history of more or less severe initial traumatic injury. The pain is localized at the *anterior* part of the shoulder; it radiates in the direction of the lateral part of the elbow, and sometimes can reach the dorsal part of the hand. The pain may occur typically with overhead activity but is often present at rest and may awaken the patient during the night. Most patients have already undergone conservative treatment with rehabilitation programs and corticosteroid injections without any success.

Active and passive motions are usually conserved. However, a pseudoparalyzed shoulder can be present (normal passive motion but active motion in forward elevation less than 60 degrees); this should lead to the suspicion of a dislocation of the long head of the biceps associated with a cuff tear.

Looking at the patient from the back, atrophy of the supra- and infraspinatus is sometimes obvious, and leads to the diagnosis of an associated massive cuff tear. Anterior palpation of the shoulder reveals a localized pain in the area of the bicipital groove, and more important, the pain is recognized by the patient as "my pain." The cross-arm test is painful with the pain being in the *anterior* part of the shoulder instead of superior such as in acromioclavicular joint pathology. The impingement signs may be positive, but they are not very specific in our experience. The testing of the cuff (e.g., Jobe, lift-off) can be positive too, depending on the presence of associated cuff lesions.

For all patients, the preoperative examination should include a radiographic evaluation with a true anteroposterior (AP) view in three rotations and a normalized supraspinatus outlet view. In case of a massive cuff tear involving the infra- and supraspinatus, the acromiohumeral distance, measured on the AP view in neutral rotation, is less than 6 mm. Computed tomography (CT arthrography) or magnetic resonance imaging (MRI) with gadolinium can demonstrate an "unstable" biceps tendon, being either subluxated or dislocated.

SURGERY

The principle of the arthroscopic biceps tenodesis is simple: After biceps tenotomy, the tendon is exteriorized and doubled on a suture and then pulled back into a humeral socket and fixed using a bioabsorbable interference screw. The fixation principle to tenodese the long head of the biceps is similar to the interference screw fixation used with success for hamstring anterior cruciate ligament reconstruction of the knee.

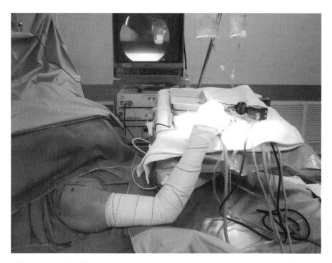

Figure 8-1. Patient in the beach-chair position with the shoulder in the position of "arthrodesis": 30 degrees of flexion, 30 degrees of internal rotation, and 30 degrees of abduction. The elbow is flexed to 90 degrees.

Patient Positioning

Although the lateral decubitus position can be used, we prefer to perform this technique with the patient in the beach-chair position, under general anesthesia and/or interscalene block. The shoulder should be placed in approximately 30 degrees of flexion, 30 degrees of internal rotation, and 30 degrees of abduction ("arthrodesis position"), allowing the anterior part of the subacromial bursa to be adequately filled with water in order to have a clear view of the superior part of the bicipital groove. When using the beach-chair position, a classic knee support (horseshoe support) is used with a Mayo stand. The elbow can be extended and flexed (Fig. 8-1).

Bony Landmarks

Draw the bony landmarks on the shoulder to identify the spine of the scapula, the acromion, the coracoid process, and the coracoacromial ligament. This procedure requires three arthroscopic portals: The classic posterior portal is created 2 cm inferior and 2 cm medial to the posterolateral corner of the acromion; two anterior portals (anteromedial and anterolateral) are created 1.5 cm on each side of the bicipital groove (Fig. 8-2). The posterior and anterolateral portals are used for the scope (viewing portals) and the anteromedial portal is used for the instruments (working portal). A pump is helpful to obtain distention of the joint and the bursa but it is important to maintain low pump pressure (30 mm Hg or less) during the procedure to prevent excessive soft-tissue distention.

Glenohumeral Exploration and Tenotomy of the Long Head of the Biceps

Explore the glenohumeral joint with the 30-degree scope through the posterior portal. Establish an anteromedial portal from inside to outside, passing the trocar of the scope through the rotator interval, lateral to the coracoid process, 1 cm distal to it, and just above the subscapularis tendon (Fig. 8-2). After insertion of a cannula, assess the deep surface of the rotator cuff and confirm the pathology of the biceps tendon: tenosynovitis, subluxation, dislocation, or prerupture. Biceps tendon pathology is very often in the intertubercular groove portion and it is important to draw this part of the biceps tendon into the joint with a probe via the anteromedial portal (Fig. 8-3). Transfix the long head of the biceps intraarticularly with a spinal needle at its entrance into the groove; this will avoid its retraction

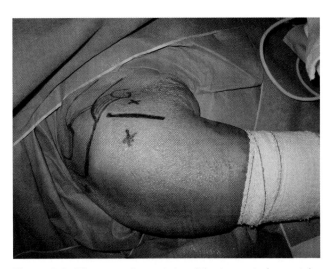

Figure 8-2. The posterior portal and the two anterior portals: anteromedial and anterolateral, on each side of the bicipital groove.

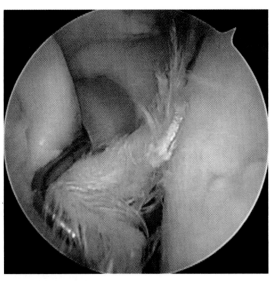

Figure 8-3. Use a probe to pull tendon into the joint to demonstrate biceps pathology.

into the groove and help identify its location during subacromial bursoscopy. Then detach the tendon from its glenoid insertion using a knife, a punch, or electrocautery (Fig. 8-4).

Location and Opening of the Bicipital Groove after Anterosuperior Bursectomy

Move the scope, still in the posterior portal, and reorient it under the acromion into the subacromial bursa. Do the same for the anteromedial cannula, which is placed into the anterosuperior bursa (lateral to the coracoacromial ligament). Begin the bursectomy with either a motorized shaver or the Mitek VAPR device (Mitek Worldwide, Norwood, Massachusetts). Create the third anterolateral portal, located 3 cm from the anterior border of the acromion and 3 cm from the anteromedial portal, to allow triangulation. Remove the arthroscope from the posterior portal and place it in the anterolateral portal. At this point, the anteromedial portal is the working portal, the anterolateral portal is the viewing portal,

A

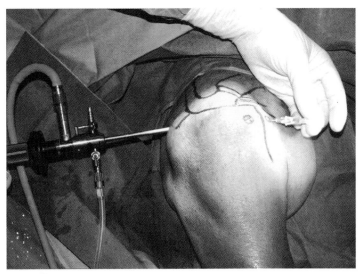

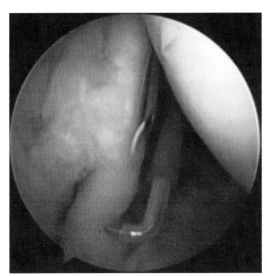

B

Figure 8-4. A, B: Do a tenotomy of the long head of the biceps after transfixion with a spinal needle to prevent distal retraction.

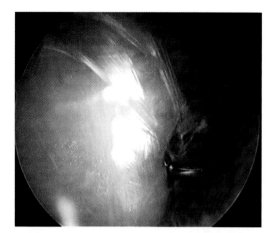

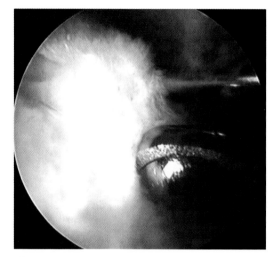

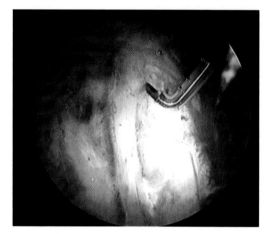

Figure 8-5. Do an anterior bursectomy and locate the spinal needle.

Figure 8-6. Locate the bicipital groove with a probe (the "soft spot"), and open the transverse humeral ligament with electrocautery. Note the vessels on the lateral border of the bicipital groove.

and the posterior portal is for outflow only. Instruments are placed in the anteromedial portal to continue the bursectomy and identify the bicipital groove. Shaving of the anterior part of the bursa is essential for visualization and is continued until the spinal needle is located (Fig. 8-5). Evaluate the superficial surface of the rotator cuff and, if no tear is found, identify its insertion into the greater tuberosity. Use a probe to palpate the "soft spot" corresponding to the bicipital groove (Fig. 8-6), which is usually just medial to the lateral part of the greater tuberosity, and feel the "roll" of the biceps tendon in its groove. Visualization of the white fibers of the transverse ligament and of the ascendant vessels on the lateral part of the groove also helps to locate the bicipital groove. Open the transverse humeral ligament in a longitudinal fashion, using an electrocautery. Stay in the middle of the groove and avoid the vessels on either border of the groove. Once the groove is open, probe the long head of the biceps and perform a careful arthroscopic synovectomy using the shaver. Now lift the biceps tendon out of the groove to free possible adhesions (Fig. 8-7). Of course, locating the groove is much easier when there is a large cuff tear, with the biceps being uncovered when it enters the superior part of the groove.

Biceps Exteriorization and Preparation

Grasp the long head of the biceps in its groove with a forceps while the spinal needle is removed. The biceps should be grasped at its most proximal end to facilitate exteriorization.

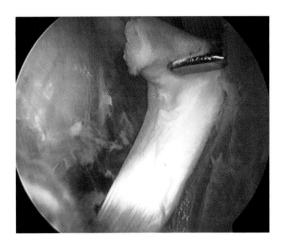

Figure 8-7. Lift the tendon out of the groove to free possible adhesions and grasp it with a forceps.

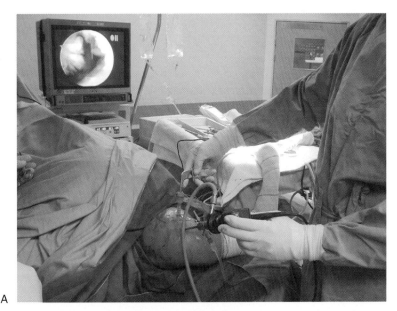

A

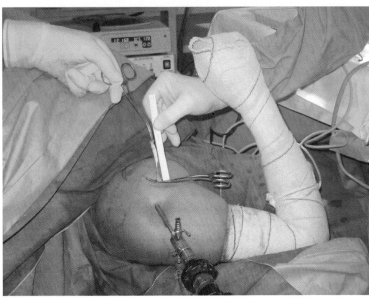

B

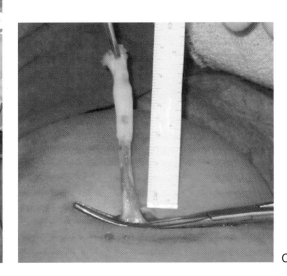

C

Figure 8-8. A: Exteriorize the tendon outside anteromedial portal. **B,C:** Flexion of the elbow allows pulling 5 or 6 cm of tendon. Use a vascular clamp to avoid any damage to the tendon. Notice the hypertrophy of the intraarticular portion and the synovitis around the biceps tendon in the grove portion.

The tendon is now exteriorized through the anteromedial portal while the cannula is temporarily removed (Fig. 8-8). Exteriorization of the tendon is facilitated by flexion of the elbow. Use a vascular clamp to grasp the tendon more distally and to keep it outside the wound; this will help to avoid tendon damage and to allow tendon preparation. About 4 to 5 cm of tendon should be exteriorized to prepare the tendon. A brief tenosynovectomy and trimming of the tendon is performed, and then the tendon is doubled over a no. 5 suture (Ethibond; Ethicon, Inc., Somerville, NJ or Flexidene; Braun, Germany) (Fig. 8-9). The tendon is evened and the end of the tendon is whip stitched using a running baseball stitch with no. 2 absorbable suture (Vicryl; Ethicon, Inc. or Dexon; Braun). The tendon should be doubled and sewn to its anterior face for a length of about 2 cm. Measure the diameter of the double tendon using the same type of graft sizer used for cruciate ligament grafts in the knee. The diameter of the double tendon should be 7 or 8 mm. If the tendon is too large (i.e., hypertrophic), a part of it must be cut in the direction of the fibers and removed to create a diameter of the doubled tendon of 8 mm. The size of the doubled tendon determines the drill diameter of the humeral socket. Reintroduce the working cannula into the anteromedial portal while the biceps tendon is kept outside the wound and outside the cannula; placing the no. 5 suture under tension by attaching it to the sterile drapes with a nonpenetrating clamp facilitates this. The rest of the procedure is done with the scope in the anterolateral (viewing) portal and the instruments inserted through the anteromedial (working) portal (Fig. 8-10).

Drilling the Humeral Socket

Clean the bicipital groove of all fibrous tissue with the shaver or the VAPR. Take care not to shave on the most lateral or medial parts of the groove because of the leash of several

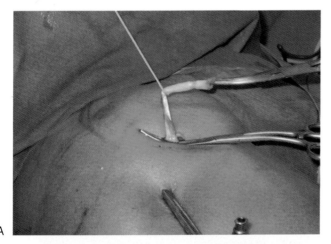

A

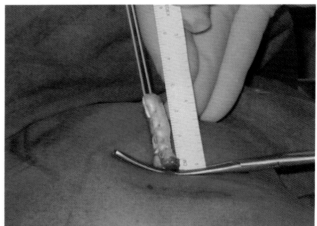

B

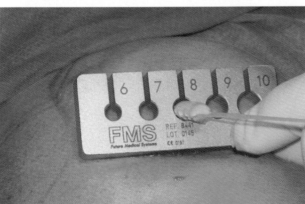

C

Figure 8-9. Tendon preparation: doubled on a traction suture **(A)**, whipstitched **(B)**, and calibrated (usually 8 or 9 mm) **(C)**.

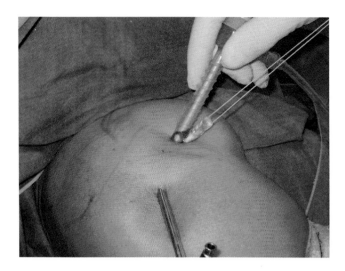

Figure 8-10. Keep the biceps tendon outside the wound while a cannula is re-introduced through the anteromedial portal.

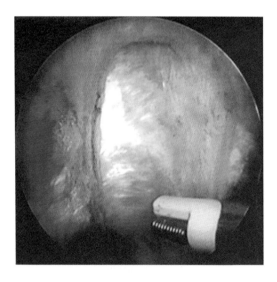

Figure 8-11. Clean the groove of synovial tissue using the VAPR (Mitek Worldwide, Norwood, Massachusetts).

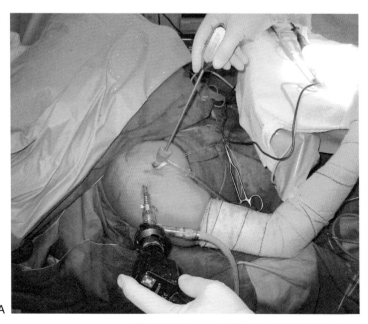

A

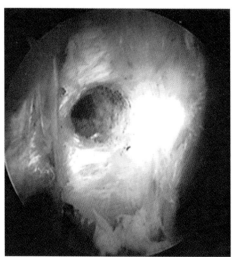

B

Figure 8-12. A,B: Make a pilot hole in the groove 1 cm from the top.

small vessels (Fig. 8-11). The socket placement is assessed with probe measurement: This is optimally placed approximately 10 mm below the top of the groove entrance to prevent any anterosuperior impingement with the acromial arch. The location for the humeral socket is chosen and the cortex penetrated with a sharp-tipped pick or awl, as the bone of the groove is quite hard. This procedure prevents skiving or sliding of the guide pin along the cortical bone of the groove when drilling (Fig. 8-12). Place a guidewire in the pilot hole and orient it strictly perpendicular to the humerus and parallel to the lateral border of the acromion (Fig. 8-13). A guide (Shoulder-Guide; Future Medical Systems, Glen Burnie, MD) can be used to perform this procedure safely, without any risk for the axillary nerve (Fig. 8-14). This makes the procedure reproducible for any surgeon. Drill the guidewire until it just penetrates the posterior cortex of the humerus. Overdrill the humeral guide pin with a 7- or 8-mm cannulated reamer, depending on the size of the double tendon, to a depth of 25 mm (Fig. 8-15). Then, remove the reamer and guide pin. Use a motorized shaver and an arthroscopic burr to chamfer smooth the entrance of the humeral socket by removing bone debris and tissues that may contribute to tendon blocking and abrasion. Most attention should be paid to the inferior part of the humeral socket, where the tendon will enter. The synovial tissue around the biceps tendon should also be removed (Fig. 8-16).

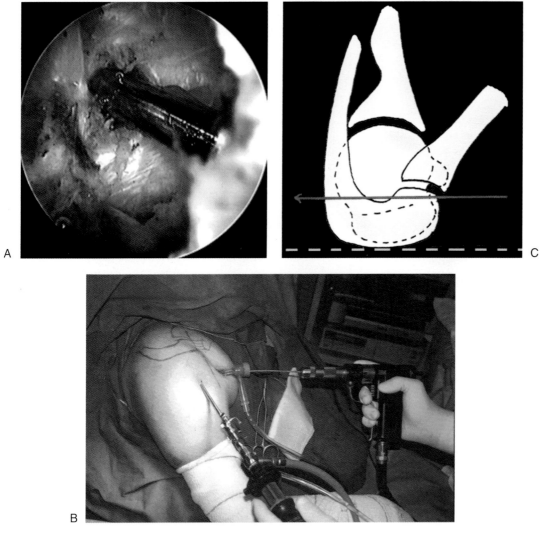

Figure 8-13. A: Place a guide pin in the pilot hole and transfix the humerus staying perpendicular to the humerus and parallel to the acromion. **B,C:** Position for drilling humeral guides pin: strictly perpendicular to humeral shaft, strictly parallel to lateral border of acromion.

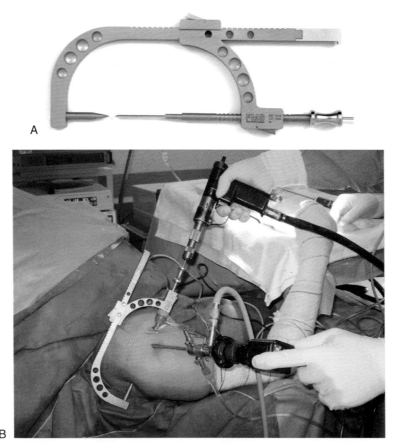

Figure 8-14. Use of a shoulder guide (Shoulder-Guide; Future Medical Systems, Glen Burnie, MD) **(A)** provides good control during all steps of the procedure **(B)**, making it easier and safer.

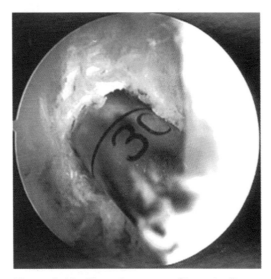

Figure 8-15. Place the reamer (8 mm in diameter in this case) over the humeral guide pin, and ream the humeral socket to a depth of 25 mm.

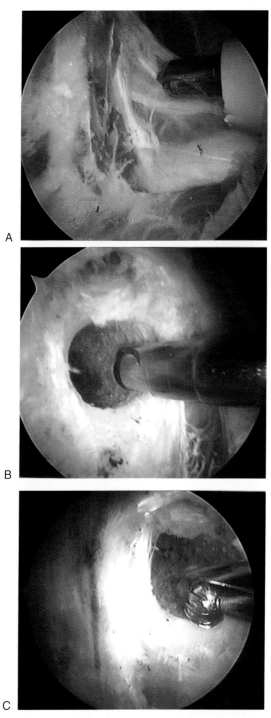

Figure 8-16. Perform a synovectomy around the biceps tendon **(A)**, clean the humeral socket from bone debris **(B)**, and ream the inferior rim using a burr **(C)**.

Passing the Transhumeral Pin

A Beath needle is used to pull-through for tendon placement. The needle has an eyelet on its trailing end and serves as a suture passer. Place the Beath pin through the anteromedial cannula into the humeral socket. Again, the direction of the transhumeral Beath pin is very important: It should be strictly perpendicular to the humerus and parallel to the lateral border of the acromion. A metallic cylinder is used to center the Beath needle. The Beath pin

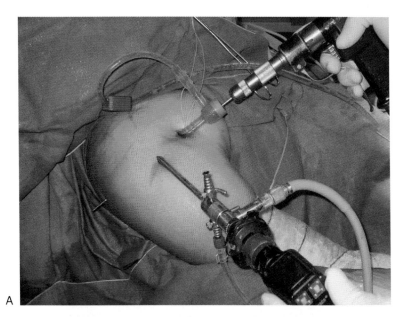

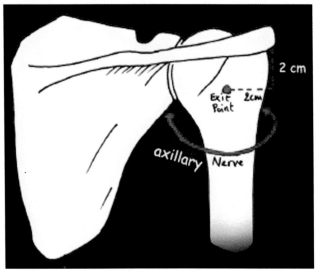

Figure 8-17. A: Transfix the humerus with the Beath needle after centering it in the humeral socket, and exiting through the posterior portal. **B:** Position of Beath needle in relation to axillary nerve.

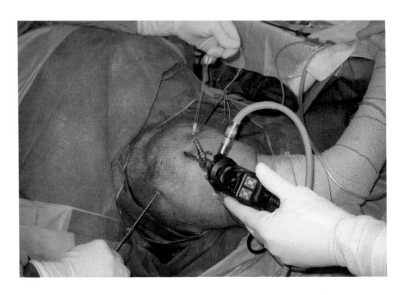

Figure 8-18. Pull the Beath needle with the suture through the humerus.

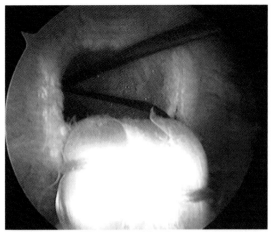

Figure 8-19. Place a guidewire in the humeral socket for interference screw before tendon placement. The biceps tendon is inserted into the socket, with a blue mark for depth guide.

is drilled until it exits the skin, which will be approximately 2 to 3 cm below the posterolateral border of the acromion, avoiding the axillary nerve. The target should be the posterior portal (Fig. 8-17). Both ends of the no. 5 suture are threaded through the eyelet of the Beath pin, and the pin/sutures are pulled through the humerus (Fig. 8-18). Before pulling the biceps tendon into the socket, insert a flexible guidewire for the interference screw to prevent screw divergence (Fig. 8-19). To facilitate placement of this guide pin in the socket, bring the anteromedial cannula into direct contact with the humeral socket entrance. Once the pin is inside the socket, pull the biceps tendon into the humeral socket. The ink mark at the base of the doubled portion of the tendon is visualized to insert it completely into the humeral socket. Take care to take the same direction for the biceps tendon with the Beath needle to avoid incarceration of deltoid fibers.

Interference Screw Fixation

The tendon is fixed in the hole using a bioabsorbable interference screw (dimensions, 8 × 25 or 9 × 25 mm). As a rule, use a screw with a diameter 1 mm larger than the humeral socket diameter: a 9-mm screw for an 8-mm socket for example. This provides a strong fixation. Not all screws can be used for this procedure. The screws we used are bioabsorbable polylactic acid (PLA98); they are smooth so as not to damage the tendon, and the resorption is very slow (2 to 5 years) to avoid any inflammatory reaction (Tenoscrew; Phusis, Tornier, Inc., USA, Stafford, TX). Apply tension on the pull-through sutures to completely insert the biceps tendon into the humeral socket before interference screw placement (Fig. 8-20). Place the screw on the superior aspect of the tendon while the elbow is still flexed at 90 degrees. Once the tip of the screw is engaged between the tendon and the socket wall, the tendon is stabilized by extending the elbow. This prevents twisting and rotation of the tendon during screw placement. After complete insertion of the tendon, the fixation is checked by probing the biceps tendon (Fig. 8-21). After flexing and extending the elbow, fixation of the tendon is rechecked. The rotator cuff is repaired if a tear is present. Doubling the biceps tendon has at least three advantages: (a) it reinforces the strength of the tendon, which is not damaged by the interference screw; (b) it prevents a possible sliding of the tendon after screw insertion ("stop-block" effect); and (c) it allows an optimal tensioning of the biceps muscle since tension is not changed.

An alternative way to place the tendon in the humeral socket is to push the tendon inside the socket (instead of pulling it) by using a fork wire (Fig. 8-22).

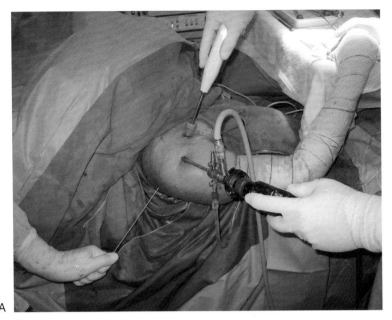

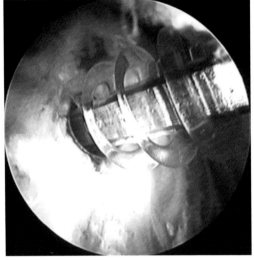

A

B

Figure 8-20. A: Place tension on pull-through sutures to completely insert biceps tendon into humeral socket prior to interference screw placement **(B)**.

Figure 8-21. A–C: Final biceps tenodesis construct with interference screw fixation.

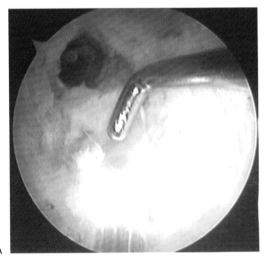

A

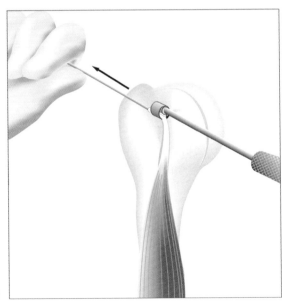

B

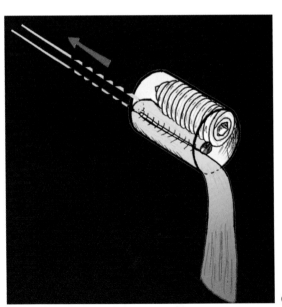

C

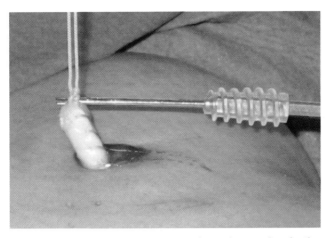

Figure 8-22. Alternative way to place the tendon in the humeral socket: the tendon is pushed inside the socket (instead of being pulled) by using a fork wire.

POSTOPERATIVE MANAGEMENT

Passive and active elbow flexion and extension are allowed the day of surgery with no restriction and no immobilization. In cases of isolated biceps tenodesis, complete passive and active motion is allowed for the shoulder. In patients with associated cuff repair, only early passive motion is allowed for the shoulder for the first 6 weeks.

RESULTS

Between 1997 and 1999, our department performed arthroscopic biceps tenodesis in 43 patients. The indication for a tenodesis of the long head of the biceps was a pathologic biceps tendon, diagnosed preoperatively with CT scan or MRI and/or intraoperatively under arthroscopy: tenosynovitis (4 cases), prerupture (15 cases), subluxation (11 cases), or dislocation (13 cases). A pathologic biceps tendon was encountered in three different clinical situations: (a) in 3 cases of arthroscopic or mini-open rotator cuff repairs; (b) in 6 cases of isolated pathology of the biceps tendon with an intact cuff (one SLAP lesion type 3) or with a partial deep cuff tear; (c) in 34 cases of massive, degenerative and irreparable cuff tears in which a tenodesis was preferred to a simple tenotomy.

Preoperatively, patients typically complained of pain in the anterior region of the shoulder, with occasional distal radiation along the anterior aspect of the upper arm and the cervical spine. Pain was more severe in overhead activities and at night. The Speed test was positive and helpful in the preoperative examination. Tenderness with palpation of the bicipital groove (approximately 2 cm distal to the anterolateral acromion with the arm in neutral rotation) was present. Tenderness with passive external rotation of the arm, as the examiner is palpating the bicipital groove, was also present, as the pathologic biceps is "rolled" under the examiner's fingers.

The mean age of the patients was 63 years (range, 25 to 78 years). All patients were reviewed with a mean follow-up of 17 months (range, 12 to 34 months). The shoulder function was evaluated using the Constant scoring system. The mobility of the elbow was measured and the strength of the biceps was measured using a spring balance with the elbow in flexion and the forearm in supination. Radiographs of the shoulder, and in 12 cases MRI, were obtained.

The Constant score averaged 43 points (range, 13 to 60 points) preoperatively and it averaged 79 points (range, 59 to 87 points) at review ($p < 0.005$). No deficit of flexion or extension of the elbow was observed compared to the contralateral side. Strength of the tenodesed biceps averaged 90% of the other side (range, 80% to 100%).

The shape and contour of the biceps was conserved in all but two cases. MRI evaluation demonstrated tight fixation of the biceps tendon in the humeral socket with no adverse reaction related to the bioabsorbable screw.

The advantages of this new arthroscopic biceps tenodesis using a bioabsorbable interference screw are multiple. First, it is a quick, safe, and reproducible technique. The humeral socket is drilled strictly perpendicular to the humeral shaft and parallel to the acromion. A guide can be used to perform this procedure safely, without any risk for the axillary nerve; this makes the procedure reproducible for any surgeon. The axillary nerve is not at risk because the transhumeral pin exits the skin through the posterior portal or just lateral to it. No neurologic or vascular complication was encountered in this series. Second, this technique is less traumatic than classic open surgery and, if no rotator cuff tear is present, this technique avoids any violation of the intact rotator cuff. Third, this technique needs only three small portals and is performed entirely under arthroscopy, contrary to other techniques that are done partially open. Exteriorization of the biceps tendon through the anteromedial portal makes its preparation easy. Fourth, interference screw fixation provides secure fixation of the biceps tendon into bone, allowing immediate mobilization of both the shoulder and the elbow. Fifth, doubling the tendon restores its functional length and an optimal tension of the biceps tendon. Sixth, bioabsorbable screw fixation does not interfere with MRI evaluation of the shoulder and allows evaluation of the cuff.

COMPLICATIONS

Two failures were encountered and were related to technical mistakes early in our experience. In both cases, the biceps tendon was friable, and the diameter of the screw (7 mm) proved to be insufficient. The screw diameter should be 1 mm larger than the socket diameter, as a rule. Because of the habitual size of the biceps tendon, we usually drill a 7- or 8-mm humeral socket and systematically use an 8- or 9-mm interference screw, respectively. No neurologic or vascular complications occurred. Four patients were diagnosed with reflex sympathic dystrophy because of persistent pain and stiffness after the operation: Rehabilitation allowed these patients to regain complete motion and all patients were pain-free at review. A possible intraoperative complication is incarceration of deltoid fibers because of divergent portals at the time of passing the Beath needle. In this case, this step should be done again. Using a screw not specifically designed for this purpose can lead to complications, such as rupture of the tendon at the time of insertion of the screw because of overaggressive manipulation of the screw, inflammatory reaction because of different polylactide or polyglycolide screws, and so forth.

In conclusion, arthroscopic biceps tenodesis using a bioabsorbable screw fixation is technically possible and gives good clinical results. This technique can be used in case of a pathologic biceps tendon (isolated or associated with a cuff tear). A very thin, fragile, almost-ruptured biceps tendon may be the technical limit of this arthroscopic technique. In such a situation, the arthroscopic procedure can be easily converted to simple tenotomy alone or open tenodesis without difficulty. We do not pretend that arthroscopic biceps tenodesis is superior to a simple tenotomy, but we consider it to be another technical option available for the arthroscopic shoulder surgeon. Interference fixation with specific absorbable screws provides strong initial fixation at least equal if not superior to those techniques that use sutures tied over soft tissue or metallic anchors placed in the bicipital groove.

RECOMMENDED READING

1. Berleman, U., Bayley, I.: Tenodesis of the long head of the biceps brachii in the painful shoulder: improving the results in the long term. *J Shoulder Elbow Surg* 4(6): 429–435, 1995.
2. Boileau, P., Krishnan, S.G., Coste, J.S., et al.: A new technique for tenodesis of the long head of the biceps using bioabsorbable screw fixation. *Tech Shoulder Elbow Surg* September, 2001.

3. Boileau P., Walch, G.: A new technique for tenodesis of the long head of the biceps using bioabsorbable screw fixation [abstract]. *J Shoulder Elbow Surg* 8(5): 557, 1999.

4. Burkhead, W.Z., Jr.: The biceps tendon. In: Rockwood, C.A. Jr, Matsen, F.A., III, eds.: *The shoulder.* Vol. 2. Philadelphia: WB Saunders; 791–836, 1990.

5. Gartsman, G., Hammerman, S.: Arthroscopic biceps tenodesis. *Arthroscopy* 16(5): 550–552, 2000.

6. Goldfarb, C., Yamaguchi, K.: The biceps tendon: dogma and controversies. In: *Sports medicine and arthroscopy review.* Philadelphia: Lippincott Williams & Wilkins; 93–103, 1999.

7. Habermeyer, P., Mall, U.: Arthroscopic tenodesis of the long head of the biceps: technique and results [abstract]. *J Shoulder Elbow Surg* 8(5): 557; 1999.

8. Patte, D., Walch, G., Boileau, P.: Luxation de la longue portion du biceps et rupture de la coiffe des rotateurs. *Rev Chir Orthop* 76[Suppl I]: 95, 1990.

9. Snyder, S.J.: Arthroscope-assisted biceps tendon surgery. In: Snyder, S.J., ed.: *Shoulder arthroscopy.* New York: McGraw-Hill; 61–76, 1994.

10. Walch, G., Nové-Josserand, L., Boileau, P., et al.: Subluxations and dislocations of the tendon of the long head of the biceps. *J Shoulder Elbow Surg* 7(2): 100–108, 1998.

9

Arthrothermal Stabilization

Edward V. Craig

INDICATIONS/CONTRAINDICATIONS

The unstable shoulder remains one of the most challenging, interesting, and common disorders in orthopaedic surgery. It has generally been believed that the pathogenesis of shoulder instability may involve bone deficits of glenoid or humeral head or both, capsular laxity, labral or capsular avulsion, capsular stripping, rotator cuff tearing, or combinations of the above. The history of treatments for the unstable shoulder has suggested that if the pathology responsible for shoulder instability is treated specifically and completely by any one of a number of methods, recurrence of shoulder instability is unusual, and the preservation of motion, strength, and function can be maximized.

While many surgeons' experiences with arthroscopic stabilization have been encouraging, numerous published studies have shown that this method of stabilization has not offered the predictability of success that open methods have provided. While there may be many reasons for this, including varied patient populations, varied outcome criteria, differences in surgical skill, different methods of assessing results, and varied pathology, most surgeons have found that the main arthroscopic limitation has centered on being able to precisely tension the capsule in patients in whom capsular laxity is an important contribution to instability. The earliest stabilization techniques thus focused on methods to repair the labral avulsion (Bankart lesion) with tacks, suture methods, and suture anchors. Experience has suggested that if clearly defined labral avulsion is the predominant pathologic mechanism, early or late repair arthroscopically is as effective as open methods of stabilization.

While a number of methods have been described to deal with concomitant or predominant capsular laxity, these methods have been, in most surgeons' hands, technically difficult and have produced inconsistent results.

E. V. Craig, M.D.: Department of Orthopaedics, Weill Medical College of Cornell University; and Hospital for Special Surgery, New York, New York.

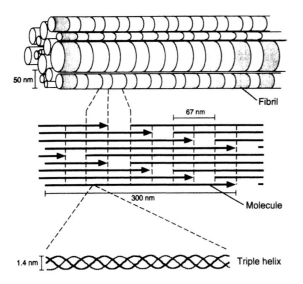

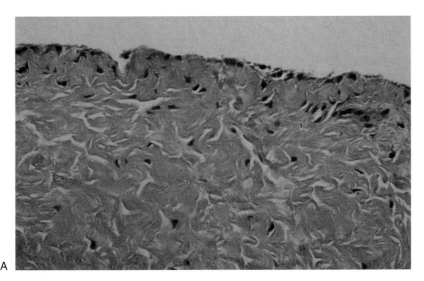

Figure 9-1. Structural orientation of type I collagen. Molecules are packed in a staggered fashion that give rise to the striated appearance in transmission electron micrographs. (From Fanton, G.S., Wall, M.S.: Thermally-assisted arthroscopic stabilization of the shoulder joint. In: Warren, R.F., Craig, E.V., Altchek, D.W., eds.: *The unstable shoulder.* Philadelphia: Lippincott–Raven Publishers, 133, 1999.)

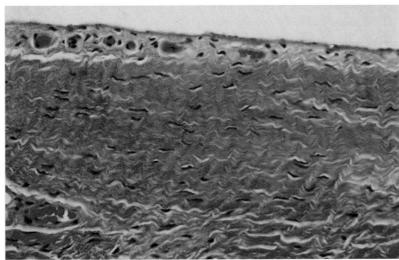

Figure 9-2. A: Untreated capsule demonstrates normal collagenous architecture. B: Treated area 9 months after thermal stabilization. Abundant and well-organized collagen fibrosis is seen with typical "crimping" that appears in type I collagen. Abundant fibroblasts are noted with no identifiable inflammatory cells. (From Fanton, G.S., Wall, M.S.: Thermally-assisted arthroscopic stabilization of the shoulder joint. In: Warren, R.F., Craig, E.V., Altchek, D.W., eds.: *The unstable shoulder.* Philadelphia: Lippincott–Raven Publishers, 340, 1999.)

It was the recognition that the known affects of heat applied to collagen might successfully be used on the shoulder capsule that gave rise to the technique of arthroscopic thermal stabilization using a radiofrequency probe as a well-controlled heat source. The challenges have been to determine whether collagen shrunk through this method can retain normal mechanical properties, whether cellular death can be avoided, and whether the technique can be performed without generating unacceptable risks and complications.

The thermal modification of collagen has long been recognized in surgical and nonsurgical disciplines. In its native state, type I collagen is present in a highly organized or "extended crystalline" structure, for which collagen stability is maintained by intramolecular and intermolecular bonds (Fig. 9-1). When heat is applied in a certain temperature range for a period of time, this conformation of collagen changes, and it "melts into an amorphous, random, coil state in which it also contracts" (4). It is this contracted property that has been used in the shoulder in an attempt to reduce capsular volume while treating clinical shoulder instability (Fig. 9-2).

A range of temperatures has been shown to be affective in shrinking collagen. Shrinkage is both temperature- and time-dependent, and the same amount of shrinkage can occur if high heat is applied for a short time as at a low heat applied for a longer period. Wall (11) have shown that the shrinkage process is extremely sensitive to time and to the temperature applied to the collagen. While shrinkage occurs rapidly (instantaneous) at high temperatures, lower rates of shrinkage ("incipient") occur at low temperature and a longer application time (Fig. 9-3). This sensitivity to small temperature changes is the reason that any device applying heat to tissue must do so within precise temperature ranges. Wall et al. also studied the mechanical properties of tissue when heat was applied. The collagen mechanical properties decreased with increasing amount of shrinkage (Fig. 9-4). The optimal amount of shrinkage should be that which does not result in significant reduction in mechanical strength. These thermal affects seem to be present no matter how the heat is applied, whether with a laser, or more recently, with a radiofrequency probe.

The use of radiofrequency to apply heat has had many uses in surgery, including coagulation, cautery, and ablation. One difference between heat applied via laser energy and via radiofrequency probe is that laser energy acts at some distance from the target tissue whereas

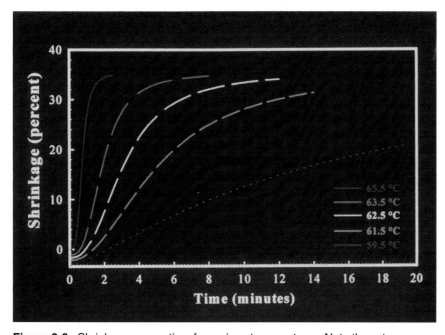

Figure 9-3. Shrinkage versus time for various temperatures. Note the extreme sensitivity of shrinkage rate to temperature change. (From Fanton, G.S., Wall, M.S.: Thermally-assisted arthroscopic stabilization of the shoulder joint. In: Warren, R.F., Craig, E.V., Altchek, D.W., eds.: *The unstable shoulder.* Philadelphia: Lippincott–Raven Publishers, 334, 1999.)

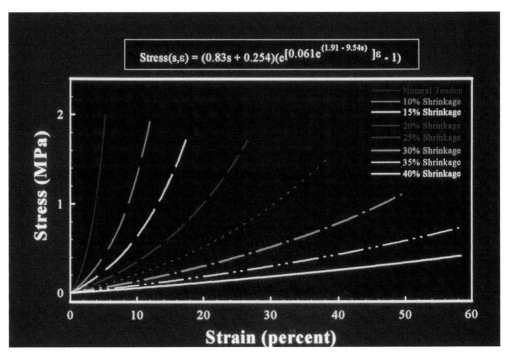

$$\text{Stress(s,}\varepsilon) = (0.83s + 0.254)(e^{[0.061e^{(1.91 - 9.54s)}]\varepsilon} - 1)$$

Figure 9-4. Relation between tissue stress and strain as a function of increasing tissue shrinkage. Note the mechanical properties decrease with increasing shrinkage. This is independent of the method used in achieving the shrinkage. (From Fanton, G.S., Wall, M.S.: Thermally-assisted arthroscopic stabilization of the shoulder joint. In: Warren, R.F., Craig, E.V., Altchek, D.W., eds.: *The unstable shoulder.* Philadelphia: Lippincott–Raven Publishers, 332, 1999.)

radiofrequency application must be in direct contact with the tissue to be modified and held there while the heat is applied to see the collagen affect (4). It is believed that the thermal affect is achieved through oscillation and excitation of electrons within and outside of the cells. One radiofrequency probe that has been developed (Fig. 9-5) (Oratek Probe, Oratek Interventions, Inc., Menlo Park, CA) can be set at specific temperatures and a built-in thermal couple controls the application of current at the probe tip. The tip itself has been developed in various sizes to more adequately increase the flexibility in application to target tissue and

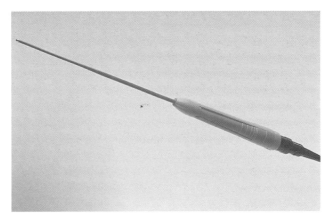

Figure 9-5. A radiofrequency thermal-feedback arthroscopic probe (Oratec Interventions, Inc., Menlo Park, CA). The radiofrequency probe can be set at a specific temperature. A built-in thermal couple controls the application at the probe tip.

Figure 9-6. Temperature-controlled probes are available in various sizes and shapes to reach different locations and different joint configurations.

is malleable for use in certain difficult-to-reach capsular areas (Fig. 9-6). Few arthroscopic procedures have had such evolving indications as radiofrequency capsular shift.

After an initial group of reports suggesting highly successful clinical application of this method, some subsequent studies reported complications with this method of instability surgery. Thus, there has been a recent, appropriate, and evolving degree of caution in this technique. Some continue to use this technique widely with broad applications, including primary capsular shrinkage and as an adjunct to arthroscopic labral repairs. My personal indications for thermal stabilization include the following:

1. *"Internal" impingement.* A condition that usually occurs in throwing athletes in which there are deep surface rotator cuff changes and labral changes usually posteriorly and superiorly and that is usually associated with anterior capsular laxity.
2. *Subtle anterior instability.* Instability without true subluxation and dislocation episodes, which may present predominately as pain associated with unidirectional capsular laxity. This is clinically confirmed intraoperatively with increased translation under anesthesia and secondary affects on glenoid articular cartilage or labrum consistent with pathologic instability.
3. *Anterior subluxation* with few episodes (and no true dislocations) due to capsular laxity.
4. *Capsular stretching and paralytic shoulders,* frequently as a result of brachialplexus injuries, in which inferior instability secondary to paralyzed muscles produces clinical symptomatology. In this group of patients, arthrodesis or open methods are frequently the surgical alternatives. Minor degrees of reduction in capsular volume may significantly improve the symptom complex related to inferior shoulder laxity.

While there are no absolute contraindications for arthroscopic thermal stabilization, my relative contraindications include the following:

1. Instability due to global capsular laxity or multidirectional shoulder instability in the athlete with normal rotator cuff and deltoid muscles.
2. Gross instability with many recurrent episodes of dislocation.
3. Instability of long duration with many episodes of subluxation or dislocation.
4. Recurrent shoulder instability after previous surgical stabilization.

PREOPERATIVE PLANNING

The patient with subtle instability who I believe is a candidate for arthroscopic thermal stabilization is a patient who has had a minor degree of instability, frequently with internal impingement. This may be a throwing athlete in whom the combined pathology of undersurface rotator cuff, posterior labral fraying, and mild capsular laxity results in abnormal anterior translation of the humerus during throwing, with resultant pain and inability to effectively compete. The history commonly includes shoulder pain with athletic activities rather than true subluxation episodes. The throwing athlete may in fact complain of nothing more than pain, easy fatigability, altered pitching mechanics, and ineffective performance.

The patient with internal impingement and subtle instability on physical examination characteristically has an excellent range of motion in all directions tested. A throwing athlete may show an increased amount of external rotation, particularly with abduction and may show a concomitant asymmetric decrease in internal rotation in the involved shoulder. The patient may have increased translatability to load-and-shift testing and may have a measurably positive "sulcus" sign. In an athlete with subtle shoulder instability, muscular guarding frequently precludes the ability to demonstrate subluxability unless the patient is anesthetized. The patients, however, may demonstrate a positive relocation test (i.e., pain in the position of abduction and external rotation), which is diminished when an anterior pressure is applied to the humerus, centering it in the glenoid. There may not be classic anterior apprehension in this group of patients. Active range of motion of the shoulder is usually normal and muscle strength is usually undiminished. Physical findings at the time of examination may reflect associated tendonopathy or partial tearing of the rotator cuff or superior labrum. These may include a classic positive impingement sign, pain with resisted contraction of the rotator cuff tendons, and pain when the arm is brought up into the throwing position of abduction/external rotation.

Findings on plain radiographs, including an anteroposterior, outlet lateral, and axillary views, are typically unremarkable.

A good quality magnetic resonance imaging (MRI) scan can be helpful as an additional study. MRI may reveal associated anterior or posterior labral pathology, capsular injury, or the findings associated with internal impingement, such as posterosuperior labral fraying and undersurface rotator cuff damage or tearing. Full-thickness tearing of the rotator cuff is unusual in the patient who has subtle instability. Associated pathology in the throwing athlete may include the presence of a superior labrum anterior and posterior (SLAP) lesion, paralabral ganglion, worn articular cartilage of the humeral head or the glenoid and biceps tendinosis, split, or tearing.

A diagnostic injection of Xylocaine (Abbott Labs, North Chicago, IL) in the subacromial space may be helpful in differentiating intraarticular from an extraarticular subacromial source of shoulder pain. If the superficial source of the rotator cuff and subacromial bursa is anesthetized with subsequent diminution of positional pain of the shoulder, this is highly suggestive that the subacromial space is the main location responsible for the patient's discomfort. It would be unusual for numbness of the subacromial space to have an anesthetic affect on intraarticular pathology such as abnormal translation associated with symptomatic instability.

SURGERY

The standard lateral decubitus or beach-chair position for shoulder arthroscopy is used. Regional anesthesia with interscalene block is the preferred block of regional anesthesia. Once anesthesia is obtained, a careful examination under anesthesia is performed with stress anteroposteriorly and anteroinferiorly. The degree of translation and the presence and direction of subluxability are documented. It is frequently helpful to test the degree of translation both with the capsular restraints relaxed and subsequently tensioned. For instance, anteroinferior shoulder instability may be demonstrable with the humeral head in neutral position. However, subsequent tensioning of the glenohumeral ligaments in abduction and external rotation may control, diminish, or eliminate the translatability of the humeral head. If subluxation of the head of the humerus is not present under anesthesia with tensioning of the normal capsular restraints, the diagnosis of clinical shoulder instability must be questioned, particularly if little intraarticular pathology is found at the time of arthroscopy.

After examination under anesthesia, a standard arthroscopic posterior portal is used, parallel to the posterior joint line. This may be identified by translating the humerus posteriorly and palpating the interval between the humeral head and glenoid. Typically, this is 2 cm inferior and 2 cm medial to the posterolateral corner of the acromion. The arthroscope is introduced to the posterior portal and an anterior portal is established in the area of the rotator interval above the subscapularis. If treatment of the anterior capsule is anticipated, including all elements of the glenohumeral ligaments, the entryway of the second portal may be slightly superior to the usual portal directly above the subscapularis edge. The glenohumeral joint is carefully examined for associated intraarticular pathology. The degree of "drive-through" is identified, that is, the ease with which the arthroscope can be directly passed from the posterior capsule to the anterior subscapularis and capsule. This reflects some degree of generalized capsular laxity as the humeral head is distracted from the glenoid. Associated labral pathology is appropriately treated by either débridement or direct repair. The rotator cuff undersurface is carefully examined and probed and areas of fraying, partial tearing, and damage are noted and treated appropriately. Associated biceps pathology can be addressed at the same time. If there is a clear-cut labral avulsion, (Bankart) stabilization of the shoulder is better and more effectively handled with direct labral repair of the Bankart lesion rather than with thermal treatment of collagen. In those patients who have more subtle instability with minor degrees of translation, once a complete and thorough diagnostic arthroscopy of the glenohumeral joint and treatment of associated labral, biceps, and rotator cuff pathologies are performed, capsular shrinkage is begun.

The radiofrequency generator is set at 35 WM (wattmeter) and 65°C (Fig. 9-7). This has been found to be the most effective way to rapidly produce instantaneous shrinkage of the collagen. While it is important to directly touch all tissue to be treated, painting the entire inferior and anterior capsule has the potential to result in excessive amount of collagen shrinkage with subsequent capsular contracture. In effect, overtreating the capsule may produce more problems just as overtightening a shoulder with open instability repairs can produce significant shoulder pathology and problems. This is particularly true if the instability itself is more subtle and of a more minor degree. It is difficult to know precisely when just enough capsule has been treated to allow control of the subtle instability without avoiding overtreating the capsule and thus producing excessive stiffness. In addition, care must be taken to avoid prolongation of the contact of the probe to the direct inferior capsular pouch, particularly if this is a poor-quality tissue or extremely thin tissue. There have been reports of heat injury to the axillary nerve after prolonged exposure of the probe on the inferior capsule. In general, if treating minor degrees of instability or subtle instability as an adjunct to internal impingement, "less is more" regarding treatment.

In general, those areas of the capsule that have increased collagen density respond most dramatically. Thus, the anterior and posterior bands of the inferior glenohumeral ligament (IGHL) may respond more dramatically than the intervening inferior capsular sling (4).

The probe is left in contact with the tissue until capsular contracture is visually observed (Fig. 9-8). Moving too quickly makes it difficult for the generator to maintain the preset heat temperature. The tip is moved slowly back and forth, as the tissue response is directly visualized, usually after a lag of a few seconds. The tissue may change color as it contracts, demonstrating response to the technique (Fig. 9-9).

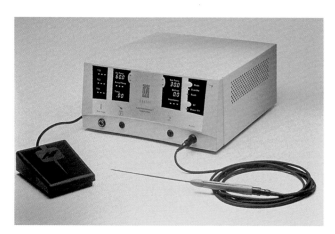

Figure 9-7. Intraoperative instrumentation for radiofrequency probe. The machine is set at a specific temperature with feedback from the probe tip.

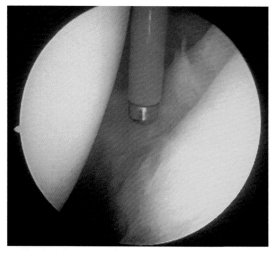

Figure 9-8. The probe is seen in direct contact with the inferior glenohumeral ligament. The probe tip must be applied directly to the area to be treated.

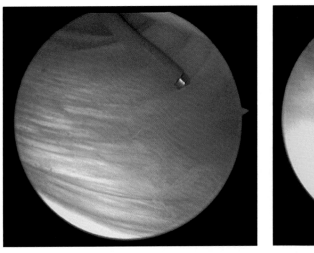
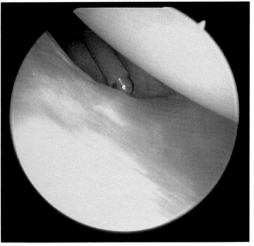

A   B

Figure 9-9. Untreated **(A)** and treated **(B)** capsular tissue. After treatment, contracted shortened collagen and a change in color can be seen. This is directly and immediately observed at the time of tissue treatment.

If anteroinferior shrinkage is being undertaken, the radiofrequency probe is introduced through the anterior portal (Fig. 9-10). The stabilization sequence for anterior instability is posterior band of the IGHL, anterior band of the IGHL, and finally the middle and superior glenohumeral ligaments (Fig. 9-11). Although there are a number of techniques for direct application of the capsule, including a painting motion, a zebra-striping technique (leaving areas of normal untreated capsule between areas of treated capsule), and selective horizontal application along each of the glenohumeral ligaments, there is little information that one is a more effective short-term or long-term means of applying heat to the capsule. The probe is kept in direct contact with the tissue until the shrinkage response is identified. The probe is then moved in a slow, steady fashion from the glenoid toward the humeral head and back toward the glenoid while observing the instantaneous effect on capsular tissue.

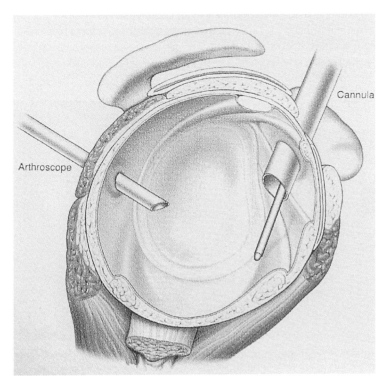

Figure 9-10. Position of imaging through an anterior position of probe and arthroscope for shrinkage of anteroinferior capsule.

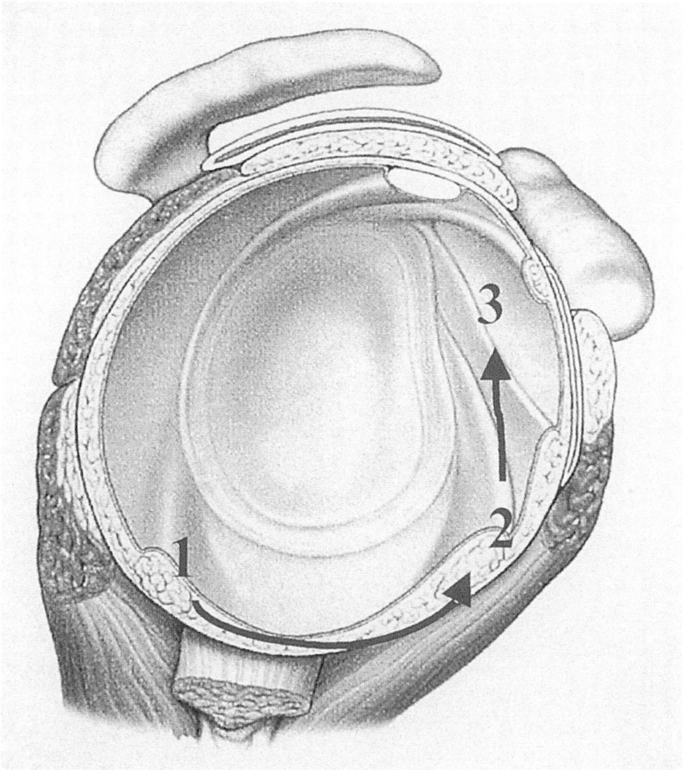

Figure 9-11. Stabilization sequence for anteroinferior capsular treatment.

With treatment, the inferior capsule contracts, the humeral head may be seen to move up in toward the glenoid, and in fact, the drive-through sign may be dramatically reduced.

Beginning at the most inferior recess of the glenohumeral joints allows the inferior capsule and IGHLs to be treated while preserving visualization of the middle and superior ligaments. Eventually, the entire capsule is treated in this fashion.

If the instability to be treated is thought to be predominately posterior, with the posterior capsule the main factor responsible for the pathologic laxity, the posterior capsule is the main source to be treated with thermal probe. The arthroscope is placed in the anterior portal and the radiofrequency probe is directed through the posterior portal to directly contact the posterior and posteroinferior capsule (Fig. 9-12). A satisfactory sequence in treating the posterior and posteroinferior capsule is to treat first the anterior band of the IGHL, the inferior sling, the posterior band of the ligament, and finally to finish with the main bulk of the posterior capsule, which may be quite thin (Fig. 9-13). On occasion, it may be effective to establish an accessory posterior portal, inferior to the standard posterior portal. This portal may be used to treat the inferior and posteroinferior capsules directly with the probe being introduced in a more horizontal fashion (Fig. 9-14).

Treatment of multidirectional shoulder instability with radiofrequency capsulorrhaphy is somewhat controversial. In one sense, access to the globally lax capsule is ideal for the radiofrequency probe, as exposure is excellent, broad areas of all parts of the capsule can be treated, and direct and immediate effects can be observed; however, although some studies have shown success in treating multidirectional shoulder instability, others believe that the patient with multidirectional shoulder instability is one of the at-risk groups for failure with this method. In my practice, use of radiofrequency treatment in a patient with multidirectional shoulder instability and global laxity is confined to the patient with a paralytic shoulder. Radiofrequency arthroscopic stabilization seems a low-risk alternative to the more drastic procedure such as shoulder arthrodesis and may have an impact on gross inferior subluxation. Because these patients frequently have axillary nerve involvement from the brachialplexus injury, resulting in atrophy of the deltoid, concern over axillary nerve injury from heat may be less important. In those patients in whom radiofrequency probe is to be

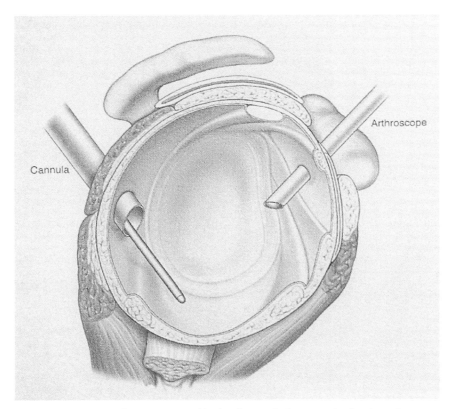

Figure 9-12. Instrument positioning for posterior capsular treatment.

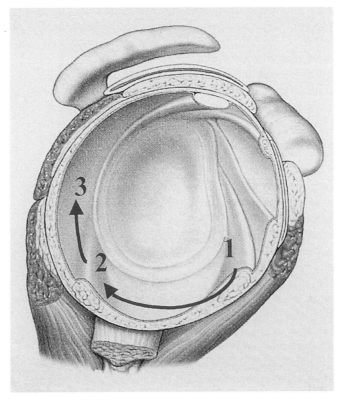

Figure 9-13. Shrinkage sequence for posteroinferior capsular treatment.

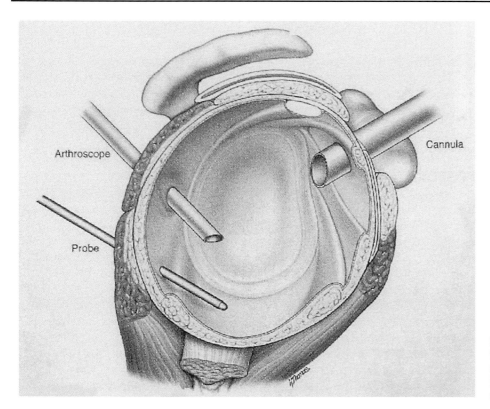

Figure 9-14. Accessory posteroinferior portal to treat inferior or posterior capsule. This is below the standard posterior arthroscopic portal.

used for global laxity, a useful sequence is as follows: First the anteroinferior capsule and inferior sling are treated, followed by the middle glenohumeral ligament, the rotator interval, and the superior glenohumeral ligament. Finally, with arthroscope in the anterior portal, the posteroinferior capsule and, subsequently, the direct posterior capsule are treated with the probe (Fig. 9-15).

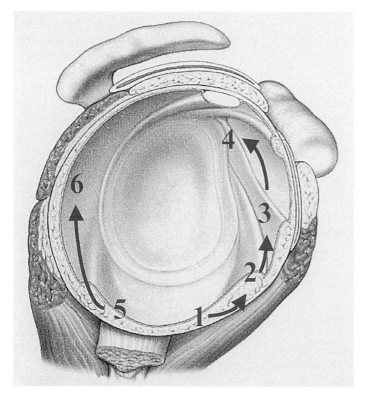

Figure 9-15. In patients with multidirectional shoulder instability, this is the proposed shrinkage sequence.

It is important that in contrast to what many surgeons will do following open stabilization or other arthroscopic stabilization techniques, such as the direct repair of the Bankart lesion, it seems to be important not to directly test the treated collagen at the time of the capsular shrinkage. In the denatured, amorphous treated phase, the collagen is extremely fragile and weak. Stressing this treated collagen may result in damage to the melted collagen in this state and may undo an otherwise successful surgical repair. The inability to immediately test the shoulder for efficacy of the stabilization procedure is one disadvantage to radiofrequency probe stabilization.

POSTOPERATIVE MANAGEMENT

Because of the nature of collagen in this "melted" state, it is initially quite weak. It is important for the patient to have a period of immobilization to permit initial capsular scarring without stretching the vulnerable capsule. Therefore, the patient is placed in a sling or immobilizer for approximately 3 weeks. During that time, shoulder range of motion is not permitted. However, elbow and hand active and passive range of motion may be initiated. The arm may be used for light activity with the arm near the side. In addition, isometric exercises for deltoid, rotator cuff, and parascapular muscles are initiated in the early postoperative period. Patients have occasionally reported that they feel the arm actually get tighter over the first week or 10 days after surgery, as the initially treated tissues undergoes scarring and further contracture.

Approximately 3 weeks after surgery, the sling is removed and gentle passive and active assistive range of motion is permitted. At 6 weeks after surgery, continued passive and assistive range of motion for flexibility is permitted and more resistive active range of motion for deltoid and rotator cuff is begun. When range of motion has returned and when 90% of the strength of the deltoid, scapula, and rotator cuff is achieved, the patient may begin to return to noncontact sports. If the patient is an overhead athlete such as a tennis player or baseball player, a return to the throwing program may be initiated at this time. Contact athletes are generally not permitted to return to their sport until approximately 6 months after surgery.

RESULTS

The initial results reported with laser-assisted and thermal-assisted capsular stabilization were extremely encouraging. The collagen could be seen "instantaneously" at the time of surgery to shrink and tighten up and, despite the fact that the long-term mechanical properties of the tissue were unknown, the early clinical results in terms of controlling instability were positive; however, in some series, these encouraging early clinical results have not been maintained. At the Hospital for Special Surgery, in a series of 130 patients who underwent arthroscopic thermal stabilization, at the 2- to 5-year follow up, there has been a 30% unsatisfactory result, either because of recurrent instability, lost range of motion, persistent pain, or low scores on the patient self-evaluation score used for outcomes assessment. The patients who consistently do the poorest with this procedure are those patients who had multidirectional shoulder instability, those patients who previously failed surgery for instability and for which arthroscopic thermal stabilization was a repeated surgery, and those patients who had the most episodes of recurrent dislocations. This procedure is now recommended only with reservation and with caution, as the results in these patients are least predictable. Thus, it appears that the failure rate in this technique may increase over time, and patients should be made aware of reservations in the use of this technique.

COMPLICATIONS

A number of complications have been reported with arthroscopic thermal stabilization. These complications have been varied and have been related to the technical aspects of the procedure itself, the postoperative immobilization, the postoperative rehabilitation, the return to activity, and the status of the tissue at the time of any necessary revision surgery.

1. *Nerve injury.* Axillary nerve heat injury has been reported to be a complication. Temperatures in the axillary nerve may be elevated in cadaver shoulders with the arm in a position of 90 degrees of abduction. The axillary nerve is in contact with the shoulder capsule almost throughout the inferior capsular range. In addition, abduction of the arm increases the distance from the glenoid to the main axillary nerve. This suggests that the surgeon should not leave the thermal probe at the most inferior portion of the shoulder capsule for a long period.

2. *Stiffness.* Excessive tightness with scarring, stiffness, and subsequent lost range of motion has been reported in a few cases. This has generally been thought to be secondary to overzealous painting of the capsule and an overly prolonged period of immobilization. This can be minimized by judiciously treating not the entire anterior and anteroinferior capsule but only the select glenohumeral ligaments. In addition, the patient should be monitored carefully and if range of motion is not being achieved in a normal fashion or if the patient's shoulder is thought to be excessively tight at the time of the initial examination, attention may be paid in the early postoperative period to range of motion exercises. Reportedly, it is rare that it becomes necessary for a second procedure to selectively release overly tightened glenohumeral ligaments, although this is an option if excessive contracture and lost range of motion persists.

3. *Recurrence.* Surgical failure has been reported in those groups most at risk, such as those with multidirectional instability, large numbers of dislocations, and previous instability surgery.

4. *Capsular destruction.* A unique complication has been reported in groups of patients undergoing thermal stabilization—that is, failure to achieve a good result with subsequent open stabilization techniques. Some reports indicate that if the capsule has been treated with the radiofrequency probe, at the time of a revision surgery the capsule has been of extremely poor quality and extremely friable, making open capsular repair difficult and challenging. It is not known how frequently this complication occurs or why this may occur. The alteration of the soft tissue at the time of the initial surgery may make revision open stabilization less predictable than if another initial stabilization technique had been used.

A high rate of unsatisfactory results in some series, whether because of recurrent instability, nerve injury, excessive tightness, or poor outcome scores, are concerning. It is important that surgeons have a better understanding of the relative indications of this procedure. Additional research is needed on surgical technique and diagnosis-specific methods of rehabilitation for this group of patients.

RECOMMENDED READING

1. Anderson, K., Warren, R.F., Altchek, D.W., et al.: Risk factors for early failure after thermal capsulorrhaphy. *Am J Sports Med* 30: 103–107, 2002.
2. Dugas, J.R., Andrews, J.R.: Thermal capsular shrinkage in the throwing athlete. *Clin Sports Med* 21: 771–776, 2001.
3. Fanton, G.S., Khan, A.M.: Monopolar radiofrequency energy for arthroscopic treatment of shoulder instability in the athlete. *Orthop Clin North Am* 32: 511–523, 2001.
4. Fanton, G.S., Wall, M.S.: Thermally assisted arthroscopic stabilization of the shoulder joint. In: Warren, R.F., Craig, E.V., Altchek, W., eds.: *The unstable shoulder.* Philadelphia: Lippincott–Raven Publishers, 1999.
5. Fitzgerald, B.T., Watson, B.T., Lapoint, J.M.: The use of thermal capsulorrhaphy in the treatment of multidirectional instability. *J Shoulder Elbow Surg* 11: 108–113, 2002.
6. Hawkins, R.J., Karas, S.G.: Arthroscopic stabilization plus thermal capsulorrhaphy for anterior instability with and without Bankart lesions: the role of rehabilitation and immobilization. *Instr Course Lect* 50: 13–15, 2001.
7. Hayashi, K., Markel, M.D.: Thermal capsulorrhaphy treatment of shoulder instability: basic science. *Clin Orthop* 390: 59–72, 2001.
8. Levy, O., Wilson, M., Williams, H., et al.: Thermal capsular shrinkage for shoulder instability: Midterm longitudinal outcome study. *J Bone Joint Surg Br* 83: 640–645, 2001.
9. Medvecky, M.J., Ong, B.C., Rokito, A.S., et al.: Thermal capsular shrinkage: basic science and clinical applications. *Arthroscopy* 17: 624–635, 2001.
10. Sperling, J.W., Anderson, K., McCarty, E.C., et al.: Complications of thermal capsulorrhaphy. *Instr Course Lect* 50: 37–41, 2001.
11. Wall, M.S., Deng, X.H., Torzilli, P.A., et al.: Thermal modification of collagen. *J Shoulder Elbow Surg* 8(4): 339–344, 2002.
12. Wallace, A.L., Hollinshead, R.M., Frank, C.B.: The scientific basis of thermal capsular shrinkage. *J Shoulder Elbow Surg* 9: 354–360, 2000.

10

Arthroscopic Capsular Release for the Stiff Shoulder

Thomas F. Holovacs, James D. O'Holleran, and Jon J. P. Warner

INDICATIONS/CONTRAINDICATIONS

The cause of primary adhesive capsulitis remains an enigma. Possible etiologies include immunologic, endocrine, and inflammatory factors, and it is often associated with systemic disorders such as diabetes mellitus (12,16). Conversely, secondary, or acquired, shoulder stiffness by definition has an identifiable cause. Acquired shoulder stiffness is most commonly encountered in the postsurgical or posttraumatic setting, frequently in the context of prolonged immobilization (7,13,16,18). Unlike adhesive capsulitis, acquired shoulder stiffness commonly results from extraarticular scar tissue. Alternatively, the anatomic characteristic of adhesive capsulitis is thickening and contracture of the joint capsule itself, resulting in decreased intraarticular volume and capsular compliance (16). These changes limit glenohumeral rotation in all planes of motion, leading to global loss of active and passive movements.

Regardless of the cause, the historic management of shoulder stiffness has been controversial since Codman first coined the term "frozen shoulder." Recommended treatments include tincture of time, oral analgesics and nonsteroidal medications, intraarticular injections, distention arthrography (brisement), closed manipulation under anesthesia, and open surgical release. Coincident with the burgeoning utility of the arthroscope, however, a new therapeutic option has evolved.

Arthroscopic capsular release for the stiff shoulder was described in the 1990s. This technique represents a specific treatment for patients with intrinsic capsular contracture re-

T. F. Holovacs, M.D.: Department of Orthopaedic Surgery, Harvard University Medical School; and Harvard Shoulder Service, Massachusetts General Hospital, Boston, Massachusetts.

J. D. O'Holleran, M.D.: Department of Orthopaedics, Harvard Combined Orthopaedic Surgery, Massachusetts General Hospital, Boston, Massachusetts.

J. J. P. Warner, M.D.: Department of Orthopaedic Surgery, Harvard Shoulder Service, Massachusetts General Hospital and Brigham and Women's Hospital, Boston, Massachusetts.

fractory to nonoperative measures (3,7,13,17,18). In our experience, arthroscopic capsular release provides a controlled, precise means to selectively and incrementally release the capsule on the basis of each patient's particular pathology.

Indications

The main indication for arthroscopic capsular release is shoulder stiffness due to capsular contracture, recalcitrant to nonoperative means.

In patients with shoulder stiffness, it is important to identify the anatomic location of the soft-tissue scarring, as arthroscopic release is most beneficial for intrinsic capsular contracture of the glenohumeral joint (16). This occurs most commonly in primary adhesive capsulitis, but it may also occur after surgery or trauma.

The mainstay of initial management for shoulder stiffness is physical therapy. The primary indication for operative treatment is failure to restore normal motion after a prolonged trial of physical therapy. Absolute measures of improvement vary, yet physical therapy is considered to be a failure if passive range of motion is not restored to within 80% of the contralateral, unaffected shoulder, and/or the patient continues to have pain and functional impairment.

The recommended duration of physical therapy varies from 3 to 36 months (2,7,12,13,16–18). It is important to differentiate between primary and secondary causes of stiffness, however, as the latter are more often resistant to conservative treatment (16,18). In the case of postoperative or posttraumatic stiffness, operative treatment is recommended if physical therapy has failed to meet the above criteria after 6 to12 months. Indeed, some patients may recover most or all of their motion after 1 year of conservative management. Alternatively, patient dissatisfaction with the progress of physical therapy can justifiably hasten operative intervention.

Stiffness after surgery for instability may represent a special case. In such circumstances, where there is severe loss of external rotation, the patient remains at risk for development of arthritis due to excessive joint compressive force that is directed across the posterior joint as a result of the anterior soft-tissue contracture (6,9). In these patients, we recommend release of their contracture if therapy has been unsuccessful for more than 1 year after their instability repair surgery.

Closed manipulation under anesthesia has historically been advocated as the next step after failure of conservative therapy (12). The large amount of force necessary to lyse the dense capsular scar tissue, however, is often extreme (especially in secondary stiffness), risking either failure to achieve sufficient mobility or fracture. Alternatively, arthroscopic capsular release provides a controlled, precise means to selectively and incrementally release the capsule on the basis of each patient's needs.

Contraindications

Not all types of shoulder stiffness are amenable to arthroscopic capsular release. Patients with shoulder stiffness resulting from contracture of the extraarticular soft tissues, such as after a Bristow or Putti-Platt procedure, would not be appropriate candidates for arthroscopic capsular release. In such cases contracture involves both the capsule and the subscapularis tendon. Open surgical release of extraarticular adhesions is the treatment of choice, and in some cases a Z-plasty lengthening of the capsule and subscapularis tendon is required.

Most intraoperative contraindications are either related to technical problems or unanticipated findings. For example, in a patient who has undergone an anterior instability repair where the subscapularis has been shortened or may even be insufficient, that tendon may not be seen during arthroscopy. Loss of this landmark is a contraindication to proceeding with an arthroscopic release as it constitutes not only the endpoint of an anterior capsular release but it is also the structure that protects the brachial plexus from injury by arthroscopic release instruments.

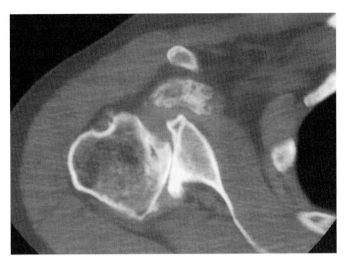

Figure 10-1. Severe degenerative arthritis with joint incongruity. Arthroscopic capsular release would not be indicated.

Rarely, the joint may be so tight as to inhibit introduction of the arthroscope. Inadequate visualization is usually the result of poor portal placement or uncontrolled bleeding from prior manipulation. In such cases, the procedure should be converted to a formal open release.

In some instances a patient may actually have instability combined with stiffness. This can occur in a situation where the patient's original multidirectional instability was treated only with a unidirectional repair such as a Bankart procedure or Putti-Platt procedure. In these cases, a formal open release of the anterior capsule is combined with a revision capsular shift to eliminate the redundancy in the inferior and posterior capsule. Description of this method is beyond the scope of this chapter but has been described elsewhere (14,19).

The presence of osteoarthritis is not an absolute contraindication to arthroscopic release provided that the humeral head remains round and congruent in the glenoid fossa. Indeed, release of a capsular contracture can mitigate the pain of osteoarthritis when combined with débridement (10,11).

If the joint is incongruous with bony blocks to rotation, an arthroplasty is the only viable alternative for restoration of motion and pain relief. (Fig. 10-1).

Finally, surgical treatment for primary adhesive capsulitis should not be considered while severe pain is a major component of the clinical picture, as this may represent the inflammatory phase of the disease. Surgery at this stage may actually exacerbate the motion loss by adding further capsular injury (12,16). In such cases, it is preferable to inject the joint with steroid and have the patient continue with gentle range-of-motion exercises.

PREOPERATIVE PLANNING

Accurate history and physical examination are prerequisites to proper treatment of the refractory stiff shoulder. Patients with adhesive capsulitis frequently report no inciting traumatic event. These patients describe the insidious and unremitting onset of shoulder pain, which predates stiffness and is unresponsive to physical therapy. Acquired shoulder stiffness, on the other hand, occurs as a result of a well-defined event, such as prolonged immobilization following trauma and anatomic (capsular shift) or nonanatomic (Putti-Platt) surgical overtightening for glenohumeral instability. Prior surgery or trauma must be clarified. For example, if a patient had a fracture and then developed stiffness after prolonged immobilization, this might indicate that there are adhesions between tissue planes as well as a capsular contracture. Radiographic imaging would then determine if there is bony incongruity around the joint. Such cases respond less reliably to arthroscopic release due to extensive extraarticular scarring and bony blocks to motion.

Another concern would be an instability procedure that has shortened or tethered the subscapularis; examples include the Magnuson-Stack, Putti-Platt, and Bristow procedures. These conditions usually require an open release as well.

Medical conditions such as diabetes must also be considered. Patients who develop a stiff shoulder without trauma or even after trauma or surgery may have this as a confounding variable. Finally, a patient who develops a stiff shoulder after rotator cuff surgery may also have a rerupture of the rotator cuff. This may affect decision making, because both stiffness and rotator cuff insufficiency must be addressed.

Physical examination of the shoulder begins with inspection of the ipsilateral and contralateral shoulders for signs of prior trauma or surgery, atrophy, and deformity. Thus always examine the patient while viewing the exposed shoulder and torso from the front and back. Assess active motion of the shoulder girdle using a goniometer with the patient seated. Document active flexion, elevation in the scapular plane, abduction, and internal/external rotation, both at the side and in abduction. Next, passively assess mobility in the same planes of motion, first with the patient seated and then supine (to stabilize the scapula and minimize scapulothoracic substitution). It should be noted that scapulothoracic substitution might give the appearance of good shoulder motion when glenohumeral motion is actually quite restricted. These patients have active and passive motion loss that is equal. If there is active motion loss but passive motion is preserved, one should think of rotator cuff insufficiency.

Patterns of motion loss are very important to recognize. Primary adhesive capsulitis tends to present with global restriction of motion, while postsurgical or posttraumatic stiffness may present with a more discretely isolated motion loss (16). For example, a patient may have good flexion but marked loss of external rotation after a Putti-Platt or Bristow procedure. Often this physical finding is important in surgical planning, as the pattern of stiffness may indicate the location of anatomic contracture. For example, diminished external rotation in adduction indicates contracture of the anterosuperior capsule and the rotator interval, while limited external rotation in abduction is associated with scarring in the anteroinferior capsule. Furthermore, limitation of internal rotation in either adduction or abduction may be associated with posterior capsular scarring.

While these patients may have pain with flexion, the impingement symptoms that seem to suggest rotator cuff disease are actually secondary due to alterations in joint mechanics as a result of the capsular contracture. This is "nonoutlet" impingement, and it occurs without alteration of the architecture of the acromion, but instead is due to a tight capsule that pushes the humeral head in a superior direction when flexion is attempted (4,5,15).

Imaging studies have a limited role in the diagnosis of the stiff shoulder. However, plain radiographs are necessary to confirm the presence of a normal glenohumeral joint by identifying arthrosis, fractures, or loose metallic implants that may contribute to motion loss.

Arthrography has been advocated by many to confirm a decreased joint capacity (12). However, it has been shown that there is no direct correlation between arthrographic findings and motion loss (8). Therefore, its use is often limited to an adjunctive role, such as in ruling out a concomitant rotator cuff tear.

Likewise, the roles of magnetic resonance imaging and contrast-enhanced computed tomography are limited to aiding in the diagnosis of additional shoulder pathology, such as a rotator cuff tear or the exact position of hardware that may be impinging on the articular surface.

SURGERY

Anesthesia/Analgesia Management

Adequate anesthesia is a prerequisite for a successful result after an arthroscopic release. Complete muscle paralysis is necessary to allow safe introduction of the arthroscope into a contracted joint. We prefer interscalene regional anesthesia using an indwelling catheter, which remains in place during the procedure and for 48 hours postoperatively. Supplemental sedation with general anesthesia can then be used if desired. Alternatively, if general anesthesia alone is used, complete muscle paralysis is necessary. Postoperative pain control can then be achieved with an intraarticular catheter, which administers long-acting local anesthetic into the joint. Commercial devices are available. In general, we have not found oral, intravenous, or intramuscular pharmacologic management of pain control to be adequate to allow early postoperative motion in most patients.

Surgical Positioning, Prepping, and Draping

We perform arthroscopic capsular release in the beach-chair position because it allows greater mobility of the arm, simple and accurate assessment of passive range of motion, and simple conversion to an open approach if necessary. Some surgeons prefer performing the procedure with the patient in a lateral decubitus position, as they believe that traction allows better visualization.

After positioning the patient on the operating room table in the beach-chair position, assess and document passive range of motion under anesthesia. This allows easy and direct comparison to the range of motion achieved after the capsular release. While the senior author (J.J.P.W.) previously performed a closed manipulation prior to introduction of the arthroscope, this step has been abandoned. Closed manipulation usually resulted in incomplete return of motion but caused hemorrhage into the joint from partial capsular rupture, making visualization difficult. Furthermore, arthroscopic release allows less forceful restoration of joint motion, thus minimizing the risk of fracture and rupture of the rotator cuff tendons, especially in patients who may have stiffness after rotator cuff repair.

Prep the entire upper extremity in a sterile fashion such that the entire shoulder girdle (including the medial border of the scapula) will be in the operative field after draping. We use a mechanical arm holder to maintain the position of the arm and shoulder without requiring an extra surgical assistant (Fig. 10-2).

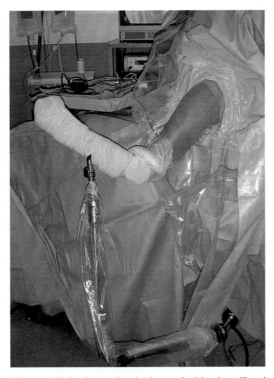

Figure 10-2. A mechanical arm holder is utilized to facilitate positioning during surgery and to minimize the number of assistants necessary.

Technique

After prepping and draping, place the shoulder in neutral rotation (or as close as possible) and palpate and outline the bony landmarks of the shoulder, including the acromion, acromioclavicular (AC) joint, clavicle, and coracoid. The posterior arthroscopic portal is slightly higher (0.5 cm) than routine. The anterior portal is consistently identified by palpating the AC joint and palpating the "soft spot" immediately anterior to it. This soft spot corresponds to the underlying rotator interval and is the preferred location for the anterior portal. Mark the anterior and posterior arthroscopic portal sites and inject them with local anesthetic/epinephrine solution.

Next, insert an 18-gauge spinal needle through the posterior portal site into the glenohumeral joint and inject saline into the joint. After injecting 10 to 15 mL of saline, remove the trocar from the spinal needle. Rapid egress of saline out of the joint confirms intraarticular placement of the needle. Slower reflux suggests placement of the needle into extraarticular soft tissues. After confirmation that the needle is intraarticular, inject 10 to 15 mL more saline. In addition to confirming the intraarticular location of the needle tip, introduction of the spinal needle also confirms the orientation of a tight joint so that the subsequently placed arthroscope can easily duplicate the same trajectory as the needle. Finally, injecting saline into the joint causes slight joint distention, moving the humeral head away from the glenoid and thus minimizing risk of articular cartilage trauma during arthroscope insertion.

Remove the spinal needle, incise the skin with a no. 11 scalpel blade, and duplicate the needle's trajectory with the arthroscope, carefully guiding it over the humeral head. In severe cases of adhesive capsulitis, only the superior portion of the anterior joint is visible because of the capsular contracture. However, the biceps and intraarticular subscapularis tendons, along with the intervening rotator interval, are typically visible (Fig. 10-3). Using the previously marked anterior portal site and under direct arthroscopic visualization, insert the 18-gauge spinal needle into the joint, directly through the rotator interval capsule inferior to the biceps and superior to the subscapularis tendon at a point halfway between the glenoid and the humeral head. Remove the needle, incise the skin with the no. 11 blade, and insert a 6-mm smooth cannula (Figs. 10-4 and 10-5).

If visualization is poor because of hypertrophic synovium, use a 4.5-mm full-radius arthroscopic shaver to clear away just enough tissue to visualize the anterior cannula.

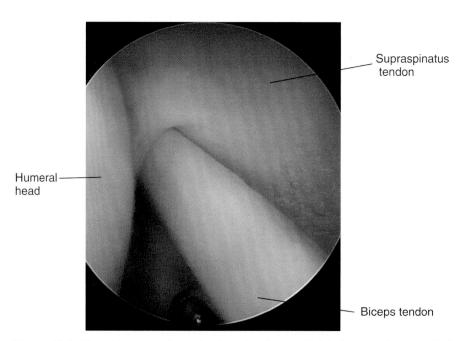

Supraspinatus
tendon

Humeral
head

Biceps tendon

Figure 10-3. Even in a severely contracted glenohumeral joint, the superior aspect of the joint, including the biceps tendon, can be visualized in beginning the release.

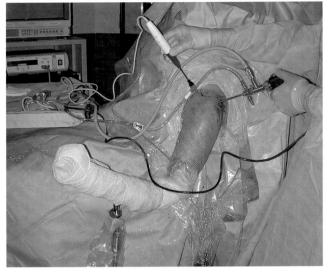

Figure 10-4. The anterior and posterior portals are established.

Avoid overaggressive use of the shaver as this may cause unintended bleeding, obscuring the view. If visualization is adequate, proceed to the capsular release.

The first step is to release the contracture of the rotator interval capsule, anatomically comprised of the superior glenohumeral and the coracohumeral ligaments. Using a hook-tip radiofrequency or electrocautery device, release the contracted capsule immediately above the cannula and below the biceps tendon (Fig. 10-6). Release scarred tissue until the overlying deltoid fibers just become visible. We recommend a "pulling" motion with the hook-tip device facing up to perform the initial release (Fig. 10-7). Next, turn the hook-tip device downward and release the capsule inferiorly to the level of the intraarticular subscapularis tendon using the pulling motion (Figs. 10-8 and 10-9).

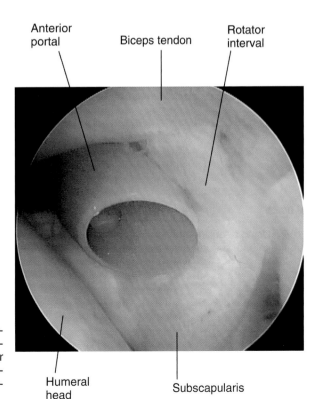

Figure 10-5. The anterior portal is visualized in the rotator interval, between the superior border of the intraarticular subscapularis and the inferior border of the biceps tendon.

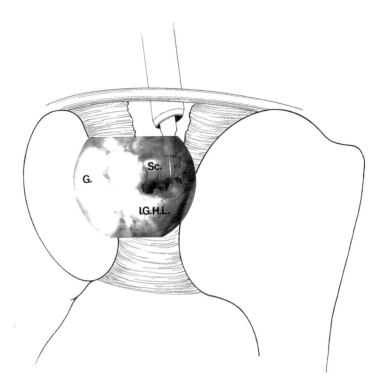

Figure 10-11. Schematic representation of the release of the capsule deep to the subscapularis. Great care must be taken to avoid damage to this tendon while performing the release. *G*, glenoid; *SC*, subscapularis; *IGHL*, inferior glenohumeral ligament.

10-11). Using a "pushing" motion, direct the hook tip away from the overlying subscapularis, turn on the device, and release the capsular scar posterior to the subscapularis. Release the thickened capsular scar until the overlying subscapularis is visualized. Continue inferiorly deep to the subscapularis until the 5-o'clock position on the glenoid (7-o'clock position for a left shoulder) (Figs. 10-12 and 10-13). This marks the lower border of the subscapularis, where the axillary nerve is in close proximity to the capsule and thus at risk for iatrogenic injury.

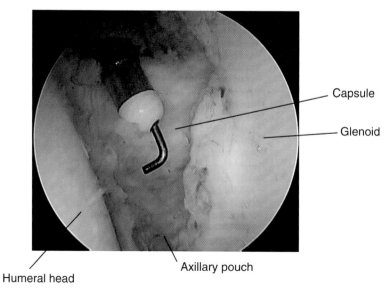

Figure 10-12. The remainder of the anterior capsule is released, to the beginning of the axillary pouch.

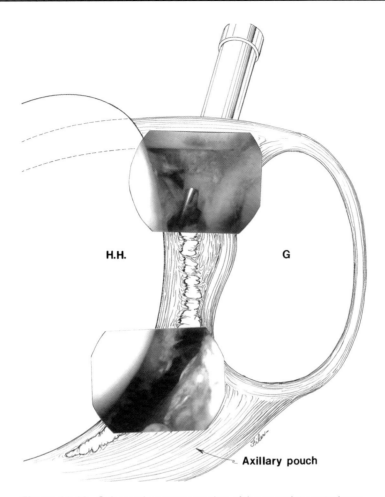

Figure 10-13. Schematic representation of the complete anterior release. Again, great care must be taken to end the release here, to avoid damage to the axillary nerve just inferior to the axillary pouch. *HH*, humeral head; *G*, glenoid.

If the capsular scar is so dense as to preclude visualization of the subscapularis tendon, use the hook-tip device to release the capsule in a posterior-to-anterior direction until the subscapularis tendon and/or muscle belly is visualized. Then, proceed with the anteroinferior release as described above.

In patients with diminished internal rotation requiring posterior capsular release, remove the arthroscopic camera, leaving the cannula inside the joint. Place the camera through the smooth anterior cannula and place the "inflow" into the side port of the anterior cannula. Place a "switching stick" through the posterior cannula and then replace the camera cannula with a smooth 6-mm cannula (Fig. 10-14).

Visualizing the posterior capsule from the anterior portal, introduce the hook-tip device through the posterior portal. Using a similar "pulling" motion with the hook tip, release the posterior capsule in a superior-to-inferior direction, beginning just posterior to the biceps tendon (Fig. 10-15). Continue with the cautery inferiorly until the overlying (posterior) infraspinatus muscle belly becomes visible (Figs. 10-16 and 10-17). Next, turn the hook tip "downward" to release the posterior capsule below the posterior portal, ending the release just posterior to the axillary pouch. The entire extent of the posterior release is from just posterior to the biceps tendon to the 7-o'clock position along the glenoid rim (5-o'clock for a left shoulder). After adequate release with the hook-tip device, use the basket forceps to resect the thickened posterior capsular scar.

After the anterior and posterior releases have been completed, remove the arthroscopic equipment and assess passive range of motion. Motion in all planes will be dramatically

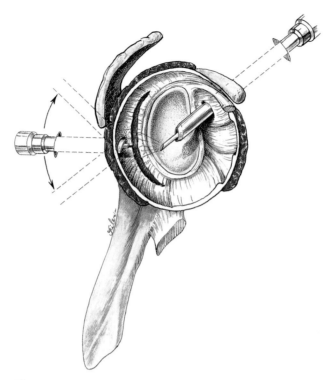

Figure 10-14. The camera and the hook-tip probe are switched in the anterior and posterior portals to begin the posterior release.

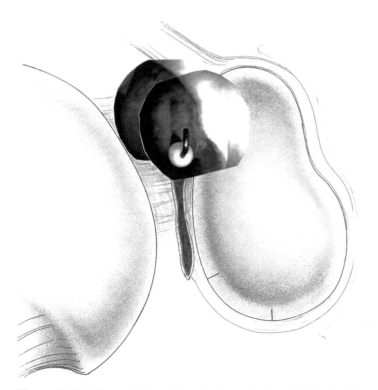

Figure 10-15. The posterior release is begun just posterior to the biceps tendon.

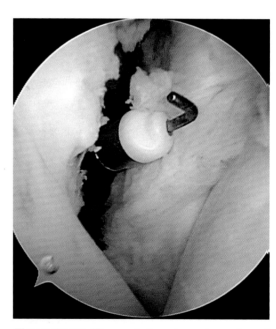

Figure 10-16. The posterior release is continued inferiorly until overlying muscle belly and infraspinatus are visible.

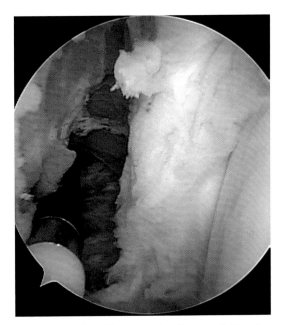

Figure 10-17. The muscle fibers of the infraspinatus are identified posterior to the capsule, indicating an adequate depth of release.

improved. Persistent stiffness may accompany passive flexion because the axillary pouch of the inferior glenohumeral ligament is still intact. However, very gentle force will release this portion of the capsule, thus restoring full range of motion.

The arthroscope is inserted into the subacromial space if the patient has any symptoms of impingement. If the patient has had a subacromial injection of local anesthetic preoperatively and this has alleviated his or her pain with flexion, it suggests irritation of the rotator cuff. Although the patient may not require an acromioplasty because this impingement may be secondary to his or her contracture, a bursectomy may help speed the recovery. Often the bursa is thickened and inflamed although there is no rotator cuff disease.

In cases where stiffness follows prior subacromial surgery, there may be dense adhesions between the acromion and the rotator cuff as well as the deltoid and the rotator cuff. The arthroscope is then introduced into the subacromial space and these adhesions are released. It is helpful to use a radiofrequency device in addition to a motorized shaver because this minimizes bleeding in addition to ablating adhesions. Usually the arthroscope is placed from the posterior portal underneath the acromion and then a radiofrequency device removes adhesions from the rotator cuff and acromion. The shoulder can be rotated to bring adhesions into view so that the radiofrequency device does not need to be moved. Finally the arthroscope can be placed in the lateral portal and either a radiofrequency device or a shaver can be placed in the anterior portal to remove adhesions while the shoulder is rotated. Care is taken to remove adhesions laterally from between the deltoid and the humerus as well as between the acromion and rotator cuff.

Reapproximate the skin edges of the arthroscopic portals and apply a sterile dressing. Place the patient's arm in a sling and apply a cryotherapy device.

POSTOPERATIVE MANAGEMENT

This step is as critical as the arthroscopic release. Adequate analgesia must be available to allow immediate range of motion. This can be accomplished by an interscalene catheter, repeated interscalene block, or intraarticular pain pump. In the recovery room, when the patients are awake, they are shown their postoperative passive range of motion. This helps them understand that now that motion has been recovered, it is their responsibility to maintain these gains. Physical therapy is commenced on the morning of the first postoperative day. The sling is removed and the patients are encouraged to move the arm. Usually they will have a partial motor blockade, and exercises can be demonstrated to perform independently, using the contralateral arm for assistance. The therapist then performs passive motion in all planes. This is done twice daily. Cold therapy in the form of a compressive device helps to control pain and to minimize swelling. It should be worn most of the time during the first 2 days after surgery. It can then be applied after each therapy session. Continuous-passive-motion devices are not usually used because we have found that they are not cost-effective. The patients are discharged on the afternoon of the second postoperative day after the interscalene catheter has been removed. They are encouraged to use their shoulder for daily activities, and no sling is worn.

Rehabilitation

Narcotic pain medicine is prescribed to last 7 to 10 days until the first scheduled follow-up. Formal physical therapy at a prescribed outpatient facility must occur once per day for the next 1 to 2 weeks, and this is supplemented with a home therapy program, which includes a pulley. If a pool or other water environment is available, we encourage water therapy where the patient performs active stretching exercises in the buoyancy of a water environment. After 2 weeks, the therapy program may be adjusted to three times each week if motion gains have been maintained. Strengthening is commenced when the shoulder is pain-free with a reasonably good range of motion. We do not recommend use of an upper bicycle ergometer because we find that it irritates the shoulder as it reproduces the movements most associated with impingement symptoms.

RESULTS

Results of the senior author have been reported elsewhere (17,18), but in general arthroscopic release for refractory idiopathic adhesive capsulitis has a success rate of 94%. Arthroscopic release for postoperative stiffness had a less satisfactory rate but was still in the range of 80% to 90%. This was due to comorbid factors such as articular injury or soft-tissue insufficiency (such as rotator cuff tear). Gerber et al. (1) have reported similar results.

COMPLICATIONS

Complications are rare after arthroscopic capsular release. The most common sequela is persistent stiffness stemming from inadequate postoperative rehabilitation for a variety of reasons, including poor compliance and interscalene block failure. In addition, failure to recognize extracapsular causes of shoulder stiffness may lead to failure of arthroscopic release.

Instability, while theoretically a risk following arthroscopic release, has not proved to be of practical concern. This is due to the overall tight soft-tissue envelope around the glenohumeral joint. Apparently, even with release of a contracted capsule, there is still sufficient joint compression from surrounding tissue tension to provide glenohumeral stability. In the last 250 cases performed by the senior author, there has been no instance of postoperative instability.

Axillary nerve neurapraxia as reported in the literature is rarely seen but has always been in the form of transient numbness or weakness. In the experience of the senior author, this complication has not been encountered.

Anesthetic complications are related to placement of the interscalene catheter and include Horner's sign, transient hemidiaphragm paralysis, pneumothorax, high cervical block with apnea, and transient or permanent causalgia from intraneural injection. It must be emphasized that these complications are directly related to the experience and skill of the anesthesiologist and in our institution there has been only one instance of bothersome burning in the extremity in one out of 500 cases. There have been no pneumothoraces and no high cervical blocks.

RECOMMENDED READING

1. Gerber, C., Espinosa, N., Perren, T.: Arthroscopic treatment of shoulder stiffness. *Clin Orthop* 390: 119–128, 2001.
2. Harryman, D.: Shoulders, frozen and stiff. *Instruct Course Lect* 42: 247–257, 1993.
3. Harryman, D., Matsen, F., Sidles, J.: Arthroscopic management of refractory shoulder stiffness. *Arthroscopy* 13(2): 133–147, 1997.
4. Harryman, D., Sidles, J., Clark, J., et al.: Translation of the humeral head on the glenoid with passive glenohumeral motion. *J Bone Joint Surg Am* 72: 1334–1343, 1990.
5. Harryman, D., Sidles, J., Harris, S., et al.: The role of the rotator interval capsule in passive motion and stability of the shoulder. *J Bone Joint Surg Am* 74: 53–66, 1992.
6. Hawkins, R., Angelo, R.: Glenohumeral osteoarthrosis: a late complication of the Putti-Platt repair. *J Bone Joint Surg Am* 72: 1193–1197, 1990.
7. Holloway, G., Schenk, T., Williams, G., et al.: Arthroscopic capsular release for the treatment of refractory postoperative or post-fracture shoulder stiffness. *J Bone Joint Surg Am* 83: 1682–1687, 2001.
8. Itoi, E., Tabata, S.: Range of motion and arthrography in frozen shoulders. *J Shoulder Elbow Surg* 1: 106–112, 1992.
9. Lazarus, M., Harryman, D.: Complications of open anterior stabilization of the shoulder. *J Am Acad Orthop Surg* 8: 122–132, 2000.
10. MacDonald, P., Hawkins, R., Fowler, P., et al.: Release of the subscapularis for internal rotation contracture and pain after anterior repair for recurrent anterior dislocation of the shoulder. *J Bone Joint Surg Am* 74: 734–737, 1992.
11. Naranja, R., Iannotti, J.: Surgical options in the treatment of arthritis of the shoulder: alternatives to prosthetic arthroplasty. *Semin Arthroplasty* 6: 204–213, 1995.
12. Neviaser, R., Neviaser, T.: The frozen shoulder, diagnosis and management. *Clin Orthop* 223: 59–64, 1987.
13. Pollock, R., Duralde, X., Flatow, E., et al.: The use of arthroscopy in the treatment of resistant frozen shoulder. *Clin Orthop* 304: 30–36, 1994.
14. Pollock, R., Owens, J., Flatow, E., et al.: Operative results of the inferior capsular shift procedure for multidirectional instability of the shoulder. *J Bone Joint Surg Am* 82: 919–928, 2000.
15. Ticker, J., Beim, G., Warner, J.: Recognition and treatment of refractory posterior capsular contracture of the shoulder. *Arthroscopy* 16: 27–34, 2000.
16. Warner, J.: Frozen shoulder: diagnosis and management. *J Am Acad Orthop Surg* 5: 130–140, 1997.
17. Warner, J., Allen, A., Marks, P., et al.: Arthroscopic release for chronic refractory adhesive capsulitis of the shoulder. *J Bone Joint Surg Am* 78: 1808–1816, 1996.
18. Warner, J., Greis, P.: The treatment of stiffness of the shoulder after repair of the rotator cuff. *J Bone Joint Surg Am* 79: 1260–1269, 1997.
19. Warner, J., Johnson, D., Miller, M., et al.: Technique for selecting capsular tightness in repair of anterior-inferior shoulder instability. *J Shoulder Elbow Surg* 4: 352–364, 1995.

11

Arthroscopic Calcium Excision

Steven Klepps, Chunyan Jiang, and Evan L. Flatow

INDICATIONS/CONTRAINDICATIONS

Calcific deposits in the rotator cuff with associated tendinitis are a common cause of shoulder pain, peaking in the fourth and fifth decades of life. Symptomatic calcifications are usually located on or within the supraspinatus tendon adjacent to the insertion on the greater tuberosity but can be associated with tendons of the subscapularis, infraspinatus, and teres minor. The etiology of this condition remains unclear. Uhthoff (17,18) have stated that the calcifications are a cell-mediated response with minimal degenerative etiology, whereas others think there is a significant degenerative component (4). Calcific tendonitis generally runs a self-limited course not requiring surgical intervention (7,10). Some patients, however, have symptoms that do not completely resolve with nonoperative treatment.

Many authors have described different stages of the calcification process, usually termed "formative," "resorptive," and "chronic" (3,5,18). In the formative phase, calcium crystals are deposited in matrix vesicles and the calcium appears chalklike if removed. The resorptive phase is characterized by spontaneous resorption of calcium with an influx of macrophages and multinucleated giant cells. In this stage, the calcium deposit can be grossly characterized as thick and creamy. It is during this phase that pain usually occurs and patients seek medical attention. The chronic phase is generally defined as persistent symptoms and radiographic evidence of calcific tendonitis that does not resolve within 6 months.

Much has been written about nonsurgical treatment of both acute and chronic calcific tendonitis. Initial treatment, regardless of stage, is frequently direct needling of the lesion

S. Klepps, M.D.: Orthopedic Associates, Yellowstone Medical Center, Billings, Montana.

C. Jiang, M.D., PH.D.: Shoulder Service, Department of Orthopedic Trauma, School of Medicine, Peking University; and Beijing Ji Shui Tan Hospital, Beijing, People's Republic of China.

E. L. Flatow, M.D.: Department of Orthopaedics, Mount Sinai School of Medicine; and Mount Sinai Hospital, New York, New York.

followed by nonsteroidal antiinflammatory drugs and physical therapy. An 18-gauge needle is used for placing multiple stabs within the calcific deposit, which is localized both by identification of the point of maximal tenderness and by plain radiography. After needling, an injection of lidocaine, Marcaine, and steroid is placed within the subacromial space to alleviate the pain and the inflammatory reaction stimulated by the release of the calcium. Multiple studies have reported success using this treatment (5,14) (Fig. 11-1). The injection may be repeated unless the patient receives no relief from the initial injection. The indications for surgical intervention differ in patients who have acute calcific tendonitis versus those with chronic calcific tendonitis. In acute calcific tendonitis, if the patient has failed to respond to direct needling and antiinflammatory medication, surgical intervention should be considered. In a patient who presents with chronic shoulder pain and evidence of chronic calcific tendonitis, nonoperative treatment, including medication, injection, and rehabilitation efforts, may be considered for a minimum of 6 months.

Another option for patients in the acute stage of disease who have failed to obtain relief from the injection is the use of shock-wave therapy (11,15,19). Although promising short-term and midterm results have been reported in acute and chronic conditions, no large series or long-term results have been described. This may be especially useful in patients in the acute phase who have failed conservative treatment.

The contraindications for surgical treatment of acute or chronic calcific tendonitis are few but include patients not considered medically stable and those whose level of symptoms do not warrant surgical treatment. In those patients in whom chronic calcific tendonitis is accompanied by a painful limitation of range of motion and who have failed nonoperative treatment, surgical treatment may include addressing the limited range of motion by manipulation, lysis of adhesions, or selective capsular releases.

Although open techniques have been successful (3,4), there are several advantages to the arthroscopic technique, including (a) better evaluation of the entire glenohumeral joint and rotator cuff status; (b) ability to assess the subacromial space for evidence of an impingement lesion as well as to perform a decompression; and (c) reduced disruption of the deltoid with less likely morbidity (1,2,8). An investigation comparing conservative treatment to surgical treatment for calcifying tendonitis was reported by Wittenberg et al. (20). In that study, 100 patients underwent a matched-pair analysis. The authors concluded that conser-

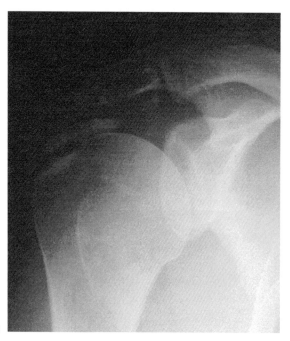 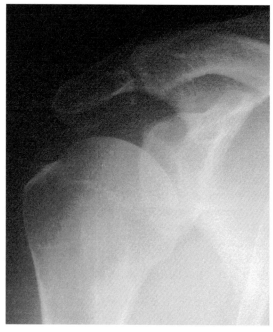

A   B

Figure 11-1. A: Anteroposterior radiograph with evidence of calcification within the supraspinatus. **B:** Calcification resolved completely 4 months after needling as shown on the anteroposterior radiograph.

vative treatment for calcifying tendonitis leads to less favorable long-term results than surgical treatment. Surgery shortens the painful period and may reduce the number of future rotator cuff ruptures.

PREOPERATIVE PLANNING

There are few conditions in orthopaedic surgery as dramatically painful as acute calcific tendonitis of the shoulder. The patient frequently gives a history of some increase in activity followed by the onset of shoulder pain, which, gradually, over a period of several hours or days, becomes progressively severe and incapacitating. The patient frequently will hold the arm in a protected position, as any voluntary movement is exquisitely painful. Range of motion is difficult to test because of the severity of pain, and there is often guarding and muscle spasm. The tendon that is involved in the acute process is usually exquisitely tender; this may be a helpful sign for localization of the involved tendon and for localization of the needle to aspirate the calcium acutely. The patient who presents with chronic shoulder pain and associated chronic calcific tendonitis is often unable to be thoroughly examined to assess range of motion, strength, and point of maximal tenderness. Patients who have chronic calcific tendonitis and who have normal passive range of motion may exhibit many of the findings of subacromial impingement, including a positive impingement sign and pain with movement of the involved tendon under the coracoacromial arch. Because of this, it is difficult to separate noncalcific subacromial impingement syndrome from that which is associated with chronic calcific tendonitis.

Diagnostic imaging is helpful in localizing the calcium deposit. A routine shoulder series is performed, including anteroposterior views in the frontal and scapular plane and, if necessary, in internal and external rotation (Figs. 11-2 and 11-3) as well as an axillary and supraspinatus outlet view (Fig. 11-4A–C). Magnetic resonance imaging (MRI) and computed tomography scans (Fig. 11-4D) may also aid in locating the calcium deposit.

If time has elapsed between the initial radiograph showing calcific deposit and surgical treatment, it is wise to repeat a radiographic series, since ongoing shoulder pain may persist from bursitis and subacromial scarring, even if no radiographic evidence of calcium exists. An up-to-date radiographic series may permit the frustrating operative search for an already-resorbed calcium deposit.

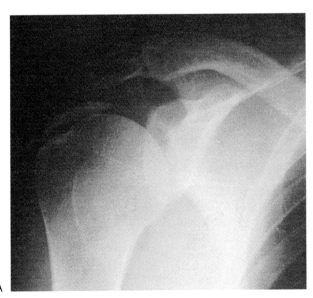 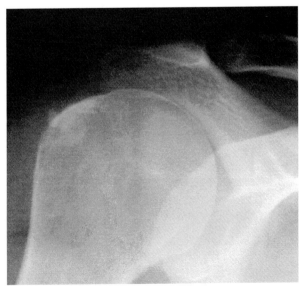

A   B

Figure 11-2. Calcification within the supraspinatus seen on the anteroposterior views in external rotation **(A)** and internal rotation **(B).**

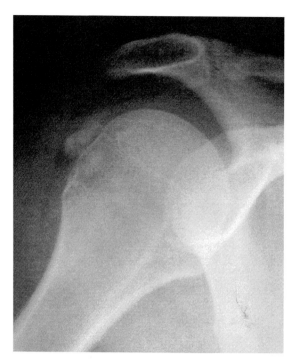

Figure 11-3. The anteroposterior view in internal rotation can also show the calcification posteriorly within the infraspinatus.

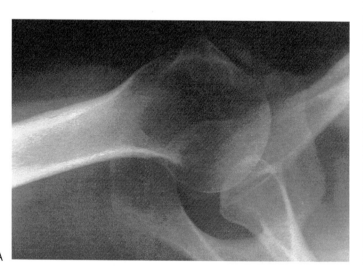

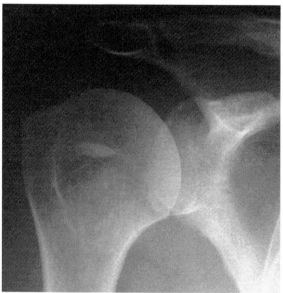

A

B

Figure 11-4. Axillary **(A)**, external rotation anteroposterior **(B)**, and outlet **(C)** views show the calcification in the subscapularis anterior to the lesser tuberosity on the axillary and outlet views and superimposed behind the center of the head on the anteroposterior view. *(continued)*

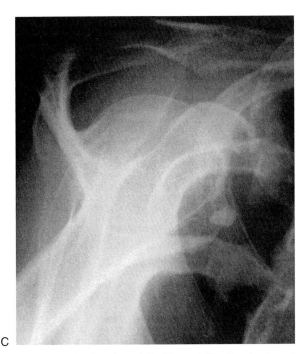

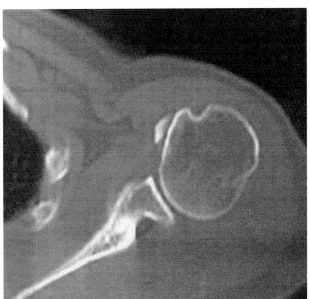

C

D

Figure 11-4. *Continued.* **D:** The calcification is also visualized in the computed tomography scan anterior to the lesser tuberosity.

The calcium deposit is evaluated for location and evidence of homogeneity (6). Most calcium deposits requiring surgery are located in the supraspinatus tendon. In addition, to localize the calcium, the outlet view is used for determining the acromial morphology and the presence of any subacromial osteophytes. Less commonly, the deposits may be located within the infraspinatus seen posteriorly.

Before the surgical procedure, the patient should undergo MRI (Fig. 11-5) or ultrasound to evaluate for associated lesions, especially rotator cuff defects, as the physical examination may be difficult to interpret. If there is concern that intraoperative localization may be difficult (i.e., the subscapularis), preoperative ultrasonographic mapping can be considered (16). However, we do not routinely perform this step in our patients and have found the combination of multiple radiographic views and an MRI provides adequate localization.

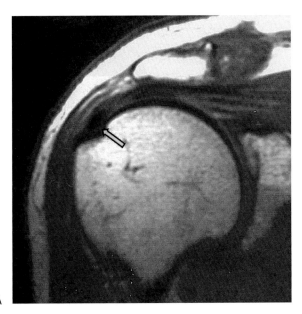

Figure 11-5. Magnetic resonance imaging shows the calcification as a blackened area on the coronal **(A)**, sagittal view. *(continued)*

A

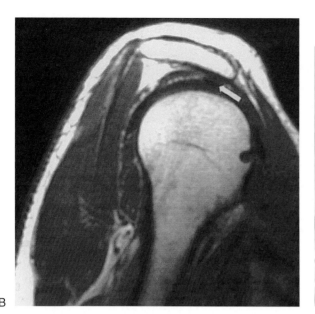

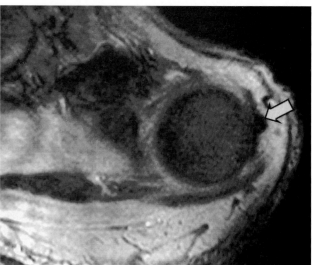

B   C

Figure 11-5. *Continued.* Magnetic resonance imaging shows the calcification as a blackened area on the sagittal **(B)**, and axial **(C)** views.

The decision to perform subacromial decompression is based on multiple factors, including the radiographic appearance of the acromion and the arthroscopic appearance of the subacromial space. We have retrospectively studied our patients undergoing this procedure and found a similar outcome for patients undergoing calcium excision alone and those undergoing both calcium excision and decompression (2). Although this may indicate that decompression is not necessary, we believe it more likely shows that based on clinical, radiographic, and arthroscopic findings, we are currently selecting the proper patients for concomitant decompression and the correct patients for calcium excision alone. Young patients with episodic flares of pain, normal rotator cuff tendons on MRI and arthroscopic inspection, and normal acromial architecture are treated by calcium excision alone. Older patients with a long, chronic history may have secondary subacromial scarring and cuff defects. These patients also undergo decompression if they have a prominent acromial spur or attritional changes on the acromial undersurface at the time of arthroscopy.

SURGERY

Instrumentation

Equipment includes the standard arthroscopic equipment along with a spinal needle, an arthroscopic knife, and a curette. If exposing the deposit results in a large or deep defect in the tendon, a repair of the tendon should be considered and the equipment for a tendon repair should be available. However, we generally prefer to not repair the tendon thus allowing further leakage and resolution of the calcium deposit.

Positioning

We perform the procedure with an interscalene regional block with the patient in the beach-chair position. All bony prominences are carefully padded. An antibiotic, usually a cephalosporin unless contraindicated, is administered preoperatively. An examination under anesthesia is documented prior to the usual preparation and draping of the extremity, specifically looking for reduced range of motion. The bony landmarks of the shoulder, including the acromion, acromioclavicular joint, and coracoid, as well as the planned portal sites, are marked on the skin with a marking pen. The skin around the portals is infiltrated with local anesthetic containing equal parts short- and long-acting local anesthetic with epinephrine. Local infiltration is also placed along the posterior axilla, over the acromioclavicular joint, and along the anterior axilla to supplement the interscalene block and assist with hemostasis. We typically use 20 mL of agent to supplement the interscalene block. In addition, 5 mL of epinephrine in a 1:1000 solution is injected into each 3-L bag of arthroscopic saline solution distributed with an arthroscopic pump, usually set at 40 mm Hg.

Surgical Technique

The posterior soft spot of the shoulder is palpated. This is approximately 2 cm inferior and 1 cm medial to the posterior lateral corner of the acromion. Because most of the work is to be carried out in the subacromial space, the posterior portal can be placed slightly more superior than normal if desired to facilitate placement of the arthroscope into this space. This allows easier maneuvering above the humeral head. The arthroscope is placed into the glenohumeral joint, and the anterior portal is placed lateral to the coracoid process. A careful inspection of the glenohumeral joint is carried out and any additional pathologic changes are identified and treated appropriately. A probe is used to allow adequate evaluation of the rotator cuff and the biceps tendon.

The undersurface of the rotator cuff, particularly in the area of the suspected calcium deposit, should be carefully inspected for any suspicious bulge, area of hyperemia, or signs of damage (Fig 11-6). If a suspicious area is identified, an 18-gauge spinal needle is inserted directly through or adjacent to this portion of the rotator cuff from a lateral entry. Frequently, flecks of calcium can be seen in the bore of the needle if correct localization is achieved (Fig. 11-7). A colored, absorbable, size 0 monofilament suture [polydioxanone synthetic (PDS) suture; Ethicon Inc., Somerville, NJ] is placed as a marking stitch (Fig. 11-8). If the deposit is not visualized, landmarks such as the biceps, acromion, and greater tuberosity can be used to locate the deposit on the basis of its position on preoperative radiographs and MRI.

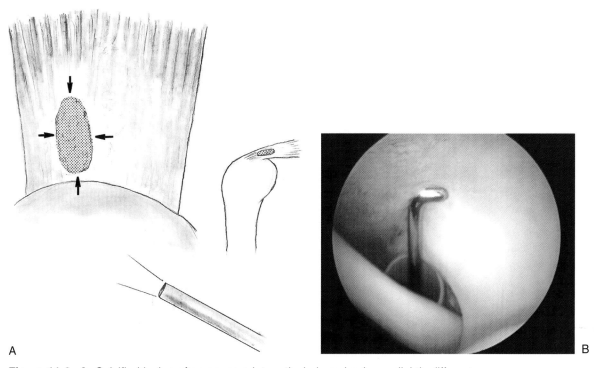

A   B

Figure 11-6. A: Calcified lesion often appears intraarticularly as having a slightly different color from the surrounding tendon. **B:** When palpated, this area may feel firmer than surrounding area.

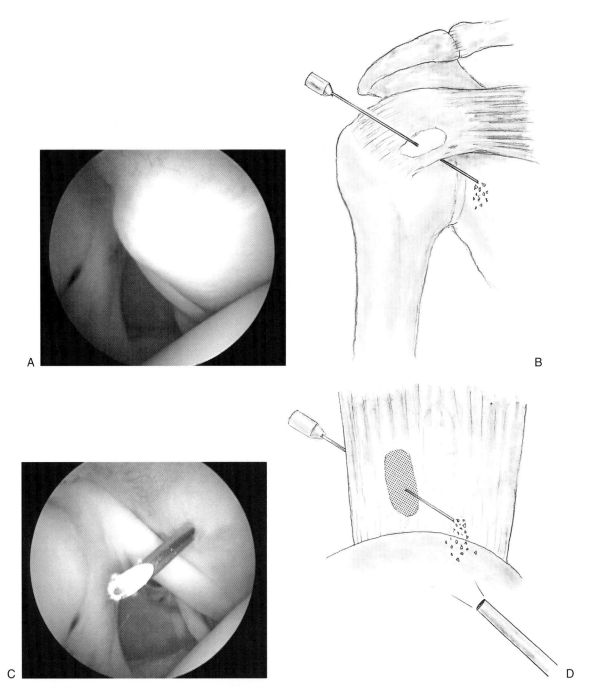

Figure 11-7. A: Hardened calcific area appears to "bulge" when viewed intraarticularly. **B:** Needle is introduced so it emerges through area of suspected calcification. If a clearcut area of abnormal tendon is not seen, multiple "trial-and-error'" passes may be helpful. **C:** Calcification is seen in the bore of entering needle. **D:** Calcium seen in suspected area. Needle is left in place for passage of marking suture.

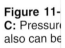

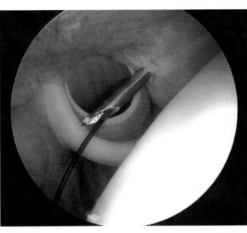

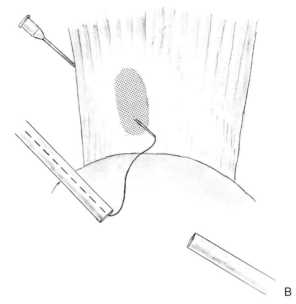

A   B

Figure 11-8. A: Polydioxanone synthetic (PDS) suture (Ethicon Inc., Somerville, NJ) is passed through bore of needle to mark calcific area for later subacromial identification. **B:** Once the intraarticular suture end is grasped and brought out anterior portal, the needle can be withdrawn because the calcific area has been marked.

A

**Figure 11-
C:** Pressure
also can be

more invol·
arthroscopi
by the teno
activity leve
depth of the
of removal
may be left
very difficu
cium remov
need to be c
preference i
the damage
mit extrava
paired; we
the greater
or with a "r

If there i
ence, consi

To deter
tively revie
than 50% e
between the
pain was re

Through the anterior portal, a grasper is used to retrieve the intraarticular limb of the suture. Careful planning is used to keep the lateral entry of the suture away from the site of the lateral portal that will be created to perform the subacromial portion of the procedure. We also take into account the confines of the bursa when placing the marking suture, as the posterior margin of the bursa is usually located near the midportion of the acromion. If the suture is placed outside the bursa, usually posteriorly, it will be more difficult to identify. If the calcific deposit is located more posteriorly, this may be unavoidable.

After the glenohumeral joint has been adequately inspected and débrided, the arthroscopic cannula is redirected into the subacromial space using the same posterior portal. Wide, sweeping motions are made to clear the bursa, particularly in the lateral subacromial and subdeltoid area, to facilitate visualization for creation of the lateral portal.

A lateral portal is established under direct visualization with the aid of an 18-gauge spinal needle. This is usually placed at the junction of the anterior and middle thirds of the lateral acromion (often in line with the posterior aspect of the acromioclavicular joint), and distally enough from the lateral edge of the acromion (2 to 3 cm) with the arm adducted, so that instruments can enter the subacromial space easily. The subacromial space is cleared of most of the bursa using a full radius shaver and a bipolar cautery unit, to ensure complete visualization.

Once the veil of bursa is removed, the rotator cuff can be evaluated for tears, calcium deposits, and suture location (Fig. 11-9). Internal and external rotation as well as abduction of the humerus may be needed to bring the involved area of the tendon into clear view and within easy access from the lateral portal. If the calcium deposit is not easily identified, an 18-gauge spinal needle is used to penetrate the rotator cuff in the region of the marking stitch until the calcium deposit become apparent. If a marking suture has not been placed, the bursal surface of the tendon is inspected for a suspicious bulge, an area of hyperemia, or any signs of damage. It is then needled to identify the calcium deposit. If a particular area is suspected, further bursa can be removed to expose more of the tendon. In addition, the preoperative imaging studies should be available in the operating room for further review.

As the deposit is opened using an arthroscopic blade or curette, calcium is liberated and will often be seen as a "snowstorm" effect. With the precise location of the calcium identified, an attempt is made to remove the entire deposit. A knife is used to make the initial tenotomy in the tendon longitudinally, directly over the deposit (Fig. 11-10). An attempt is tioned the need for calcium excision and recommend only subacromial decompression. However, we believe that as much calcium as possible should be removed, and other studies have shown better results when the entire calcification is removed (9,13). When no calcium is identified, we strongly consider performing subacromial decompression, again depending on the patient's age and acromial appearance.

As a final step, the subacromial space is irrigated to flush out any remaining calcium crystals that could potentially cause inflammation. The arthroscopic instruments are removed, and the portals are closed with absorbable sutures. Sterile dressings are applied, and the arm is placed in a sling.

POSTOPERATIVE MANAGEMENT

Appropriate analgesia is important to diminish pain during the early postoperative period as well as during rehabilitation. A series of radiographs are obtained at the first postoperative visit to demonstrate the removal of the calcium.

Unless a rotator cuff tear has been repaired, rehabilitation is much the same as that following an arthroscopic acromioplasty. Full passive range-of-motion exercises as well as active-assisted range-of-motion exercises using a stick or pulleys are begun immediately. Patients with calcific tendonitis are especially prone to stiffness and must be encouraged to perform these exercises frequently (four or five times daily). These exercises are progressively increased as tolerated to restore full range of motion as promptly and as comfortably as possible. In general, patients are encouraged to use the arm as normally as possible, within the range of comfort. Patients who undergo rotator cuff repair are not allowed active motion for the first 6 weeks.

When full range of motion has been restored and pain is controlled, active exercises are initiated with progression to a resistive strengthening exercise program. The goal is to have the patient using the arm for light activities of daily living by 2 to 3 weeks and involved in normal activities by 2 to 3 months. Return to upper-extremity sports or activities may require additional time for specific strengthening and functional rehabilitation. Occasionally, postoperative inflammation limits a patient's progress. When this occurs, nonsteroidal antiinflammatory medications and/or, in certain cases, a subacromial injection with a steroid may be beneficial.

COMPLICATIONS

Complications specific to calcium release include failure to provide relief, rotator cuff tendon disruption or damage, deltoid damage, and postoperative capsulitis. All can be avoided or managed with meticulous attention to detail, surgical technique, and appropriate rehabilitation.

Bicipital tendonitis may complicate calcifying tendonitis. Depalma and Kruper (5) reported biceps symptoms in 16 of 136 patients treated for calcific tendonitis. Frozen shoulder may also occur in association with calcific tendonitis. Therefore, it is important to achieve near-normal motion intraoperatively whether by associated manipulation, arthroscopic lysis of lesions, or limited capsular releases. In addition, the patient should undergo an aggressive program of postoperative exercises to maintain range of motion. Recurrence of calcific lesion is rather rare: Uhthoff and Loehr (17) reported only one case in a series of 127 patients who underwent surgery.

RECOMMENDED READING

1. Ark, J.W., Flock, T.J., Flatow, E.L., et al.: Arthroscopic treatment of calcific tendonitis of the shoulder. *Arthroscopy* 8: 183–188, 1992.
2. Arroyo, J., Flatow, E., Bigliani, L.: Calcific tendonitis of the rotator cuff: long term follow-up of arthroscopic excision. Arthroscopy Association of North America annual proceedings, 1997.

A

A

3. Bosworth, D.M.: The supraspinatus syndrome: symptomatology, pathology and repair. *JAMA* 1177: 422–428, 1941.
4. Codman, E.A.: *The shoulder: rupture of the supraspinatus tendon and other lesions in or about the subacromial bursa.* Boston: Thomas Todd, 1934.
5. Depalma, A., Kruper, J.: Long term study of shoulder joints afflicted with and treated for calcific tendinitis. *Clin Orthop* 20: 61–72, 1961.
6. Gazielly, D.F., Gleyze, P., Montagnon, C., et al.: Functional and anatomical results after surgical treatment of ruptures of the rotator cuff, II: postoperative functional and anatomical evaluation of ruptures of the rotator cuff. *Rev Chir Orthop Reparatrice Appar Mot* 81: 17–26, 1995.
7. Geschwend, N., Patte, D., Zippel, J.: Therapy of calcific tendinitis of the shoulder. *Arch Orthop Unfallchir* 73: 120–135, 1972.
8. Gleyze, P., Kempf, J.: Clinical and anatomic results of a series of 20 rotator cuff ruptures treated with endoscopic stapler. *Acta Orthop Belg* 61[Suppl 1]: 32–36, 1995.
9. Jerosch, J., Strauss, J.M., Schmiel, S.: Arthroscopic treatment of calcific tendinitis of the shoulder. *J Shoulder Elbow Surg* 7: 30–37, 1998.
10. Litchman, H.M., Silver, C.M., Simon, S.D.: The surgical management of calcific tendinitis of the shoulder: an analysis of 100 consecutive cases. *Int Surg* 50: 474–479, 1968.
11. Loew, M., Daecke W., Kusnierczak D., et al.: Shock-wave therapy is effective for chronic calcifying tendinitis of the shoulder. *J Bone Joint Surg Br* 81: 863–867, 1999.
12. Marra, G., et al.: Calcific tendinitis of the rotator cuff in long term follow-up of arthroscopic excision. *Orthop Trans* 22: 6–7, 1998.
13. Mole, D., Kempf, J.F., Gleyze, P., et al.: Results of endoscopic treatment of non-broken tendinopathies of the rotator cuff, II: calcifications of the rotator cuff. *Rev Chir Orthop Reparatrice Appar Mot* 79: 532–541, 1993.
14. Pfister, J., Gerber, H.: Chronic calcifying tendinitis of the shoulder-therapy by percutaneous needle aspiration and lavage: prospective open study of 62 shoulders. *Clin Rheumatol* 16: 269–274, 1997.
15. Rompe, J.D., Zoellner, J., Nafe, B.: Shock wave therapy versus conventional surgery in the treatment of calcifying tendinitis of the shoulder. *Clin Orthop* 387: 72–82, 2001.
16. Rupp, S., Seil, R., Kohn, D.: Preoperative ultrasonographic mapping of calcium deposits facilitates localization during arthroscopic surgery for calcifying tendinitis of the rotator cuff. *Arthroscopy* 14: 540–542, 1998.
17. Uhthoff, H.K.: Calcifying tendinitis, an active cell-mediated calcification. *Virchows Arch Pathol Anat Histol* 66: 51–58, 1975.
18. Uhthoff, H.K., Loehr, J.W.: Calcific tendinopathy of the rotator cuff: pathogenesis, diagnosis, and management. *J Am Acad Orthop Surg* 5: 183–191, 1997.
19. Wang, C.J., Ko, J.Y., Chen, H.S.: Treatment of calcifying tendinitis of the shoulder with shock wave therapy. *Clin Orthop* 387: 83–89, 2001.
20. Wittenberg, R.H., Rubenthaler, F., Wolk, T., et al.: Surgical or conservative treatment for chronic rotator cuff calcifying tendinitis: a matched-pair analysis of 100 patients. *Arch Orthop Trauma Surg* 121: 56–59, 2001.

12

Arthroscopic Repair of Labral and SLAP Lesions

Stephen J. Snyder and Earl J. Kilbride

INDICATIONS/CONTRAINDICATIONS

Superior labrum anterior and posterior (SLAP) lesions of the shoulder are defined as injuries to the superior glenoid labrum anterior and posterior to the biceps. Before the advent and common usage of magnetic resonance imaging (MRI) and shoulder arthroscopy, superior labral lesions were difficult to diagnose and even harder to successfully treat. The indications for arthroscopic repair of SLAP lesions can be somewhat ambiguous.

1. *Mechanical symptoms and MRI diagnosis of labral pathology.* Classically, labral involvement occurs after a fall on an abducted arm, causing compression or twisting of the joint. When patients exhibit this specific mechanism of injury, mechanical symptoms, and MRI findings suggestive of a labral tear, arthroscopy will often confirm the pathology and allow arthroscopic repair techniques.
2. *Suspected labral pathology in the face of known coexisting shoulder abnormalities.* In this group of patients, superior labral tears may not be suspected preoperatively but are visualized intraoperatively. The concurrent shoulder pathology must be addressed to ensure satisfactory results.
3. *Refractory intraarticular symptoms with inconclusive diagnostic studies.* Unfortunately, this situation occurs commonly. The history, physical examination, and radiographic studies fail to confirm any particular diagnosis. These patients are often treated with injections and/or sent for a trial of therapy, with unacceptable results. The decision to proceed with diagnostic arthroscopy is a result of continued symptoms.

S. J. Snyder, M.D.: Center for Learning Arthroscopic Skills, Southern California Orthopedic Institute; Southern California Orthopedic Research and Education; and Center for Orthopedic Surgery, Inc., Van Nuys, California.

E. J. Kilbride, M.D.: Department of Orthopaedics, Southern California Orthopaedic Institute, Van Nuys, California.

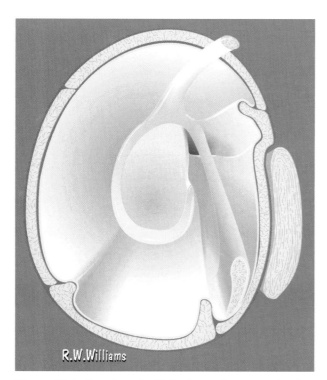

Figure 12-1. Drawing of a Buford complex, a rare but important anatomic formation. It is often mistaken for a pathologic labral detachment. (From Snyder, S.J.: Diagnostic arthroscopy of the shoulder: normal anatomy and variations. In: *Shoulder arthroscopy,* 2nd ed. Philadelphia: Lippincott Williams & Wilkins, 22–38, 2003.)

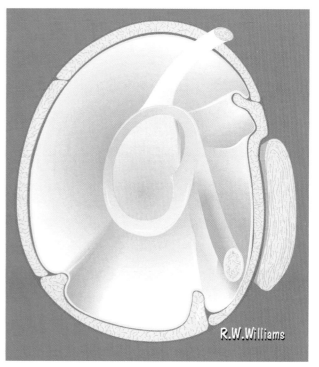

Figure 12-2. Drawing of a sublabral foramen. The cordlike middle glenohumeral ligament may attach to the superior labrum, often with an underlying sublabral hole. (From Snyder, S.J.: Diagnostic arthroscopy of the shoulder: normal anatomy and variations. In: *Shoulder arthroscopy,* 2nd ed. Philadelphia: Lippincott Williams & Wilkins, 22–38, 2003.)

The relative contraindications to arthroscopic SLAP repair are as follows:

1. Arthroscopic repair of labral lesions will not give consistent long-term successful results in the face of concurrent untreated shoulder pathology such as instability.
2. Patients with anatomic variants such as a Buford complex (Fig. 12-1) or a sublabral foramen (Fig. 12-2) must be identified. Preoperative MR arthrography can facilitate their recognition. When these conditions are treated as pathologic entities rather than anatomic variants, the results are always suboptimal.
3. True SLAP lesions are a disease of the young adult. Although repairable SLAP lesions can exist in the older population, arthroscopic repair of these abnormalities as an isolated diagnosis should be undertaken with caution because their symptoms are most likely due to other etiologies.

PREOPERATIVE PLANNING

The labrum performs multiple functions. As a result, it can be injured by a multitude of mechanisms such as compression, traction, avulsion, and attrition. Typically, patients with symptomatic labral pathology are young. There may be a history of trauma, either acute such as a fall or chronic as in throwers. SLAP lesions often coexist with other shoulder pathology such as instability, impingement, rotator cuff tear, or acromioclavicular (AC) joint arthropathy.

A comprehensive physical examination is essential. The examiner should begin with inspection from both anterior and posterior. Muscle atrophy, especially in the supraspinatus or infraspinatus muscle locations, should be documented. Palpation for tenderness should include the bony anatomy, soft tissues, and musculature. A thorough cervical spine examination must be performed. Range of motion and strength must be tested.

Superior labral pathology can often be revealed by a variety of tests. The biceps tension test is performed by resisting shoulder flexion with the shoulder forward flexed at 90 degrees, the elbow extended, and the forearm supinated. A painful response is suggestive of biceps involvement. The compression rotation test described by Andrews et al. (1) is essentially the McMurray test of the shoulder. While the shoulder is abducted to 90 degrees and a compressive load is applied to the glenohumeral joint, the humerus is internally and externally rotated in an attempt to catch a loose labral fragment. Kibler (6) described the anterior slide test, which is performed with the patient's hands on the hips. The examiner applies a superior force to the patient's elbow while the patient resists. A positive test elicits pain or popping. O'Brien et al. (9) report that the active compression test has a high sensitivity. The patient places his or her shoulder in 90 degrees of flexion, 15 degrees of adduction, and maximal internal rotation. The examiner then applies a downward force, which is repeated with the arm in supination. Pain that decreases in supination is a positive finding. Mimori et al. (8) reported a test similar to that of O'Brien et al., but the arm is abducted 90 degrees and the shoulder is externally rotated. A downward force is applied with maximal forearm pronation and supination. Like the test of O'Brien et al., an increase in pain with pronation is a positive finding.

Berg and Ciullo (2) recently described the SLAPprehension test, which was 87.5% sensitive for unstable SLAP tears. In that test, the arm is adducted across the chest with the elbow extended and the forearm fully pronated. It is then repeated in full forearm supination. A positive result is present when popping, clicking, or pain is demonstrated to a greater extent in full pronation.

Finally, the examination must contain tests for concurrent shoulder pathology. Specific tests for impingement, AC involvement, instability, and biceps tendonitis should be performed and judicious use of injections is encouraged.

As with most shoulder pathology, conventional radiographs are often performed on patients with labral lesions. The images must be evaluated for coexisting shoulder disease such as arthritis, impingement, AC arthropathy, dislocation, neoplasms, and calcific tendonitis. Ianotti and Wang demonstrated an uncommon entity of superior glenoid tubercle fracture in patients with SLAP lesions. Otherwise, plain radiographs are not specific for labral involvement. Computed tomography scans, even without intraarticular contrast, better reveal bony anatomy. Ultrasonography plays no role in the diagnosis of labral disease. MRI is useful in soft-tissue evaluation of the shoulder. The intraarticular injection of gadolinium enhances the ability to visualize labral pathology and normal anatomic variants. In short, the usual course of evaluation includes plain radiography and MRI with or without gadolinium. However, definitive diagnosis most often is performed arthroscopically.

SURGERY

Preparing the Patient

With the patient placed in the lateral decubitus position, the anesthesiologist turns the table to a 45-degree angle. The arthroscopic video equipment tower is on the anterior side of the table, in clear view of the surgeon. The irrigation tower, arthroscopy pump, and electrosurgical power unit are also located on the anterior side of the patient, where the surgeon can clearly see them. We routinely put these items toward the feet of the patient (Fig. 12-3).

We use two Mayo stands and a back table for instruments. Mayo stand number one contains the instruments needed to delineate the surgical anatomy and enter the joint. Mayo stand number two has the mechanical and electrical operating equipment to be used in the procedure. Also on it are the remote controls for the video and arthroscopic equipment as well as some of the more commonly used instruments such as a probe, a grasper, and baskets. The back table contains the remainder of surgical equipment and instruments.

Unless medically contraindicated, we prefer to use general anesthetic with most arthroscopic shoulder procedures. After administration of the anesthetic, the patient is placed in the lateral decubitus position. We are diligent in the padding of all bony prominences, ensuring safe cervical alignment, and using an axillary roll. The patient is then tilted posteriorly approximately 15 degrees and the beanbag is deflated to hold this position.

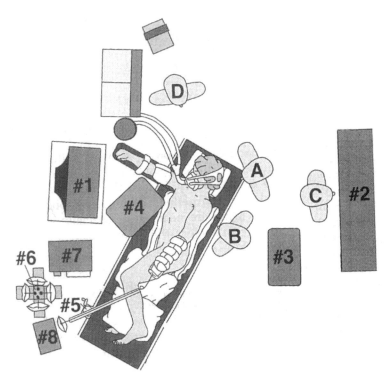

Figure 12-3. Overview of the operating room layout for should arthroplastic surgery with the patient in the lateral decubitus position. *A,* surgical assistant; *B,* surgeon; *C,* scrub nurse; *D,* anesthesiologist; *1,* video cart with television monitor, video recorder, camera and light source, and shaver power system; *2,* auxiliary instrument table; *3,* Mayo stand no. 1; *4,* Mayo stand no. 2; *5,* traction apparatus for arm support; *6,* adjustable irrigation tower; *7,* electrosurgical power unit; *8,* arthroscopic pump. (From Snyder, S.J.: Diagnostic arthroscopy of the shoulder: normal anatomy and variations. In: *Shoulder arthroscopy,* 2nd ed. Philadelphia: Lippincott Williams & Wilkins, 22–38, 2003.)

An electrosurgical grounding pad is placed on the patient's lateral thigh. Nonsterile drapes are then used to isolate the surgical field. We apply a plastic U-drape first with the base of the "U" at the upper part of the patient's chest. A second barrier drape running across the patient's mid thorax completes the field.

The relaxed examination under anesthesia is an essential part of any surgical procedure. Range of motion and stability are carefully assessed and videotaped.

At the Southern California Orthopedic Institute, we suspend the arm using an overhand traction device. A sterile suspensory traction arm-holding device is placed and connected to the nonsterile overhead device by a sterile S-hook, which is applied by the surgeon. The upper extremity is then supported in a position of approximately 70 degrees' abduction and 10 degrees' forward flexion. For average-sized patients, we are able to hold this position with 10 lb of weight suspended from the traction device.

Anatomy and Portals

Once the traction is applied and the patient is in a stable position, we outline the shoulder anatomy with a surgical pen. The acromion, clavicle, AC joint, and coracoid are all drawn. We use an additional line that begins at the posterior aspect of the AC joint. This line is marked laterally to cross perpendicular to the lateral edge of the acromion. This orientation line divides the acromion into an anterior two fifths and a posterior three fifths. Under the anterior portion lies the subacromial space and bursa. The line is also helpful in creating a lateral portal for subacromial or rotator cuff pathology.

The posterior portal is established first. On average, it is situated 2 cm inferior and 1 cm medial to the posterolateral acromial edge. However, the "soft spot" should be palpated. A small stab is made through the skin and subcutaneous tissues only with a no. 11 scalpel blade. A blunt obturator in an arthroscopic sheath is then used to enter the joint.

Next, the anterosuperior (AS) portal is placed just superior to the biceps tendon in the rotator interval. An outside-in technique can be used, using a spinal needle first to confirm proper location high in the rotator interval.

The third and final portal used in arthroscopic labral repairs is the anterior mid-glenoid (MG) portal. This portal is made using the outside-in method as well. Intraarticularly, the portal is located at the superior edge of the subscapularis tendon, whereas the skin incision is typically placed 2 cm inferior to the AS portal.

Technique

As originally described by Snyder et al. (12), lesions of the superior labrum that begin posteriorly and extend anteriorly stopping before or at the MG notch were termed "SLAP" lesions. They were then categorized into four types. Type I has a frayed superior labrum but its attachment and biceps anchor are intact. Type II lesions have pathologic detachment of the labrum and biceps anchor from the superior glenoid with or without fraying of the superior labrum. Type III SLAPs consist of a bucket-handle tear in the superior labrum that may or may not be displaced; however, the biceps anchor remains intact. Type IV is similar to type III with a bucket-handle labral tear, but the tear progresses into the biceps tendon. In these, the biceps anchor remains intact. Type V SLAP lesions are any combination of the above, most commonly type II and type IV.

Because type I SLAP lesions (Fig. 12-4) do not involve the biceps anchor, they can be simply débrided back to stable tissue with care to leave the biceps intact. Type III lesions

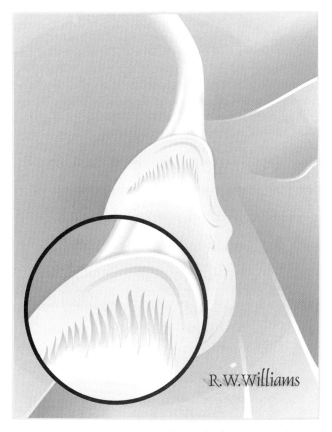

Figure 12-4. Drawing of type I superior labrum anterior and posterior (SLAP) lesion.

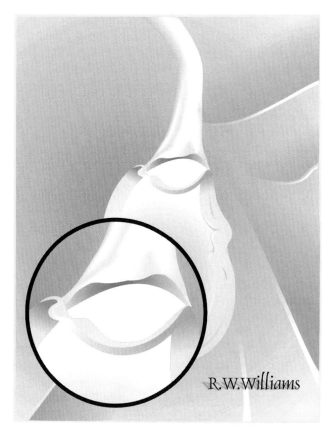

Figure 12-5. Drawing of type III superior labrum anterior and posterior (SLAP) lesion.

(Figs. 12-5 and 12-6) can also be resected back to normal, stable labrum much like a bucket-handle tear of a knee meniscus. Sometimes the anterior attachment of the bucket-handle tear includes the attachment sight of the middle glenohumeral ligament rendering it unstable. These situations require reattachment of the middle glenohumeral ligament to the glenoid to ensure stability of the shoulder (Fig. 12-7).

Type II labral injuries (Figs. 12-8 and 12-9) involve the biceps anchor with detachment of the labrum/anchor from the superior glenoid tubercle. Arthroscopically, this diagnosis must be confirmed. Often, the superior labrum is meniscoid in appearance with a bony at-

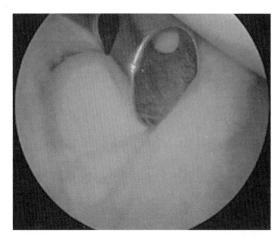

Figure 12-6. Intraoperative arthroscopic photograph of type III superior labrum anterior and posterior (SLAP) lesion.

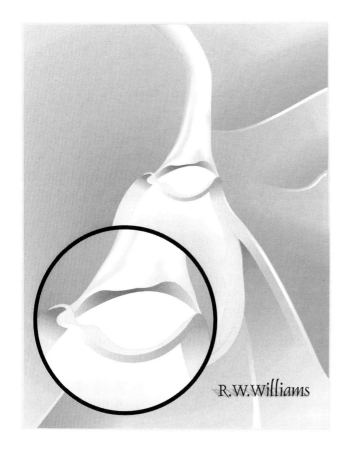

Figure 12-7. The middle glenohumeral ligament is sometimes attached to the bucket-handle tear of a type III superior labrum anterior and posterior (SLAP) lesion.

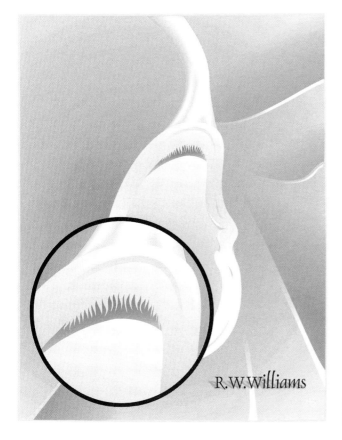

Figure 12-8. Drawing of type II superior labrum anterior and posterior (SLAP) lesion.

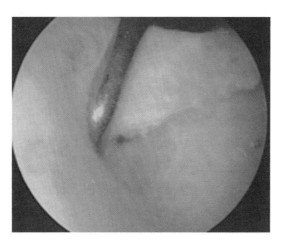

Figure 12-9. Intraoperative arthroscopic photograph of type II superior labrum anterior and posterior (SLAP) lesion.

tachment medial to and below the glenoid surface. This commonly leads to an erred diagnosis of labral avulsion. In an acute injury, the hemorrhagic accumulation of healing cells is visualized. This acute healing process changes into fibrous tissue as the lesion ages. Probing the biceps anchor enhances the confirmation of a type II SLAP lesion. Normally, the articular surface of the glenoid extends to the anchor/ labral tissue, even in instances when the meniscoid labrum is attached medial to and below the glenoid surface. In chronic type II SLAPs, a space exists between the articular cartilage and the anchor. Moreover, a 3- to 12-mm gap with arching of the anchor can be seen with traction on the biceps. In addition, when the biceps tendon is pulled away from the glenoid, tension is transmitted to the attached middle and inferior ligaments indicating that they too have a deficient anchor point. If a Buford complex exists in association with a SLAP lesion, traction on the cord-

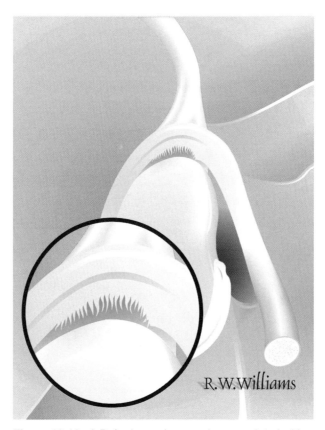

Figure 12-10. A Buford complex may be associated with a type III superior labrum anterior and posterior (SLAP) lesion.

like middle glenohumeral ligament will cause the biceps anchor to arch away from the glenoid (Fig. 12-10).

Type II SLAP Lesions. At the Southern California Orthopedic Institute, we prefer to fix type II lesions with a titanium 12-mm screw-in type suture anchor loaded with two strands of nonabsorbable braided no. 2 suture.

Superior Glenoid Preparation and Anchor Insertion. After arthroscopic diagnostic confirmation, the fibrous tissue over the superior glenoid neck is débrided with a shaver through the AS portal. The labral and biceps tissues are similarly débrided (Fig. 12-11). The arthroscopic punch is used to create the pilot hole for the Revo anchor (Linvatec Corp., Largo, FL). It is placed through the AS portal and maneuvered posterior to the biceps tendon where the tip is positioned in the center of the biceps attachment sight at an angle of 45 degrees medial and 45 degrees posterior and inserted down to the horizontal seating line (Fig. 12-12).

The screw-in 12-mm big-eye Revo suture anchor is loaded with two sutures, one green, and one white. To facilitate suture management, half of each suture strand is colored purple with a marking pencil and that strand is oriented to exit the anchor eyelet on the side closest to the biceps when the anchor is completely seated. By convention, the green suture is located at the upper end of the eyelet and the white suture is at the lower portion of the eyelet nearer to the screw threads. (Figs. 12-13 and 12-14). The anchor is then inserted into the pilot hole until the horizontal seating line is below the bone. When using the 12-mm big-eye Revo anchor, the long axis of the eyelet should be parallel to the biceps to allow better sliding of the suture.

Suture Staging before SLAP Repair. The following sequence of steps is important to allow precise suture management throughout the procedure, avoiding twisting or tangling sutures. The arthroscope is first placed in the AMGP (anterior mid-glenoid portal) and the undyed limb of white suture is retrieved out of the posterior portal with a crochet hook (Fig. 12-15). The suture is then placed outside the cannula using a switching rod. The

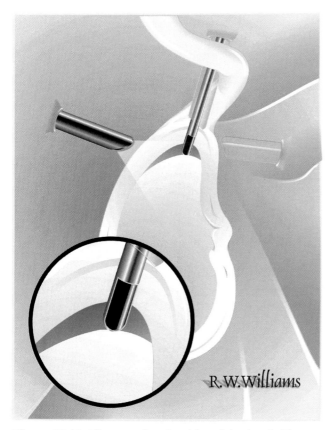

Figure 12-11. The superior glenoid neck is abraded to promote healing of the detached labrum.

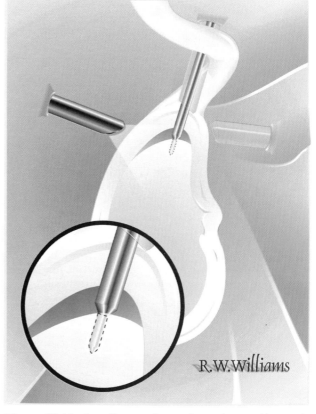

Figure 12-12. An arthroscopic punch can be used to create a pilot hole for the anchor.

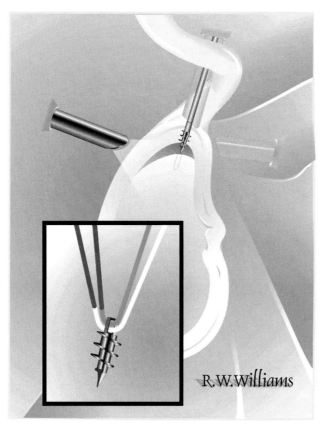

Figure 12-13. The double-loaded suture anchor and intraoperative placement of the suture anchor through the anterosuperior portal.

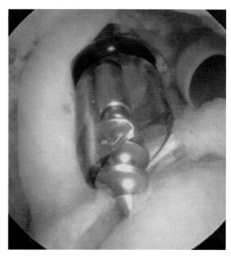

Figure 12-14. Intraoperative arthroscopic photograph of suture anchor placement.

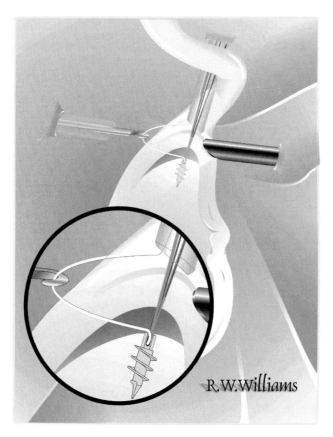

Figure 12-15. The white suture is retrieved out the posterior portal using a crochet hook. This suture is placed outside the cannula using a switching rod.

scope is repositioned in the posterosuperior (PS) portal for the remainder of the case. Next, the undyed green suture limb is retrieved into the MG portal and repositioned outside the cannula with a switching rod. The purple–green suture is retrieved into and left inside the MG cannula. Lastly, the purple–white suture is placed outside the cannula in the AS portal but moved to the anterior side of the tendon (Fig. 12-16).

Lesion Repair. A crescent-shaped suture hook is placed through the AS cannula and passed through the labrum at the corner of the biceps-labral aimed toward the Revo anchor. (Fig. 12-17). The Suture Shuttle Relay (Linvatec) is advanced into the joint, retrieved with a grasper, and carried into the anterior mid-glenoid cannula. The purple–green suture is then loaded into the Shuttle eyelet and carried through the superior labrum and out the AS cannula (Fig. 12-18). The undyed green suture is then retrieved from the MG portal around the labrum posterior to the biceps tendon and into the AS cannula with a crochet hook (Fig. 12-19). The suture is tied using a sliding knot and two half-hitches (Fig. 12-20).

Next, the purple–white suture is retrieved from the AS portal into the MG cannula with a crochet hook. The crescent-shaped suture hook is again passed through the superior labrum via the AS cannula. This time, however, it passes through the anterior edge of the biceps tendon and under the labrum (Fig. 12-21). Again the Shuttle Relay is fed into the joint and retrieved with a grasper through the MG cannula. It is loaded with the suture and pulled through the labrum and out the AS cannula. The undyed limb of white suture is retrieved from the posterior portal and carried anterior to the biceps tendon and into the AS cannula (Fig. 12-22). The suture is tied with a sliding knot and three half-hitches (Fig. 12-23). The repair is then probed and checked for tension and stability (Fig. 12-24).

Type IV SLAP Lesions. A type IV SLAP lesion is a bucket-handle–type tear of the superior labrum that extends into the biceps tendon (Figs. 12-25 and 12-26). Most often, the

(text continues on page 204)

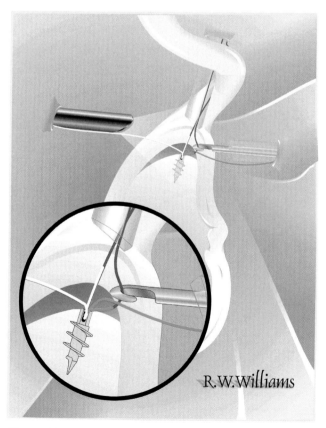

Figure 12-16. The sutures are separated into a star pattern to ease suture management.

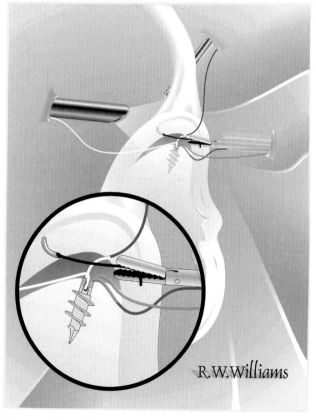

Figure 12-17. The suture passer is introduced under the labrum posterior to the biceps, and the Shuttle (Linvatec, Inc., Largo, FL) is retrieved out the mid-glenoid portal using an arthroscopic grasper.

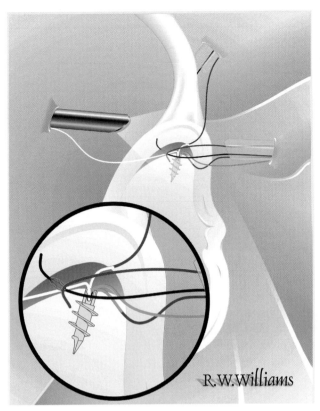

Figure 12-18. The purple limb of the green suture is passed through the tissue using the Shuttle (Linvatec, Inc., Largo, FL).

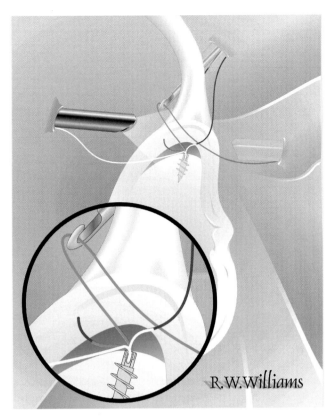

Figure 12-19. The other limb of the green suture is retrieved from the mid-glenoid portal. It should be brought on the articular side of the biceps tendon/anchor.

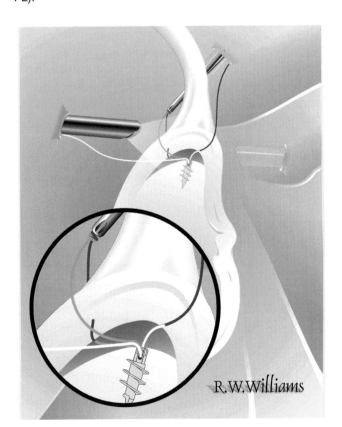

Figure 12-20. The suture is tied posterior to the biceps.

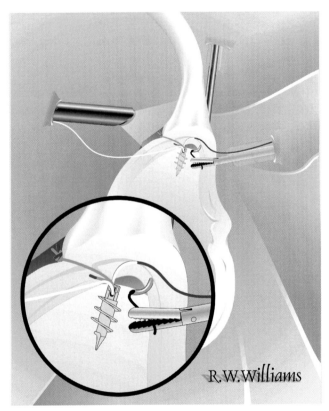

Figure 12-21. The purple limb of the white suture is brought back inside the mid-glenoid cannula using a switching stick and the suture passer is introduced under the labrum anterior to the biceps tendon, grasped, and brought out the mid-glenoid portal. The purple limb of the white suture is then loaded and passed.

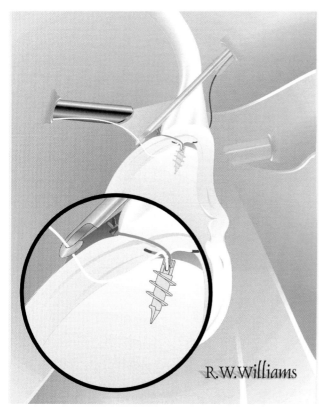

Figure 12-22. The undyed limb of the white suture is retrieved anterior to the biceps tendon out the anterior superior cannula on the articular side of the biceps tendon/anchor.

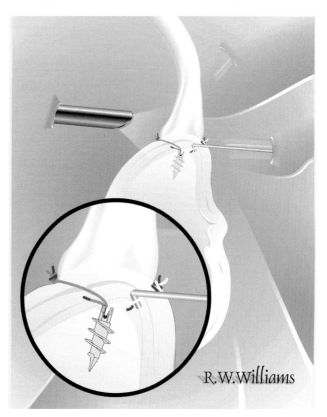

Figure 12-23. The white suture is tied and the repair is completed.

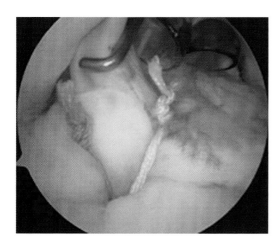

Figure 12-24. Probing the repair for stability and tension.

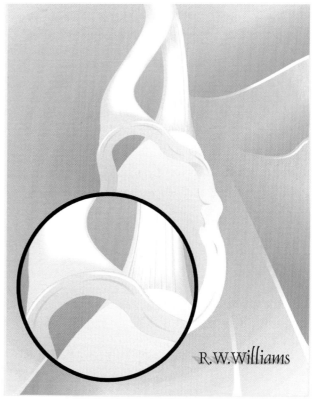

Figure 12-25. Drawing of type IV superior labrum anterior and posterior (SLAP) lesion.

203

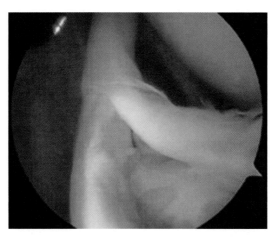

Figure 12-26. Intraoperative arthroscopic photograph of type IV superior labrum anterior and posterior (SLAP) lesion.

biceps anchor remains firmly attached. The extent of biceps involvement determines the treatment plan. If the tear involves less than 30% of the biceps, usually the biceps and the labrum can simply be débrided. If a larger biceps tear is present, age becomes a factor. An older individual commonly does well with a biceps tenodesis, especially if the remaining tendon is degenerative. Younger patients represent a unique subgroup. It is often advisable in this group to repair both the labrum and biceps with simple suture techniques. Because the anchor remains stable in most cases, bone anchors are usually not necessary.

Superior Glenoid Preparation and Anchor Insertion. Suture repair for a type IV SLAP begins with the arthroscope in the posterior portal. A 20-mm crescent hook is passed through the AS cannula into the biceps tendon across the split tear. A Suture Shuttle Relay is passed through the needle and retrieved anteriorly. A nonabsorbable suture is loaded into the Shuttle and pulled anteriorly, leaving a limb in the AS cannula. A second stick is performed 4 mm from the first, through the biceps and labral tissue. A shuttle is again passed and retrieved out the front. The anterior suture limb from the first stick is loaded into the Shuttle from the second stick and pulled out the AS cannula. This gives a mattress suture through the biceps with both limbs now inside the AS cannula, where they are then tied using arthroscopic knot tying. This suturing is continued until the split is adequately and securely closed. Occasionally, switching the viewing portal to the AS portal is necessary if the tear extends posteriorly.

Complex SLAP Lesions. Complex lesions are a combination of SLAP subgroups, most often types II and IV.

POSTOPERATIVE MANAGEMENT

After the patient is discharged from the recovery unit, pain is controlled with oral pain and/or antiinflammatory medications to supplement the intraarticular lidocaine injection performed at the end of the operation. The dressings are changed at 24 hours by the patient, followed by a physician's examination at 1, 3, and 6 weeks postoperatively. With no coexisting shoulder pathology, the patient should undergo a progressive rehabilitation to a painless, fully functional shoulder.

Postoperatively, the patient is immobilized in a sling for 3 weeks. We use the Ultrasling (DJ Ortho, Vista, CA), which is a neutral rotation sling. Active use of the hands, wrist, and elbow is encouraged immediately, along with pendulum exercises, as long as the biceps is not strained. When the sling is discontinued, the patient begins gentle shoulder exercises including isometric internal and external rotation and pulley flexion. The patient is to strictly avoid external rotation beyond neutral and extension of the shoulder and elbow

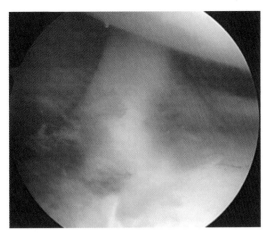

Figure 12-27. Healed superior labrum anterior and posterior (SLAP) repair on second-look arthroscopy.

behind the body. At 4 to 5 weeks postoperatively, therapy is advanced to include shoulder range of motion and protected biceps strengthening. Resistance and motion are progressed gradually. Only after 3 months is stressful biceps activity allowed and the patient permitted to begin sport-specific rehabilitation.

RESULTS

As mentioned earlier, superior labral lesions often coexist with other shoulder pathology. As a result, the outcome of labral repair or débridement often depends on the concurrent pathology and the treatment rendered. Isolated labral lesions do occur and these patients can expect a full recovery to preinjury activities within a few months after surgery (Fig. 12-27).

COMPLICATIONS

Fortunately, complications of arthroscopic repair of SLAP lesions using the single anchor–double suture technique are rare. Like other arthroscopic shoulder techniques, there is a small but definite risk of infection, bleeding, transient traction injury to nervous structures, equipment failure, or breakage.

The main complications specific to labral repairs relate to missed coexisting shoulder pathology. In these situations, patients generally do well for an initial period only to have recurrent shoulder symptoms later. This is prevented by accurate diagnostic examinations, injections, and radiographic studies and concurrent treatment of these additional diagnoses.

Another source of suboptimal outcomes relates to the technical placement of the fixation device. Care must be taken to place the anchor off the articular surface at the biceps anchor at the proper angle 45 degrees posterior and medial. Failure to do so often results in damage to articular surface, fracture of the glenoid, or inadequate fixation. This is best avoided by careful, meticulous soft-tissue débridement at the anchor site. Moreover, because these are young healthy patients with good-quality bone, a punch can be used to develop a starting hole at the desired site.

A final source of morbidity can be related to a failure to recognize anatomic variants. Repairing a Buford complex or a sublabral foramen to the glenoid commonly results in an unacceptable decrease in shoulder motion. To avert this unwanted consequence, careful examination of preoperative studies and familiarity with arthroscopic anatomy are required.

In summary, undesirable results from labral surgery are uncommon. However, all preoperative suspicions must be confirmed during surgery prior to any repair. Furthermore, attention to the technical points is important to ensure optimal chance of recovery.

RECOMMENDED READING

1. Andrews, J.R., Carson, W.G. Jr., McLeod, W.D.: Glenoid labrum tears related to the long head of the biceps. *Am J Sports Med* 13: 337–341, 1985.
2. Berg, E.E., Ciullo, J.V.: A clinical test for superior glenoid labral or SLAP lesions. *Clin J Sport Med* 8(2): 121–123, 1998.
3. Burkhart, S.S., Morgan, C.D.: The peel-back mechanism: its role in producing and extending posterior type II SLAP lesions and its effect on SLAP repair rehabilitation *Arthroscopy* 14(6): 637–640, 1998.
4. Cordasco, F.A., Steinmann, S., Flatow, E.L., et al.: Arthroscopic treatment of glenoid labral tears *Am J Sports Med* 21(3): 425–431, 1993.
5. Handelberg, F., Williams, S., Shahabpour, M., et al.: SLAP Lesions: a retrospective multicenter study *Arthroscopy* 14(8): 856–862, 1998.
6. Kibler, W.B.: Specificity and sensitivity of the anterior slide test in throwing athletes with superior glenoid tears. *Arthroscopy* 11: 296–300, 1995.
7. Mileski, R.A., Snyder, S.J.: Superior labral lesions in the shoulder: pathoanatomy and surgical management *J Am Acad Orthop Surg* 6(2): 121–131, 1998.
8. Mimori, K., Muneta, T., Nakagawa, T., et al.: A new pain provocation test for superior labral tears. *Am J Sports Med* 27(2): 137–142, 1999.
9. O'Brien, S.J., Paganani, M.J., Fealy, S.: The active compression test: a new and effective test of diagnosing labral tears and acromioclavicular abnormalities. *Am J Sports Med* 26: 610–613, 1998.
10. Rodosky, M.W., Harner, C.D., Fu, F.H.: The role of the long head of the biceps muscle and superior glenoid labrum in anterior stability of the shoulder *Am J Sports Med* 22(1): 121–130, 1994.
11. Snyder, S.J., Banas, M.P., Karzel, R.P.: An analysis of 140 injuries to the superior glenoid labrum *J Shoulder Elbow Surg* 4(4): 243–248, 1995.
12. Snyder, S.J., Karzel, R.P., DelPizzo, W., et al.: SLAP lesions of the shoulder. *Arthroscopy* 6: 274–279, 1990.
13. Warner, J.J., Kann, S., Marks, P.: Arthroscopic repair of combined Bankart and superior labral detachment anterior and posterior lesions: technique and preliminary results *Arthroscopy* 10(4): 383–391, 1994.

PART II

Instability

13

Bankart Repair of Anterior Shoulder Dislocation and Subluxation

Bertram Zarins

INDICATIONS/CONTRAINDICATIONS

Although Perthes (15) first proposed reattachment of an avulsed anterior shoulder capsule, this lesion has most commonly been named after Bankart ("Bankart lesion") (1,2). The Bankart procedure consists of reattachment of an avulsed anterior glenohumeral capsule, with or without its glenoid labrum, directly to the bone of the anterior glenoid rim. A modified Bankart repair is an anterior shoulder capsulorrhaphy in which a stretched capsule is overlapped and secured to a stable glenoid labrum (20). Perhaps more than anyone else, Rowe refined and popularized this technique and has shown that the results have stood the test of time (7,18–21).

The Bankart procedure is indicated for symptomatic recurrent anterior shoulder dislocations and subluxations that persist despite nonoperative measures. The operation is most clearly indicated for the shoulder in which the etiology of the instability is traumatic. Post-traumatic shoulder instability is commonly associated with an avulsion of the anterior glenoid labrum from the glenoid rim by the inferior glenohumeral ligament (12). The patient for whom this operation is ideal is the one who has unidirectional anterior shoulder instability.

A second indication for this procedure is in a patient who has had failed prior instability surgery, in which that prior surgery did not specifically address the presence of a Bankart lesion. Whatever the prior surgical procedure, if a persistent Bankart lesion exists, the patient may benefit tremendously by a direct repair of that lesion.

This surgical repair is not indicated in patients who have voluntary shoulder instability and who have emotional or psychological problems that contribute to their shoulder condition. These patients, of course, are not surgical candidates for any type of repair. A relative contraindication for this operation is the presence of multidirectional shoulder instability.

B. Zarins, M.D.: Department of Orthopaedic Surgery, Harvard Medical School; and Sports Medicine Service, Massachusetts General Hospital, Boston, Massachusetts.

209

The Bankart procedure effectively tightens the anterior capsule to the glenoid rim. In the patient who has multidirectional instability, failure to address the other directions of laxity can lead to persistent instability and, in fact, a fixed subluxation in the direction opposite the anterior repair. In the patient who has multidirectional instability, a Bankart repair may be combined with other capsular procedures to correct all directions of laxity.

Another relative contraindication to performing this procedure alone is the presence of significant glenohumeral arthritis. In a patient who has advanced glenohumeral arthritis, repair of the Bankart lesion would not be expected to provide significant benefit; however, the presence of severe degenerative changes in the glenohumeral joint is not commonly associated with symptomatic anterior shoulder instability.

PREOPERATIVE PLANNING

A Bankart lesion can be prepared as an open procedure or as an arthroscopically assisted operation (6,8,11,14,22). The principle is the same: to reattach the avulsed capsule to the

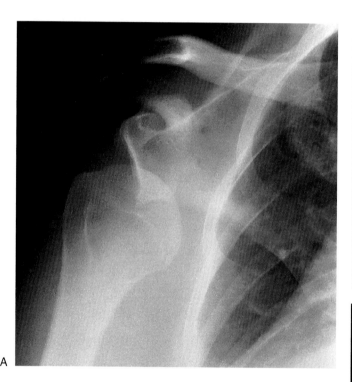

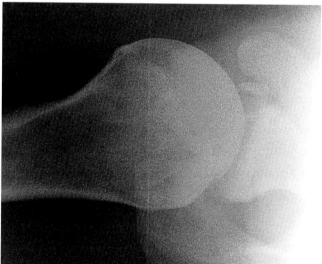

B

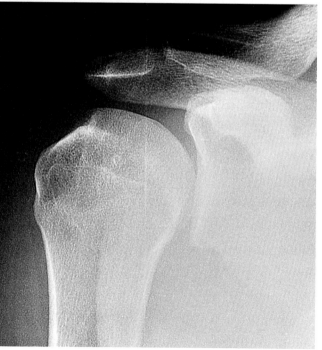

A

Figure 13-1. A: Anterior right shoulder dislocation. **B:** Axillary view of the reduced shoulder shows bony fracture of the anterior glenoid rim seen at surgery. **C:** Postoperative radiograph shows good position of the humerus relative to the glenoid. The Hill-Sachs lesion is visible in this view.

C

anterior glenoid rim. This chapter describes the open approach. The most important component of preoperative planning is to correctly diagnose the direction of instability. It is easy to arrive at the correct diagnosis if radiographs document the shoulder in a dislocated state (Fig. 13-1A). Correctly diagnosing shoulder subluxation can be more difficult. A typical symptom of anterior subluxation is pain during forceful throwing or other overhead activities (20). Rowe (20) coined the term "dead arm syndrome" for recurrent transient subluxation of the shoulder. Positive physical findings in patients who have anterior subluxation are a positive apprehension sign when the shoulder is externally rotated in a position of 90 degrees' abduction and anterior translation of the humeral head in this position of the arm. A momentary subluxation or click sometimes can be elicited.

A patient who has unidirectional instability may have a positive relocation test in which the pain or sense of apprehension is eliminated as posterior pressure on the humeral head centers the humeral head into the glenoid fossa. Although it is unusual to be able to elicit specific subluxation or dislocation of the shoulder on examination because of intense muscle guarding in the threatened position, subluxability may be present and painful when the arm is at the side if direct pressure is applied on the posterior humeral head increasing the translation in an anterior direction. Range of motion of the shoulder is typically not limited other than by apprehension. Strength of the rotator cuff and deltoid is usually normal. The most helpful radiographs are an anteroposterior view in internal rotation, a Stryker notch view, and a West Point axillary view (Fig. 13-1B). The first two radiographs are most helpful in identifying the presence of an associated Hill-Sachs lesion (Fig. 13-1C), and the last view can show bone reaction, rounding off, erosion, or separation of the anterior glenoid rim. In addition, mild arthritic changes may be present on the humeral head.

Additional imaging studies have proven helpful in identifying the presence of a Bankart lesion. These include computed tomography arthrography, magnetic resonance imaging (MRI), and MRI arthrography. While plain MRI is of limited value, the addition of contrast material more clearly defines the pathology in the glenoid labrum area. In addition, all of these studies can show the presence of even small Hill-Sachs lesions.

However, if the presence or absence of a Bankart lesion is to be determined with a high degree of accuracy, diagnostic arthroscopy gives the best direct view of intraarticular pathology. The advantage of this is that it can be combined with a careful examination under anesthesia to ensure that the instability is truly unidirectional.

SURGERY

Patient Positioning

General anesthesia is induced and both shoulders are examined to determine excessive laxity. An intravenous dose of antibiotic is administered. The supine patient is positioned flat on the table (Fig. 13-2). Nothing is placed under the scapula. An arm board is placed close to the side of the operating room table so that the patient's elbow is level with one end of the arm board. This allows the surgeon to stand close to the patient's body and to place a large bolster under the patient's elbow. The shoulder, hemithorax, and upper extremity up to the wrist are prepared and draped in a sterile manner (Fig. 13-3). Before a SteriDrape (3M Worldwide, St. Paul, MN) is applied over the skin, the arm is adducted across the body to define the natural axillary skin folds; these folds are marked using a skin marker (Fig. 13-4). Lines are drawn perpendicular to the skin marks (to act as guides for reapproximating the skin edges) and the SteriDrape is applied to seal the skin. The surgeon stands at the patient's side just distal to the flexed elbow that is supported by the large bolster.

Technique

Make a vertical skin incision in the anterior axillary fold along the line previously marked (Fig. 13-5). The proximal end of the incision is located near the coracoid process. The incision can be placed in the axilla if cosmesis is a concern. Infiltrate the subcutaneous tis-

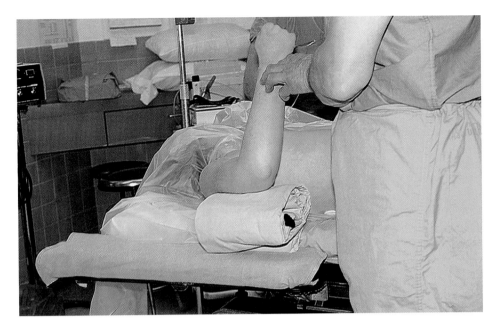

Figure 13-2. Patient positioning for Bankart procedure of the right shoulder. The patient is positioned flat on the table in a supine position. Nothing is placed under the scapula. The arm board is placed so that the surgeon can stand close to the patient's body, and a bolster can be placed on the arm board to elevate the elbow.

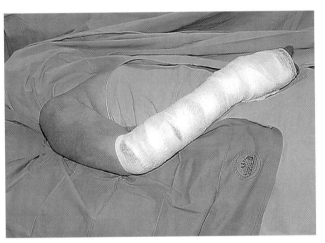

Figure 13-3. The right shoulder is prepped and draped. A sterile towel covers the forearm and hand and is wrapped with a sterile gauze.

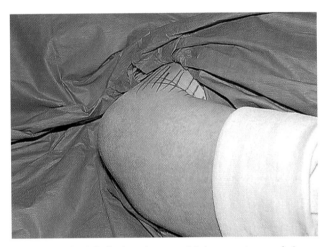

Figure 13-4. A hole has been cut into a waterproof drape and the arm placed through the hole. A vertical skin line is drawn to mark the axillary fold. Lines are drawn perpendicular to the skin folds to act as guides for later approximation of the skin.

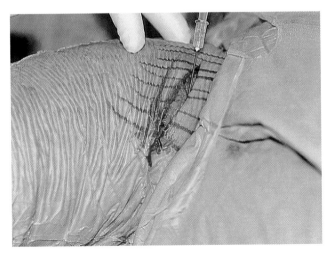

Figure 13-5. A sterile drape has been applied to the skin. A vertical skin incision is made along a line previously marked. Bupivicaine with epinephrine is being injected along the edges of the incision.

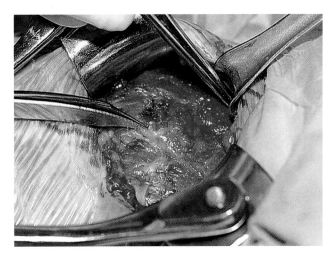

Figure 13-6. The subcutaneous tissues have been dissected to create skin flaps. A Kolbel self-retaining retractor (Link Orthopaedics, Pinebrook, NJ) has been inserted. The Richardson retractor retracts the tissues proximally. Forceps mark the coracoid process (right shoulder). The tip of the scissors marks the line of fat that is a guide to the deltopectoral interval.

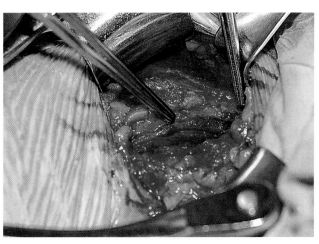

Figure 13-7. The cephalic vein has been identified on the deltoid muscle (forceps). The cephalic vein is retracted laterally.

sues with a solution containing bupivacaine 0.5% and epinephrine 1:200,000. Dissect the superficial fascial layer to create skin flaps. Do not carry the dissections as deep as the deep fascial layer or the muscle. If muscle is visible, the dissection is deep to the deep fascial layer and it will be difficult to find the deltopectoral interval. The deltopectoral interval is marked by a fine line of fat within the muscular layer just deep to the deep fascia (Fig. 13-6). The upper end of this line is close to the coracoid process, which should be palpated. Dissect in this fatty layer into the deltopectoral interval, retracting the cephalic vein and deltoid muscle laterally and the pectoralis major muscle medially (Fig. 13-7). Palpate the coracoid process and do not extend the dissection further proximally (unless the rotator cuff needs to be explored) or medially (to avoid injuring the musculocutaneous nerve). Retract the deltoid muscle laterally and the pectoralis major muscle medially using a self-retaining Kolbel retractor (Link Orthopaedics, Pinebrook, NJ) (Fig. 13-8). A single-spike retractor (Bankart Shoulder Repair Kit, Kirwan Surgical Products, Inc., Marshfield, MA) can be placed on the superior aspect of the humeral head below the coracoacromial ligament to im-

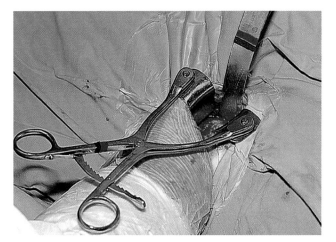

Figure 13-8. A self-retaining Kolbel retractor (Link Orthopaedics, Pinebrook, NJ) is placed deeper to retract the deltoid muscle laterally and the pectoralis major muscle medially. The single-spike retractor is placed in the superior aspect of the wound under the coracoacromial ligament.

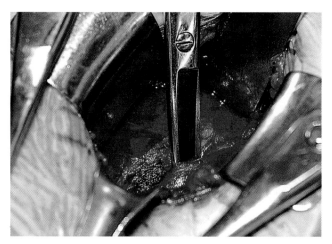

Figure 13-9. The lateral border of the conjoined tendon (to include the coracobrachialis muscle) has been dissected and is being lifted up using dissecting scissors.

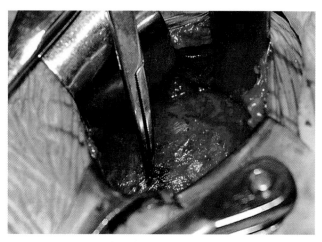

Figure 13-10. A curved snap points to the blood vessels that mark the inferior edge of the subscapularis tendon. Several small vessels have been electrocoagulated (*dark marks*).

prove visualization proximally. Incise the clavipectoral fascia, and identify the medial edge of the conjoined tendon. Do not mistake the edge of the tendon itself as the proper location to dissect: Several millimeters of coracobrachialis muscle are located lateral to the tendinous part of the conjoined tendon, and the lateral edge of the muscle is the proper site of dissection (Fig. 13-9). Move the Kolbel retractor deeper to retract the conjoined tendon medially. The subscapularis tendon is now exposed.

Internally and externally rotate the shoulder to define the subscapularis muscle and tendon. Note the several blood vessels that mark the inferior edge of the subscapularis tendon (Fig. 13-10). Palpate the superior margin of the subscapularis tendon and feel for enlarge-

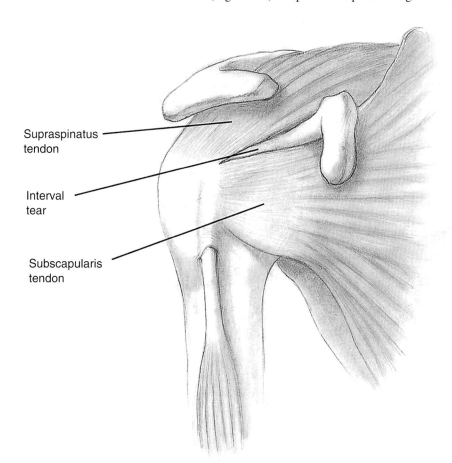

Supraspinatus
tendon

Interval
tear

Subscapularis
tendon

Figure 13-11. A common pathologic lesion in shoulders that have recurrent anterior glenohumeral dislocation is an enlargement of the seam separating the supraspinatus and subscapularis tendons. The humeral head can be palpated in this interval. This interval should be closed as part of the repair. (From Rowe, C.R., Zarins, B.: Recurrent transient subluxation of the shoulder. *J Bone Joint Surg Am* 63: 863–872, 1981, with permission.)

ment of the seam that separates the subscapularis and the supraspinatus tendons (20) (Fig. 13-11). Repair this interval laterally with no. 0 Dexon sutures if the interval is enlarged. Do not repair the interval medially or the shoulder motion will be limited postoperatively.

There are several ways of dividing the subscapularis tendon (25,26) (Fig. 13-12):

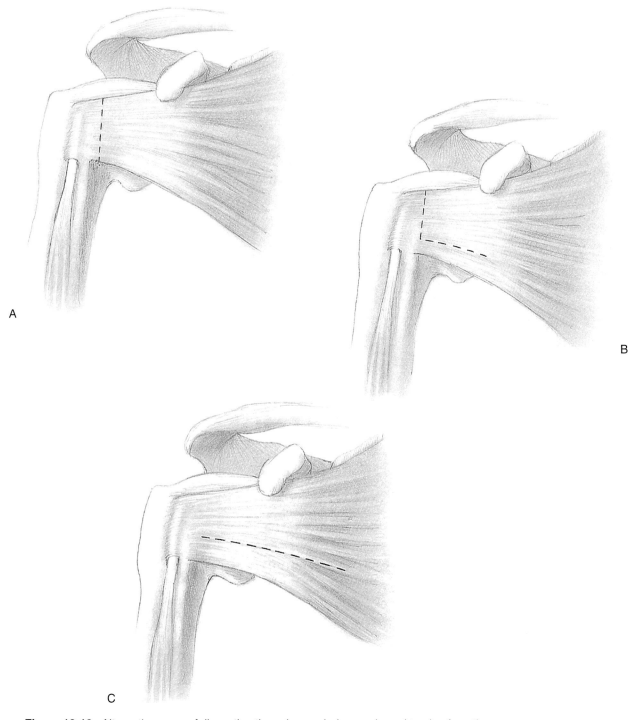

Figure 13-12. Alternative ways of dissecting the subscapularis muscle and tendon from the anterior capsule. **A:** The entire subscapularis tendon is sharply dissected off the anterior capsule and retracted medially. **B:** The lower one fourth of the subscapularis tendon is left intact to protect the anterior humeral circumflex artery and axillary nerve. **C:** The subscapularis muscle and tendon are split in a horizontal direction and retracted superiorly and inferiorly to expose the underlying capsule.

1. The entire tendon can be sharply dissected from the anterior capsule; the blood vessels at the inferior border of the subscapularis tendon are ligated (19). This method gives the best visualization.
2. The superior 75% of the tendon can be dissected, leaving the inferior fibers of the subscapularis tendon and vessels intact (17). This method allows a very good view.
3. The subscapularis tendon and muscle can be divided transversely in line with the fibers. This method was originally described by McLaughlin (R. J. Neviaser, personal oral communication, 1989) and popularized by Jobe (10). The exposure using the transverse method is not as good as the others, but it is adequate in many patients; however, special long, angled Gelpe retractors are needed.

To divide the subscapularis transversely, select a line parallel to the fibers of the subscapularis muscle that is slightly below the middle, measuring from the superior border to the inferior border of the subscapularis tendon. Make an incision through the subscapularis muscle near the musculotendinous junction and carry the dissection down to the capsule. Laterally, the subscapularis tendon blends with the capsule into a single layer near its insertion. The plane between the two structures can be more easily identified medially near the musculotendinous junction of the subscapularis. Once the proper depth has been determined, continue the dissection laterally and dissect the subscapularis tendon from the anterior capsule. The lateral extent of the incision should end halfway between the biceps tendon groove and the musculotendinous junction of the subscapularis. The transverse incision can be connected to a 1-cm-long vertical incision, creating a T-shaped incision in the subscapularis tendon to give additional exposure. A small Cobb elevator can be used to push the subscapularis muscle away from the anterior capsule. The capsule is left intact at this time. Reposition the single-spike retractor medially, placing the tip of the retractor in the midportion of the glenoid rim, slightly medial to the rim.

With the anterior capsule thus exposed, the capsule can now be incised. There are three ways of incising the capsule:

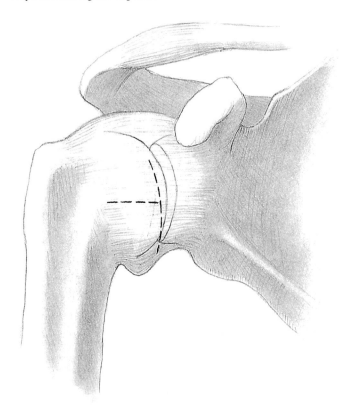

Figure 13-13. A transverse incision has been made in the mid capsule. This is connected to a vertical incision 0.5 cm lateral to the glenoid rim creating a T-shaped incision in the anterior shoulder capsule.

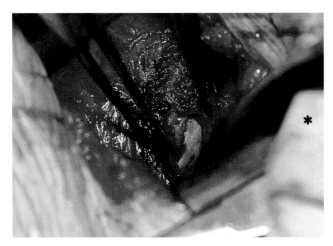

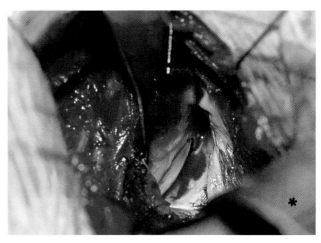

Figure 13-14. Right shoulder. A T-shaped capsular incision has been made showing a glimpse of the glenoid cavity (*). The upper and lower corners of the capsule are being held with forceps. Sutures will be placed to mark these corners.

Figure 13-15. A single-spike retractor (*) has been placed below the avulsed glenoid labrum (Bankart lesion). A modified Rowe humeral head retractor (Kirwan Surgical Products, Inc., Marshfield, MA) retracts the humeral head laterally.

1. Make a vertical incision in the capsule 0.5 cm lateral to the glenoid rim (19,20).
2. Make a transverse incision in the mid capsule and convert it to a T-shaped incision by making a vertical incision 0.5 cm lateral to the glenoid rim (24) (Fig. 13-13). Another way of making a T-shaped capsular incision (Fig. 13-14) and overlapping repair laterally was described by Protzman and colleagues (4,16).
3. Make a transverse capsule incision (26).

If a medial T-shaped capsular incision was made, tag the corners of the capsule where they meet at the T. Insert a Fukuda humeral head retractor or a modified Rowe humeral retractor (Kirwan) into the joint and retract the humeral head laterally. Reposition the single-spike retractor under the avulsed glenoid labrum (Bankart lesion) (Fig. 13-15). Use a curette or small Cobb elevator to scrape the anterior glenoid rim, creating an exposed bleeding bony surface.

Three holes are made through the corner of the glenoid rim at the 2-, 4-, and 6-o'clock positions for a right shoulder, or at the 10-, 8-, and 6-o'clock positions for a left shoulder (3) (Fig. 13-16). First, perforate the cortex of the glenoid neck with a small drill or scaphoid gouge. A curved spike (Kirwan) is then used to deepen the hole on the anterior (nonarticular) aspect of the glenoid rim. Make corresponding holes in the rim using the curved spike

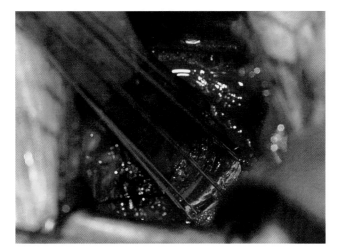

Figure 13-16. Three holes have been made in the anterior glenoid rim of the left shoulder at the 2-, 4-, and 6-o'clock positions. Double strands of no. 0 Polydex suture have been passed through each hole.

or curved awl (Kirwan). Using a no. 5 Mayo needle (Richards), pass two strands of no. 0 Polydex suture through each hole (Fig. 13-17).

An alternative method of securing the sutures to the bone is to use Mitek anchors. Polydex sutures are attached to the anchors that are located at the aforementioned positions. However, if there is sufficient space to make holes through the bone, we prefer making holes to using anchors. The holes provide a larger surface area for bone contact when the capsule is sewn down, and they eliminate the need for implanting metal.

The method of capsule closure is determined by the method of incision. If a vertical capsular incision was made, the humeral head retractor is removed and the sutures are passed through the edge of the lateral capsule using the no. 5 Mayo needles (19,20). The inferior part of the repair is most important. The capsule at the 6-o'clock position should be pulled upward to eliminate the axillary fold of capsule. The shoulder is adducted and internally rotated as the sutures are securely tied, anchoring the capsule to the glenoid rim. One end of the pair of suture strands is cut, and the second (single) strand is passed through the medial flap of the capsule; this strand is tied to an adjacent single strand that was also passed through the medial flap. This reinforces the repair in a double-breasted manner (19,20). The shoulder is externally rotated gently with the elbow at the patient's side. If the shoulder can be externally rotated 30 degrees, the repair is not too tight.

If the capsule was incised in a T-shaped manner, the corner of the inferior flap is pulled upward to be secured to both the middle and lower holes that were placed in the glenoid rim (Fig. 13-18). The sutures are passed through the inferior flap of the capsule with the

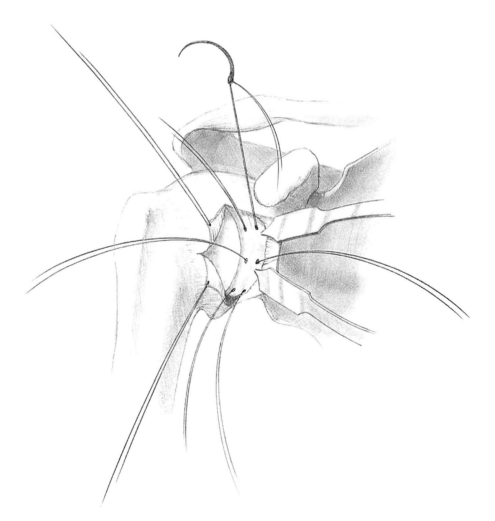

Figure 13-17. Right shoulder showing three holes and a T-shaped capsular incision in preparation for securing the capsule to the glenoid rim.

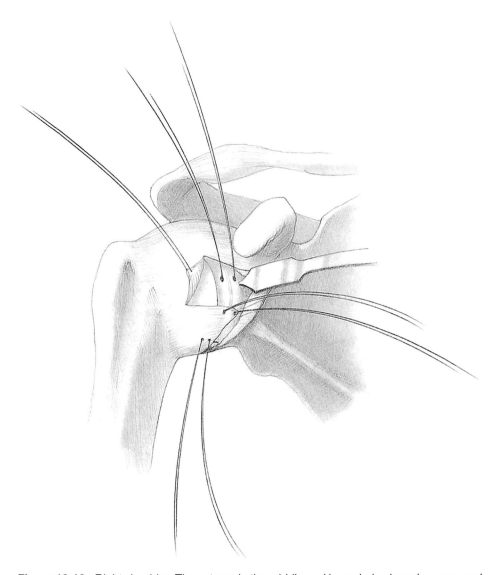

Figure 13-18. Right shoulder. The sutures in the middle and lower holes have been passed through the inferior flap of the capsule, to be securely tied.

humeral head retractor still in place (Fig. 13-19). The retractor is then removed and the sutures are tied with the arm held in adduction and internal rotation. The superior flap of the capsule is then overlapped over the inferior flap (Fig. 13-20): The sutures that were passed through the middle hole (that have already been tied) and upper hole are passed through the superior flap of capsule. With the arm held internally rotated and adducted, the sutures are tied securely, thereby overlapping the capsule. One strand of each of the upper and lower pairs of sutures and both strands of the middle pair of sutures are further passed through the medial flap of capsule. Adjacent strands of the upper and middle sutures and middle and lower sutures are tied together, reinforcing the repair (Fig. 13-21). The transverse limb of the T-shaped capsule incision is closed using interrupted no. 0 Dexon sutures. The shoulder is rotated with the elbow at the side to be sure 30 degrees of external rotation can be achieved (Fig. 13-22).

Closure

The subscapularis tendon and muscle are repaired using interrupted no. 0 Dexon sutures. If the subscapularis tendon was divided vertically or in an L-shaped manner, the free end of

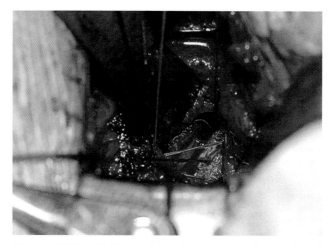

Figure 13-19. Right shoulder. Sutures have been placed into the middle and lower holes in preparation for being tied. The humeral head retractor will be removed prior to tying the sutures.

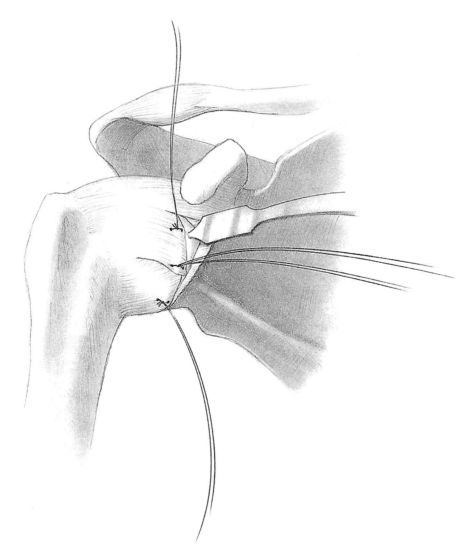

Figure 13-20. The sutures passed through the upper and middle holes are now passed through the upper flap of the capsule. These will be tied to secure the upper capsule to the rim, overlapping the inferior capsule that has already been repaired to the rim. The middle sutures thus pass through the lower flap as well as the upper flap of the capsule where they overlap.

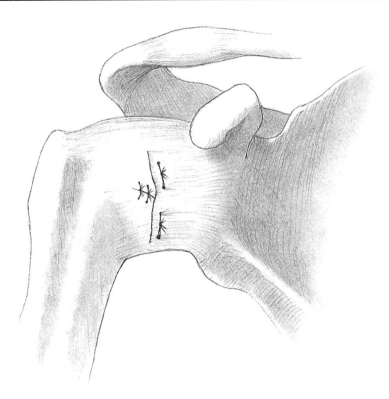

Figure 13-21. Sutures have been further passed through the medial flap of the capsule and tied, reinforcing the repair in a double-breasted manner.

the tendon is reattached to its prior location using interrupted no. 0 Dexon sutures (Fig. 13-23). The subscapularis tendon is not advanced laterally. If the subscapularis muscle and tendon were divided horizontally, the defect is repaired using interrupted no. 0 Dexon sutures. Hemostasis is meticulously achieved before complete closure. The fascia at the edges of the deltopectoral groove is repaired using interrupted absorbable sutures (Fig. 13-24). The subcutaneous tissues are closed using interrupted buried absorbable sutures (such as 3-0 plain catgut). The skin is closed using interrupted 3-0 nylon sutures. Sterile dressings are applied and the arm is placed in a sling.

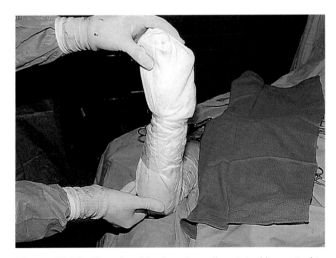

Figure 13-22. The shoulder is externally rotated in neutral to be sure 30 degrees of external rotation can be achieved.

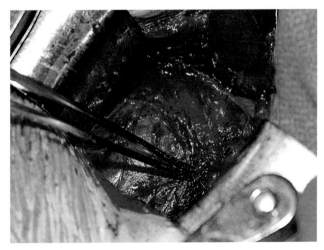

Figure 13-23. A subscapularis tendon is reattached to its normal anatomical location using interrupted Dexon sutures.

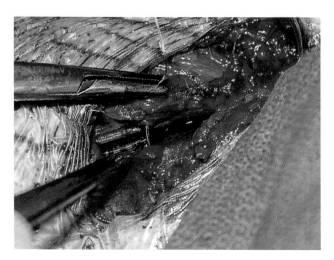

Figure 13-24. The fascia of the deltopectoral interval is repaired using interrupted Dexon sutures. The cephalic vein is deep to the repair.

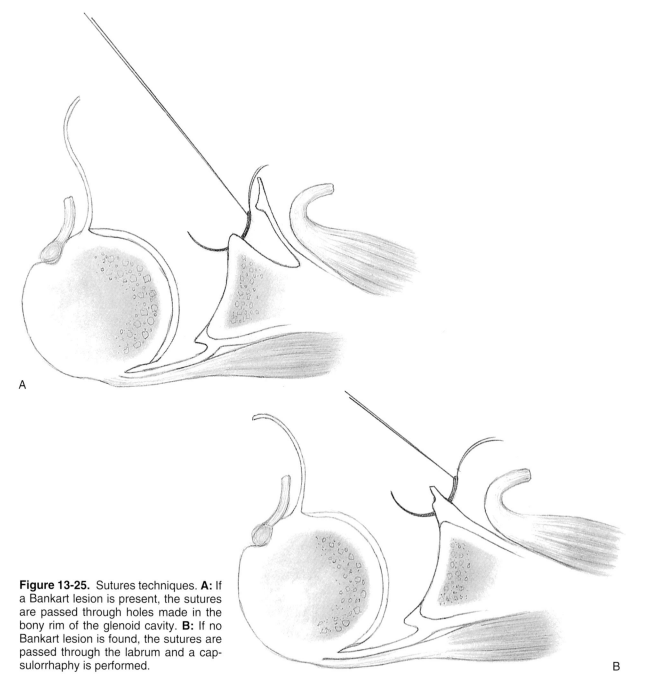

A

B

Figure 13-25. Sutures techniques. **A:** If a Bankart lesion is present, the sutures are passed through holes made in the bony rim of the glenoid cavity. **B:** If no Bankart lesion is found, the sutures are passed through the labrum and a capsulorrhaphy is performed.

Technique Modification for Capsulorrhaphy

If the anterior capsule and labrum have not been avulsed from the glenoid rim, that is, if there is no Bankart lesion present, the sutures can be passed through the intact glenoid labrum instead of through the bone (Fig. 13-25). This procedure is identical to that described for the Bankart repair, except holes are not made through the glenoid bone but rather the sutures are passed through the glenoid labrum adjacent to the glenoid rim.

POSTOPERATIVE MANAGEMENT

The operation can be performed on an outpatient basis (13). The sling is removed on the first postoperative day. Gentle passive pendulum exercises are begun. The patient is encouraged to use the hand and elbow normally and to reach up to the face. The patient is instructed to keep the arm anterior to the coronal plane of the body, that is, not to move the elbow behind the midline of the body. The patient should use the sling in public or in situations in which there is risk of injury, such as when using public transportation or going to school. Sutures are removed 1 week after surgery. At 3 weeks after surgery, the patient should be able to flex the shoulder 90 degrees and externally rotate to 0 degrees with the arm at the side. The shoulder is allowed to regain motion naturally through the use of the limb. Formal physiotherapy is rarely indicated. At 3 months, the shoulder should have achieved 90% of its full motion. The patient works on resisted exercises to increase strength and does stretching exercises to achieve full motion between 3 and 6 months. By 6 months after surgery, the shoulder should have full strength and range of motion, permitting the patient to return to unrestricted activity.

COMPLICATIONS

Nerve Injuries

The musculocutaneous nerve is at risk for injury from excessive pressure of the Kolbel self-retaining retractor on the conjoined tendon. The nerve can also be injured by dissecting medial to the conjoined tendon and the coracoid process. The axillary nerve can easily be injured as it passes below the inferior capsule in the 6-o'clock position. Care must be taken when dissecting the lower border of the subscapularis tendon and inferior capsule. Special care must be exercised when passing sutures through the inferior capsule to prevent incorporating the axillary nerve in the repair.

Limited Motion

Sometimes the patient can have difficulty regaining full motion following a Bankart repair. The most common reason is that the vertical capsule incision was made too far lateral to the glenoid rim. Another reason is excessive overlapping of the corners of a T-shaped capsule incision in an inferosuperior direction. Closing the rotator cuff interval too much will also limit shoulder rotation. The incidence of arthrofibrosis can be reduced by not making the repair too tight and by initiating passive range-of-motion exercises immediately after surgery. By allowing the patient to use the arm for activities of daily living as tolerated during the first week postoperatively, the frequency of limited motion is minimized.

Recurrent Dislocation

The incidence of recurrent dislocation following Bankart repair has been reported to be 3% (19). If a large Hill-Sachs lesion is present, the recurrence rate is 6%. Methods of treating recurrent dislocation in a shoulder that has had a prior repair have been described by Rowe et al. (21).

RECOMMENDED READING

1. Bankart, A.S., Cantab, M.C.: Recurrent or habitual dislocations of the shoulder joint: 1923 [classical article]. *Clin Orthop* 291: 3–6, 1993.
2. Bankart, A.S.B.: Recurrent or habitual dislocation of the shoulder. *BMJ* 2: 1132, 1923.
3. Black, K.P., Schneider, D.J., Yu, J.R., et al.: Biomechanics of the Bankart repair: the relationship between glenohumeral translation and labral fixation site. *Am J Sports Med* 27: 339–344, 1999.
4. Cofield, R.H., Kavanagh, B.F., Frassica, R.J.: Anterior shoulder instability. *Instr Course Lect* 34: 210–227, 1985.
5. Flannigan, B., Kursunoglu-Brahme, S., Snyder, S., et al.: MR arthrography of the shoulder: comparison with conventional MR imaging. *AJR* 155: 829–832, 1990.
6. Gartsman, G.M., Roddey, T.S., Hammerman, S.M.: Arthroscopic treatment of anterior-inferior glenulohumeral instability. *J Bone Joint Surg Am* 82: 991–1003, 2000.
7. Gill, T.G., Micheli, L.J., Gebhard, F., et al.: Bankart repair for anterior instability of the shoulder. *J Bone Joint Surg Am* 79: 850–857, 1987.
8. Guanche, C.A., Quick, D C., Sodergren, K.M., et al.: Arthroscopic versus open reconstruction of the shoulder in patients with isolated Bankart lesions. *Am J Sports Med* 24: 144–154, 1996.
9. Hajek, P.C., Baker, L.L., Sartoris, D.J., et al.: MR arthrography: anatomic–pathologic investigation. *Radiology* 163: 141–147, 1987.
10. Jobe, F.W.: Unstable shoulder in athletes. *Instr Course Lect* 34: 228–231, 1985.
11. Koss, S., Richmond, J.C., Woodward, J.S.: Two- to five-year followup of arthroscopic Bankart reconstruction using a suture anchor technique. *Am J Sports Med* 25: 809–812, 1997.
12. Levine, W.N., Flatow, E.L.: The pathophysiology of shoulder instability. *Am J Sports Med* 28: 910–917, 2000.
13. Levy, H.J., Mashoof, A.A.: Outpatient open Bankart repair. *Am J Sports Med* 28: 377–379, 2000.
14. O'Neill, D.B.: Arthroscopic Bankart repair of anterior detachments of the glenoid labrum. *J Bone Joint Surg Am* 81: 1357–1366, 1999.
15. Perthes, G.: Uber Operationen bei habitueller Schulterluxation. *Deutsch Ztschr Chir* 85: 199–227, 1906.
16. Protzman, R.R.: Anterior instability of the shoulder. *J Bone Joint Surg Am* 62: 909–918, 1980.
17. Rockwood, C.A. Jr.: Fractures and dislocations of the shoulder, II: subluxations and dislocations about the shoulder. In: Rockwood, C.A. Jr., Green, D.P., eds.: *Fractures in adults,* 2nd ed. Philadelphia: Lippincott, 1984.
18. Rowe, C.R.: *The shoulder.* New York: Churchill Livingstone, 1988.
19. Rowe, C.R., Patel, D., Southmayd, W.W.: The Bankart procedure: a long term end-result study. *J Bone Joint Surg Am* 60: 1–16, 1978.
20. Rowe, C.R., Zarins, B.: Recurrent transient subluxation of the shoulder. *J Bone Joint Surg Am* 63: 863–872, 1981.
21. Rowe, C.R., Zarins, B., Ciullo, J.: Recurrent anterior dislocation of the shoulder after surgical repair: apparent cause of failure and treatment. *J Bone Joint Surg Am* 66: 159, 1984.
22. Steinbeck, J., Jerosch, J.: Arthroscopic transglenoid stabilization versus open anchor suturing in traumatic anterior instability of the shoulder. *Am J Sports Med* 26: 373–378, 1998.
23. Thomas, S.C., Matsen, F.A. III: An approach to the repair of avulsion of the glenohumeral ligaments in the management of traumatic anterior glenohumeral instability. *J Bone Joint Surg Am* 71: 506–512, 1989.
24. Warren, R.F.: Instability of the shoulder in throwing sports. *Instr Course Lect* 34: 337–348, 1985.
25. Zarins, B.: Bankart repair for anterior shoulder instability. *Techn Orthop* 3: 23–28, 1989.
26. Zarins, B., Rowe, C. R.: Modifications of the Bankart procedure. In: Post, M., Morrey, B.F., Hawkins, R.J., eds.: *Surgery of the shoulder.* New York: Mosby–Year Book, 174–177, 1990.

14

Anterior Capsulolabral Reconstruction for Instability in the Overhead-throwing Athlete

Larry R. Stayner and Frank W. Jobe

There are many procedures to choose in the surgical treatment of the unstable shoulder. Careful diagnosis and patient selection is imperative in selecting the appropriate procedure. The purpose of this chapter is to describe the main causes of pathology in the overhead-throwing shoulder. The diagnosis and treatment will be discussed as well as the operative steps in the anterior capsulolabral reconstruction. The postoperative rehabilitation will be described emphasizing its importance in the treatment of the overhead-throwing athlete. This chapter includes our expectations for the procedure and our published results of the surgery. As is the case in many surgical procedures, multiple pitfalls and pearls can affect the surgery. These pitfalls and pearls are described in the chapter.

INDICATIONS/CONTRAINDICATIONS

The overhead-throwing athlete places tremendous stresses on the glenohumeral joint and surrounding stabilizing structures such as the rotator cuff and glenohumeral ligaments.

The internal rotation of the shoulder during the acceleration phase of pitching has been calculated at 100 degrees in 0.05 second (9). Repetitive stresses of this magnitude placed on the glenohumeral joint can lead to several areas of injury in the shoulder joint, including the superior labrum, rotator cuff tendons, greater tuberosity, inferior glenohumeral ligaments, and superior glenoid bone (3) (Fig. 14-1).

Common areas of injury in the glenohumeral joint from repetitive overhead throwing are the posterosuperior labrum and the articular undersurface of the rotator cuff tendons (12).

L. R. Stayner, M.D.: Kerlan-Jobe Orthopaedic Clinic, Los Angeles, California; and Department of Orthopedic Surgery, Missoula Community Medical Center, Missoula, Montana.

F. W. Jobe, M.D.: Department of Orthopaedic Surgery, University of Southern California Keck School of Medicine; and Kerlan-Jobe Orthopaedic Clinic, Los Angeles, California; and Orthopaedic Consultant, Los Angeles Dodgers, PGA Tour, and Senior PGA Tour.

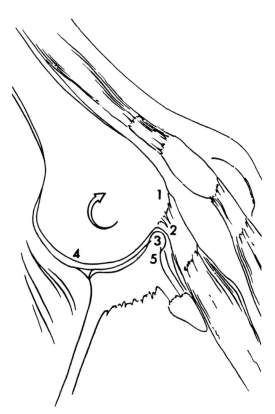

Fig. 14-1. Five areas prone to injury in overhead-throwing athlete: *1.* greater tuberosity, *2.* rotator cuff tendon, *3.* superior labrum, *4.* inferior gleno-humeral ligament and labrum, *5.* superior glenoid bone. (Modified from Jobe, C.M.: Posterior superior glenoid impingement: expanded spectrum. *Arthroscopy* 11: 530–536, 1995, with permission.)

The process whereby these two structures become impinged and injured has been termed "internal impingement" (1,8).

The cause of internal impingement is multifactorial in throwers (Fig. 14-2). Overuse, poor mechanics, and poor endurance can lead to stretching of the anterior shoulder structures and hyperangulation of the arm during throwing that can ultimately lead to anterior

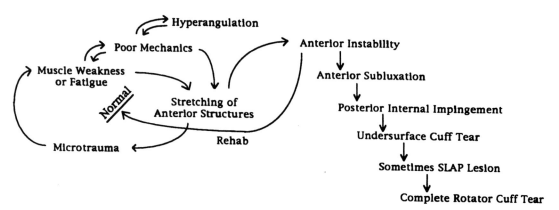

Figure 14-2. Continuum of shoulder injury in the overhead-throwing athlete. (Modified from Pink, M.M., Jobe, F.W.: Concept of overhead athletic injuries. In: Garrett, W.E., Speer, K.P., Kirkendall, D.T., eds.: *Principles and practices of orthopedic sports medicine.* Philadelphia: Lippincott Williams & Wilkins, 551–567, 2000.)

instability of the glenohumeral joint (5,10). Poor strength and poor flexibility can also contribute to this continuum. If left untreated, this instability can lead to the internal impingement and rotator cuff tearing.

Other disease processes can manifest themselves in the overhead-throwing athlete but are much less common than internal impingement. These include external or outside impingement and traumatic dislocation. Older patients are more prone to external or outside impingement, which occurs as the humeral head impinges on the coracoacromial arch. This is a rare event in the overhead-throwing athlete and a diagnosis of instability with internal impingement must first be ruled out to entertain this diagnosis.

Traumatic dislocation is not associated with impingement and does not follow the pathology continuum for internal impingement. Patients with hyperelasticity and multidirectional instability can also get internal or inside impingement during overhead throwing.

Most patients with subtle instability and secondary internal impingement can be successfully rehabilitated without surgical intervention. The inflammatory aspect of the disease can be treated with rest, antiinflammatory medication, and icing. The instability aspect of the disease process can be treated with aggressive rotator cuff and scapular stabilizer strengthening as well as sport-specific training.

Patients who do not respond to this treatment protocol over a 3- to 6-month period will need anterior capsulolabral reconstruction to stabilize their shoulders. As will be discussed in the results section of this chapter, this procedure is very successful in returning overhead athletes to their prior athletic form.

PREOPERATIVE PLANNING

Signs and symptoms in the overhead thrower can often be subtle. The primary symptom of the overhead thrower with this problem will be pain, which can be located either anterior or posterior around the shoulder. Decreased performance and the inability of the thrower to warm up the shoulder before throwing are both indications of this process. A complete evaluation of the overhead thrower must include a thorough evaluation of mechanics. Poor mechanics, including opening up too soon, elbow dropping down, and hyperangulation, are important factors in the pathology continuum (4) (Fig. 14-3).

The physical examination is an important contributor to diagnosis along with the history. A standard evaluation of the cervical spine and neurologic system is mandatory. Along with a standard shoulder examination, careful attention must be paid to the rotator cuff and labrum. The modified relocation test is the cornerstone of diagnosis in the overhead-throwing athlete with subtle anterior instability and secondary internal impingement (2). As Fig. 14-4 shows, the patient is placed supine on an examination table and the affected shoulder is placed over the edge of the table. An anteriorly directed force is then applied to the gleno-

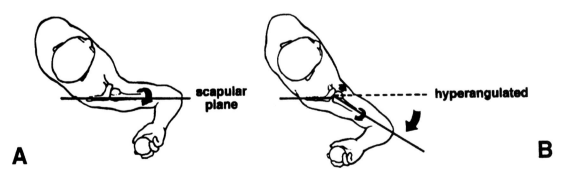

Figure 14-3. A: In normal shoulder, the humerus is abducted in the scapular plane during cocking phase of throwing. **B:** Hyperangulation occurring as the humerus moves into the coronal plane. (Modified from Jobe, C.M., et al. Anterior shoulder instability, impingement, and rotator cuff tear: theories and concepts. In: Jobe, F.W., ed. *Operative techniques in upper extremity sports injuries.* St. Louis: Mosby—Year Book, 164–176, 1996, with permission.)

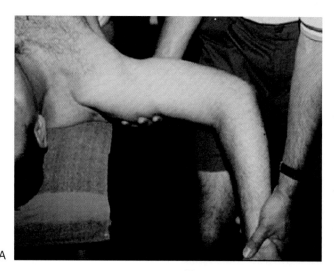
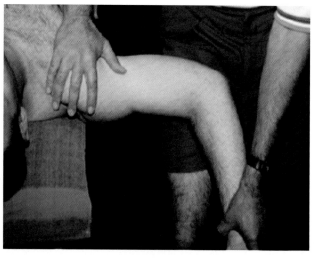

A   B

Figure 14-4. A: Part 1 of modified relocation test: anteriorly directed force applied to posterior, proximal humerus with arm in maximal external rotation. **B:** Part 2 of modified relocation test: posteriorly directed force applied to anterior, proximal humerus with arm in maximal external rotation.

humeral joint placed at 90 degrees of abduction and external rotation. This will cause posterior shoulder pain as the humeral head is brought anteriorly, impinging the rotator cuff on the posterior superior labrum. A posteriorly directed force is then applied in the second step of the test. This will alleviate the pain by keeping the humeral head centered in the glenoid and thus avoiding impingement of the rotator cuff on the posterosuperior glenoid rim. These maneuvers are repeated at 110 and 120 degrees for greater detection of a positive re-

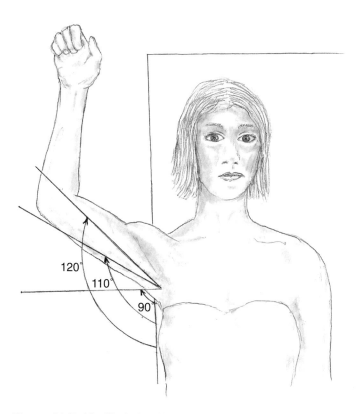

Figure 14-5. Modified shoulder relocation test performed at 90, 100, and 110 degrees of shoulder abduction.

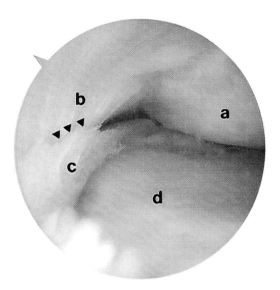

Figure 14-6. Posterosuperior glenoid impingement: *(a)* anteriorly translated humeral head, *(b)* undersurface rotator cuff fraying, *(c)* posterosuperior glenoid labrum/rim (*arrowheads* indicate site of impingement), *(d)* glenoid fossa.

location test (Fig. 14-5). Arthroscopic depiction of the modified relocation test is shown in Figs. 14-6 and 14-7.

Radiographic evaluation includes a standard shoulder series including anteroposterior, axillary lateral, and supraspinatus outlet views. In the overhead-throwing athlete with subtle instability, these radiographs will often be normal in appearance and will rarely reveal fracture, neoplasm, or other pathology. Magnetic resonance imaging is often part of the routine workup to rule out rotator cuff tear and/or labral injury. Newer techniques using gadolinium enhancement are much improved over previous techniques in revealing undersurface rotator cuff tears and labral injuries.

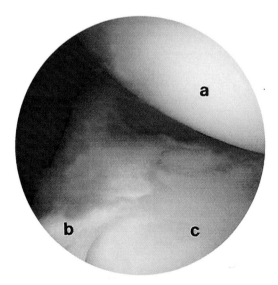

Figure 14-7. Reduced position of glenohumeral joint: *(a)* humeral head reduced, *(b)* posterosuperior labral fraying, *(c)* glenoid fossa.

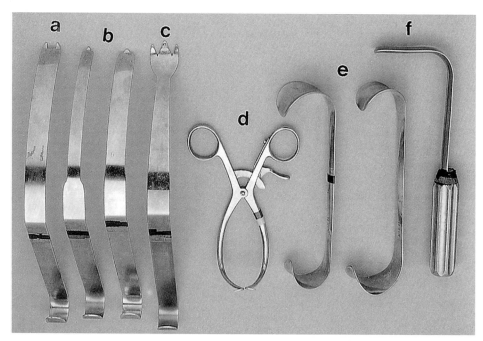

Figure 14-8. Anspach shoulder instruments (The Anspach Effort, Inc., Palm Beach Gardens, FL): **(A)** double-pronged humeral head retractor, **(B)** single-pronged humeral head retractors, **(C)** pitchfork retractor, **(D)** modified Gelpi retractor, **(E)** modified Goulet retractors, **(F)** long, narrow Richardson retractor.

SURGERY

Special instruments needed to perform the surgery are shown in Figs. 14-8 and 14-9. An examination under anesthesia is first performed with the patient in the supine position. The patient is then placed in the lateral decubitus position and a standard diagnostic arthroscopy is performed. After a diagnosis of instability is clearly verified, the arthroscopic wounds are closed and sealed with an Op-site (Smith and Nephew, Inc., Memphis, TN) or other sterile dressing. The patient is placed in the supine position with the arm resting on the Parker arm board. Towel rolls are placed under the scapula and the arm is prepped and draped in sterile fashion.

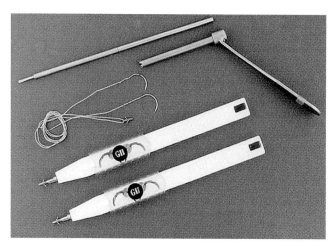

Figure 14-9. Ethibond sutures (Ethicon, Inc., Somerville, NJ) preloaded onto second-generation G-II MITEK anchors (Mitek Worldwide, Norwood, MA).

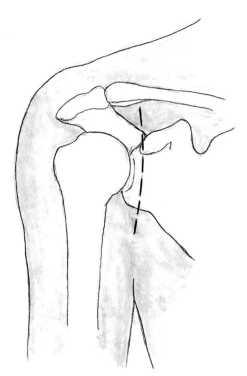

Figure 14-10. Anterior axillary skin incision in Langer lines.

A standard anterior approach to the shoulder is made using an incision in the axillary crease for cosmesis (Fig. 14-10). After skin incision and undermining of subcutaneous tissues over the muscular layer, the interval between the pectoralis major and the deltoid is found (Fig. 14-11). The cephalic vein marks it. The cephalic vein is retracted laterally as the interval is bluntly defined. Goulet retractors are placed under the pectoralis major and

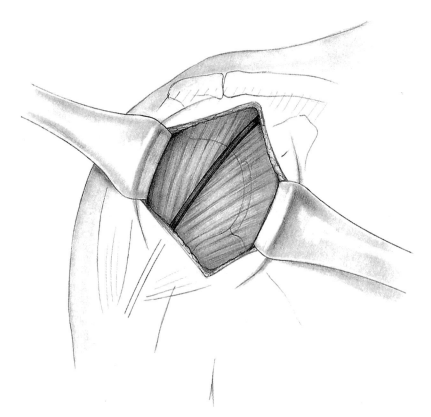

Figure 14-11. Interval betwaen pectoralis major and deltoid marked by cephalic vein.

under the deltoid. The conjoined tendon is then identified running vertically in the wound. The lateral aspect of the conjoined tendon is bluntly dissected off the underlying subscapularis (Fig. 14-12). It is important to find the most lateral border of the conjoined tendon, which is usually marked by the edge of muscular tissue rather than its obvious tendinous border. After carefully freeing up the conjoined tendon, a long narrow Richardson retractor is used to retract this tendon medially. It must be noted that overly aggressive retraction medially can cause stretch injury to the musculocutaneous nerve as it enters the coracobrachialis muscle. The subscapularis tendon is now identified in the depth of the wound. Its insertion site on the lesser tuberosity should be traced while noting the biceps tendon in the bicipital groove. The axillary nerve should also be identified by placing a finger inferiorly and medially on the subscapularis muscle belly and tracing its course. Visualization of the nerve is not needed.

The arm is externally rotated to bring the subscapularis muscle and tendon into full view. The junction of the upper two thirds and lower third of the subscapularis muscle is split horizontally in the direction of the muscle fibers (Fig. 14-13). A fine-tipped Bovie cautery is used in this maneuver. Kocher clamps are placed on the edges of the subscapularis tendon to facilitate retraction. Sharp dissection is used to free the adherent subscapularis muscle from the underlying joint capsule (Fig. 14-14). The plane of dissection between the subscapularis and the joint capsule is facilitated by starting medially under the muscular portion rather than the tendinous portion. Sharp dissection in this plane is essential in freeing up both the upper and lower portions of the subscapularis to fully visualize the joint capsule. A modified Gelpi retractor is used to keep open the subscapularis tendon split. The Kocher clamps are removed before placing the Gelpi retractor.

A three-pronged pitchfork retractor is placed on the anterior glenoid rim just medial to the glenoid rim. An incision is made in the joint capsule at the junction of the upper two thirds and lower one third (Fig. 14-15). The humeral head is manually distracted and a one- or two-pronged humeral head retractor is placed to retract the humeral head laterally. Stay sutures are placed in the superior and inferior joint capsule flaps at the level of the glenoid rim. The capsular incision is brought medially onto the glenoid rim and neck. It is impera-

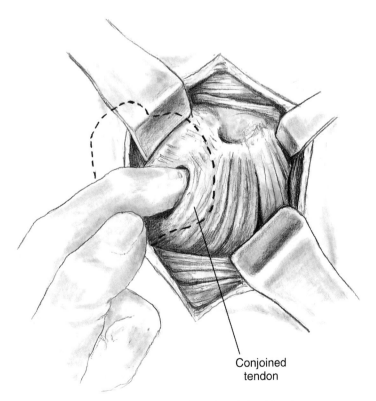

Conjoined
tendon

Figure 14-12. Retraction of conjoined tendon.

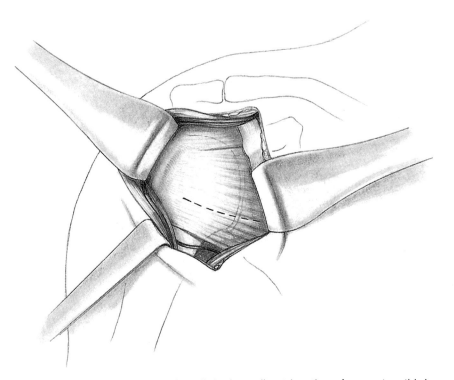

Figure 14-13. Subscapularis muscle split horizontally at junction of upper two thirds and lower one third.

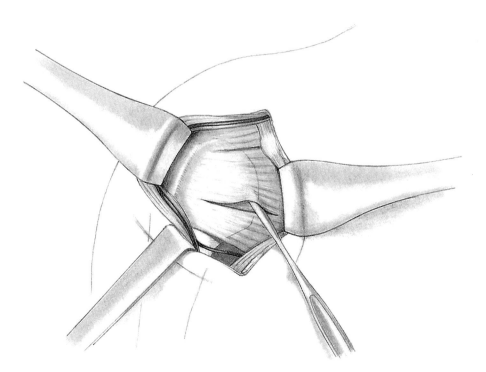

Figure 14-14. Dissection of subscapularis muscle from the underlying capsule.

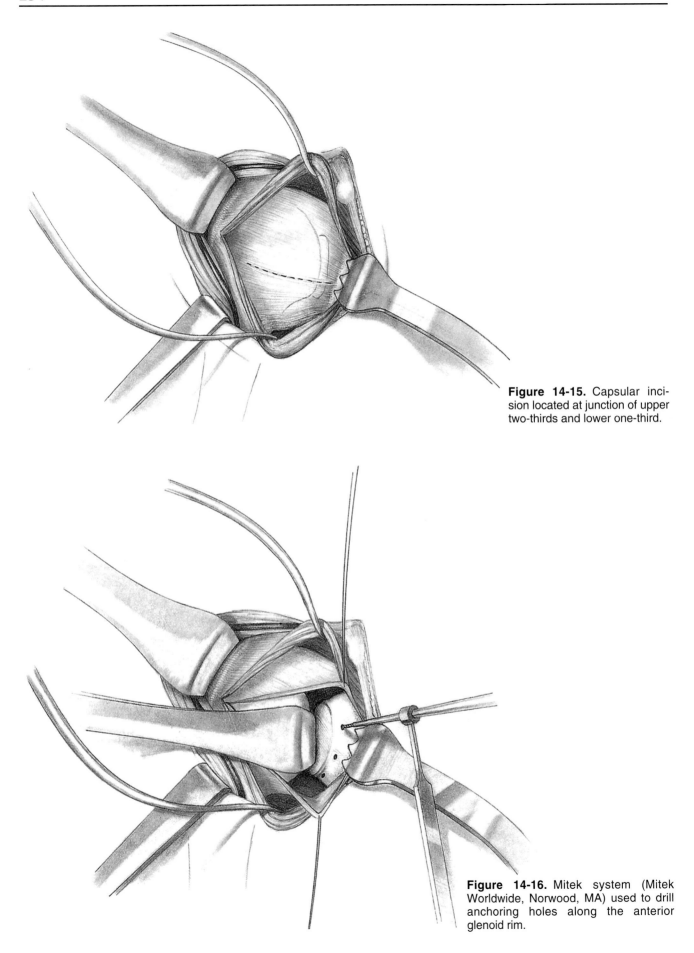

Figure 14-15. Capsular incision located at junction of upper two-thirds and lower one-third.

Figure 14-16. Mitek system (Mitek Worldwide, Norwood, MA) used to drill anchoring holes along the anterior glenoid rim.

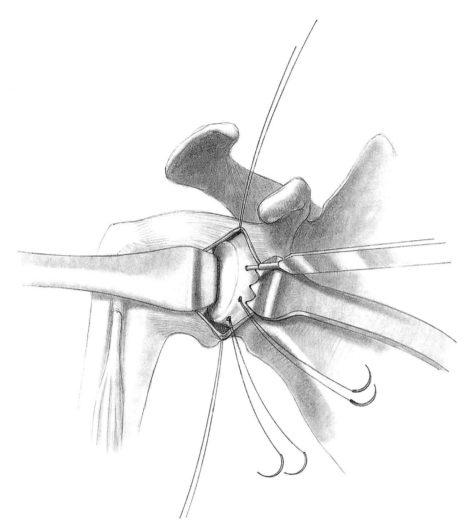

Figure 14-17. Preloaded no. 2 Ethibond (Ethicon, Inc., Somerville, NJ), double-limbed sutures inserted into drill holes.

tive to avoid injuring the underlying glenoid labrum. The capsule should be elevated off the glenoid rim and neck subperiosteally. If a Bankart lesion is discovered, the labrum must be elevated with the capsule to be later incorporated into the repair. The capsule should be elevated down to the 6-o'clock position to allow shifting of the redundant inferior capsule. The glenoid rim is débrided of overlying tissue. The drill holes are created just medial to the glenoid articular margin (2 mm) (Fig. 14-16). Suture anchors are placed at the 3-, 4-, and 5:30-o'clock positions (Fig. 14-17). The inferior capsular limb is tensioned with the stay suture to shift it superiorly. The two limbs of the suture anchors are used to secure the inferior limb to the glenoid (Fig. 14-18). It is important to place the sutures medial to the stay sutures in order to avoid excessive horizontal shifting of the tissues. This can lead to excessive tightening, postoperative shoulder tightness, and decreased range of motion. The superior capsular limb is shifted inferiorly, passing the middle and the superior suture limbs through both the superior and inferior limbs in a pants-over-vest orientation (Fig. 14-19). To avoid overtightening the capsule the shoulder is placed in an abducted and externally rotated position prior to completely tightening the capsule. Do not suture the overlap of the capsule over the last inch laterally (Fig. 14-20). This gives a chance for the capsule to adjust to the correct amount of tightening. The subscapularis muscle is closed along with a standard wound closure (Fig. 14-21). If excessive bleeding is encountered, a drain may be placed before closure.

(text continues on page 238)

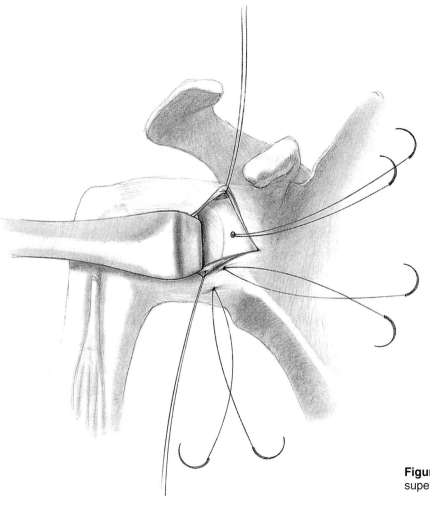

Figure 14-18. Inferior capsular flap advanced superiorly and anchored into position.

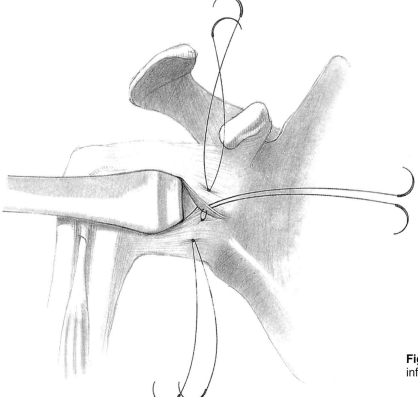

Figure 14-19. Superior capsular flap advanced inferiorly, overlying inferior capsular flap.

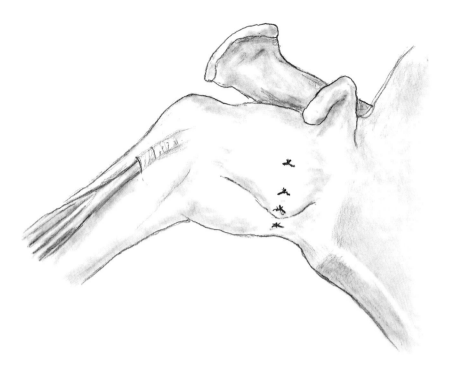

Figure 14-20. Closure of the capsule in a "pants-over-vest" fashion. Capsular split laterally is not sutured closed.

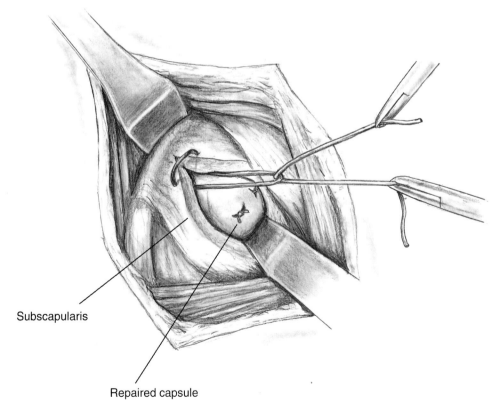

Subscapularis

Repaired capsule

Figure 14-21. Subscapularis closure.

POSTOPERATIVE MANAGEMENT

After surgery, the patient is immediately immobilized in a sling. Pain management includes the use of an intraoperative wound injection, oral narcotics, and a scalene block. Most patients are discharged to home on the day of surgery. If a drain is placed at the time of surgery, it is removed on the first postoperative day. This can be done in the clinic setting. Sutures are removed on the seventh postoperative day.

Rehabilitation

Movement of the wrist and elbow is started on the first day after surgery. Active forward flexion is also started after surgery and continued daily. Active external rotation is started gradually after surgery and is increased to full range of motion over the first 4 weeks after surgery. At 4 weeks, muscular strengthening of the rotator cuff muscles and scapular stabilizers is begun. Key exercises in strengthening these muscles in addition to a standard rotator cuff protocol include scaption with thumbs down to approximately 70 degrees of elevation, rowing, push-ups with a plus, press-ups, and flexion and horizontal abduction with arms externally rotated (7,11). Fine-motor tuning is started in supervised therapy sessions along with the strengthening exercises.

Gentle ball tossing is allowed at 4 to 6 months if the rotator cuff muscles and scapular stabilizers have regained substantial strength. This can be assessed by isokinetic testing. If the strength of the shoulder musculature has regained approximately 80% of the normal shoulder, then ball tossing is begun. Pitchers gradually increase their frequency and duration of throwing over the next 6 months while continuing strength and fine-motor work with a therapist. Total body conditioning is also stressed during this time period. At 12 months, the overhead thrower will have regained full range of motion and muscle strength with appropriate muscle synchrony to protect the shoulder. Full activities without restriction are allowed. Resumption of full pitching is allowed at this point with continued emphasis on strengthening, conditioning, proper throwing mechanics, and the avoidance of overuse (5).

RESULTS

Montgomery and Jobe (6) showed 97% good/excellent results and an 81% return to high-level overhead athletics in 31 of 32 recreational, collegiate, and professional athletes at more than a 24-month follow-up. The average loss of range of motion in external rotation and forward flexion in this study was 1 degree. As this study illustrates, we have been able to regain most of the range of motion in patients with minimal losses of external rotation.

Anterior capsulolabral reconstruction in the proper setting with the correct indications has been shown to be highly effective in achieving stability of the shoulder joint. It has also been shown to allow highly skilled, overhead-throwing athletes to resume athletics at their premorbid level of competition (6).

COMPLICATIONS

Loss of range of motion postoperatively is a problem that can interfere with return to high-level overhead athletics. Proper technique during the surgical intervention is key in avoiding loss of range of motion. Two important points during the procedure must be kept in mind. First, overtightening of the capsule medially onto the glenoid must be avoided. This can lead to excessive horizontal shifting of the capsule and a corresponding loss of external rotation. Second, the lateral aspect of the capsule must not be closed. This allows for some forgiveness in the repair, allowing earlier and better range of motion.

ACKNOWLEDGMENTS

We thank Marilyn Pink, Ph.D., for her help in preparing the manuscript for publication.

RECOMMENDED READING

1. Davidson, P.A., El Attrache, N.S., Jobe, C.M., et al.: Rotator cuff and posterior-superior glenoid labrum injury associated with increased glenohumeral motion: a new site of impingement. *J Shoulder Elbow Surg* 4: 384–390, 1995.
2. Hamner, D.L., Pink, M.M., Jobe, F.W.: A modification of the relocation test: arthroscopic findings associated with a positive test. *J Shoulder Elbow Surg* 9: 263–269, 2000.
3. Jobe, C.M.: Posterior superior glenoid impingement: expanded spectrum. *Arthroscopy* 11: 530–536, 1995.
4. Jobe, C.M., et al.: Anterior shoulder instability, impingement, and rotator cuff tear: theories and concepts. In: Jobe, F.W., ed.: *Operative techniques in upper extremity sports injuries.* St. Louis: Mosby–Year Book, 164–176, 1996.
5. Kauffman, J., Jobe, F.W.: Anterior capsulolabral reconstruction for recurrent anterior instability. *Sports Med Arthros Rev* 8: 272–279, 2000.
6. Montgomery, W.H., Jobe, F.W.: Functional outcomes in athletes after modified anterior capsulolabral reconstruction. *Am J Sports Med* 22: 352–358, 1994.
7. Moseley, J.B., Jobe, F.W., Pink, M.M., et al.: EMG analysis of the scapular muscles during a shoulder rehabilitation program. *Am J Sports Med* 20: 128–134, 1992.
8. Paley, K.J., Jobe, F.W., Pink, M.M., et al.: Arthroscopic findings in the overhand throwing athlete: evidence for posterior internal impingement on the rotator cuff. *Arthroscopy* 16: 35–40, 2000.
9. Pappas, A.M., Zawacki, R.M., Sullivan, T.J.: Biomechanics of baseball pitching. *Am. J. Sports Med* 13: 216–222, 1985.
10. Pink, M.M., Jobe, F.W.: Concept of the overhead athletic injuries. In: Garrett, W.E., Speer, K.P., Kirkendell, D.T., eds.: *Principles and practice of orthopaedic sports medicine.* Philadelphia: Lippincott Williams & Wilkins, 551–567, 2000.
11. Townsend, H., Jobe, F.W., Pink, M.M., et al.: Electromyographic analysis of the glenohumeral muscles during a baseball rehabilitation program. *Am J Sports Med* 19: 264–272, 1991.
12. Walch, G., Goileau, P., Noel, E., et al.: Impingement of the deep surface of the supraspinatus tendon on the posterior glenoid rim: an arthroscopic study. *J Shoulder Elbow Surg* 1: 238–245, 1992.

15

Anteroinferior Capsular Shift for Involuntary Multidirectional Instability

Steven P. Kalandiak, R. Stacy Tapscott, Michael A. Wirth, and Charles A. Rockwood, Jr.

INDICATIONS/CONTRAINDICATIONS

Multidirectional instability (MDI) is a common problem that is frequently misdiagnosed or improperly treated. Since the classic description of this condition by Neer and Foster (18), a higher index of suspicion and a better understanding of MDI have led to increased recognition of this condition and improved surgical outcomes. Most patients with MDI will respond favorably to a rigorous, physician-directed, home exercise program (3). Involuntary multidirectional shoulder instability rarely requires surgical intervention, but when surgery is necessary, methods of operative intervention that provide satisfactory results for traumatic instability have not typically worked for patients with MDI. In these patients, an anteroinferior capsular shift, designed to tighten the capsule, decreasing its overall volume, has proven successful when a properly directed rehabilitation program fails to stabilize the shoulder (18).

The primary indication for operative treatment of MDI is symptomatic, involuntary, global glenohumeral instability in a patient who has no psychological impairment and has failed a course of at least 6 months of conservative treatment in a physician-directed therapy program aimed at strengthening the rotator cuff, deltoid, and scapular stabilizers. The two essential components of the reconstruction involve closure of the rotator interval capsule and reduction of the excessive joint volume through symmetric and anatomic plication of the redundant anterior, inferior, and posteroinferior aspects of the capsule. Patients with

S. P. Kalandiak, M.D.: Department of Orthopaedics and Rehabilitation, University of Miami School of Medicine; and Jackson Memorial Hospital, Miami, Florida.

R. S. Tapscott, M.D.: Shoulder/Sports Medicine, Decatur Orthopaedic Clinic, Decatur, Alabama.

M. A. Wirth, M.D. and C. A. Rockwood, Jr., M.D.: Department of Orthopaedics, The University of Texas Health Science Center at San Antonio, San Antonio, Texas.

traumatic initial episodes are less likely to respond to a conservative treatment program and are more likely to have a Bankart-Perthes lesion noted on radiographic examination or at surgery.

Contraindications to this procedure relate primarily to patient selection. Absolute contraindications include documented emotional or psychological disturbances, glenoid aplasia or hypoplasia (28), and noncompliance with previous preoperative therapy regimen. Relative contraindications include motivation by secondary gain (e.g., some workman's compensation cases) and significant neurologic injury to the axillary or suprascapular nerves. Although a history of multiple prior surgeries does decrease the likelihood of a good result, it is not a contraindication to performing an anteroinferior capsular shift. We have obtained good results in most revision cases using this technique, although extra attention to details is of paramount importance (25).

Patients who have involuntary MDI and have completed at least a 6-month course of conservative management with no improvement are candidates for anteroinferior capsular shift, although we may continue patients with atraumatic instability in their rehabilitation program for a full year before opting for surgical intervention. A major benefit of a lengthy preoperative conservative treatment program is the opportunity to evaluate the patient's character, which plays a significant role in the eventual outcome of any management strategy. We stress to patients that a significant portion of the success or failure of their treatment is dependent upon their willingness to participate in and direct their preoperative and postoperative rehabilitation. This gives the patients a sense of control over their outcome and encourages an active role in their treatment.

PREOPERATIVE PLANNING

Together, the history, physical examination, and radiographic examinations create a picture of the unstable shoulder that allows accurate preoperative planning. In contemplating surgical treatment for MDI of the shoulder, it is essential to determine whether the primary direction of instability is anterior, inferior, or posterior. This particular information is generally gleaned from the history given by the patient. Patients with predominantly anterior instability will describe symptoms that occur when their arm is in the apprehension position of abduction and external rotation, such as when they cock their arm to throw a ball. Patients with predominantly posterior instability will complain that their shoulder tends to "slip out of place" when their arm is forward flexed and internally rotated, such as when they remove a book from an overhead shelf. Inferior instability will most often be demonstrated when patients carry objects at their side, such as a heavy suitcase.

Patients with MDI often give a history of shoulder complaints beginning in childhood, and initial episodes of subluxation or dislocation that were atraumatic or occurred with minimal trauma. Involuntary, symptomatic instability results gradually from multiple recurrences or begins after a traumatic event. Dislocations in patients with MDI are frequently transient and often do not require the assistance of a physician or another person to obtain a reduction. Painful subluxation is generally associated with global instability secondary to traumatic events rather than with MDI of an entirely atraumatic origin.

Physical examination of the patient with MDI usually reveals generalized ligamentous laxity as evidenced by hyperextension of the elbows, knees, and metacarpophalangeal joints; hyperabduction of the thumb (passive abduction of the thumb to the forearm with the wrist flexed); and patellofemoral laxity. Many patients with MDI can voluntarily sublux their shoulders, usually in a posterior direction. This ability does not absolutely contraindicate surgical intervention, but patients with voluntary subluxation should undergo psychiatric evaluation. Instability testing, by definition, shows laxity in both the anteroposterior (AP) and inferior directions, manifested by a positive sulcus sign (a dimple created between the humeral head and the acromion when the humeral shaft is pulled distally), a positive anterior or posterior drawer (load and shift) test (anterior or posterior subluxation noted when directly pushing the humeral head anteriorly or posteriorly, after centering the head in the glenoid fossa), and a positive push–pull test (more than 50% posterior translation of the shoulder in the supine patient when the wrist is pulled up while the proximal humerus is pushed downward). Rotator cuff and deltoid strength are typically normal, although patients with MDI can often differentially contract the heads of the deltoid, causing subluxation. Even if strength is normal, added strength, coordination, and endurance, particularly in the rotator cuff and scapular stabilizers, help to control dynamic instability by improving scapular positioning and increasing and centering the joint reaction force in the glenoid, thus improving stability through increased concavity-compression.

Although patients with MDI often have normal radiographic findings, an instability series consisting of AP views in internal and external rotation, an axillary lateral view, a Stryker notch view, and an apical oblique view should be obtained. These patients can have traumatic episodes superimposed on a background of generalized ligamentous laxity, and the presence of a Bankart-Perthes lesion has implications for the outcome of a conservative treatment program. It is also important to recognize the presence of these lesions preoperatively, as all Bankart-Perthes lesions and extremely severe Hill-Sachs lesions should be addressed at the time of surgery. The axillary lateral view should be scrutinized for evidence of glenoid hypoplasia or aplasia or excessive glenoid retroversion, as both conditions are poorly treated by anterior capsular reconstructions alone. Patients with glenoid retroversion abnormalities should undergo computed tomography scanning of both shoulders to further delineate the condition.

An examination under anesthesia is not necessary to make the diagnosis of MDI, but it can be performed in the operating room before anteroinferior capsular shift.

Although we recognize the growing enthusiasm of the orthopaedic community for arthroscopic instability repair, we continue to believe that the best way to address MDI is with an open procedure. Excessive capsular laxity is the primary pathology in MDI, and it is difficult to treat arthroscopically. Open repair allows intraoperative assessment of the amount of capsular redundancy and adjustment of the capsular tension according to the patient's individual needs. In addition, anterior labral pathology, if present, is easily addressed at the time of open capsular shift. Although the history, physical examination, and radiographic studies for MDI are generally clear, in rare situations, when the diagnosis remains obscure, diagnostic arthroscopy may help clarify treatment decisions. Posterior and superior labral pathologies are also being recognized with increasing frequency, and, if present, may be addressed arthroscopically before performing capsular shift.

SURGERY

The anteroinferior capsular shift procedure described below was developed and used by the senior author (C.A.R.) beginning in 1970, and was first described in 1984 (15). The technique incorporates aspects of the methods of Bankart and Putti-Platt, as well as the classic inferior capsular shift described by Neer and Foster in 1980 (18). In addition, there are several important alterations in this procedure:

- Only the upper two thirds of the subscapularis tendon is reflected from the capsule; the lower one third of the muscle–tendon unit is left intact, which may spare some proprioceptive capacity, in addition to preserving the primary blood supply to the humeral head, the anterior humeral circumflex vessels;
- Elevation and retraction of the lower one third of the subscapularis tendon from the capsule provides protection of the axillary nerve while incising and shifting the inferior capsule;
- The capsule is freed from the overlying subscapularis tendon from top to bottom;
- The capsular incision is made halfway between the glenoid rim and the attachment of the capsule to the humeral neck and extends from the rotator interval down to, and if necessary, beyond the 6-o'clock position; division of the capsule in this fashion allows the thin anterior capsule to be strengthened by double-breasting it in the midportion rather than shifting it medially on the glenoid or laterally on the humerus;
- The rotator interval, increasingly recognized as contributing to posterior and inferior instability, is plicated at the beginning of the capsular repair to reduce overall capsular volume;

- When the shift is completed, the detached medial upper two thirds of the subscapularis tendon is repaired to its lateral stump in an end-to-end fashion without shortening, minimizing the risk of internal rotation contracture.

We have found that these simple modifications of the procedure provide us with satisfactory, predictable, and reproducible results.

Preparing the Patient

We prefer to perform the procedure under general anesthesia with the patient in a semi-Fowler, or beach-chair position. We remove the headrest from the standard operative table and replace it with a special headrest. In the past we have used a Mayfield headrest (Ohio Medical Instrument Co., Inc., Cincinnati, OH), but we are currently using a McConnell headrest (McConnell Orthopedic Manufacturing Co., Greenville, TX), which provides better access to the shoulder for the assistant at the head of the table and allows the patient to be moved toward the edge of the table (Fig. 15-1). The patient's head is secured to the headrest with 2-in. cloth tape, and two towels are secured to the forehead to prevent injury by the first assistant's elbow. The shoulder is prepped and the arm draped free (Fig. 15-2), affording the primary surgeon or a second assistant a comfortable position in the axilla to perform the procedure. It is critical that the surgeon have a minimum of two able assistants to perform the procedure properly. In general, antibiotic prophylaxis is given for 24 hours for primary and 48 hours for revision cases.

The Incision and Approach

The standard axillary incision extending from the coracoid process into the axilla following the anterior axillary fold is used for the approach (Fig. 15-3). If necessary, this incision can be extended proximally toward the clavicle in large, muscular males. For a more cosmetic scar in females, the incision can be modified in the manner described by Leslie and Ryan (13), with the incision in the axilla. This pure axillary incision necessitates more ex-

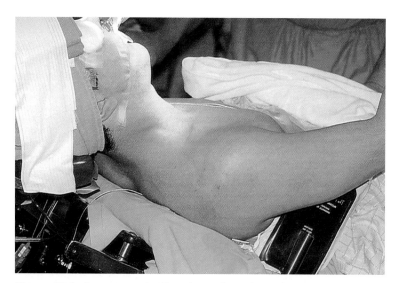

Figure 15-1. A neurosurgical headrest allows the patient to be positioned safely at the edge of the table, giving the surgeon and surgical assistants easy access to the shoulder. Two towels are placed on the forehead, and the head is secured to the headrest to prevent inadvertent injury to the patient by the elbow of the assistant standing at the head of the table. This position maintains the patient's head in a stable position throughout the procedure.

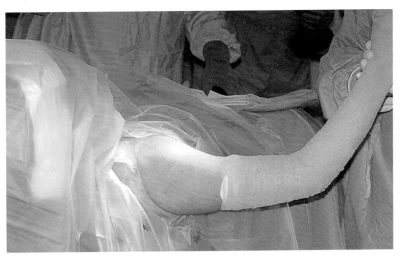

Figure 15-2. The shoulder is prepped and draped with the entire arm free.

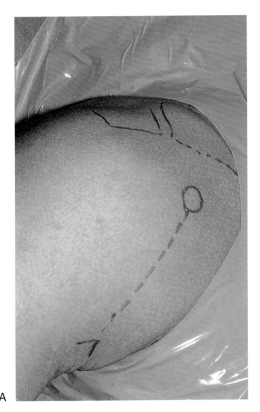

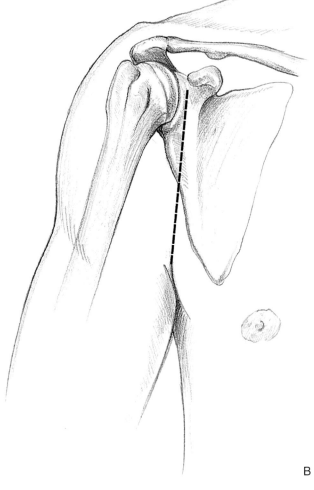

A

Figure 15-3. An anterior axillary incision from the coracoid process to the axilla, following Langer skin lines, is used. **A:** Superomedial view. **B:** Relationship of incision to shoulder girdle anatomy.

B

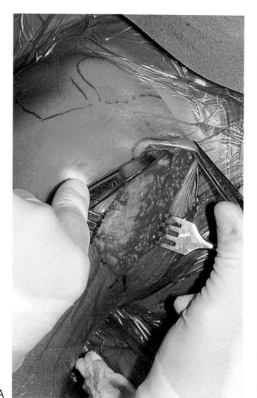

A

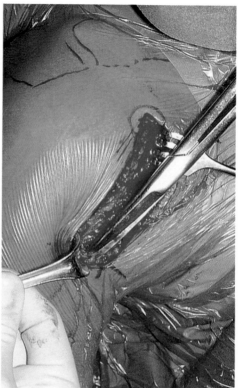

B

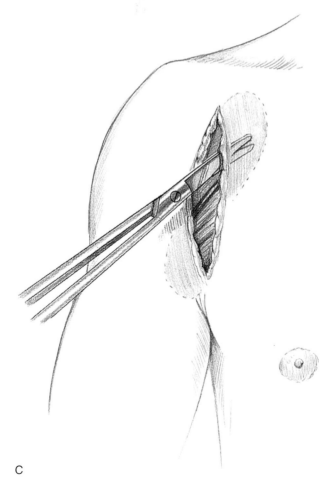

C

Figure 15-4. The deltopectoral interval is identified and exposed by subcutaneous dissection **(A)** superomedially and **(B)** inferolaterally in the axillary incision. **C:** Region of subcutaneous dissection in shaded area to expose the cephalic vein and the deltopectoral interval.

tensive proximal subcutaneous dissection to the level of the clavicle for exposure of the deltopectoral interval. The incision through the dermis is performed with a no. 10 blade, then Bovie electrocautery is used in the cutting mode to complete the incision down through the subcutaneous tissue. Curved Mayo scissors are used to undermine the subcutaneous tissue superomedially and inferolaterally (Fig. 15-4). This effectively exposes the deltopectoral interval, which crosses the incision diagonally and can be identified by the presence of the cephalic vein (Fig. 15-5). Occasionally, the cephalic vein is not readily identifiable, as it may be absent or deep within the deltopectoral interval. When this is the case, the interval is more easily identified proximally where there is greater divergence of the muscle fibers of the deltoid and pectoralis major, which are also separated by the easily palpated coracoid process. The cephalic vein is carefully preserved and taken laterally with the deltoid, preserving all feeders from the deltoid. Because we have seen increased venous congestion and postoperative discomfort in patients with cephalic vein disruption, we do not recommend ligation of the cephalic vein and will even repair small inadvertent perforations in the vein with interrupted 8-0 nylon sutures. Blunt fingertip dissection can then define the deltopectoral interval from the clavicle down to the insertion of the pectoralis major tendon just lateral to the bicipital groove. There is no need to detach any portion of the deltoid from its origin on the clavicle or its insertion on the humerus. Releasing the proximal 1 to 2 cm of the pectoralis major insertion can be helpful for improving visualization of the inferior capsule, but care must be taken not to injure the tendon of the long head of the biceps, which lies in the bicipital groove just medial to the pectoralis major insertion. We do not recom-

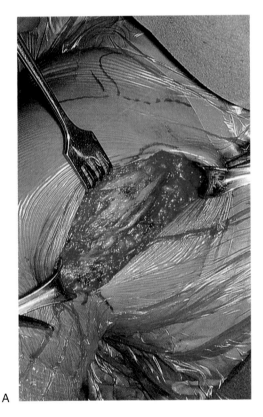

A

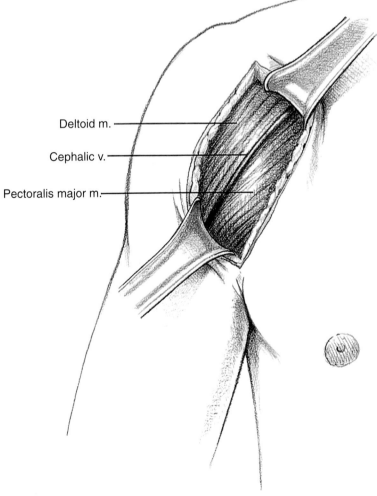

Deltoid m.

Cephalic v.

Pectoralis major m.

Figure 15-5. A: The cephalic vein demarcates the deltopectoral interval. **B:** The cephalic vein is retracted laterally with the deltoid.

B

mend detachment of the coracoid process or the conjoined tendon. Narrow Richardson retractors retract the deltoid laterally and the pectoralis major medially. The clavipectoral fascia, which overlies the subscapularis and the conjoined tendon and is continuous with the coracoacromial ligament proximally (Fig. 15-6), is then divided vertically just lateral to the muscle belly of the short head of the biceps, which generally projects laterally from beneath the conjoined tendon. The conjoined tendon is freed from its investing fascia, and the clavipectoral fascia is released proximally to the level of the coracoacromial ligament attachment to the lateral aspect of the coracoid.

The musculocutaneous and axillary nerves are then located, palpated, and protected. The entry point of the musculocutaneous nerve into the conjoined tendon complex is quite variable, though ordinarily it is approximately 5 cm distal to the tip of the coracoid (5). Digital palpation just dorsal and medial to the conjoined tendon and muscles will reveal the region of penetration of the musculocutaneous nerve (Fig. 15-7). The axillary nerve is at higher risk during the inferior capsular shift procedure (Fig. 15-8) and can be palpated by sliding the index finger down along the anterior border of the subscapularis until it reaches the 6-o'clock position, where the axillary nerve can be hooked with the index finger as it dives posteriorly and lies inferior to the capsule as it approaches the quadrangular space (Figs. 15-9 and 15-10). A large Richardson or a self-retaining Kolbel retractor is placed beneath the conjoined tendon to expose the underlying subscapularis muscle and tendon (Fig. 15-11A). It is extremely important that retraction on the conjoined tendon not be overly vigorous, as a transient musculocutaneous palsy may result.

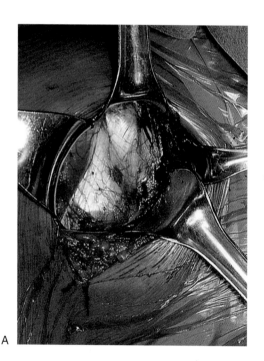

A

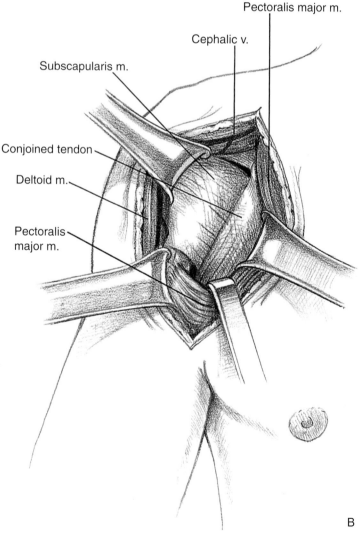

B

Figure 15-6. A: Muscle fibers from the short head of the biceps can be seen just lateral to the conjoined tendon when the deltoid is retracted laterally and the pectoralis major medially. The clavipectoral fascia is incised just lateral to these muscle fibers so the Richardson retractor can be placed beneath the conjoined tendon. **B:** The conjoined tendon of the short head of the biceps and the coracobrachialis overlies the subscapularis tendon and muscle. It is not necessary to detach the coracoid process.

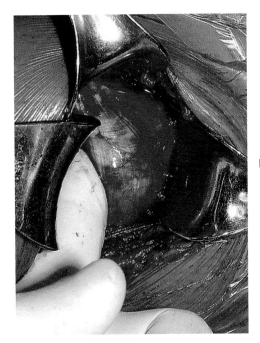

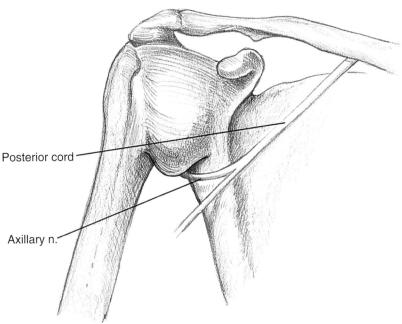

Figure 15-7. Sliding the index finger posterior to the conjoined tendon, the surgeon can locate and then protect the cord of the musculocutaneous nerve. The nerve is usually on the posteromedial edge of the tendon, but it has a variable course and is occasionally even seen on the lateral border of the tendon.

Figure 15-8. The axillary nerve is at high risk during the capsular shift. The nerve hugs the scapular neck and is intimately opposed to the joint capsule as it moves from anterior to posterior to exit the quadrangular space.

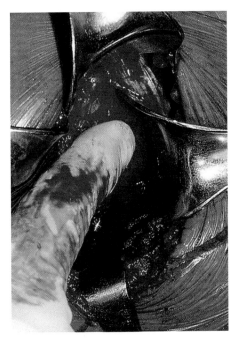

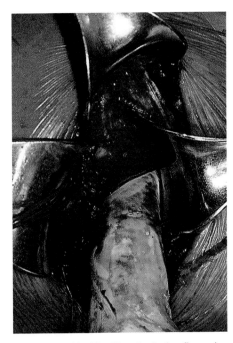

Figure 15-9. The axillary nerve must be protected. It can be identified by sliding the index finger along the anterior surface of the subscapularis tendon beneath the conjoined tendon.

Figure 15-10. Hooking the index finger inferiorly, the cord (the axillary nerve) is readily palpated.

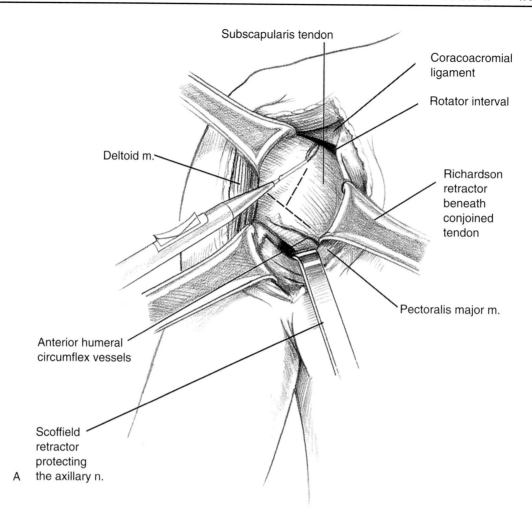

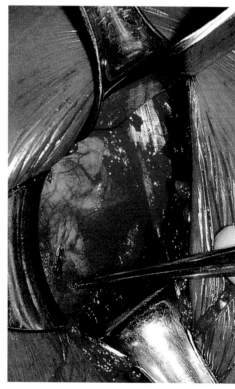

Figure 15-11. A: The anterior humeral circumflex vessels are found on the inferior third of the subscapularis tendon and should be spared when freeing the upper two-thirds of the subscapularis from the underlying capsule. **B:** The anterior humeral circumflex vessels (the "three sisters") provide the primary blood supply to the humeral head and are readily identifiable.

Technique

After sweeping the remaining fascia from the surface of the subscapularis and irrigating the wound, the upper and lower borders of the subscapularis tendon are identified. The "soft spot" of the rotator interval (i.e., the natural demarcation between the tendons of the supraspinatus and subscapularis) marks the superior border of the subscapularis tendon, and the "three sisters" (i.e., the anterior humeral circumflex artery and its two accompanying veins) can routinely be identified just proximal to the inferior border of the subscapularis tendon (Fig. 15-11B). The rotator interval is often patent in patients with MDI. If not, a small Darrach retractor is placed in the rotator interval to help define the superior border of the subscapularis tendon, and if necessary, a ball-tipped pusher can be used to push the humeral head posteriorly to enhance exposure. With the arm externally rotated to expose the entire tendon (Fig. 15-11B), the upper two thirds of the subscapularis tendon is vertically transected with electrocautery approximately 1.5 to 2 cm medial to its insertion on the lesser tuberosity (Figs. 15-12 to 15-14). Care is taken to avoid penetration of the underlying anterior capsule while separating the subscapularis tendon from the adherent capsule. A small portion of the subscapularis tendon may be left attached to the capsule, as this may supply some extra strength to the capsular repair. The inferior one third of the subscapularis tendon is not transected. This maintains the integrity and some proprioception of the muscle–tendon unit and preserves the anterior humeral circumflex vessels, which provide the vast majority of the blood supply to the humeral head. Once the vertical transection is completed, electrocautery is used to create a horizontal incision in line with the fibers of the subscapularis tendon and muscle between the upper two thirds and lower one third of the subscapularis tendon. Mayo scissors are used to cautiously reflect the upper two thirds of the subscapularis from the underlying capsule, until that portion of the subscapularis muscle and tendon are a free, dynamic unit (Fig. 15-15). Again, it is important to avoid injury to the underlying capsule. Several nonabsorbable no. 1 cottony Dacron sutures are placed as stay sutures in the lateral edge of the medial portion of the subscapularis tendon

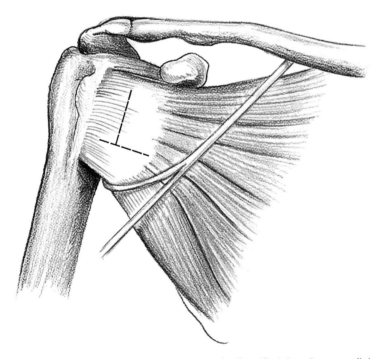

Figure 15-12. The subscapularis is vertically split 1.5 to 2 cm medial to the biceps tendon, extending from the rotator interval superiorly to a point proximal to the anterior humeral circumflex vessels, in line with its fibers, leaving approximately two thirds superior and one third inferior.

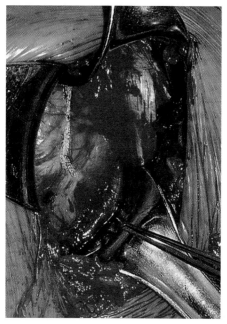

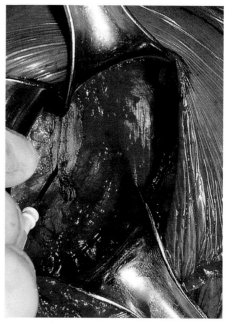

Figure 15-13. A preliminary mark made with electrocautery showing the incision of the subscapularis. Note the vessels inferior to the horizontal portion of the incision.

Figure 15-14. The incision is carried down through the subscapularis utilizing electrocautery, being careful not to violate the underlying capsule that is intimately adherent to the undersurface of the subscapularis. The plane between the subscapularis and the capsule is extremely difficult to define, and it is better to leave a few fibers of the subscapularis tendon with the capsule than to excessively thin out the capsule or make numerous punctures.

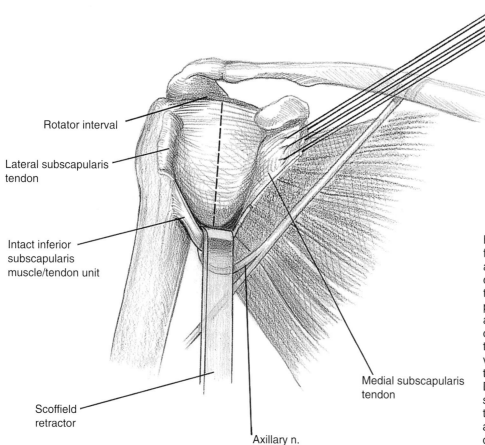

Rotator interval

Lateral subscapularis tendon

Intact inferior subscapularis muscle/tendon unit

Scoffield retractor

Axillary n.

Medial subscapularis tendon

Figure 15-15. The stump and free tendon of the subscapularis are freed from the underlying capsule and retracted to expose the anterior capsule. The intact portion of the subscapularis must also be dissected free from the capsule to allow visualization of the capsule from the rotator interval to at least the 6-o'clock position. Several no. 1 cottony Dacron sutures are placed as stay sutures in the free edge of the medial subscapularis tendon and will later be utilized for repair of the free tendon to its stump.

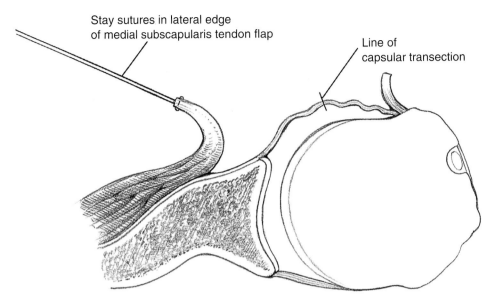

Figure 15-16. A transverse depiction of the subscapularis dissected free from the underlying capsule showing the vertical line of transection of the capsule half-way between the glenoid rim and the capsular attachment to the humeral head (see also Fig. 15-15).

for use in retraction and later repair (Fig. 15-16). One-millimeter cottony Dacron tapes can be used in the subscapularis if the patient is large, strong, and extremely active. A no. 15 blade is used to free the lateral stump of the subscapularis from the capsule to facilitate the final tendon repair (Figs. 15-17 and 15-18). A periosteal elevator is used to gently strip the intact inferior portion of the subscapularis from the anteroinferior capsule until the entire capsule can be visualized from the 12- to the 6-o'clock positions (Fig. 15-19). A Scoffield retractor can then be placed inside the lower third of the subscapularis to expose the inferior capsule and protect the axillary nerve during the capsular shift (Figs. 15-20 and 15-21). This is followed by copious wound irrigation.

The anterior capsule is divided midway between its glenoid and humeral attachments in a vertical fashion from the rotator interval (Fig. 15-22) to the 6-o'clock position or just be-

(text continues on page 256)

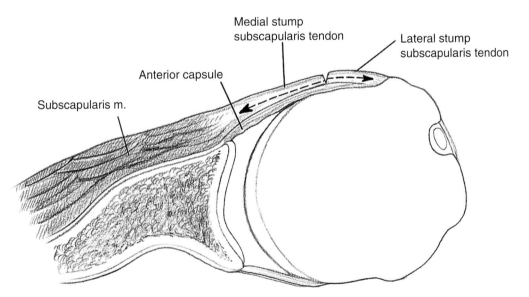

Figure 15-17. A periosteal elevator, a knife blade, Mayo scissors, or electrocautery can be used to reflect the subscapularis tendon from the adherent capsule beneath both the medial tendon and the lateral stump.

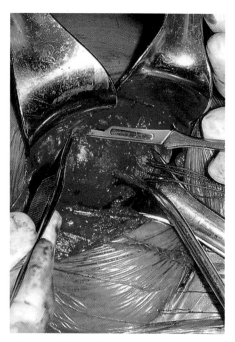

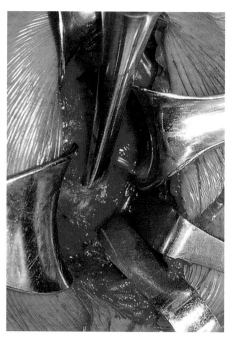

Figure 15-18. The medial tendon has been freed from the capsule with sharp dissection and is retracted medially with stay sutures. The lateral stump is liberated from the underlying capsule using a no. 15 knife blade to expose the remainder of the anterior capsule.

Figure 15-19. Working from medial to lateral, the inferior third of the subscapularis is gently stripped from the inferior capsule until the entire anterior capsule can be visualized from the 12-o'clock position to at least the 6-o'clock position.

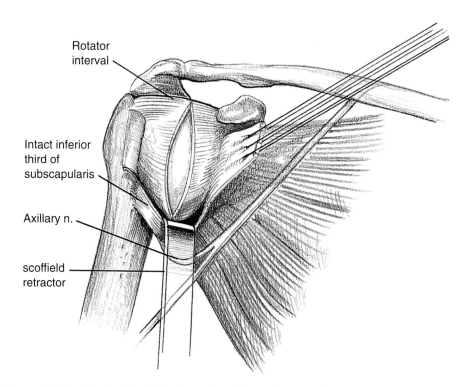

Figure 15-20. After the intact inferior portion of the subscapularis is dissected free from the capsule, a Scoffield retractor is placed inferiorly to protect the axillary nerve when the capsular incision is made.

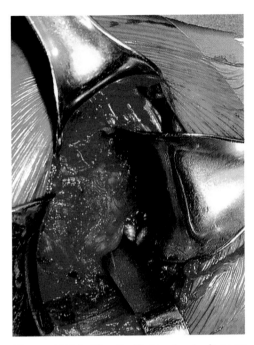

Figure 15-21. The Scoffield retractor is seen in its proper position between the inferior portion of the subscapularis and the inferior capsule medially, where it will protect the axillary nerve while we perform the capsular shift.

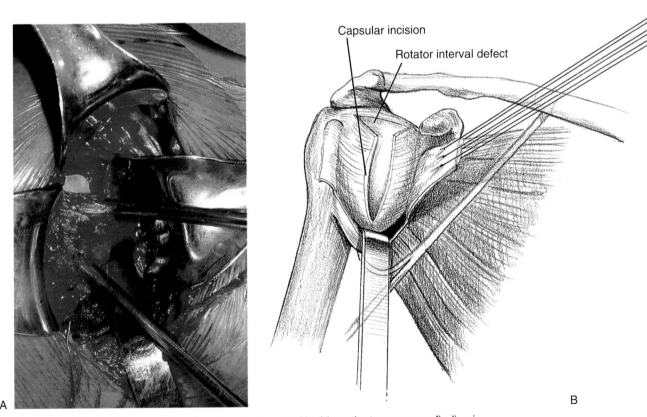

Figure 15-22. A: A large rotator interval defect is noted in this patient, a common finding in multidirectional instability. This will serve as the superior extent of the capsular incision. **B:** This defect must be repaired prior to performing the capsular shift, so that there is a foundation upon which the inferior capsular shift can be performed.

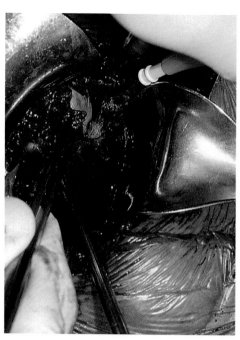

Figure 15-23. The vertical capsular incision is made with electrocautery from the rotator interval down to at least the 6-o'clock position midway between the glenoid rim and the capsular attachment to the humeral head.

yond (Fig. 15-23). This allows for the double-breasted repair, while still allowing for visualization and repair of any existing Bankart-Perthes lesion. A no. 2 cottony Dacron suture is placed in the inferomedial corner of the capsule immediately upon completing the capsular incision, followed by the placement of several similar sutures, progressing superiorly along the medial capsular border to the rotator interval. These sutures are all placed in a horizontal mattress fashion with the free ends of the sutures exiting the extraarticular side of the capsule. These sutures will be used later to secure the medial capsular leaf beneath the lateral

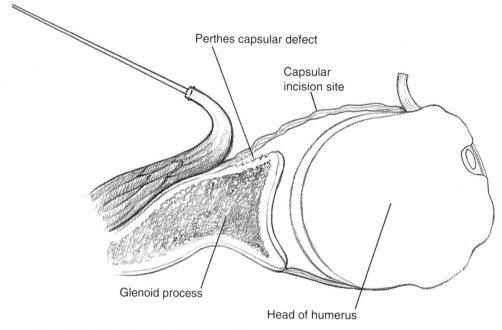

Figure 15-24. It is important to inspect for a Bankart-Perthes lesion or anterior capsular stripping once the capsule is opened.

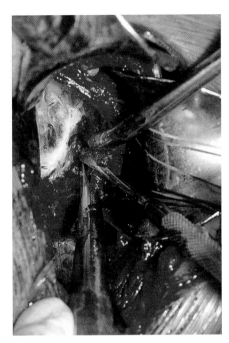

Figure 15-25. A large Bankart-Perthes lesion is noted on examination of the anterior labrum, and the anterior glenoid neck is exposed with a Cobb elevator.

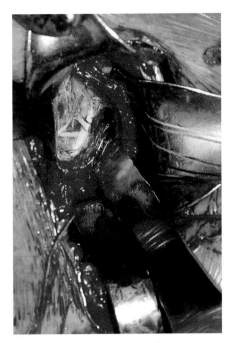

Figure 15-26. A dinner fork retractor is placed anteriorly beneath the capsule to allow the anterior neck of the glenoid to be decorticated with a bur or rose-petaled with a small osteotome.

leaf of the capsule. Occasionally, in patients with flimsy or deficient anterior capsules, 1-mm Dacron tapes can be placed in the inferior capsule to provide a stronger repair when performing the capsular shift. These sutures are used to retract the medial capsule, facilitating joint exploration and examination of the anterior glenoid rim for evidence of a Bankart-Perthes lesion or anterior capsular stripping (Figs. 15-24 to 15-27). In most patients with MDI, the anterior capsule is lax and redundant with a large inferior pouch, but it is firmly at-

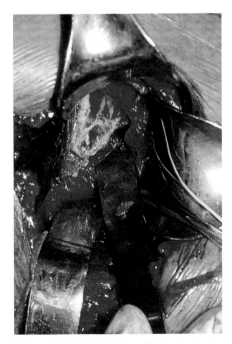

Figure 15-27. The decorticated anterior neck of the glenoid is ready for suture fixation of the Bankart-Perthes lesion.

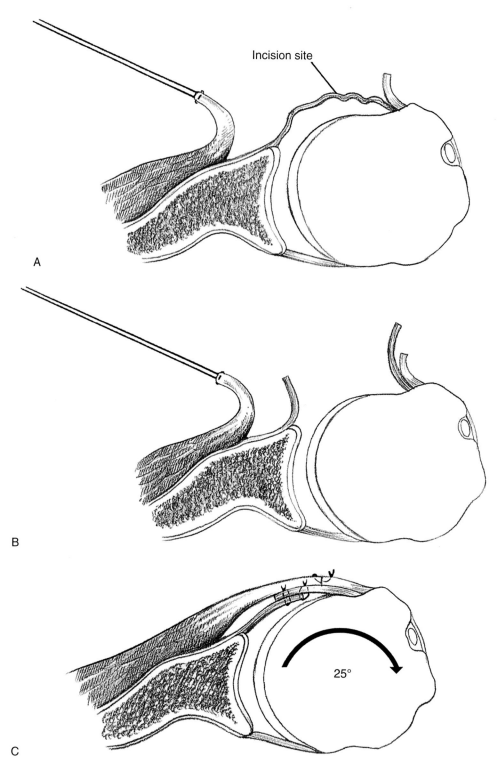

Figure 15-28. If no Bankart-Perthes lesion exists, the subscapularis is dissected free from the capsule medially and laterally **(A)**, the capsule is divided halfway between the glenoid rim and its humeral attachment **(B)**, and the shift is performed (in 25 to 30 degrees of external rotation with the arm at the side) just prior to reapproximating the subscapularis tendon **(C)**. If the subscapularis is too long to develop significant tension, it can also be double breasted when repaired.

tached to the glenoid rim, and the labrum appears normal. In addition, the rotator interval defect may be pronounced (Fig. 15-22). It is important to remember, however, that patients with MDI can have traumatic injuries to their shoulders that create Bankart-Perthes lesions. If the capsule and labrum are securely fixed to the glenoid rim, we proceed with the capsular shift (Fig. 15-28). If the anterior labrum, capsule, or both have been stripped or avulsed from the rim and scapular neck, attention should be directed to repairing the defect before commencing the capsular reconstruction. Decortication of the anterior glenoid neck is necessary to allow solid healing of the detached capsule and labrum (Figs. 15-27 and 15-29). In some cases, it may be necessary to T the capsular incision with a horizontal cut to provide adequate visualization and exposure to decorticate the scapular neck and glenoid rim with a small osteotome or motorized burr. This extension of the capsular incision must be repaired before executing the capsular shift. Several retractors designed by Rowe and Jobe look like dinner forks and are ideal for retracting the medial capsule while preparing the anterior glenoid neck (see Figs. 15-26 and 15-27). A number of different methods and instruments are available to the surgeon for resecuring the labrum and anterior capsule. We have changed our technique for repair of the Bankart-Perthes lesion in recent years and now use biodegradable suture anchors to anchor the capsule back to the glenoid rim instead of using bone tunnels, which reattach the capsule somewhat more medially on the glenoid neck. This technique offers several advantages over the bone tunnel method:

- Suture anchor application is generally faster and more reproducible than creating bone tunnels, with less chance of fracturing through the glenoid rim.
- Suture anchors permit reattachment of the capsule to the edge of the glenoid rim, rather than a few millimeters medial on the neck.
- Placement of suture anchors at the glenoid rim allows some of the redundant capsule to be gathered at the glenoid rim, creating a "capsulolabral augmentation" that effectively deepens the glenoid. Augmentation created in the direction of instability may enhance stability by the mechanism of concavity-compression (5).

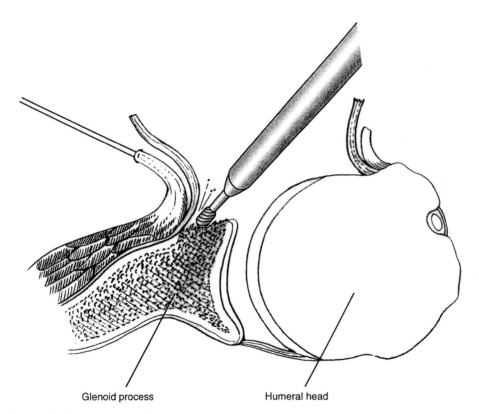

Glenoid process   Humeral head

Figure 15-29. If a Bankart-Perthes lesion is present, after the capsular incision is made and a burr, sharp osteotome, or curette is used to decorticate the glenoid neck and prepare a bleeding bed for repair of the lesion.

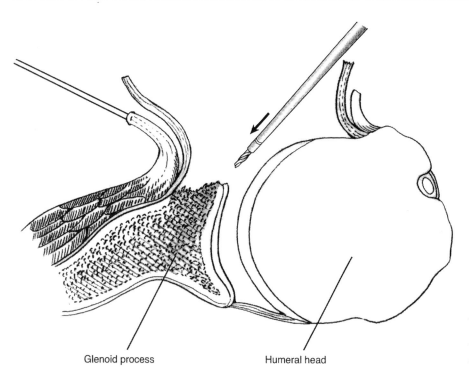

Figure 15-30. After the starting point is formed with a needle-nosed rongeur along the articular edge of the glenoid rim, a small drill creates a hole at approximately 45 degrees to the articular surface in preparation for suture anchor placement.

We place two or three anchors at the articular margin of the glenoid between the 2- and 6-o'clock positions in a right shoulder or the 10- and 6-o'clock positions in a left glenoid rim (Figs. 15-30 to 15-32). The anchors are loaded with no. 2 braided nonabsorbable sutures. Use of a Rowe or Fukuda humeral head retractor to push the head posteriorly facilitates placement of the sutures in the anterior glenoid rim.

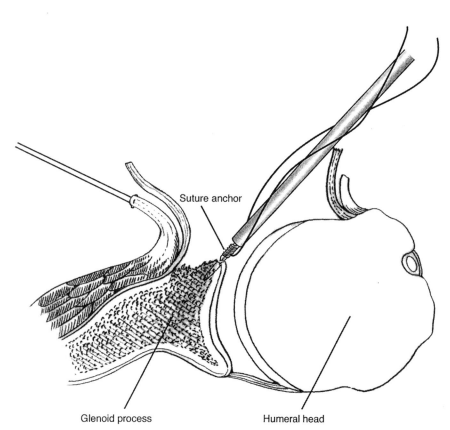

Figure 15-31. After tapping the drill hole, a biodegradable suture anchor is placed and secured into position.

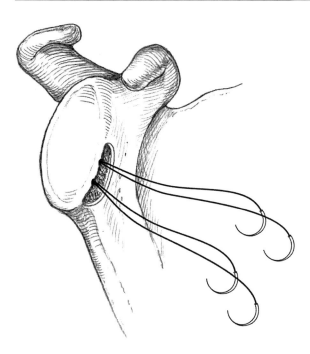

Figure 15-32. When completed, the suture anchors should be evenly spaced 6 to 8 mm apart *(shaded area).*

Once the anchors are placed, the anteromedial capsule is pulled laterally, the sutures are passed up through the appropriate site in the medial capsule and tied, firmly reattaching the capsule and labrum to the rim (Figs. 15-33 to 15-35). If an additional "bumper" at the articular margin is desired, the anchor is used to "gather" some additional capsule at the glenoid rim.

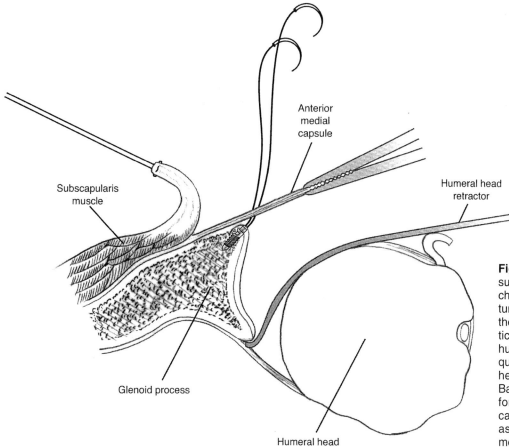

Figure 15-33. Double-armed sutures extending from the anchor are used to place the sutures from inside out, so that the knots will be tied extraarticularly, over the capsule. A humeral head retractor is required to displace the humeral head posteriorly while the Bankart-Perthes repair is performed. The anteromedial capsule is pulled laterally to assure proper suture placement through the capsule.

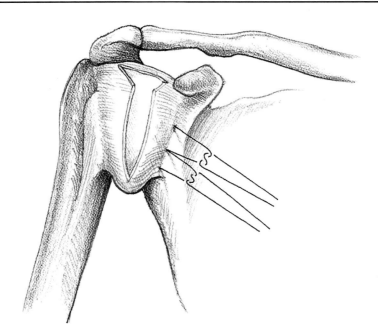

Figure 15-34. With the medial capsule pulled into anatomic position the Bankart repair sutures are pulled through the appropriate spot in the medial capsule. Placing the sutures too lateral will inhibit external rotation. The Bankart-Perthes lesion is repaired before performing the capsular shift.

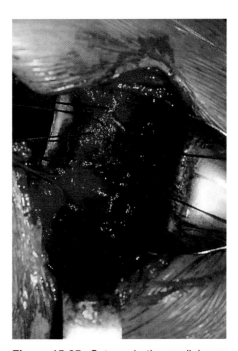

Figure 15-35. Sutures in the medial capsule facilitate the Bankart repair, allowing for atraumatic positioning of the medial capsule. The most medial suture is the repair suture, and corresponds to a spot just medial to the glenoid labrum (so that repair provides restoration of the anatomy, with the labrum sitting on the rim of the glenoid).

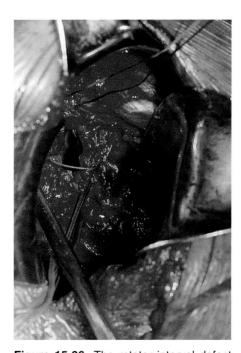

Figure 15-36. The rotator interval defect must be closed prior to performing the capsular shift, otherwise the shift exaggerates the defect without tightening the inferior and posterior capsule. This suture is placed in the superior capsule and the medial and lateral leafs, taking care not to include the supraspinatus in the repair. The medial leaf should be brought underneath the lateral leaf.

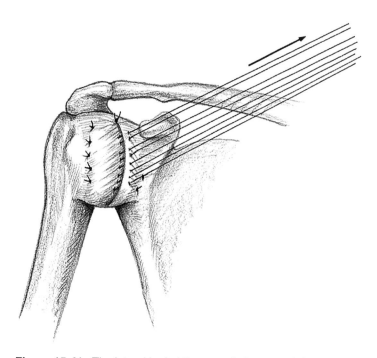

Figure 15-41. The lateral leaf of the capsule is sutured down on top of the medial leaf. The amount of overlap is dependent upon the quantity of free lateral capsule and the capsular laxity remaining.

sized. If the anterior capsule is tightened excessively, functional limitation of external rotation may be seen, with the potential long-term effect of posterior glenohumeral subluxation and eventual capsulorraphy arthropathy with posterior glenoid erosion.

The lateral capsule is then shifted medially and superiorly over the medial capsule and held in place with no. 2 cottony Dacron sutures (Figs. 15-41 to 15-44). Again, it is critical

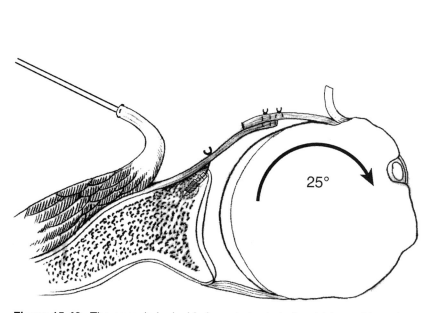

Figure 15-42. The capsule is double-breasted anteriorly, which provides a buttress against anterior displacement.

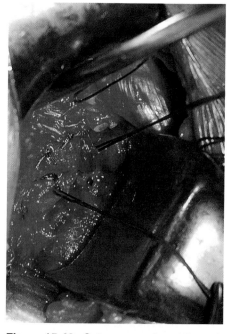

Figure 15-43. Sutures are placed through the leading edge of the lateral leaf and attached to the medial leaf while the arm is externally rotated approximately 25 to 30 degrees.

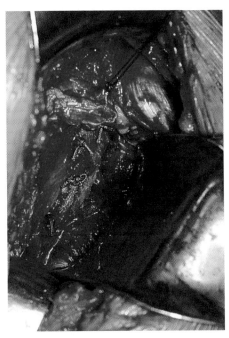

Figure 15-44. The final double-breasted capsular repair.

to ensure that the desired amount of external rotation can be achieved after these sutures are tied. The wound is then irrigated copiously.

Having completed the capsular shift, the subscapularis is repaired. The previously placed stay sutures are used to reattach the tendon to its lateral stump without shortening the muscle–tendon complex (Figs. 15-45 to 15-48). The horizontal division of the subscapularis tendon is closed with interrupted no. 2 cottony Dacron sutures. The wound is then irrigated generously with antibiotic solution. At the completion of the procedure, elimination of the anteroinferior capsular laxity should be visually demonstrable (Fig. 15-49), and palpation of the axillary nerve should reveal it to be intact (Figs. 15-9 and 15-10).

Prior to closure, the soft tissues, including the deltoid and pectoralis major muscles, are infiltrated with 25 to 30 mL of 0.25% Marcaine to decrease immediate postoperative pain. The deltopectoral interval does not routinely need to be closed, as it generally falls back together.

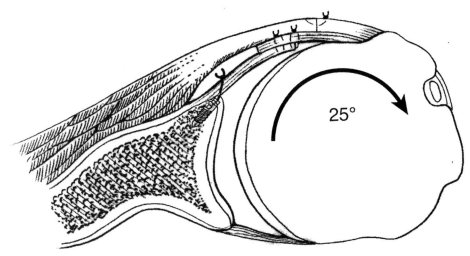

Figure 15-45. The subscapularis tendon is repaired in an end-to-end fashion to the lateral stump without shortening, providing a double-layered closure.

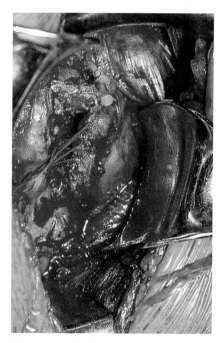

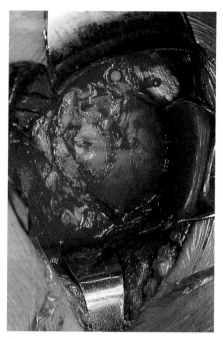

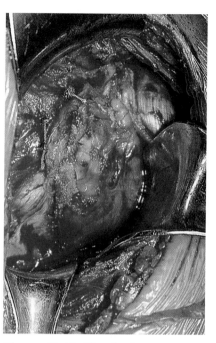

Figure 15-46. The stay sutures in the lateral edge of the retracted subscapularis tendon are reattached to the lateral stump in an end-to-end fashion.

Figure 15-47. Tension on the stay sutures after passing them through the lateral stump shows a nice, smooth repair. With the subscapularis in this position, the arm should still easily externally rotate 30 degrees.

Figure 15-48. The final repair of the subscapularis. Several interrupted sutures are used to close the horizontal split in the subscapularis.

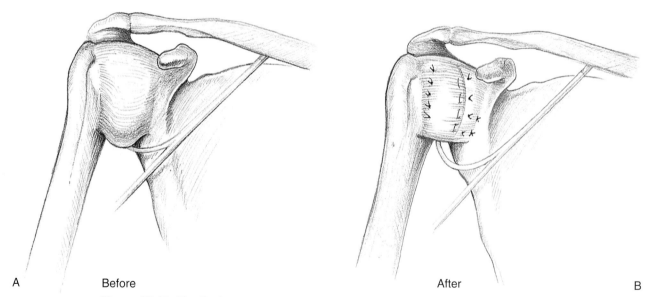

A   Before   After   B

Figure 15-49. The final effect of the repair is a tightening of the anterior and posterior capsule, as well as a diminution of the redundancy in the inferior pouch. The volume changes from the voluminous capsule seen in multidirectional instability **(A)** to a more normal capsular volume **(B)**.

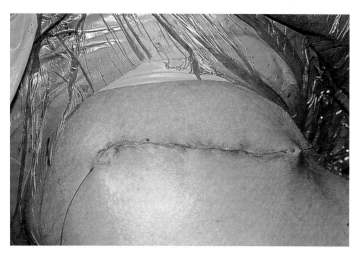

Figure 15-50. The only part of the surgery the patient sees is the wound closure; therefore, we perform a subcuticular skin closure that leaves a nice, thin-line scar.

A drain is placed in the wound if bleeding is likely to cause hematoma formation. We have recently used a percutaneous pain control catheter placed under the conjoined tendon near the axillary nerve so that the patient receives an additional slow infusion of Marcaine for the first postoperative day. Wound closure is achieved with interrupted 2-0 absorbable sutures in the deep fascia and the subcutaneous layer, and a running 2-0 Prolene subcuticular suture for skin closure (Fig. 15-50). The wound is then cleaned, dried, and covered with an Adaptic dressing, gauze, abdominal pad, and tape (we tie the Prolene suture over the dressing to hold it in place) (Fig. 15-51). An additional abdominal pad is placed in the axilla, and the operated upper extremity is placed in a commercial shoulder immobilizer (sling and swathe) prior to awakening the patient (Fig. 15-52). The patient is then delivered to the recovery room.

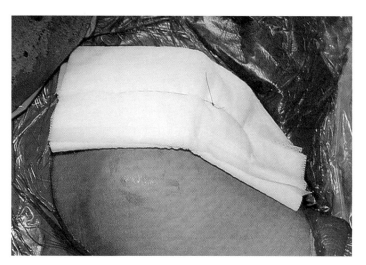

Figure 15-51. The suture ends are left long and tied over the dressing. Wound dehiscence cannot occur unless the suture is cut.

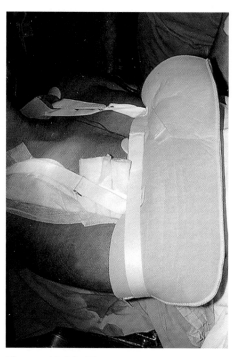

Figure 15-52. The operated extremity is placed in a commercial shoulder immobilizer before the patient is awakened from anesthesia.

POSTOPERATIVE MANAGEMENT

Postoperative pain is managed with morphine in a patient-controlled analgesia (PCA) pump, which has been very effective for us in regulating postoperative pain. The Marcaine injected during wound closure provides adequate pain relief in the recovery room for most patients and generally covers them until the PCA is connected to the intravenous line. The PCA is continued for 24 to 36 hours, after which patients are generally comfortable enough that oral medications suffice for pain control. In addition, we have found that meticulous handling and sparing of the cephalic vein intraoperatively, with repair if necessary, prevents a noticeable amount of the postoperative swelling and pain that can be associated with ligation of the vein.

In the recovery room, a shoulder-cooling unit, or an ice pack, is placed over the dressing on the operated shoulder to minimize swelling, reduce bleeding, and aid in pain management. This is maintained while the patient is in bed for the initial 24 to 48 hours.

The important items to address postoperatively include neurovascular status, swelling, drainage, pain, and postoperative instructions. We like to perform a neurovascular check in the recovery room, and then again in the evening when the patient is more alert after returning to his or her hospital room. It is important to document the status of pulses, but it is even more critical to assess the status of the axillary, musculocutaneous, radial, ulnar, and median nerves. When we perform postoperative rounds in the late afternoon, the shoulder immobilizer is removed, and the patient's arm is placed at the side with the elbow in extension. This allows the patient to move the hand, wrist, and elbow, which invariably afford relief of generalized arm and shoulder discomfort. We encourage the patient to relax the operated extremity completely while we perform gentle passive supine forward flexion up to 90 to 120 degrees. The main purpose of this maneuver is to demonstrate to the patient, while the Marcaine is still effective, that the shoulder can be moved without causing harm to the repair. Patients find this astonishing and reassuring. We discuss our expectations and the projected course of rehabilitation and return to activities, including work, with the patient and the family. It is important to relate how the pathology noted at surgery may have differed from the expected findings and describe how the pathology affects the projected outcome and course of rehabilitation.

The operative dressing is changed at 48 hours or before discharge, and the patient is given a supply of dressings at the time of discharge. We allow our patients to begin taking brief showers at 5 to 6 days postoperatively if there is no wound drainage, and we ask them to replace their dressing after each shower. The subcutaneous skin suture is removed at 2 weeks.

The goal of the surgery is to create stability in the globally unstable joint without significant compromise to the functional range of motion. Postoperatively, patients should achieve 160 or more degrees of forward flexion, internal rotation to T-8 or higher, and external rotation should be limited to approximately 30 degrees. Most patients have a supernormal range of motion preoperatively, especially with regard to external rotation. It is important not to severely restrict external rotation to prevent problems with posterior glenoid erosion and posterior subluxation. However, it is equally important to limit external rotation to the functional range described above. Although stability is greatly improved, the patient must be aware that mid-range dynamic stability is predominantly due to muscular balance and coordination, and that muscle strength must be regained and maintained postoperatively to achieve a satisfactory result. It is the surgeon's responsibility to inspire the patient to participate in the recovery by reinforcing the gravity of a lifelong rehabilitation program. A small percentage of patients with ligamentous laxity will gradually regress postoperatively until evidence of MDI returns, but persistence with the rehabilitation program makes this an extremely rare occurrence.

Rehabilitation

The postoperative rehabilitation program actually begins preoperatively, when patients are instructed in a physician-directed stretching and strengthening program. The day following surgery, under our supervision, patients begin gentle Codman pendulum exercises, passive forward flexion with an overhead pulley, and gentle passive external rotation with a 3-ft stick. We instruct them to swing their shoulder gently through a few degrees of flexion–extension, abduction–adduction, and circumduction. Pendulum exercises are performed a minimum of four to six times daily. Initially, patients perform passive forward flexion with an overhead pulley while supine and progress to sitting in a chair on postoperative day two or three. The limit of passive external rotation allowed is determined at the time of surgery. The passive forward flexion and external rotation exercises are performed three times daily with five repetitions and holding for a count of five seconds at the point of stretching. Patients are encouraged to get up and out of bed on the first postoperative day, and to use their operated extremity for simple tasks that primarily involve elbow flexion, such as feeding themselves. The sling is used for 2 to 3 weeks while outside the home, and the patients are instructed to increase the use of their operated extremity for daily living activities. These activities can include dressing, combing hair, brushing teeth, and eating.

When patients return at 6 to 8 weeks, most have a reasonable range of motion. Those patients with stiffness are advanced to a more comprehensive stretching. We ask patients to perform these exercises a minimum of six times daily, and emphasize that they are responsible to a large degree for the final outcome of the surgery by their participation in the exercise program. Once patients have achieved 140 degrees of forward flexion and a minimum of 15 to 20 degrees of external rotation, they can add a gentle, progressive strengthening program to the stretching program. We use Therabands of gradually increasing resistance to strengthen the deltoid and rotator cuff muscles. We also teach patients exercises to strengthen their scapular stabilizers. Once patients have progressed through the Therabands, a weight program using pulleys and weights can be undertaken to maintain and improve deltoid and rotator cuff strength.

We allow patients to return to activities commensurate with their strength. Patients should not be allowed to return to heavy manual labor or sports until they have regained a range of motion similar to that of the opposite side and have approximately 85% to 90% of the strength in their opposite extremity, which generally takes between 5 and 8 months. We caution patients, especially those in their second and third decade of life, that maintenance of shoulder stability and strength necessitates a commitment to continuing their exercise program two or three times per week once their formal rehabilitation is completed.

RESULTS

Most patients with involuntary MDI respond well to a physician-directed rehabilitation program aimed at strengthening their deltoid, rotator cuff, and scapular stabilizers (3). Successful surgical treatment of patients with MDI of the glenohumeral joint can be elusive, with some authors reporting failure rates up to 70% (19). The high rates of failure are due to posterior reconstructions of a flimsy capsular structure, poor recognition of the multidirectional components of posterior laxity, and inadequate rehabilitation. Posterior reconstructions have not been gratifying in our hands, because of the tissue-paper–thin, weak posterior capsule. We have performed inferior capsular shifts from an anterior approach for the past three decades with good success for patients with MDI, including many whose primary direction of symptomatic instability was posterior (26). Attention to the details presented will allow the shoulder surgeon to safely perform this procedure and produce reliable, effective results.

COMPLICATIONS

The best method for treating the complications of any surgical procedure is prevention. Careful attention to the details of the technique described above, and a sound knowledge of the anatomy of the shoulder are essential for ensuring optimal results. Listed below are some of the more serious complications that can occur with this procedure.

Neurovascular Injury

Careful identification of the axillary and musculocutaneous nerves is critical. The musculocutaneous nerve has a highly variable course, and occasionally it can be noted on the lateral border of the conjoined tendon (5). Palpation or visualization of this nerve, along with gentle retraction of the conjoined tendon, will prevent serious injury. The axillary nerve is at risk during mobilization of the subscapularis inferiorly and during the division and shift of the inferior capsule. It is critical to palpate and then protect this important nerve when working on the inferior aspect of the joint. A tight capsule and stable shoulder will do the patient absolutely no good if they have no deltoid function postoperatively. The axillary artery and brachial plexus can often be visualized or palpated deep and medial to the conjoined tendon. Deep retractors in this area can cause neuropraxic injury. Sensory neuropraxias are not uncommon, while motor neuropraxias are relatively rare. We have not experienced any permanent neurologic or any vascular injuries with this procedure, though these certainly could occur.

Loss of External Rotation

Excessive tightening of the anterior capsule can result in loss of external rotation and eventual iatrogenic degeneration of the glenohumeral joint. This is characterized by progressive posterior displacement of the head of the humerus and subsequent erosion of the posterior glenoid, associated with a gradual increase in pain and further limitation of range of motion in all planes (14). Checking in the operating room to ensure that adequate external rotation can be obtained passively will ensure against this complication. Consideration should be given to returning patients to the operating room for subscapularis lengthening and anterior capsular release if, at 6 months, their external rotation is limited to the neutral position. Patients with moderate to severe degenerative changes can be salvaged successfully with an anterior capsular release and shoulder arthroplasty plus subscapularis lengthening if needed (27).

Recurrent Multidirectional Instability

If the capsular incision is not extended far enough inferiorly, if the Bankart-Perthes lesion is not repaired, if an inadequate anterosuperior shift of the capsule is performed, or if the anterior capsular incision is closed without placing the stabilizing suture in the rotator interval, recurrent MDI can result. Attention to intraoperative details and good preoperative planning can prevent this complication. Although surgery is more difficult with each revision and results are less predictable, we have obtained excellent results in many revision cases using the same technique outlined above. Furthermore, it must be emphasized that patients with MDI may also sustain traumatic injuries with resultant Bankart-Perthes lesions. Reconstruction of a redundant, patulous capsule without regard for this lesion can result in recurrent instability.

Posterior Instability

Posterior instability can occur if the anterior capsule is overlapped excessively and external rotation is limited, or if the shift is not extended far enough inferiorly to remove the inferior and posterior capsular bulge. This can be corrected by performing a posterior capsular shift if the patient still has good external rotation, or by revision of the anterior reconstruction, paying specific attention to inferior extension of the capsular incision and superior shift of the inferior capsule, while minimizing the lateral displacement of the medial capsule during the shift.

Subscapularis Retraction

Fortunately, subscapularis retraction is a rare complication of the inferior capsular shift when care is taken to free the subscapularis from the underlying capsule, and heavy Dacron tapes or sutures are used for the repair. Retraction of the subscapularis can present as recurrent anterior instability. If recognized acutely, surgical repair is usually possible. Chronic subscapularis retraction is more difficult to treat. If the tendon can be located and dissected free, direct repair should be performed, making use of lengthening techniques as needed. If the tendon cannot be located or mobilized, we transfer a portion of the pectoralis major tendon to a position lateral to the lesser tuberosity. This provides a new dynamic buttress to anterior displacement of the humeral head and effectively replaces the subscapularis.

RECOMMENDED READING

1. Arendt, E.A.: Multidirectional shoulder instability. *Orthopedics* 11: 113–120, 1988.
2. Bell, R.B., Noble, J.S.: An appreciation of posterior instability of the shoulder. *Clin Sports Med* 10: 887–899, 1991.
3. Burkhead, W.Z., Rockwood, C.A.: Treatment of instability of the shoulder with an exercise program. *J Bone Joint Surg Am* 74: 890–896, 1992.
4. Field, L.D., Warren, R.F., O'Brien, S.J., et al.: Isolated closure of rotator interval defects for shoulder instability. *Am J Sports Med* 23: 557–563, 1995.
5. Flatow, E.L., Bigliani, J.U., April, E.W.: An anatomic study of the musculocutaneous nerve and its relationship to the coracoid. *Clin Orthop Rel Res* 244: 166–171, 1989.
6. Garth, W.P., Slabbey, C.E., Och, C.W.: Roentgenographic demonstration of instability of the shoulder: The apical oblique projection: a technical note. *J Bone Joint Surg Am* 66: 1450–1453, 1984.
7. Hall, R.H., Isaac, F., Booth, C.R.: Dislocations of the shoulder with special reference to accompanying small fractures. *J Bone Joint Surg Am* 41: 489–494, 1959.
8. Harryman, D.T., Sidles, J.A., Harris, S.L., et al.: The role of the rotator interval capsule in passive motion and stability of the shoulder. *J Bone Joint Surg Am* 74: 53–66, 1992.
9. Hawkins, R.J., Angelo, R.L.: Glenohumeral osteoarthrosis: a late complication of the Putti-Platt operation. *J Bone Joint Surg Am* 72: 1193–1197, 1990.
10. Hawkins, R.J., Koppert, G., Johnston, G.: Recurrent posterior instability (subluxation) of the shoulder. *J Bone Joint Surg Am* 66: 169–174, 1984.
11. Koppert, G., Hawkins, R.J.: Recurrent posterior dislocating shoulder. *J Bone Joint Surg Br* 62: 127–128, 1980.
12. Lebar, R.D., Alexander, H.: Multidirectional shoulder instability: clinical results of inferior capsular shift in an active-duty population. *Am J Sports Med* 20: 193–198, 1992.
13. Leslie, J.T., Ryan, T.J.: The anterior axillary incision to approach the shoulder joint. *J Bone Joint Surg Am* 44: 1193–1196, 1962.
14. Lusardi, D.A., Wirth, M.A., Wurtz, D., et al.: Loss of external rotation following anterior capsulorrhaphy of the shoulder. *J Bone Joint Surg Br* 75: 1185–1192, 1993.
15. Matsen, F.A., Thomas, S.C., Rockwood, C.A.: Anterior glenohumeral instability. In: Rockwood, C.A., Matsen, F.A., eds.: *The shoulder.* Philadelphia: WB Saunders, 526–622, 1990.
16. McLaughlin, H.L.: Posterior dislocation of the shoulder. *J Bone Joint Surg Am* 34: 584, 1952.
17. Metcalf, M.H., Pond, J.D., Harryman, D.T. II, et al.: Capsulolabral augmentation increases glenohumeral stability in the cadaver shoulder. *J Shoulder Elbow Surg* 10: 532–538, 2001.
18. Neer, C.S., Foster, C.R.: Inferior capsular shift for involuntary, inferior and multidirectional instability of the shoulder: a preliminary report. *J Bone Joint Surg Am* 62: 897–907, 1980.
19. Rockwood, C.A., Gerber, C.: Analysis of failed surgical procedures for anterior shoulder instability. *Orthop Trans* 9: 48, 1985.
20. Rockwood, C.A., Wirth, M.A.: Subluxations and dislocations about the glenohumeral joint. In: Rockwood, C.A., Green, D.P., Bucholz, R.W., et al., eds.: *Rockwood and Green's fractures in adults,* 4th ed. Philadelphia: Lippincott–Raven Publishers, 1193–1339, 1996.
21. Rowe, C.R.: Prognosis of dislocations of the shoulder. *J Bone Joint Surg Am* 38: 957, 1956.
22. Schwartz, R.E., O'Brien, S.J., Warren, R.F., et al.: Capsular restraints to anterior-posterior motion of the shoulder. *Orthop Trans* 12: 727, 1988.
23. Tibone, J.E., Prieto, C., Jobe, F.W., et al.: Staple capsulorrhaphy for recurrent posterior shoulder dislocation. *Am J Sports Med* 9: 135–139, 1981.
24. Wilson, J.C., McKeever, F.M.: Traumatic posterior (retroglenoid) dislocation of the humerus. *J Bone Joint Surg Am* 31: 160, 1949.
25. Wirth, M.A., Blatter, G., Rockwood, C.A., Jr.: The capsular imbrication procedure for recurrent anterior instability of the shoulder. *J Bone Joint Surg Am* 78: 246–259, 1996.
26. Wirth, M.A., Groh, G.I., Rockwood, C.A.: Capsulorraphy through an anterior approach for the treatment of atraumatic posterior glenohumeral instability with multidirectional laxity of the shoulder. *J Bone Joint Surg Am* 80: 1570–1578, 1998.
27. Wirth, M.A., Kalandiak, S., Rockwood, C.A.: Loss of external rotation following anterior capsulorraphy of the shoulder: emphasis on surgical management. Video presentation at American Academy of Orthopaedic Surgeons, Dallas, Texas, Feb. 13–17, 2002.
28. Wirth, M.A., Lyons, F.R., Rockwood, C.A.: Hypoplasia of the glenoid: a review of sixteen patients. *J Bone Joint Surg Am* 75: 1175–1184, 1993.

16

Capsular Repair for Recurrent Posterior Instability

James E. Tibone

INDICATIONS/CONTRAINDICATIONS

Posterior instability is not as common as its anterior counterpart. It usually occurs in a young athletic population (1,2) and presents as a recurrent posterior subluxation rather than as a true recurrent posterior dislocation, which is rare.

Posterior instability itself is not an indication for surgical repair. Approximately two thirds of patients with posterior instability respond to a proper exercise program (3) consisting of exercising the external rotators of the shoulder (the infraspinatus, teres minor, and posterior deltoid muscles) and the scapula stabilizers. Such a program will usually decrease the symptoms, but the instability may remain. No patient with instability who has not had 6 months of a structured exercise program should have surgery.

Athletes commonly present with posterior instability that interferes with their athletic endeavors (1,2). Surgical procedures geared solely to enabling them to perform at a high athletic level are usually unsuccessful. An athlete who does not respond to a conservative program will rarely be improved by operative repair if his or her only goal is to return to a high level of overhead activity. Thus, the indications for surgical repair in the athlete are pain and instability that interfere with activities of daily living. The primary indication for surgical repair is the demonstration of recurrent, symptomatic, unidirectional subluxation that has failed to respond to a comprehensive nonoperative program.

Two other clinical syndromes merit discussion and caution. True unidirectional posterior subluxation may not be as common as multidirectional instability with demonstrable posterior subluxation. Each patient with posterior subluxation should be evaluated for multidirectional or global instability, and if this is present, rehabilitation should be aimed at all directions of laxity. If nonoperative treatment fails, the operative technique must include stabilizing all directions of laxity and may require an extensive inferior capsular shift from

J. E. Tibone, M.D.: Department of Orthopaedics, University of Southern California Keck School of Medicine; and Kerlan-Jobe Orthopaedic Clinic, Los Angeles, California.

either posterior or combined anterior and posterior directions. In addition, there are some patients, often with multidirectional instability, who have had an overly tight anterior repair that leads to gradually increasing symptomatic posterior instability. In these patients, especially if external rotation has been limited by the prior surgery and anterior tightness seems to be the predominant pathology, an anterior approach with subscapularis lengthening to restore humeral head centralization on the glenoid may be more effective than a posterior approach to tighten the soft tissue.

The second clinical syndrome that should be addressed is seen in the patient with a (suprascapular) nerve injury and weakness of the supra- and infraspinatus. Posterior subluxation in this patient may be related to weakness of the dynamic muscular stabilizers. Attention should be paid to the primary nerve injury and subsequent rehabilitation of the muscle groups rather than to tightening the posterior capsule, because without posterior muscular stabilization, the capsular repair will likely stretch out over time.

A posterior capsular repair is contraindicated in a ligamentously lax individual or in a patient with multidirectional instability. If surgery is indicated, these patients need a capsular shift procedure. Bony abnormalities are rare in the shoulder with posterior instability, but a congenital hypoplastic glenoid with abnormal version would be another relative contraindication to a capsular repair. In addition, any individual with significant degenerative arthritis of the glenohumeral joint is often made symptomatically worse by a capsular repair, which would overconstrain the shoulder and increase the degenerative changes. In line with this, the apparent posterior subluxation associated with osteoarthritis is secondary to asymmetric glenoid wear and should not be confused with recurrent posterior subluxation.

A relative contraindication is seen in a patient who although lax and able to posteriorly subluxate the shoulder, does not have enough symptoms to warrant surgical repair, or in a patient who has not undergone a supervised formal trial of rehabilitation. Additionally, a patient who has had prior posterior surgery with attendant damage to either the posterior cuff muscles or the suprascapular nerve is unlikely to benefit from further soft-tissue surgery posteriorly.

PREOPERATIVE PLANNING

A typical patient with posterior subluxation has had a traumatic event with an injury occurring while the arm is in a position below shoulder level. Often there is a direct blow from the anteroposterior (AP) direction followed by recurrent symptomatic subluxation. The patient, having suffered a significant single traumatic episode, may have had repeated episodes of microtrauma with gradually progressive stretching of the soft-tissue structures until the shoulder begins to subluxate.

A patient with posterior shoulder instability feels the shoulder slip, pop, or "click out and click in." These instability episodes often occur with the arm in the frontal plane and may occur dynamically. Dynamic subluxation occurs as the patient begins to raise the arm upward, it reaches a point in the arc where the shoulder slips posteriorly, and as the arc of elevation is continued, relocation occurs. Thus the patient may be able to demonstrate the posterior subluxation when asked. The posterior instability may or may not be painful.

In some patients with this type of dynamic posterior subluxation and relocation, the scapula may appear to "wing" as the humerus subluxates posteriorly. This is not true scapula winging such as that accompanying long thoracic nerve palsy and serratus anterior paralysis. Rather, it appears to be a type of scapula muscle dysfunction, of which the patients may have some control. The medial border of the scapula separates slightly from the chest wall as the head subluxates. In fact, manual stabilization of the scapula against the chest wall may actually prevent this dynamic subluxation from occurring. Thus, there may be a role for scapula muscle rehabilitation or even biofeedback techniques to "teach" the scapula to "set" properly against the chest wall. While formal surgical procedures to fix the scapula to the chest wall might theoretically appear an attractive option, these are unpredictable as procedures to control posterior subluxation in this small subset of patients with dynamic subluxation and scapula mechanic alteration.

The most important preoperative assessment is to document that the patient has an isolated posterior instability rather than a posterior instability as a component of multidirectional instability (4). On examination, care should be taken to elicit signs of generalized ligamentous laxity, which may be a clue to the presence of multidirectional shoulder instability. Hyperextensibility of the elbows, hyperflexibility of the wrist and metacarpophalangeal joints of the hand, and laxity of the contralateral shoulder all may indicate the presence of global laxity. Attempts should be made to center the humeral head in the glenoid by a load-and-shift test and to subluxate the shoulder anteriorly, posteriorly, and inferiorly. The hallmark physical finding of multidirectional instability is a sulcus sign. These findings may be elicited either in the office or under anesthesia, when less patient guarding occurs, and are an additional argument for a complete examination under anesthesia and arthroscopy before an instability reconstruction, whether open or arthroscopic.

The patient who has isolated posterior instability often can be subluxated in a posterior direction by the examiner who grasps the humeral head and pulls directly backward, with the muscles of the shoulder relaxed. This load-and-shift test, or posterior drawer test, is positive in the posterior direction but negative in the contralateral shoulder. The examiner may also be able to demonstrate posterior subluxation as the arm is brought into the frontal plane at 90 degrees and internal rotation force is applied.

Posterior apprehension, although uncommon, should be tested. The arm is brought into forward elevation with internal rotation, and posterior stress is applied (Fig. 16-1). A sense of instability, significant pain, or painful subluxation is suggestive of the diagnosis. Range of motion of the shoulder is usually not limited either passively or actively in the patient with isolated posterior subluxation. Strength of the rotator cuff muscles may be normal, but it is not uncommon to see significant external rotation weakness when manually tested, a finding that may emphasize the need for further rehabilitation.

The diagnosis of posterior instability may be confusing, and the athlete with posterior subluxation may have other causes of shoulder pain. Therefore, before considering posterior capsular repair, it is most helpful if the patient identifies the pain while the shoulder is being subluxated as the precise pain leading to the disability of the shoulder. If posterior subluxation by the examiner can be elicited but does not produce pain in the shoulder or a sense by the patient of "that's it; that is what I feel," the diagnosis should be questioned and an alternative cause of the pain should be considered.

Shoulder radiographs for instability include an AP in internal and external rotation, a lateral, and a West Point axillary view. While these views rarely show any bony changes in the glenoid, there may be some bone reaction along the posterior rim, which will increase the clinician's comfort level with the diagnosis. It is unusual to have a reverse Hill-Sachs

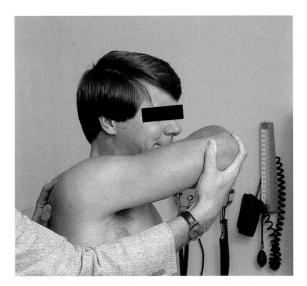

Figure 16-1. Testing posterior apprehension.

lesion. Occasionally a dynamic radiograph may be taken as the patient voluntarily subluxes the shoulder, and this film may show the humeral head in a posteriorly subluxed position. Additional imaging studies include computed tomography, arthrography, and magnetic resonance imaging (MRI). A well-done, excellent-quality MRI, however, may show labral changes, capsular damage, or abnormalities of glenoid cartilage that may aid in the diagnosis. In some patients, a detachment of the posterior labrum may be identified through an imaging study, such as a gadolinium-enhanced MRI, after a particularly significant traumatic event.

If there is any doubt about the direction or extent of instability, an examination under anesthesia with arthroscopy may clarify the predominant direction of instability and address the presence or absence of intraarticular labral pathology. If arthroscopic evidence of an anterior Bankart lesion exists, the diagnosis of isolated posterior instability must be questioned.

SURGERY

The patient is placed under general anesthesia and positioned in the lateral decubitus position with the operative shoulder superior (6). The patient is held in this position with a beanbag and kidney rests. The down leg is padded to prevent pressure on the peroneal nerve (Fig. 16-2). Arthroscopy is performed before the posterior reconstruction to assess the articular cartilage and to rule out an associated anterior labral tear, which would contraindicate the posterior procedure. A sterile shoulder wrap is used and the patient is placed in 10 lb of traction with a conventional shoulder holder. The arthroscopy is performed through a conventional posterior and/or anterior portal. The rotator interval capsule can also be treated arthroscopically, which can help decrease posterior translations and augment the open repair. After the arthroscopy is completed, the patient is released from traction and the arm is rested at the side with the patient in the same lateral decubitus position. Reprepping and draping are usually not necessary.

The landmarks for the skin incision are the posterior aspect of the acromioclavicular (AC) joint, an area just medial to the posterior lateral corner of the acromion, and the posterior axillary fold (Fig. 16-3). A 10-cm saber-cut incision is made beginning at the posterior aspect of the AC joint, proceeding approximately 2 cm medial to the posterolateral corner of the acromion, and continuing inferior toward the posterior axillary fold. The skin flaps are raised, exposing the underlying deltoid muscle (Fig. 16-4). The deltoid muscle is split in line with its fibers from the spine, in an area 2 to 3 cm medial to the posterior cor-

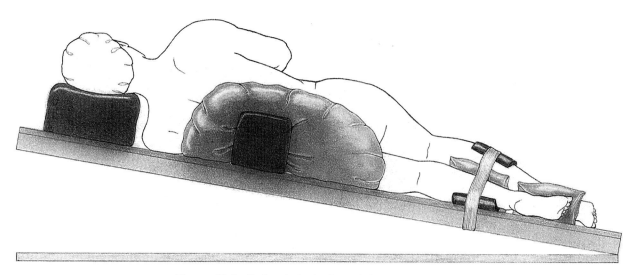

Figure 16-2. Patient is in the lateral decubitus position and held securely with a beanbag and kidney rests with padding to protect the peroneal nerve.

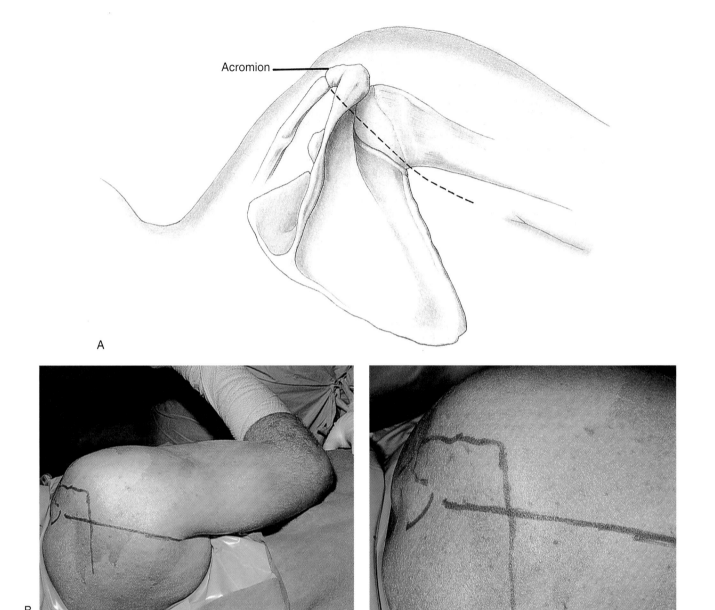

Acromion

A

B

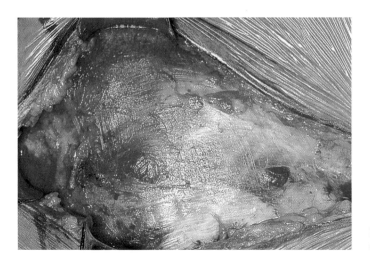

C

Figure 16-3. A–C: Skin incision from the posterior aspect of the acromioclavicular joint toward the posterior axillary fold.

Figure 16-4. The flaps are undermined, exposing the fascia over the deltoid and trapezius muscles.

ner of the acromion, distally approximately 5 cm. It is not necessary to remove any deltoid from the spine or the acromion (Fig. 16-5). The deltoid is retracted with Goulet retractors or a self-retaining Balfour retractor. This exposes the underlying teres minor and infraspinatus (Fig. 16-6). There is a heavy fascia layer covering these muscles, and this needs to be divided to better visualize the muscles. The interval between the teres minor and the infraspinatus is poorly defined. We have used the interval between the two heads of the infraspinatus as a better landmark (5). The infraspinatus is a bipennate muscle with a fat stripe between its two heads. This landmark is an excellent area for exposure of the underlying capsule. The infraspinatus is divided between its two heads from its lateral tendinous insertion to just medial to the glenoid. Care is taken not to divide the muscle more than 1.5 cm to the glenoid to avoid damage to the branches of the suprascapular nerve to the infraspinatus. The infraspinatus is dissected free from the capsule using sharp dissection laterally and a blunt elevator medially (Fig. 16-7A). The infraspinatus must be completely separate from the capsule to allow the capsule to be mobilized. Gelpi retractors laterally between the two heads of the infraspinatus and a pitchfork retractor on the glenoid neck aid in exposure of the underlying capsule. The capsule is divided from lateral to medial in its midportion to the edge of the posterior glenoid labrum. In most cases (approximately 95%),

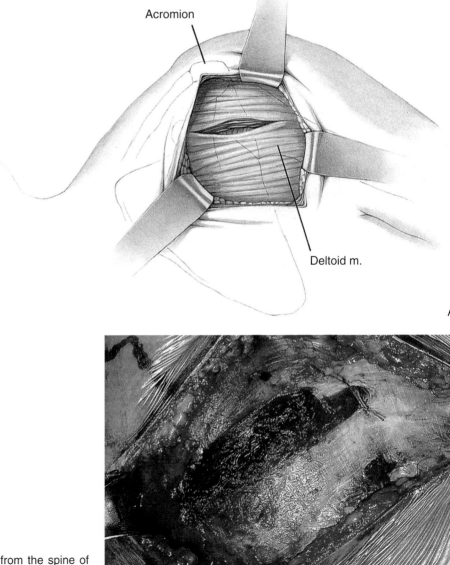

Acromion

Deltoid m.

A

B

Figure 16-5. The split in the deltoid from the spine of the scapula distally 5 to 6 cm.

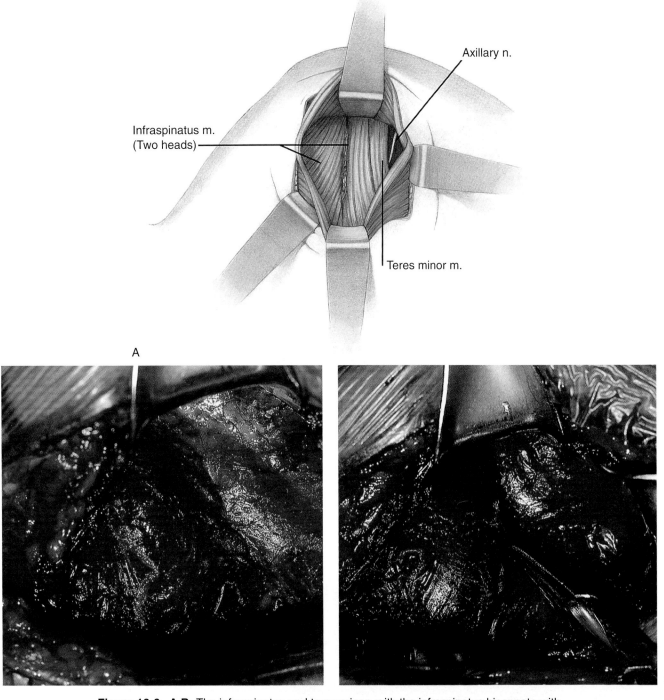

Figure 16-6. A,B: The infraspinatus and teres minor, with the infraspinatus bipennate with a fat stripe dividing the muscle. **C:** The clamp identifies the middle of the bipennate muscle.

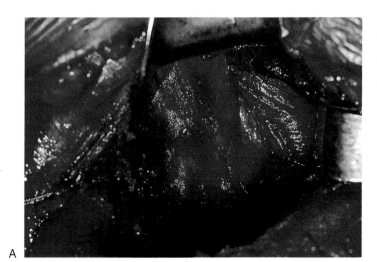

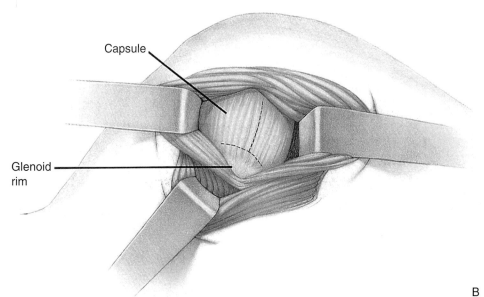

Figure 16-7. A: The interval beneath the infraspinatus is dissected, carefully separating the infraspinatus from the underlying capsule. **B,C:** Demonstration of the T capsular incision, with a horizontal capsulotomy extending laterally, then a vertical capsulotomy adjacent to the glenoid.

Capsule

Glenoid
rim

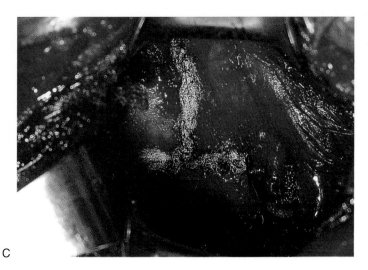

the labrum is intact. It can be used to hold sutures when advancing the capsule. Next, a T incision is made in the capsule medially along the edge of the glenoid labrum, creating a superior and an inferior flap (Fig. 16-7B,C). These are then tagged with sutures for further immobilization and for retraction. In a case where the labrum is damaged and there is a reverse-Bankart lesion present, the procedure is carried out in a similar fashion except that

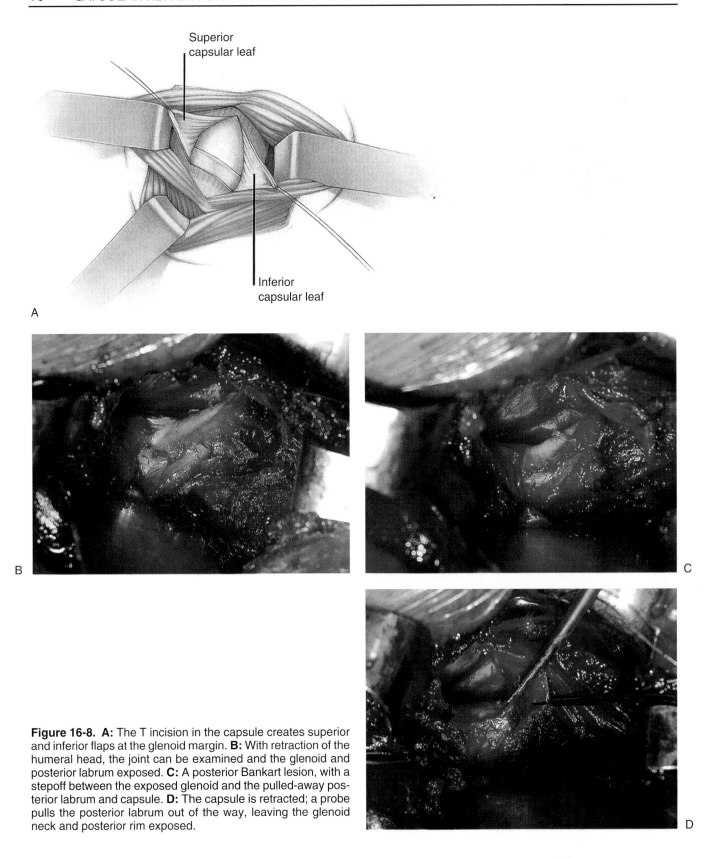

Figure 16-8. A: The T incision in the capsule creates superior and inferior flaps at the glenoid margin. **B:** With retraction of the humeral head, the joint can be examined and the glenoid and posterior labrum exposed. **C:** A posterior Bankart lesion, with a stepoff between the exposed glenoid and the pulled-away posterior labrum and capsule. **D:** The capsule is retracted; a probe pulls the posterior labrum out of the way, leaving the glenoid neck and posterior rim exposed.

the labrum is repaired with suture anchors to the glenoid rim, as in a conventional Bankart repair (Figs. 16-8 and 16-9). Three or four no. 1 Ethibond sutures (Ethicon, Inc., Somerville, NJ) are used for the repair, and these are passed through the glenoid labrum from inferior to superior. The inferior capsular flap is advanced superiorly and medially,

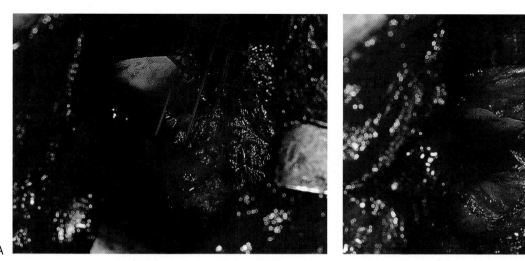

Figure 16-9. Repair of the posterior Bankart lesion with suture anchors. **A:** The suture anchors are placed, or sutures can be passed directly through the posterior glenoid labrum rim. **B:** Suture knots are tied intraarticularly or extraarticularly, reapproximating the posterior labrum and capsule to the posterior glenoid rim.

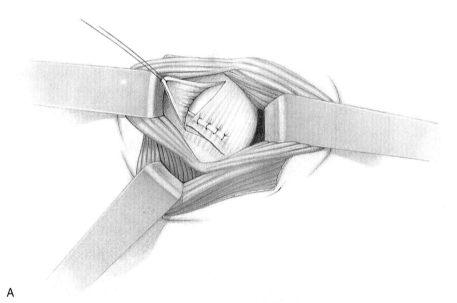

A

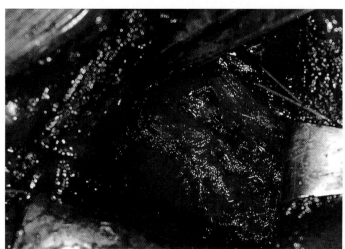

B

Figure 16-10. A,B: The advancement of the inferior capsular flap superiorly, eliminating the inferior pouch and anchoring the inferior pouch to the posterior glenoid labrum. Preparation is made to advance the superior flap inferiorly.

and the Ethibond sutures are mattressed through the capsule beginning inferiorly and pro-ceeding superiorly (Fig. 16-10). The sutures are tied with the arm in neutral rotation. The superior flap is brought over the inferior flap and advanced distally and medially (Fig. 16-11). The same Ethibond sutures that were previously tied are then mattressed through the superior flap. This creates a double layer at the rim of the glenoid. The lateral split in the

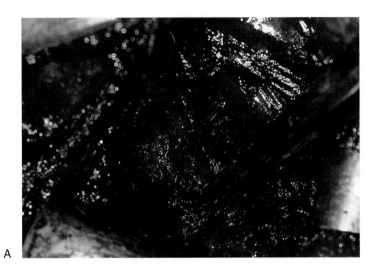

A

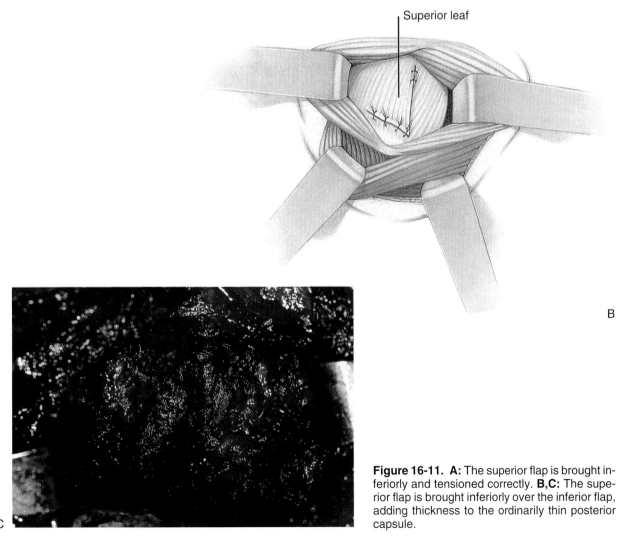

B

C

Figure 16-11. A: The superior flap is brought in-feriorly and tensioned correctly. **B,C:** The supe-rior flap is brought inferiorly over the inferior flap, adding thickness to the ordinarily thin posterior capsule.

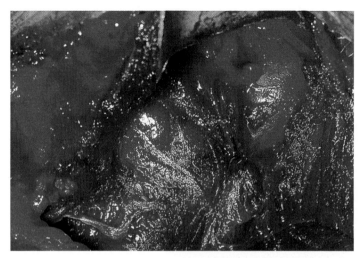

Figure 16-12. The split in the infraspinatus is reapproximated.

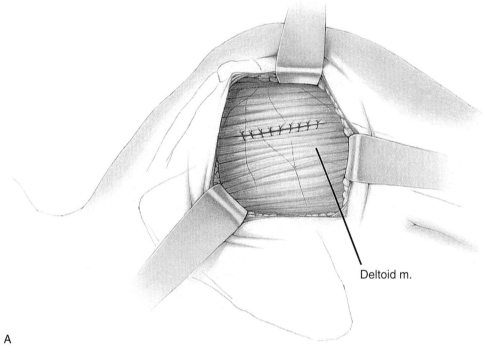

Deltoid m.

A

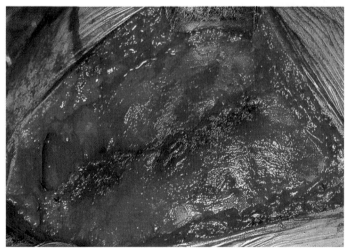

B

Figure 16-13. A,B: The split in the deltoid is closed.

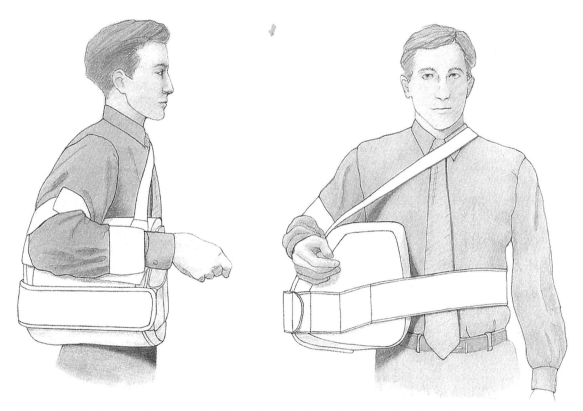

Figure 16-14. Postoperative immobilization in the abduction pillow. The elbow is positioned posterior to the coronal plane of the body.

capsule is repaired in a side-to-side fashion with no. 1 absorbable suture, and if necessary, the split in the infraspinatus is closed (Fig. 16-12). The split in the deltoid is closed with a no. 1 absorbable stitch through the superficial fascia (Fig. 16-13). The subcutaneous tissue and skin are closed in a routine fashion. A subcuticular stitch on the skin leaves a cosmetically acceptable scar. A sterile dressing is applied and the patient is placed in an abduction pillow used for rotator cuff surgery. The elbow is kept posterior to the coronal plane of the body to take the stress off the repair. With the elbow in this position, the pillow keeps the shoulder in neutral rotation (Fig. 16-14).

POSTOPERATIVE MANAGEMENT

The patient is kept in the abduction pillow for 3 weeks. The arm should be kept in neutral rotation to keep tension off the repair. At 3 weeks, the arm is brought down to the side and the patient is allowed to internally rotate the shoulder at the side. Gentle range-of-motion exercises with an overhead pulley in the plane of the scapula, external rotation with the arm at the side, and Codman exercises are begun. Because the deltoid has not been detached, and because the infraspinatus has not been violated, active external rotation exercises can begin within 3 weeks, initially with submaximal isometric exercises and then progressing to more resistive exercises. No forward flexion in the frontal plane or forward flexion combined with internal rotation is permitted until 6 weeks postoperatively.

By 6 months, range of motion is usually normal, but deficits may continue to exist in external rotation strength. Any residual tightness to internal rotation may be addressed by specific stretching exercises. By 9 months postoperatively, there is usually full range of motion and near-normal strength. Patients are usually without apprehension and feel that the shoulder is stable. By 1 year after surgery, full motion, strength, stability, and return to normal function and sports have occurred. The return of the throwing athlete to a competitive level may be delayed if necessary. Athletes should be informed at the time of surgery that

1 year is required for a return to sports activities, and that 18 months may be required in the throwing athlete.

COMPLICATIONS

The most common complication of this procedure is recurrence, with reports of 30% in some series (7). In part, this may be a result of poor posterior capsular tissue. In some series, multiple operations by multiple surgeons have created difficulty in interpreting the results of surgical treatment. In other series, ligamentous laxity and multidirectional instability may not have been specifically excluded; thus, poor patient selection for isolated capsular repair may be one reason for increased failure rate. However, by reinforcing the posterior capsule, minimum interference with the infraspinatus, adequate postoperative immobilization and support, and careful attention to and supervision of the rehabilitation, recurrence can be minimized and the success rates of this surgery can approach those of anterior repair.

A second, not infrequent complication results from an overly tightened repair. This usually occurs when, because of the poor posterior capsular tissue, the surgeon decides to detach and advance the infraspinatus or overly tighten the posterior capsule, and an overly long immobilization period is recommended postoperatively. The likelihood that this complication will occur can be minimized by intraoperative attention to how tight the posterior capsule is repaired. At the conclusion of the posterior capsule repair, the patient's head should be able to rest comfortably on the anterior chest without much tension on the posterior capsule or sutures. If it appears that there is difficulty in restoring postoperative internal rotation, earlier stretching exercises in this direction should be considered.

A third complication that has been reported is injury to the suprascapular or axillary nerve. The suprascapular nerve innervates the infraspinatus within 1.5 cm from the posterior glenoid rim. Care must be taken to limit the split of the infraspinatus to 1.5 cm medial to the glenoid. Although the axillary nerve is not commonly encountered if the teres minor is left intact, this nerve is in jeopardy as the inferior capsular flap is developed. Adequate visualization of the inferior capsule must be achieved and the axillary nerve retracted before any dissection is performed in that area.

Finally, hardware complications may occur if staples are used in any part of this capsular repair and their positions are not identified precisely (7). As with other surgical procedures around the shoulder, hardware complications can be eliminated only by alternative forms of fixation of the soft tissue, such as suture or absorbable fixation devices.

RESULTS

In our hands, capsular repair for recurrent posterior instability has not been as successful as an anterior repair. There has been a 30% incidence of recurrence of posterior instability. However, the patients with ligamentous laxity and a multidirectional component to their instability were eliminated from the series after a more thorough analysis of results. Reanalysis indicated that the results of a capsular repair for recurrent posterior instability approach 90%. The return to the same level of sports competition is based on the level of competition with the high-level athlete having the most guarded prognosis. In addition, the throwing athlete is the most difficult to return to the same level of performance after this procedure. Most recreational athletes can return to their sports, however, the high-level collegiate or professional athlete will return in only approximately 50% of the cases. The results of any series in the literature will be determined by careful patient selection, eliminating patients with multidirectional instability. The other factor that determines the results in the literature is the patient population, with the higher-level athletes having the worse results.

RECOMMENDED READING

1. Bigliani, L.U., Pollock, R.G., McIlveen, S.J., et al.: Shift of the posteroinferior aspect of the capsule for recurrent posterior glenohumeral instability. *J Bone Joint Surg Am* 77: 1011–1020, 1995.
2. Fronek, J., Warren, F.R., Bowen, M.: Posterior subluxation of the glenohumeral joint. *J Bone Joint Surg Am* 71: 205, 1989.
3. Hawkins, R.J., Koppers, G., Johnston, G.: Recurrent posterior instability (subluxation) of the shoulder. *J Bone Joint Surg Am* 66: 169, 1984.
4. Hurley, J.A., Anderson, T.E., Dear, W., et al: Posterior shoulder instability: surgical vs. conservative results with evaluation of glenoid version. *Am J Sports Med* 20: 396–400, 1992.
5. Neer, C.S. II, Foster, C.F.: Inferior capsular shift for involuntary interior and multidirectional instability of the shoulder. *J Bone Joint Surg Am* 62: 897, 1980.
6. Shaffer, B.S., Conway, J.E., Jobe, F.W., et al.: Infraspinatus splitting incision in posterior shoulder surgery: an anatomic and electromyographic study. *Am J Sports Med* 22: 113, 1994.
7. Tibone, J.E.: Posterior capsulorrhaphy for posterior subluxation. In: Paulos, L.E., Tibone, J.E., eds.: *Operative techniques in shoulder surgery*. Gaithersburg, MD: Aspen, 143–147, 1991.
8. Tibone, J.E., Bradley, J.P.: The treatment of posterior subluxation in athletes. *Clin Orthop Rel Res* 291: 124–137, 1993.
9. Tibone, J.E., Ting A.: Capsulorrhaphy with a staple for recurrent posterior subluxation of the shoulder. *J Bone Joint Surg Am* 12: 999, 1990.
10. Wirth, M.A., Groh, G.I., Rockwood, C.A.: Capsulorrhaphy through an anterior approach for the treatment of posterior glenohumeral instability with multidirectional laxity of the shoulder. *J Bone Joint Surg Am* 80: 1570–1580, 1998.

17

McLaughlin Procedure for Acute and Chronic Posterior Dislocations

Joseph D. Zuckerman

INDICATIONS/CONTRAINDICATIONS

Posterior glenohumeral dislocations can result in anteromedial humeral head impression fractures. These impression fractures occur as a result of contact between the posterior rim of the glenoid and the anteromedial portion of the humeral head (Fig. 17-1). They are often referred to as reverse Hill-Sachs defects (the posterolateral humeral head defects commonly found in association with anterior glenohumeral dislocations).

The size of the anteromedial defects can be quite variable. Acute posterior dislocations that are reduced properly will usually result in small and often insignificant defects (Fig. 17-1A). However, multiple episodes of posterior dislocation, even if reduced promptly, can result in a larger defect. In addition, prolonged contact between the posterior glenoid and the humeral head, as occurs in chronic unreduced dislocations, may result in defects that encompass a significant portion of the humeral head (Fig. 17-1B). In both situations, the bony defect can become a factor causing recurrent instability. When this occurs, operative management is often directed at correcting the anteromedial humeral head defect.

The McLaughlin procedure is defined as a transfer of the subscapularis tendon into an anteromedial humeral head defect that resulted from either an acute or a chronic posterior glenohumeral dislocation. The modified McLaughlin procedure consists of a transfer of the lesser tuberosity with the subscapularis attached, into the anteromedial humeral head defect.

In acute dislocations, defects of less than 20% will probably not contribute to recurrent instability. However, in chronic dislocations, a defect of even this size may require subscapularis transfer at the time of open reduction (Fig. 17-2A). Defects of 20% to 40% are usually found in association with chronic dislocations (Fig. 17-2B). Following open reduction of these injuries, a subscapularis transfer or a lesser tuberosity transfer will be re-

J. D. Zuckerman, M.D.: Department of Orthopaedic Surgery, New York University School of Medicine; and NYU-Hospital for Joint Diseases, New York, New York.

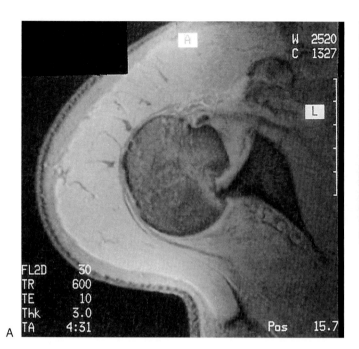

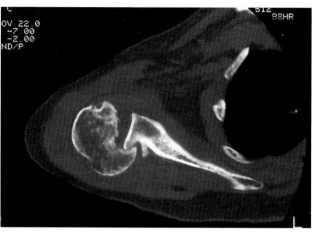

Figure 17-1. Anteromedial humeral head impression fractures associated with posterior dislocations can vary significantly in size. Relatively small defects **(A)** may be of limited clinical significance. However, larger defects **(B)** may represent a significant factor in the ability to maintain a stable reduction.

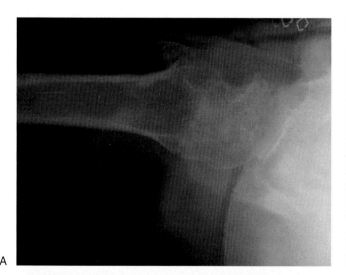

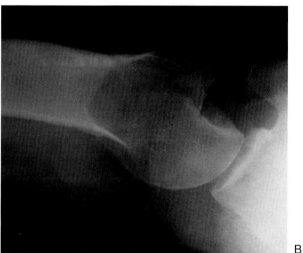

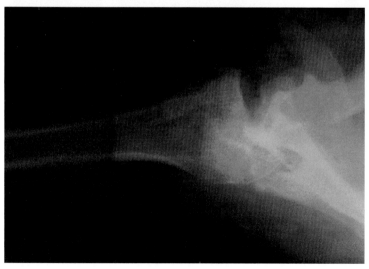

Figure 17-2. The size of the anteromedial humeral head defect is an important factor in determining the preferred treatment. Defects that encompass approximately 20% of the articular surface **(A)**, particularly when associated with chronic dislocations, will generally require subscapularis transfer to fill the defect. Defects that encompass 20% to 45% of the humeral head **(B)** will usually require a lesser tuberosity transfer because of the larger size of the defect. Impression fractures that encompass more than 45% of the humeral head **(C)** will generally require prosthetic replacement to achieve a stable reduction.

quired to maintain stability. Defects encompassing more than 40% of the humeral head will usually require prosthetic replacement (Fig. 17-2C).

The indications for the subscapularis transfer as opposed to the lesser tuberosity transfer are important to understand. In general, subscapularis transfer alone is sufficient for small humeral head defects (up to 20%) in which the soft tissue alone is sufficient to fill the defect. However, larger defects (greater than 20%) will require lesser tuberosity transfer with the subscapularis attached to adequately fill the bony defect and prevent recurrent instability.

There are two important contraindications to the McLaughlin and modified McLaughlin procedures. These include (a) an anteromedial humeral head defect that encompasses more than 40% of the articular surface, and (b) cases of long-standing dislocation in which there is significant deterioration of the remaining articular cartilage of the humeral head or glenoid. In both these situations, subscapularis transfer or lesser tuberosity transfer is contraindicated and prosthetic replacement is preferred.

PREOPERATIVE PLANNING

The preoperative evaluation of the patient should include a careful assessment of the etiology of the posterior instability. An underlying seizure disorder is often present and will require consultation with a neurologist. The goal of this consultation is first to adequately control the seizures to avoid additional episodes during the postoperative period, and second to identify any treatable or correctable etiology of the seizure disorder.

The chronicity of the dislocation should also be assessed preoperatively, because this will have a few important implications. First, it will indicate the chance of achieving a successful closed reduction. Second, it will provide some indication of the difficulty of achieving an open reduction. Third, it will indicate the status of the remaining articular cartilage. A careful history from the patient and relatives will generally provide a reasonably accurate estimation of the duration of the dislocation.

The patient with a locked posterior dislocation presents with characteristic findings. There is a history of trauma, either recognized by the patient or unrecognized, as may occur with a seizure. The patient may have been seen in an emergency department and may have had radiographs taken. Up to 70% of acute posterior dislocations are unrecognized by the initial examiner, usually because radiographs have been inadequate for diagnosis or have been interpreted incorrectly. In many cases, an axillary radiograph has never been obtained. This diagnosis will not be overlooked if a well-done axillary radiograph is obtained and interpreted correctly (Fig. 17-3).

The patient frequently presents with pain and virtually always notes loss of motion. Whatever the history, the presenting physical findings are classic. Because of the locked position of the humeral head posteriorly, there is frequently a flattened appearance to the anterior shoulder and a fullness posteriorly. The hallmark physical finding, however, is the inability to externally rotate the humerus because of the locked posterior position of the humeral head posteriorly. These findings are seen whether the dislocation is acute or longstanding and chronic. A locked posterior dislocation, if unrecognized, may result in chronic clinical and radiographic changes.

The most important aspect of the examination is the determination of the size of the humeral head defect. The size of the defect (expressed as a percentage of the humeral head articular surface) is the key factor in determining treatment and can be determined radiographically. The standard trauma series, including most importantly the axillary view (Fig. 17-2), provides a reliable indication of the size of the defect. However, a computed tomography scan is particularly helpful for accurate determination of the size of the defect (Fig. 17-1B).

Based on the information provided, the first decision is whether a transfer procedure is indicated. Generally, for defects that involve less than 40% of the articular surface, a transfer procedure is preferred. If this is the case, the second decision is whether a subscapularis transfer or a lesser tuberosity transfer is preferred. This decision is based primarily on the size of the defect as noted previously.

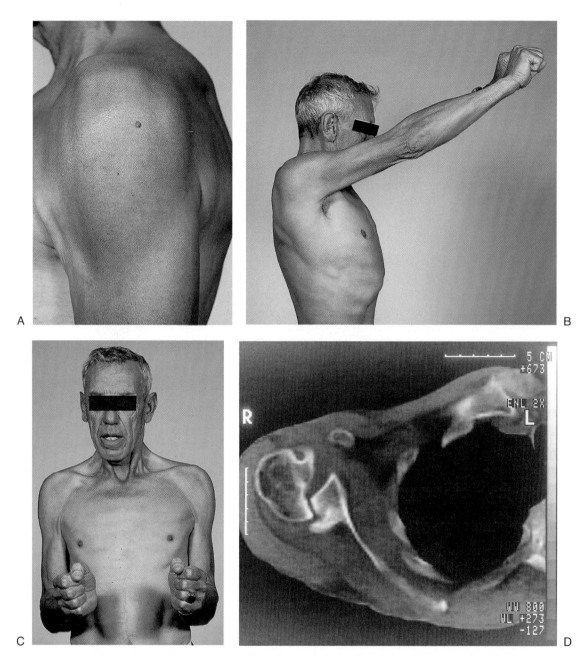

Figure 17-3. Clinical presentation of chronic locked posterior dislocation. **A:** Flattened anterior shoulder with coracoid prominence and fullness posterior from locked position of the humeral head. **B:** The patient may exhibit a surprising amount of arm elevation, particularly if range-of-motion exercises have been instigated to achieve motion. **C:** However, because of the locked posterior position of the head behind the glenoid, external rotation is lost. **D:** Computed tomography scan showing loss of humeral head and apparent new "articulation" along neck of scapula because of forced range of motion while the head was dislocated.

SURGERY

This procedure can be performed under general or regional anesthesia as long as optimal muscle relaxation can be achieved. The operating table should be placed in a beach-chair position with the head elevated approximately 30 degrees (Fig. 17-4). Use of a shoulder arthroscopy positioner facilitates proper positioning of the patient. The mobility of the involved shoulder and upper extremity should not be limited by the operating table. The area of skin preparation should include the entire upper extremity and as much of the shoulder

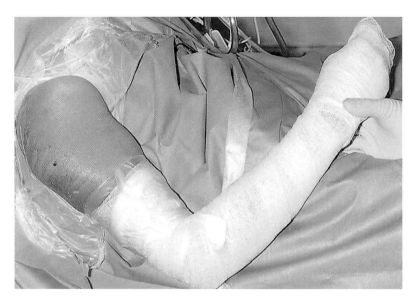

Figure 17-4. The beach-chair position is preferred with the head of the bed elevated 30 degrees and the patient moved off the side of the table for complete access to the anterior and posterior portions of the shoulder and for unrestricted mobility of the shoulder.

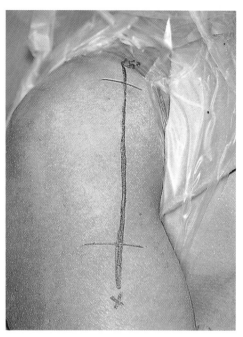

Figure 17-5. An anterior deltopectoral approach is preferred with the skin incision oriented obliquely starting just medial to the acromioclavicular joint and extending distally and laterally to the insertion of the deltoid muscle.

girdle as possible. The preparation should extend to the base of the neck as well as anteriorly and posteriorly to allow complete access to the glenohumeral joint.

An anterior deltopectoral approach is preferred. The skin incision is oriented obliquely starting just medial to the acromioclavicular joint and extending distally and laterally to the insertion of the deltoid muscle (Fig. 17-5). An anterior axillary incision can also be used; it is placed in line with the axillary skin crease. The skin and subcutaneous tissues are divided, and medial and lateral flaps are developed at the muscle layer. Preparation of these flaps will improve the surgical exposure. The deltopectoral interval is then determined by identifying the junction of the fibers of the deltoid, which run in a lateral and distal direction, and distinguishing them from the fibers of the pectoralis major, which run in a more transverse direction. The interval is also marked by a fat stripe that covers the cephalic vein. Careful dissection in this area will allow identification of the cephalic vein. Retraction of the vein medially or laterally is generally a matter of the surgeon's preference. Most of the muscle branches enter the vein from the deltoid side; therefore, mobilization laterally with the deltoid is often preferred. However, in this situation, the cephalic vein crosses the interval superiorly, which puts it at risk for injury from retraction during the procedure. For this reason, some surgeons prefer medial mobilization. I have found that the initial dissection of the cephalic vein usually indicates that the vein is more easily mobilized in one direction or the other, based on the specific anatomy encountered. Regardless of which direction the vein is retracted, care should be taken to preserve the vein during the procedure.

The deltopectoral interval should be developed from its origin superiorly at the clavicle to its distal extent at the insertion of the pectoralis major. Both the subdeltoid and the subpectoralis spaces should be mobilized. Release of the upper 1 cm of the pectoralis major insertion will facilitate exposure. I prefer a self-retaining retractor with blades of variable size to maintain the deeper exposure. At this point, important anatomic landmarks should be identified, including the coracoid process, the coracoacromial ligament, the lesser tuberosity with attached subscapularis tendon, and the bicipital groove. With chronic dislocations, the anterior soft tissues are more difficult to differentiate because of postinjury fibrosis. The conjoined tendon and muscles are usually adherent to the underlying subscapularis and should be mobilized by careful blunt dissection. It is important to recognize that the neurovascular structures are located medial to the coracoid process and conjoined tendon muscles, and any dissection in this area should be performed carefully using blunt instruments. The self-retaining retractor should be repositioned to retract the conjoined tendon muscles medially. The coracoacromial ligament should then be dissected off the underlying rotator cuff to which it is frequently adherent. Resection of the coracoacromial ligament is usually not necessary. Lysis of subacromial adhesions can be performed using a blunt Darrach-type elevator.

At this point, the rotator interval should be identified. This may be difficult because of postinjury fibrosis. The upper end of the bicipital groove and the anterosuperior edge of the glenoid are important landmarks. Opening the rotator interval between these two points (with care taken to avoid the biceps tendon) and placement of an angled retractor allows the inside of the joint to be palpated and visualized (Fig. 17-6). Information concerning the size and location of the humeral head defect can be obtained. This is particularly important in planning the direction of the lesser tuberosity osteotomy.

If a subscapularis transfer alone is planned, the insertion of the upper two thirds to three fourths of the subscapularis tendon should be outlined (Fig. 17-7). The most inferior aspect of the subscapularis tendon and muscle insertion should remain intact for two reasons: First, because the axillary nerve passes just below the most inferior edge of the subscapularis tendon, leaving this portion of the muscle undisturbed affords some protection of the axillary nerve; second, leaving this portion undisturbed may enhance internal rotation function after the transfer procedure. Using sharp dissection or the electro-cutting instrument, the subscapularis tendon should be dissected off its insertion into the lesser tuberosity (Fig. 17-8). The dissection should be carried medially into the defect until the subscapularis is completely released. The edge of the tendon should be tagged with no. 1 nonabsorbable suture and retracted medially.

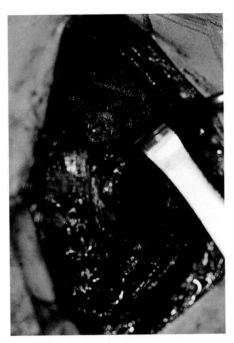

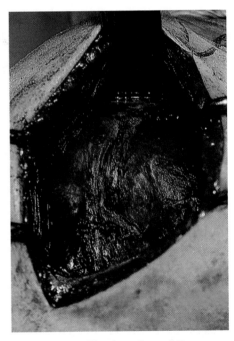

Figure 17-6. After opening the rotator interval, use of an angled retractor allows visualization of the joint. The humeral head defect can be both palpated and visualized before making a final decision between subscapularis transfer and lesser tuberosity transfer.

Figure 17-7. The insertion of the upper two thirds of the subscapularis and its insertion is outlined with the electrocautery.

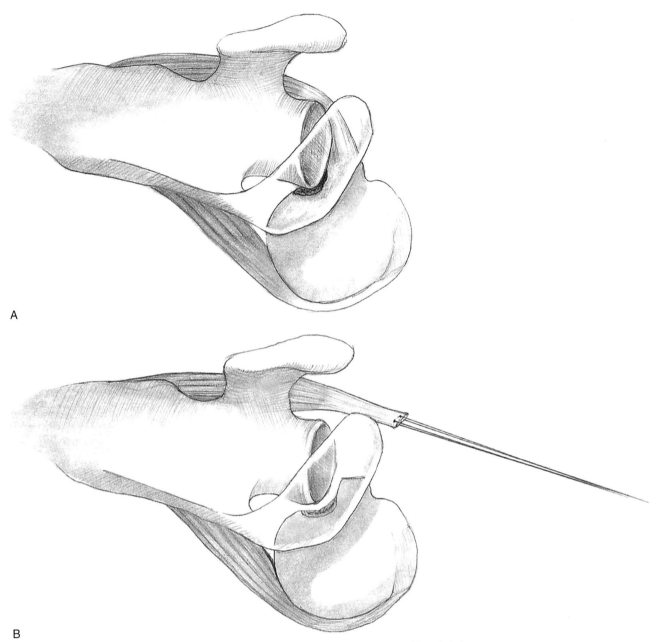

A

B

Figure 17-8. Posterior dislocation with relatively small anteromedial humeral head defect **(A)**. The subscapularis tendon is dissected off its insertion into the lesser tuberosity and tagged with suture for ease of mobilization **(B)**.

If a lesser tuberosity transfer is to be performed, a different technique is used. In this situation, the upper two thirds to three fourths of the subscapularis tendon is also outlined. The portion of the lesser tuberosity just medial to the bicipital groove should be identified, because this will be the osteotomy site. For a larger defect, osteotomy of a sufficient amount of bone may result in compromise of the most medial aspect of the bicipital groove. If this is necessary, the biceps tendon should be exposed and mobilized, and a tenodesis of the intact tendon should be performed at the completion of the procedure. This will prevent problems of biceps tendon subluxation that could result from disruption of the medial insertion of the transverse humeral ligament.

Palpation of the humeral head defect through the rotator interval will assist in determination of the angle and direction of the osteotomy. The goal is to osteotomize a sufficient amount of bone to fill a large portion of the defect without further compromise of the humeral head. The osteotomy should be directed to exit through the lateral portion of the defect just anterior to the deepest portion of the defect (Fig. 17-9). The osteotomy can be performed with either a sharp ³/₄-in. osteotome or a microsagittal saw (Fig. 17-10). I think the saw provides a greater consistency in performing the osteotomy. With either instrument, levering is to be avoided to prevent fracture of the lesser tuberosity fragment or the humeral head if the osteotomy is misdirected or deeper than desired. With completion of the osteotomy, no. 1 nonabsorbable sutures are placed in the subscapularis tendon and the lesser tuberosity is retracted medially.

At this point the humeral head defect and the joint can be visualized. In chronic dislocations, fibrous tissue often covers the glenoid and obstructs visualization of the humeral head. This tissue should be carefully removed to avoid injury to the glenoid articular surface. Fibrous tissue within the defect should also be removed to facilitate visualization of the area

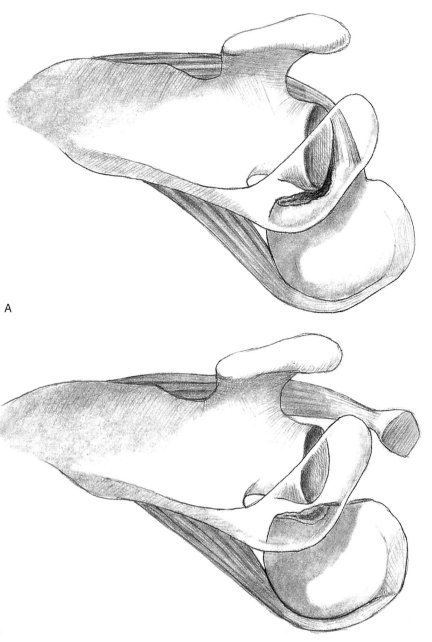

A

B

Figure 17-9. Posterior dislocation with a larger anteromedial defect **(A)**. When a larger anteromedial defect is present, the lesser tuberosity should be osteotomized just lateral to the bicipital groove **(B)**.

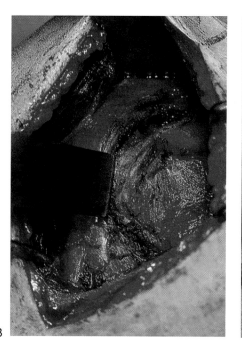
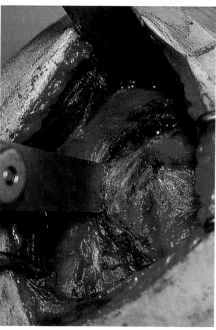

A, B

Figure 17-10. The lesser tuberosity can be osteotomized with either a sharp ³/₄-in. osteotome **(A)** or a microsagittal saw **(B)**.

of contact between the posterior glenoid rim and the defect. When proper visualization is obtained, the reduction can be attempted. All reduction maneuvers must be performed gently to avoid damage to the humeral head or the glenoid (Fig. 17-11). With gentle internal rotation, a blunt-ended elevator can be placed in the interval between the humeral head and the posterior glenoid. With the elevator in place, the humeral head should be externally rotated

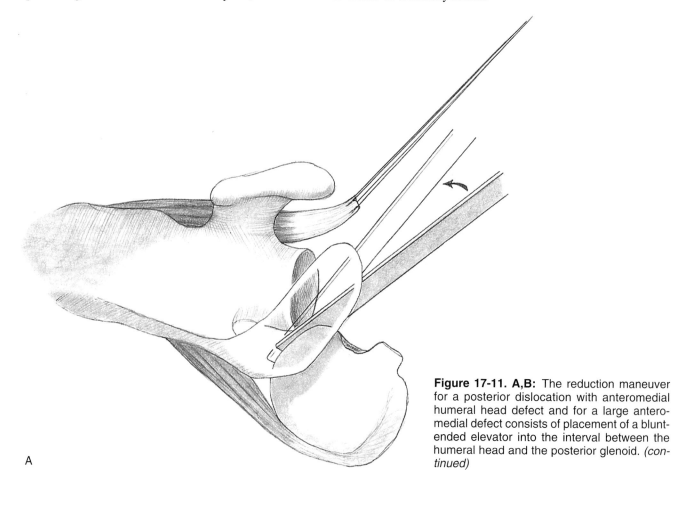

Figure 17-11. A,B: The reduction maneuver for a posterior dislocation with anteromedial humeral head defect and for a large anteromedial defect consists of placement of a blunt-ended elevator into the interval between the humeral head and the posterior glenoid. *(continued)*

A

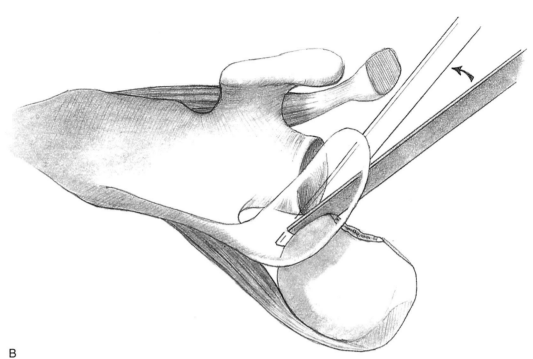

B

Figure 17-11. *Continued.* The elevator is then used to gently lever the humeral head laterally to clear the posterior rim of the glenoid.

so the elevator can be used to lever the humeral head laterally to clear the posterior rim of the glenoid. This shoehorn maneuver should be performed gently to avoid injury to the remaining portion of the humeral head. If it is difficult to reduce the humeral head using this maneuver, additional soft-tissue releases may be necessary. This generally consists of careful release of the capsular attachments to the inferior and superior glenoid. These releases will generally allow sufficient displacement of the humeral head from the glenoid for the blunt-ended elevator to be properly placed and the reduction to be achieved.

When the humeral head is reduced on the glenoid, the remaining articular cartilage should be carefully inspected to assess the degree of degenerative changes. At this point, the entire humeral head defect can also be visualized (Fig. 17-12). Fibrous tissue should be

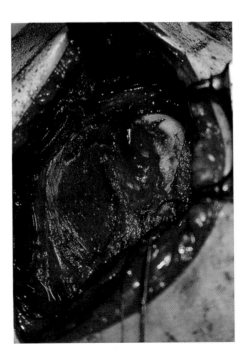

Figure 17-12. Following reduction, the humeral head defect should be carefully inspected. Fibrous tissue should be removed to expose bleeding cancellous bone.

removed to expose all surfaces of the defect. In long-standing dislocations, the bone at the base of the defect may be osteoporotic. In this case, care must be taken to avoid removal of additional bone during resection of the fibrous tissue. However, in less chronic cases, the bone can be sclerotic and often there is a portion of the articular cartilage embedded in the defect. The goal of preparing the defect is to expose a bleeding bony surface that will facilitate healing of either the lesser tuberosity or the subscapularis tendon.

I believe that it is important to understand the pathologic changes that have occurred because of the chronic dislocation. Under direct visualization, I internally rotate the humeral head to identify the position of internal rotation where posterior dislocation occurs. This provides information that will be used to assess stability after the subscapularis or lesser tuberosity transfer. Reduction of the humeral head can be easily achieved and should not be a concern as long as all maneuvers are performed gently.

Following this evaluation, the actual transfer is performed. When the subscapularis alone is being transferred, I prefer a tendon-to-bone repair using horizontal mattress sutures of a no. 5 nonabsorbable material (Fig. 17-13). Drill holes should be placed through the base of the defect and brought out through the humeral cortex. Four holes will allow placement of three horizontal mattress sutures, which should be sufficient. It is essential that the transferred subscapularis be in close contact with the articular edge of the defect. This is the critical area in which to achieve a buttress effect. To accomplish this, I prefer to secure the tendon to the edge of the articular surface as well (Fig. 17-13). Two or three no. 2 nonabsorbable sutures should be passed through the bone at the edge of the articular surface. The bone tunnels can be easily prepared with a tenaculum or awl from the Bankart instruments; a small-caliber power drill is also an option. These sutures are then passed in a horizontal mattress fashion through the tendon. The lateral anchoring sutures are tied first to secure the tendon in place, followed by these more medial buttressing sutures.

If a lesser tuberosity transfer is being performed, the osteotomized fragment should be placed into the defect (Fig. 17-14). The medial edge of the fragment should be positioned at the edge of the articular surface (Fig. 17-15). In almost all situations, the superoinferior dimension of the fragment is smaller than the superoinferior dimension of the defect. Therefore, the fragment should be placed superiorly in the defect, as well as at the medial edge of the articular surface. This is the position that provides the best defect-filling effect. Proper positioning of the fragment can be confirmed by palpation through the rotator interval. Once the position is confirmed, the fragment should be securely fixed in place. I prefer screw fixation using two screws (Fig. 17-15). Either 4.0-mm or 6.5-mm cancellous bone

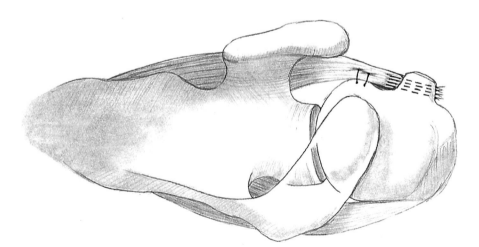

Figure 17-13. After preparation of the bed of the anteromedial humeral head defect, drill holes are placed through the lesser tuberosity to secure the subscapularis tendon into the base of the defect. Additional sutures are also placed to secure the tendon to the edge of the defect formed by the articular surface.

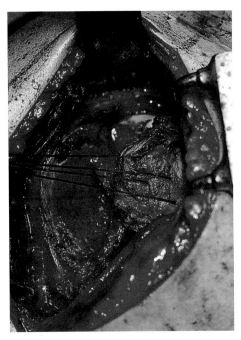

Figure 17-14. The lesser tuberosity is then transferred into the defect.

screws are acceptable and should be chosen on the basis of the size of the fragment (Fig. 17-16). Smaller fragments can usually accommodate only two 4.0-mm screws; larger fragments may be able to accommodate two 6.5-mm screws. However more commonly, one of each screw size is used. This provides secure fixation and is easily accommodated by most fragments. A washer should be used with each screw to decrease the risk of fracturing the fragment. When placing the screws, I use the following sequence: After the fragment is reduced, a drill bit is placed through the fragment into the humeral head. This drill bit remains in place for provisional fixation. A second drill bit is then placed and removed, and the screw is inserted after appropriate depth measurement and tapping. The initially placed drill bit is then removed and a second screw is inserted in a similar fashion.

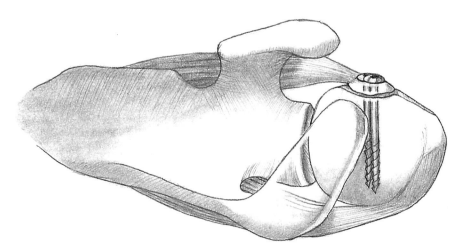

Figure 17-15. Following preparation of the bed of the humeral defect, the lesser tuberosity should be transferred into the defect. It should be positioned to fill the superior portion of the defect and to be as close to the articular surface as possible. The transferred lesser tuberosity should be fixed to the proximal humerus with screws and washers.

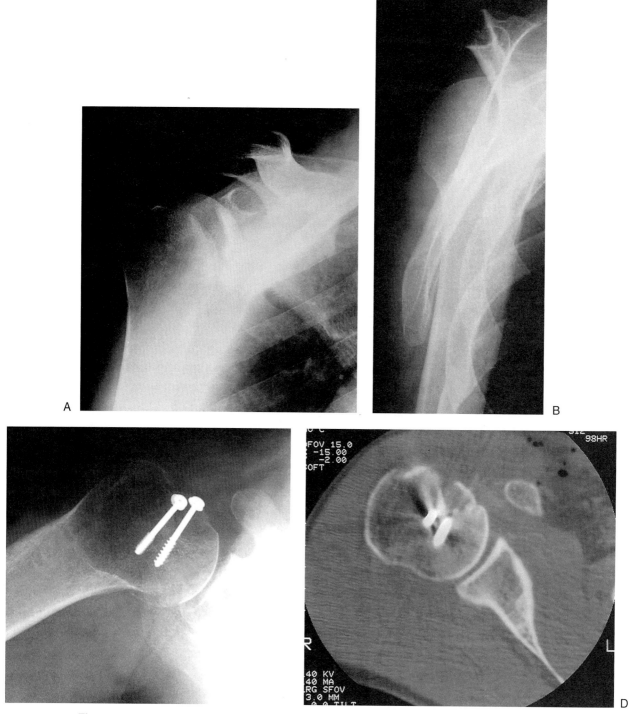

Figure 17-16. This 52-year-old man sustained a posterior dislocation of the shoulder following a grand mal seizure. Anteroposterior **(A)** and scapular lateral **(B)** radiographs show subtle findings of a posterior dislocation. An axillary view obtained following closed reduction under anesthesia shows the size of the defect (Fig. 17-2B). A lesser tuberosity transfer was performed. The lesser tuberosity should be fixed using either 4.0-mm or 6.5-mm cancellous screws with washers. Postoperative axillary view **(C)** and computed tomography scan **(D)** confirm reduction of the humeral head on the glenoid and proper positioning of the transferred lesser tuberosity. *(continued)*

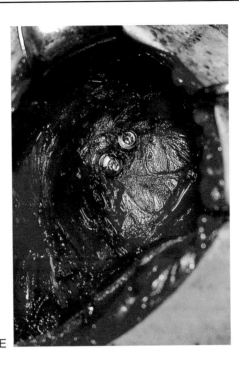

Figure 17-16. *Continued.* **E:** Proper positioning of the lesser tuberosity can also be confirmed by palpation through the rotator interval.

When the transfer portion of the procedure is complete, it is important to assess stability. With the elbow at the side, the arm should be internally rotated. Internal rotation should progress beyond the point at which dislocation occurred before the transfer (as previously assessed). A gentle posteriorly directed force can be applied to the humerus to further assess stability. Posterior translation usually occurs and is acceptable. However, if the humeral head dislocates posteriorly, the integrity of the transfer should be carefully assessed, particularly its position with respect to the articular edge of the defect. If proper position is confirmed, the instability is most likely secondary to significant redundancy of the

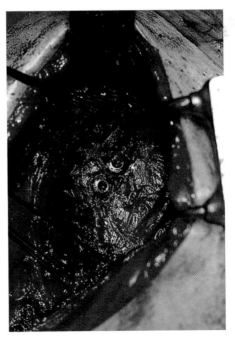

Figure 17-17. Following completion of the transfer, the rotator interval is closed with no. 1 nonabsorbable sutures. Sutures are also placed across the inferior defect in the subscapularis.

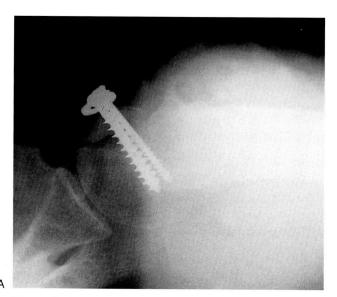
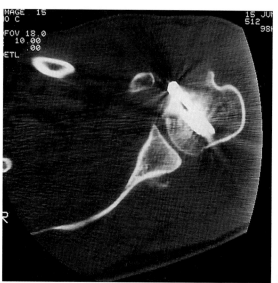

Figure 17-18. A: Radiographs obtained in the operating room confirm the reduced position of the humeral head on the glenoid, and the proper position of the lesser tuberosity at the edge of the defect. **B:** A computed tomography scan obtained on postoperative day 1 also confirms proper position of the graft at the edge of the defect with adequate filling of the defect.

posterior capsule. In this situation, I elect for a longer period of immobilization in external rotation. This can be expected to restore stability.

The closure is begun by assessing the rotator interval. This interval can be closed with two or three simple no. 1 nonabsorbable sutures (Fig. 17-17). I place the sutures with the arm in external rotation to minimize the possibility that closure of the interval will significantly limit external rotation. If a drain is necessary, it should be placed deep to the deltopectoral interval exiting the skin inferior and lateral to the end of the incision. During the remainder of the closure, the arm should be maintained in external rotation to position the humeral head on the glenoid. The deltopectoral interval is closed with interrupted sutures of 0 Vicryl (Ethicon, Inc., Somerville, NJ), with care taken to preserve the cephalic vein. The subcutaneous tissue is closed with 2-0 Vicryl and the skin can be closed with either staples or a subcuticular closure with 3-0 Prolene (Ethicon, Inc.) and Steri-Strips (3M Worldwide, St. Paul, MN). A dressing is then applied.

Radiographs should be obtained following removal of all the drapes. I prefer to maintain the sterility of all instruments until I have confirmed that radiographs show satisfactory position of the humeral head on the glenoid, the position of the lesser tuberosity, and the location of the screws. Three radiographs are obtained: an anteroposterior (AP) view with the arm in maximum external rotation, an AP view with the arm in neutral rotation, and an axillary view (Fig. 17-18).

With the patient still under anesthesia, the upper extremity is placed in a prefabricated orthosis that has been set for proper position of the upper extremity. The shoulder is positioned in 20 degrees of external rotation, 10 to 15 degrees abduction, and 10 to 15 degrees extension. When the patient is awake, a thorough neurovascular examination of the extremities should be performed and documented in the record.

POSTOPERATIVE MANAGEMENT

The patient is generally quite comfortable by the first postoperative day and can be discharged at that time. Before discharge, additional radiographs should be obtained to confirm the position of the humeral head on the glenoid. Scapular AP and lateral radiographs are easily obtained with the shoulder orthosis in place. The patient is allowed movement of the elbow, wrist, and hand as long as humeral motion does not occur and is encouraged to use a rubber ball for gripping exercises to maintain muscle tone. The patient is also instructed in isometric deltoid exercises.

The first postoperative visit is 10 to 14 days after surgery. Sutures or staples are removed at this time and repeated radiographs are obtained. The duration of immobilization varies from 4 to 6 weeks depending on different factors.

Patients with longer-standing chronic dislocations are immobilized for 6 weeks; those with shorter-duration chronic dislocations are immobilized for 4 to 5 weeks. Patients who exhibit some degree of generalized ligamentous laxity are immobilized for 6 weeks. When I am concerned about the potential for significant stiffness to develop, the duration of immobilization is usually 4 weeks. Persistent significant posterior translation or instability after the transfer (as noted intraoperatively) is an indication for 6 weeks of immobilization.

At the completion of the period of immobilization, the patient returns to the office. A trauma series of radiographs is obtained; however, I prefer to position the arm for the axillary view. If the radiographic findings confirm proper position of the humeral head on the glenoid, the patient is then placed in a sling for an additional 10 days during which time active range-of-motion exercises for the elbow, wrist, and hand and grip-strengthening and deltoid-isometric exercises are continued. When the sling is discontinued, the patient is instructed to use the upper extremity for activities of daily living with avoidance of any lifting, pushing, or pulling equivalent to more than 5 lb. The patient is also started on an active range-of-motion program for the shoulder, consisting of forward elevation, external rotation, and internal rotation. Isometric internal and external rotator–strengthening exercises are also added. At 10 weeks after surgery, if recovery of range of motion is slower than anticipated, the patient is instructed in gentle stretching exercises. Resistive strengthening is added at 12 weeks. As the patient progresses, he or she is instructed to increase activities gradually.

I expect patients to recover 90% of their range of motion by 3 to 4 months after surgery. However, range of motion can be expected to increase during the first 6 to 9 months after surgery. At 6 months, patients can perform virtually all activities except strenuous manual labor and contact sports. Return to full, unrestricted activity is allowed at 1 year.

COMPLICATIONS

The complications of primary concern are recurrent instability and shoulder stiffness. Recurrent dislocation can occur as a result of (a) improper placement of the transfer and failure to achieve the desired defect-occupying effect; (b) incorrect postoperative immobilization, either because of inadequate duration or improper position; (c) performance of a transfer procedure for humeral head defect greater than 40% of the humeral head circumference; and (d) complications due to failure to eliminate the cause of the dislocation, such as grand mal seizure. Recurrent dislocation requires treatment based on the etiology. Improper placement of the transfer will require additional surgery for repositioning. Generally, instability secondary to incorrect immobilization can be treated by closed reduction under anesthesia followed by the proper type and duration of immobilization. If the size of the humeral head defect is judged the problem, revision to a prosthetic replacement will be necessary.

Failure to recover range of motion following surgery can be due to (a) excessive duration of immobilization and (b) patient noncompliance in the postoperative rehabilitation program. The duration of immobilization should be chosen carefully on the basis of the factors discussed previously. Patients should be carefully instructed in the importance of their rehabilitation program in achieving a successful result. When compliance is an issue, the patient should be involved in a supervised therapy program with visits to the therapist three to five times per week and frequent follow-up visits.

RECOMMENDED READING

1. Engelhart, M.B.: Posterior dislocation of the shoulder: report of six cases. *Southern Med J* 71(4): 425–427, 1978.

2. Finkelstein, J.A., Waddell, J.P., O'Driscoll, S.W. et al.: Acute posterior fracture dislocations of the shoulder treated with the Neer modification of the McLaughlin procedure. *J Orthop Trauma* 9(3): 190–193, 1995.
3. Hawkins, R.J., McCormack, R.G.: Posterior shoulder instability. *Orthopedics* 11(1): 101–107, 1988.
4. Hawkins, R.J., Neer, C.S., Pianta, R.M., et al.: Locked posterior dislocation of the shoulder. *J Bone Joint Surg Am* 69: 9–18, 1987.
5. McLaughlin, H.L.: Locked posterior subluxation of the shoulder: diagnosis and treatment. *Surg Clin N Am* 43: 1621–1628, 1963.
6. McLaughlin, H.L.: Posterior dislocation of the shoulder. *J Bone Joint Surg Am* 34: 584–590, 1952.
7. Neer, C.S.: Dislocations. In: *Shoulder reconstruction.* Philadelphia: WB Saunders, 393–396, 1990.
8. Oyston, J.K.: Unreduced posterior dislocation of the shoulder treated by open reduction and transposition of the subscapularis tendon. *J Bone Joint Surg Br* 46(2): 256–259, 1964.
9. Rowe, C.R., Zarins, B.: Chronic unreduced dislocations of the shoulder. *J Bone Joint Surg Am* 64: 494–505, 1982.
10. Schultz, T.J., Jacobs, B., Patterson, R.L.: Unrecognized dislocations of the shoulder. *J Trauma* 9: 1009–1023, 1969.

PART III

Rotator Cuff

18

Mini-open and Open Techniques for Full-thickness Rotator Cuff Repairs

Edward V. Craig

INDICATIONS/CONTRAINDICATIONS

The ultimate failure of the terminal fibers of the rotator cuff and subsequent full-thickness tearing is multifactorial in its etiology and includes intrinsic degeneration of tendon, poor potential for healing, vascular insufficiency, repetitive trauma, and extrinsic mechanical pressure from the surrounding coracoacromial arch. Whatever the factors that produced the tear, surgical treatment aimed at decompressing the rotator cuff from impingement by the overlying acromion and distal clavicle, in combination with direct surgical repair of the tendons, offers the most predictable means of relieving pain and restoring movement, strength, and function to the shoulder (Fig. 18-1).

The primary indication for operative treatment of subacromial impingement syndrome and full-thickness tear is pain associated with documented subacromial impingement that has failed nonoperative treatment, or a symptomatic, documented full-thickness tear of the tendon. The rationale for surgical treatment of the full-thickness tear, in combination with an anterior acromioplasty, is that removal of the offending structure producing mechanical wear and restoration of tendon integrity can be expected to relieve the pain, minimize the likelihood of tear extension, and maximize the strength and motion of the shoulder. Lack of strength alone is much less often an indication for surgical repair. I tell the patient the most predictable result of surgical treatment is pain relief. However, return of strength is unpredictable and depends on many factors, including the size of the tear, the length of time the tendon has been torn, the adequacy of the soft tissue and quality of the tendon, the extent of associated muscle atrophy or damage, associated deltoid problems, maintenance of the repair of the tendon over time, and adequacy of the rehabilitation. For this reason, unless a patient is absolutely incapacitated by arm weakness from the rotator cuff tear, I have been reluctant to suggest surgical treatment in the absence of significant pain symptoms.

E. V. Craig, M.D.: Department of Orthopaedics, Weill Medical College of Cornell University; and Hospital for Special Surgery, New York, New York.

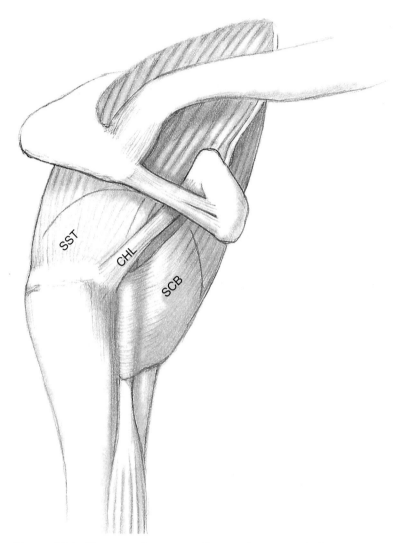

Figure 18-1. The normal rotator cuff emerging beneath the unyielding coracoacromial arch. The coracohumeral ligament (*CHL*) may be responsible for scarring of the retracted supraspinatus tendon (*SST*) to the base of the coracoid process. *SCB*; subscapularis.

An exception to this is the case of severe rotator cuff weakness from a tear following acute trauma. If the patient had no weakness before a traumatic event, and then clearly had a traumatic event that produced the tendon tear, I often elect to repair the tendon even in the absence of pain, particularly if magnetic resonance imaging (MRI) suggests good-quality muscle and tendon. This is because the tendon is usually not retracted or scarred, and a good-quality repair usually can be achieved.

The indications for resection of the acromioclavicular (AC) joint in the surgical treatment of cuff tears include clinical tenderness or radiographic changes of arthritis in the AC joint, inferior protruding osteophytes contributing to the impingement syndrome, and a need for additional exposure of a retracted supraspinatus tendon.

There are really no absolute contraindications for surgical treatment of symptomatic full-thickness rotator cuff tear. Symptoms insufficient to warrant the risks of surgery would be a relative contraindication. Likewise, a patient's medical condition may preclude surgery or anesthesia. Another consideration is the presence of a medical condition, such as the uncontrolled muscle activity of Parkinson disease and paraplegia of the weight-bearing shoulder, which have been associated with a high failure rate of surgical repair of the rotator cuff. Perhaps the most common contraindication to surgical treatment is the inability or unwillingness of the patient to participate postoperatively in protection of the tendon repair and in the rehabilitation program, both critical to the success of surgery.

There are many surgical treatments available for systematic rotator cuff tears, including open and partial repair, arthroscopic and partial repair, and débridement without rotator cuff repair. (Arthroscopic rotator cuff surgery is covered elsewhere.) With a mini-open rotator cuff repair, the bony work (anterior acromioplasty, bursectomy, lysis of adhesions, preparation of greater tuberosity area and tendon edges) is accomplished arthroscopically. A small "split" in the deltoid without deltoid detachment is used to repair and suture the rotator cuff tendon. This can be done through a separate skin incision (as with an open rotator cuff repair) or an extension of one of the arthroscopic portals. In a true open repair, both the anterior acromioplasty and the rotator cuff repair are done as open procedures. The advantage of arthroscopic decompression and mini-open repair is that there is no deltoid detachment, which may produce less postoperative pain. In addition, extensive dissection is avoided and there is minimal interference with muscle groups. Arthroscopy also allows a more complete examination of the glenohumeral joint than is typically done with an open rotator cuff repair. If other pathologies are encountered [SLAP (superior labrum anterior and posterior) lesion, labral detachment, or tearing], these can be dealt with more easily arthroscopically than with an open procedure.

My indications for arthroscopic decompression and mini-open repair of the tendon are those cases in which minimal exposure of the rotator cuff is needed, the tendon is not retracted, the tendon tear does not involve the subscapularis, the biceps is not dislocated, and significant mobilization of the rotator cuff is not required for repair. In my opinion, a prerequisite for a mini-open repair is an "expeditious acromioplasty," as a lengthy arthroscopic decompression and débridement can create significant swelling from fluid extravasation, making it difficult to expose and repair the rotator cuff through a small deltoid split. The ideal candidate for the mini-open rotator cuff repair is a patient with an isolated supraspinatus tendon tear or a nonretracted supraspinatus and infraspinatus tear, if the arthroscopic decompression can be accomplished relatively quickly.

My indications to do the entire procedure as an open procedure, including an open anterior acromioplasty and cuff repair, include the following:

1. A large or massive retracted rotator cuff tear, which requires the releases of soft tissue, adhesions, capsule, rotator interval, and coracohumeral ligament for mobilization and secure repair of the tendon.
2. A large isolated subscapularis repair with or without medial biceps dislocation since it is often difficult to retrieve the subscapularis through a portal extension of a mini-open technique.
3. If there is any consideration of arthroplasty in the presence of glenohumeral arthritis.
4. Revision rotator cuff surgery, as the muscle planes are often obscured; separation of both healthy rotator cuff tissues and surrounding soft tissue is difficult, as more extensive exposure of deltoid and rotator cuff is usually necessary.
5. If elaborate coverage methods for rotator cuff deficiency are considered, such as tendon transfers, patch reconstruction, allograft reconstruction.
6. Deltoid avulsion, retraction, or insufficiency from prior surgery requiring extensive repair or mobilization of deltoid muscle.

The advantages of performing the entire procedure as an open procedure are increased exposure, the ability to better define healthy rotator cuff and deltoid tissue, the better ability to release a contracture and adhesions, and thus better ability to mobilize the tendon. In addition, an open anterior acromioplasty as part of a surgical approach in some instances may be done more rapidly than the arthroscopic portion of the mini-open repair.

PREOPERATIVE PLANNING

The patient with subacromial impingement syndrome usually presents with a gradually progressive history of pain aggravated with use of the arm above shoulder level. As the symptoms persist and progress, the pain, initially present only with activity, may become present at rest and especially at night, awakening the patient from a sound sleep. The patient with a full-thickness rotator cuff tear may or may not notice weakness in the arm. With small cuff tears, strength may be maintained surprisingly well, although the patient may notice diminished endurance and fatigability of the arm when it is used in the overhead position. Patients with cuff tears often note that the pain affects such activities as opening doors, reaching behind the back to do bra straps, reaching high shelves, or participating in sports such as tennis, racquetball, and swimming. On physical examination, inspection often reveals few abnormalities. A patient with a rotator cuff tear may have a rupture of the long head of the biceps or muscle atrophy in the supraspinatus fossa, although atrophy generally accompanies larger tears of long duration. There may be fullness in the subdeltoid area as joint fluid fills the subacromial space. Occasionally a patient with a full-thickness tear will present with an AC joint "ganglion." This is, in fact, glenohumeral joint fluid that has leaked out into the subacromial space and through the eroded inferior capsule of the AC joint. This fluid sac gradually enlarges superiorly to present as a ganglion on top of the AC joint. It is important to recognize that the underlying pathology is not localized to the AC joint, but reflects the more difficult problem of a full-thickness tear that is usually large. Palpation of the affected shoulder not uncommonly reveals AC tenderness especially if AC arthrosis is present. There is usually a palpable subdeltoid soft crepitation, which may represent a subacromial bursal fluid, a thickened bursa, or a torn tendon moving under the coracoacromial arch. A patient with subacromial impingement syndrome without rotator cuff tearing may have normal passive range of motion; however, it is not uncommon for a mild frozen shoulder to accompany this syndrome. In the latter case, there is usually some restriction of motion passively in forward elevation, external rotation, and internal rotation. In the presence of a full-thickness rotator cuff tear, passive range of motion is often remarkably normal, as joint fluid leaks out and lubricates the subacromial space.

On physical examination, a number of impingement signs are usually positive and are very helpful in documenting the diagnosis of subacromial impingement. These include a positive painful arc as the arm is lowered to the side from the fully overhead position, the classic impingement sign, pain with abduction in the plane of the scapula, and pain with internal rotation up behind the back. There may or may not be pain with resisted external rotation and resisted abduction. Active range of motion may be normal or may be reduced. A discrepancy between active and passive motion is highly suggestive of full-thickness disruption of the rotator cuff. A classic and most convincing clinical sign of a full-thickness cuff tear is weakness with external rotation. This is tested with the arm at the side and the elbow flexed to 90 degrees. Both arms may be tested simultaneously. It is common, even in the presence of an isolated supraspinatus tear, to have demonstrable weakness of external rotation. The patient often can distinguish between lack of strength and the need to "let go" secondary to pain. In the larger tears of the rotator cuff, the patient often has so much external rotation weakness that he or she can neither initiate active motion of the arm nor maintain the arm in a position of external rotation in which it has been passively placed. In addition, a "lift-off" test has been described: The arm is brought behind the back, and an attempt is made to lift the hand off the small of the back. Inability to do this is highly suggestive of a subscapularis tear.

An alternative lift-off test for subscapularis insufficiency is the abdominal compression test, in which the hand is placed on the abdomen, the elbow is placed away from the side of the body and paramount to the hand, and the hand is pressed on the abdomen. Subscapularis insufficiency will result in the failure to maintain the elbow in the frontal plane, as the elbow folds into the side because of lack of internal rotation strength.

One of the most helpful radiographs in the diagnosis of subacromial impingement syndrome is an anteroposterior (AP) view of the shoulder in external rotation, which often reveals cystic changes, sclerosis, or bone reaction in the area of the greater tuberosity of the humerus. In addition, a subacromial traction spur may be identified and associated AC joint pathology may be present, as reflected by cystic changes, joint narrowing, or osteophyte formation. In the larger tears, this view often shows changes in the acromiohumeral interval, and in the most massive tears of long-standing duration, arthritic changes may be identified. Another AP view, with a 30-degree caudal tilt, will often more specifically show the anterior acromial spur; this view is used to outline the amount of acromion that projects anterior to the anterior edge of the AC joint, thought to be that amount of acromion pathologically projecting inferiorly. A lateral radiographic view of the scapula and acromion, with a 20-degree caudal tilt, has been termed the "outlet" view. This is intended to identify any bone projecting downward into the supraspinatus outlet, that space through which the supraspinatus passes. This view often identifies inferior protrusion of the acromion and the undersurface of the clavicle, and it may outline the shape of the acromion or an unfused acromial epiphysis. A supine axillary view is perhaps best to identify glenohumeral joint narrowing and the presence of an unfused acromial epiphysis. In a patient who has undergone previous surgery, this view also can reveal the amount of acromion that remains (Fig. 18-2).

If a rotator cuff tear is suspected, any one of a number of imaging studies may be utilized. The most common are arthrography, ultrasonography, and MRI. Arthrography is easily interpretable and can clearly define the presence or absence of a rotator cuff tear. Its disadvantages include that it is invasive, its helpfulness is usually limited to the identification of full-thickness tears only, and it rarely gives information about the quality of the tendon or the precise location of the tendons that are torn. Ultrasonography has been used to identify full-thickness tears, but it may have difficulty revealing small tears. In addition, small tears, partial tears, and even degenerative and scarred tissue may look similar. The reproducibility and high degree of accuracy that have been reported at some centers in this country and in Europe have not been uniformly reproduced in community hospitals and centers with less experience.

Although an MRI scan clearly gives the highest quality image of the shoulder and precise information about the extent and location of the tendon tear (Fig. 18-3), and may give information about associated biceps instability and associated muscle atrophy or fatty infiltration, its disadvantages include the fact that the patient may become claustrophobic and movement may interfere with MRI quality. In addition, the cost of an MRI scan is substantially greater than either of the other two imaging methods. However, for the most information and the clearest prognosis about surgical treatment and anticipated results, I prefer an MRI scan of the shoulder to identify the cuff pathology.

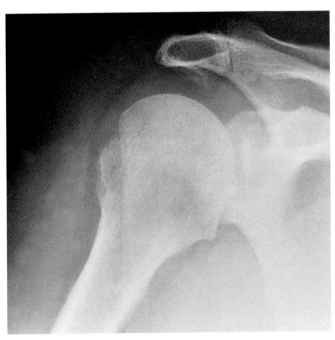
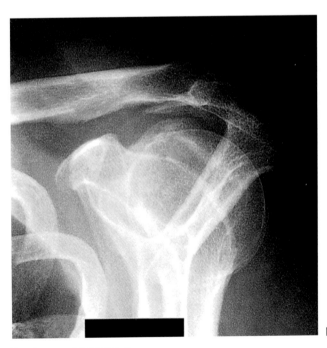

A   B

Figure 18-2. A: An anteroposterior radiograph illustrating a small subacromial spur projecting inferiorly. **B:** A lateral outlet view radiograph revealing the traction spur within the substance of the coracoacromial ligament extending into the subacromial space.

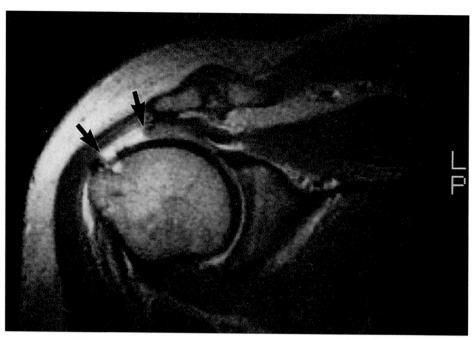

Figure 18-3. Magnetic resonance imaging scan revealing the full-thickness tear with modest tendon retraction.

If a full-thickness rotator cuff tear has been documented, I tell the patient the following:

1. There is no evidence that once a full-thickness tear occurs, there is potential to heal with exercise, immobilization, or medication.
2. Although the acuteness of the pain associated with a rotator cuff tear may subside in time, most patients remain symptomatic if they continue to try to use the arm, especially above chest or shoulder level.
3. Small tears often become larger over time. Although larger tears may not be more painful, they usually are associated with progressive weakness.
4. A small percentage of patients with untreated rotator cuff tears may develop arthritis of the shoulder, the so-called cuff tear arthropathy. It is unknown how great this risk is.
5. If nonoperative treatment fails, and if symptoms warrant taking the risk of surgery, the best chance of successfully controlling the symptoms and restoring function is with surgical repair.
6. The results of surgical repair are much more predictable for pain relief than they are for return of strength. Even with surgical repair, patients who have high demand for use of the shoulder, such as the overhead worker or manual laborer, may not be able to return to that type of job.
7. A certain percentage of surgically repaired tendons will rupture again, with the estimates being anywhere from 5% to 15%. Most times, even if there is a rerupture of a tendon, if adequate decompression has been done, the symptoms do not require further surgery.

SURGERY

The operation is done under either interscalene regional anesthesia or endotracheal anesthesia. Interscalene regional anesthesia can also be used in combination with endotracheal anesthesia for postoperative pain management.

In a mini-open rotator cuff repair, standard arthroscopic positioning, portals, and techniques are used for the complete glenohumeral joint inspection, as well as débridement of loose and torn tendon edges, greater tuberosity preparation, and arthroscopic subacromial decompression. After completion of the arthroscopic decompression, if minimal exposure is required, the standard lateral portal may be extended, subcutaneous flaps developed, and the deltoid split without detachment. With the rotation of the humerus, the torn supraspinatus can be brought into view and the standard repair accomplished with bone tunnels or suture anchors. My preference, however, even if a mini-open repair is going to be done using a deltoid split, is to use a standard anterior oblique incision similar to that described for the open technique. This places the incision in Langer line and is more cosmetic than the extension of one of the arthroscopic portals.

Once anesthetized, the patient is placed in a beach-chair position. The head is secured to the operating table and tilted slightly away from the affected shoulder, which helps provide space for retractors. A rolled-up towel is placed along the medial border of the scapula to stabilize it. The patient is positioned so that a line along the superior cortex of the acromion is perpendicular to the floor. In this way, during the acromioplasty the osteotome or oscillating saw will be directed perpendicular to the floor, thus ensuring that the undersurface of the acromion will indeed be flat. The arm is draped free (Fig. 18-4). The hand is usually the only part of the extremity that is not sterile; it can be covered with a waterproof bag, elastic bandage, and stockinette, up to the elbow. Prominent anatomic landmarks, such as the coracoid process, AC joint, posterolateral corner of the acromion, and lateral edge of the acromion, are identified.

The skin incision extends from just lateral to the coracoid process over the anterolateral corner of the acromion, ending just lateral to the acromion at a point halfway between the anterior and posterolateral corners of the acromion (Fig. 18-5). The length of the skin incision is typically 6 cm. The skin and subcutaneous tissue are infiltrated with a 1 to 500,000 concentration of epinephrine, which will minimize skin and subcutaneous bleeding (Fig. 18-6). Injecting the epinephrine solution in the area of the coracoacromial ligament and the AC joint also helps control troublesome bleeding in these areas. The subcutaneous tissue is divided down to the fascia investing the deltoid muscle (Fig. 18-7). It is helpful to avoid cutting into the fascia of the deltoid muscle, as this fascial envelope helps hold sutures for secure deltoid reattachment and minimizes fragmentation of the deltoid muscle during retraction. Flaps are developed in such a way that the entire superior AC joint may be palpated superiorly. They are undermined as far as the posterolateral corner of the acromion, and the anterior flap is undermined to a distance of at least 5 cm, which is the distance the deltoid muscle will be split. At this point the AC joint is palpated. The deltoid muscle is split in line with its fibers beginning at a point on the anterior surface of the AC joint, and extending distally a distance of approximately 5 cm (Fig. 18-8). Limiting the distance of

(text continues on page 319)

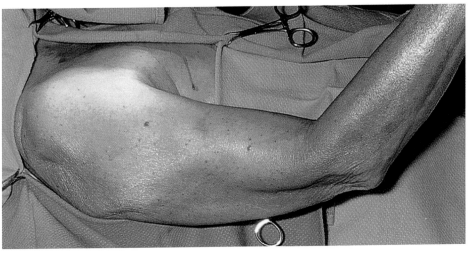

Figure 18-4. The arm is draped free, and the operative field is squared off with sterile towels.

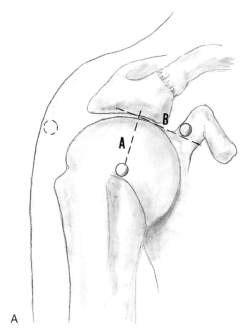

A

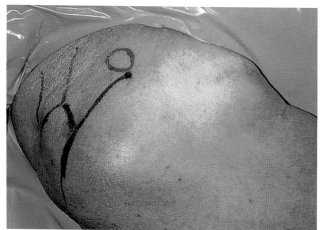

B

Figure 18-5. A,B: The skin incision extends from a point lateral to the coracoid process and passes over or adjacent to the anterolateral corner of the acromion, ending lateral to the acromion.

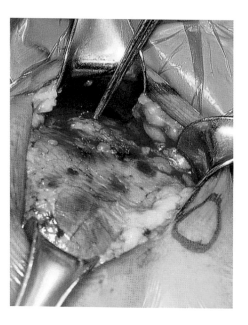

Figure 18-6. A dilute epinephrine solution in the subcutaneous region minimizes bleeding during the surgical approach.

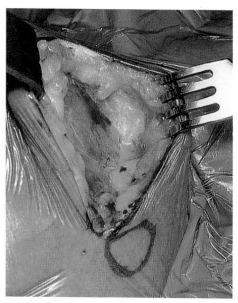

A, B

Figure 18-7. A,B: The subcutaneous tissue is divided in line with the skin incision to the level of the fascia investing the deltoid muscle.

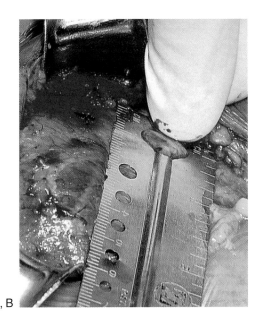

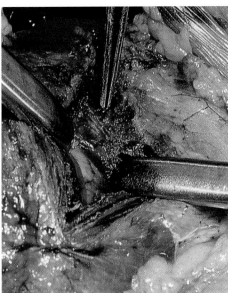

A, B

Figure 18-8. A: A sterile ruler may be used to measure the length of the 5-cm deltoid split. **B:** The deltoid muscle is split, beginning at the acromioclavicular joint, and the distal-most extent of the split marked with a stay suture. **C:** The coracoacromial ligament may be identified before or after detachment of the anterior deltoid. **D:** In a "mini" open approach, in which acromioplasty has been done arthroscopically, the split originates at the anterolateral corner of the acromion and extends distally 4 to 5 cm. This "mini" approach is used if a large area of exposure of tendon tear is not needed.

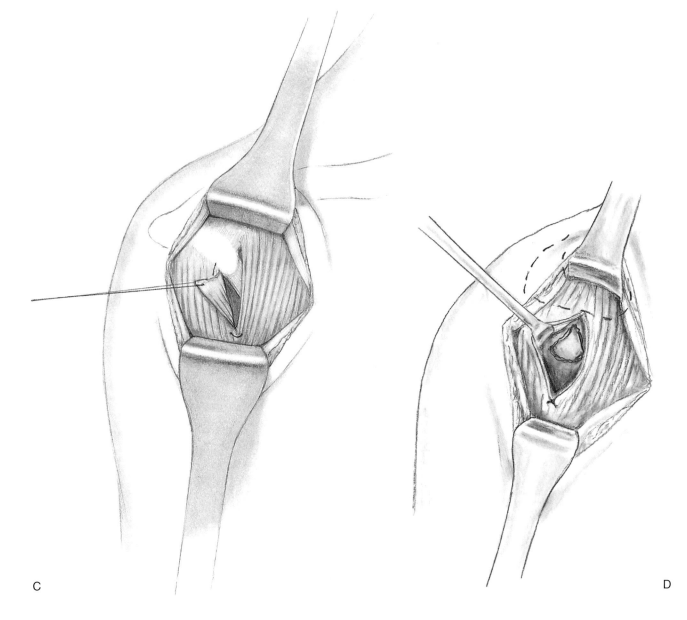

C   D

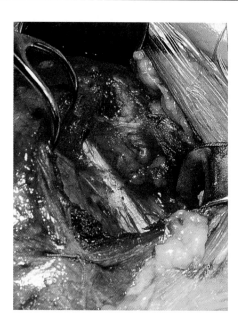

Figure 18-9. The extent of the cora-coacromial ligament is identified. Both anterior and posterior bands are removed during surgical decompression.

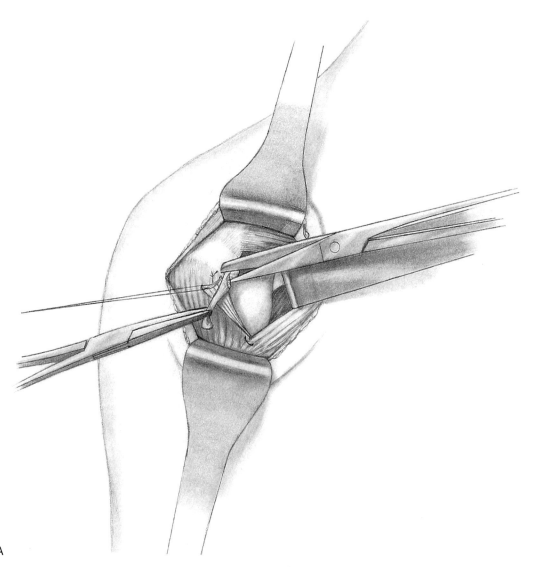

A

Figure 18-10. A: Excision of the coracoacromial ligament. (*continued*)

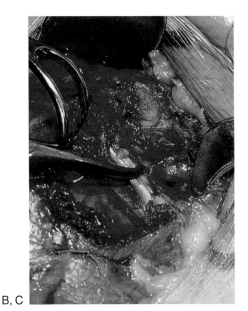
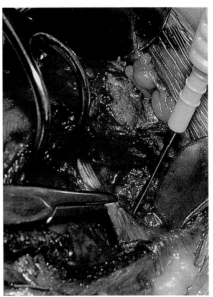
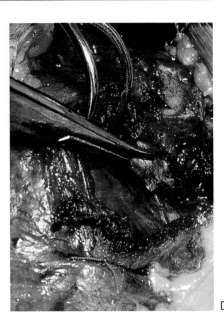

B, C   D

Figure 18-10. *Continued.* **B–D:** The coracoacromial ligament is grasped with a clamp, divided with electrocautery at its coracoid attachment, and completely removed by dividing its acromial attachments.

the deltoid split to 5 cm avoids injuring the terminal branches of the axillary nerve. A no. 1 Tevdek suture marks the distal-most split in the deltoid so that during deltoid retraction the split will not be propagated. The deltoid muscle is bluntly dissected in line with its fibers through this 5-cm distance, until the whitish yellow bursa layer is identified. Bleeding is often present in the most proximal portion of the wound and is usually easily handled with electrocauterization. Adhesions under the deltoid often prevent insertion of retractors. It is usually helpful to use a blunt instrument or an index finger to break up adhesions under the medial and lateral deltoid flaps, so that retractors can be placed beneath the deltoid muscle. Deep fasciae of the deltoid often invest and adhere to the superior surface of the coracoacromial ligament. Using a sponge and a blunt retractor to sweep this off the coracoacromial ligament will isolate and identify this ligament for clear division or excision (Fig. 18-9). The acromial branch of the thoracoacromial artery crosses the top portion of the coracoacromial ligament. Identification and cauterization of this troublesome bleeder before division of the ligament is helpful. The ligament is identified, isolated, and completely excised. Care must be taken to make sure that both anterior and posterior bands of the coracoacromial ligament are removed. This is done by clamping the coracoacromial ligament and using electrocautery or scissors along the lateral edge of the coracoid process to divide this ligament all the way to the base of the coracoid process (Fig. 18-10). Removal of the coracoacromial ligament can then be completed by retracting the deltoid out of the way and removing the ligament from the undersurface of the acromion.

At this point, a decision is made about the deltoid: It must be elevated or detached from the anterior acromion so adequate anterior acromioplasty may be performed, particularly at the anterolateral corner. Many surgeons prefer to lift the deltoid origin with its periosteal attachment off the anterior acromion. My preference is to detach a small amount of anterior deltoid extending from the AC joint to the anterolateral corner of the acromion. The total amount of deltoid detachment is usually approximately 2 cm. This is done by palpating the anterolateral corner of the acromion and using electrocautery from the AC joint directly down on the anterosuperior edge of the acromion, ending at the anterolateral corner of the acromion (Fig. 18-11). When detaching the anterior deltoid from the anterior acromion, care must be taken to include both the superior and inferior fasciae of the deltoid, as these are important soft-tissue structures that aid in holding the suture when the deltoid is reattached at the end of the procedure. The corner of the deltoid that has been detached is marked with a stay suture and the anterolateral corner is marked with a figure-eight suture

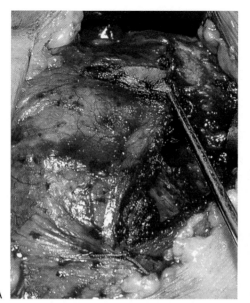
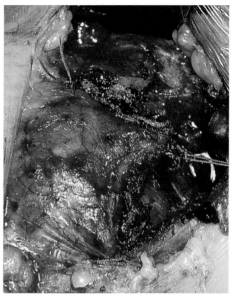

Figure 18-11. A: The deltoid is detached from the acromioclavicular joint, seen here marked by a clamp, to the anterolateral corner of the anterior acromion. **B:** The anterolateral extent of detachment is marked with a stay suture, and the small area of detached deltoid is elevated completely from the acromion.

to prevent further splitting of the deltoid laterally as the deltoid is retracted. The tendinous origin of the deltoid left behind on the acromion is then elevated slightly with a knife or electrocauterization, which aids in securing deltoid reattachment. The deltoid is retracted laterally and medially. Alternatively, the deltoid can be split at the anterolateral corner of the acromion and then detached from lateral to medial toward the AC joint capsule.

At this point, putting traction on the arm helps open up the subacromial space, and the undersurface of the acromion can be palpated to identify osteophytes, irregular bone, and the general slope or shape of the acromion. In addition, it is helpful at this point to attempt to move the acromion, because a very mobile, unfused acromial epiphysis not infrequently accompanies a full-thickness tear of the rotator cuff. If the unfused acromial epiphysis is quite a small amount of the anterior acromion, it can be excised. If it is a third of the acromion or more, it is best left alone. While some consideration may be given to grafting and fixation, this is usually not necessary, particularly if the superior AC joint ligaments and trapezius fasciae are left undisturbed, providing stability to the acromion. A blunt finger is then swept underneath the acromion and deep deltoid fossa, from posterior to anterior, to break up further subacromial adhesion and sweep some adhesions and bursa to a more anterior location for removal.

At this point, an anterior acromioplasty is performed. This is done by using a blunt retractor, such as a Darrach (George Tiemann and Co., Hauppauge, NY), to sweep periosteal attachments, bursal adhesions, and even the adherent, leading edge of the cuff from the undersurface of the acromion, and to lever the humeral head inferiorly, exposing the full undersurface of the anterior acromion (Fig. 18-12). The anterior acromioplasty is performed with an osteotome. Since the intent of the acromioplasty is to remove a wedge of bone that tapers toward the midportion of the acromion, leaving the undersurface of the acromion flat, a point on the anterior acromion has to be chosen to begin the wedge resection of the acromion (Fig. 18-13). In general, the thickness of the anterior wedge of the acromion is usually 0.8 to 0.9 cm, but this will vary according to the extent of the acromial spur and the shape and thickness of the acromion. Another landmark used to identify the starting point of the acromioplasty is the amount of bone protruding from the anterior portion of the AC joint. That amount of acromion protruding anterior to the AC joint may be safely removed if the remaining acromion undersurface is flat.

Once the starting point for the wedge acromioplasty is identified, the osteotome is directed perpendicular to the floor, so that the end result of the acromioplasty produces a to-

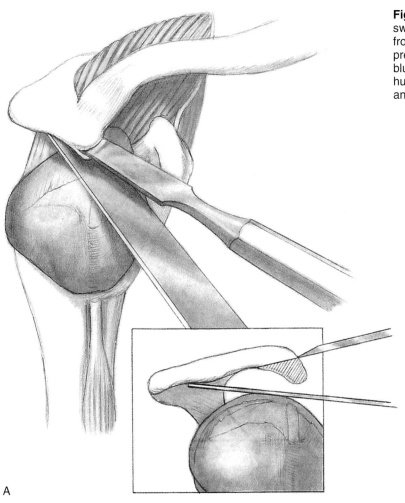

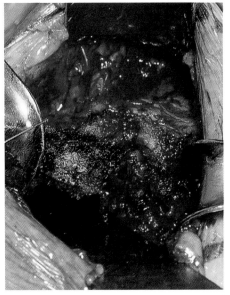

Figure 18-12. A,B: A blunt retractor is used to sweep bursa, adhesions, and retracted cuff from the undersurface of anterior acromion in preparation for the acromioplasty. By using the blunt retractor to gently lever downward on the humeral head, the whole undersurface of the anterior acromion can be exposed.

A

B

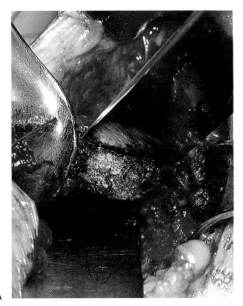

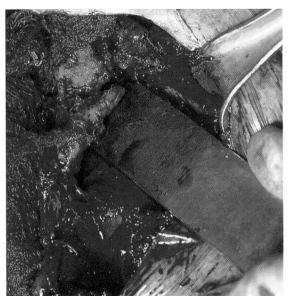

A

B

Figure 18-13. A: The anterior acromioplasty, performed with an osteotome, extends from the anteromedial to the anterolateral acromion, and removes a wedge of bone, which tapers toward the midportion of the acromion. **B:** Intraoperative photograph showing the subacromial spur.

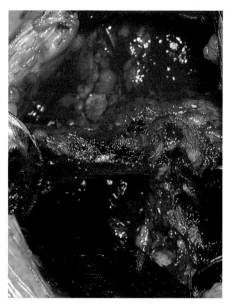

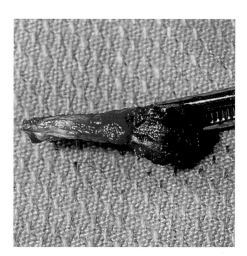

Figure 18-14. At the completion of the acromioplasty, the entire undersurface of the anterior acromion should be flat from anterior to posterior and medial to lateral.

Figure 18-15. The wedge of bone removed at the time of anterior acromioplasty, measuring 0.8 to 0.9 cm at its maximal thickness.

tally flat undersurface of the acromion. The acromioplasty is performed from the anteromedial edge to the anterolateral edge of the anterior acromion, making sure that the osteotome emerges at about the midportion or juncture of the middle and anterior thirds of the acromion. It is helpful to have an assistant use a mallet while the surgeon directs the osteotome and palpates the superior cortex of the acromion to ensure that the osteotome is not directed superiorly, minimizing the risk of superior fracture.

To ensure the anterior acromioplasty is complete from anteromedial to anterolateral, it is helpful to remove a small portion of the inferior AC joint capsule, so that the acromial facet of the AC joint may be palpated and included in the acromioplasty if prominent. At the conclusion of the acromioplasty, the undersurface of the acromion is irrigated, traction is put on the arm, the humeral head is retracted downward, and the undersurface of the acromion is inspected. If the undersurface of the acromion is flat from anterior to posterior, the acromioplasty is complete. There should be no ridges, anterior overhang of the acromion, or sharp spikes of bone at the anterolateral and anteromedial corners. While the acromio-

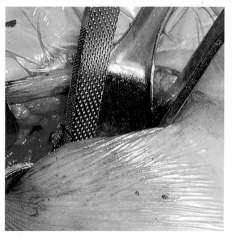

Figure 18-16. A file may be used to smooth any residual irregularities from the undersurface of acromion.

plasty is performed with an osteotome, a flat file may be used to smooth off any residual anterior ridges, ensuring the flatness of the undersurface (Figs. 18-14 to 18-16). Adequacy of the anterior acromioplasty is then checked by bringing the arm into forward elevation and observing that the rotator cuff and bursa pass beneath the residual leading edge of the acromion. Care must be taken when completing the osteotomy not to lever on the remaining anterior edge of the acromion, as this may be quite thin.

Once the wedge of acromion is removed, the undersurface of the AC joint is then palpated. Often, associated AC joint pathology accompanies the impingement syndrome. If so, a partial or complete AC joint resection is added. In general, only the inferior undersurface of the clavicle needs to be removed in an AC arthroplasty for outlet impingement. This may be done by retracting the anterior deltoid or by lifting up a small portion of the deltoid and its periosteal attachments from the distal clavicle (Fig. 18-17). The inferior AC joint ligaments, anterior AC joint capsule, and inferior AC joint capsule are removed. A blunt retractor behind the clavicle will bring the clavicle forward and help expose this difficult area. An osteotome is angled from anterior to posterior and from superolateral to inferomedial, so that a triangular portion of distal clavicle is removed. More clavicle is removed inferiorly than superiorly, so that the superior AC joint ligaments, deltoid origin, and trapezius insertion are not disturbed (Fig. 18-18). Care is also taken during AC joint excision to remove more of the clavicle posteriorly than anteriorly, as the curve of the acromion is such that adduction can bring a residual posteroinferior corner of the clavicle into contact with the acromion. If the entire distal clavicle is to be resected, a rib cutter or bone cutter can be utilized (Fig. 18-19). My indications for a more extensive AC joint resection (coplaning or shaving of inferior osteophytes) include the following:

1. Pain and tenderness at the distal clavicle and AC joint
2. Significant arthritis of the AC joint
3. Inferior and superior osteophytes significant enough to be troublesome to the patient
4. Presence of a "Geyser" sign indicating significant AC joint pathology, larger rotator cuff tear, AC capsular insufficiency, and AC joint arthrosis
5. Need for increased exposure to a very massive cuff tear

At this point, the subacromial bursa is identified and a complete subdeltoid bursectomy is performed. The actual bursal tissue can usually be identified by rotating the arm externally and internally. The tendon underlying the bursa rotates with the tuberosity and the humerus, while the bursa, adherent to the deltoid muscle, moves independently of the un-

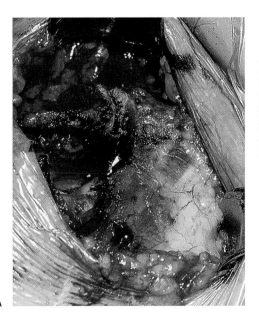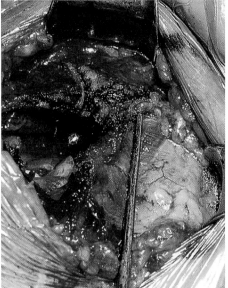

A   B

Figure 18-17. A,B: In preparation for the distal clavicle excision, the acromioclavicular joint capsule is incised, and a small portion of anterior deltoid is detached from the distal clavicle.

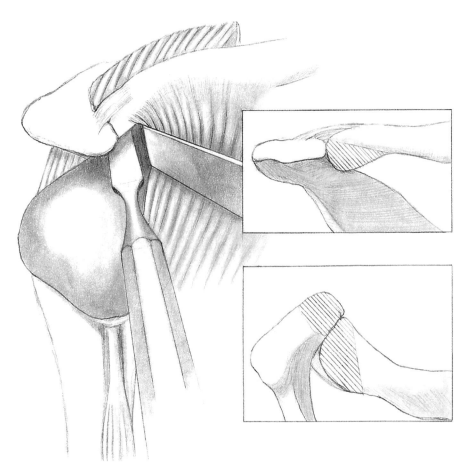

Figure 18-18. The deltoid origin may be left undisturbed if only a portion of the distal clavicle is excised. A partial distal clavicle excision removes more bone inferiorly than superiorly, more bone posteriorly than anteriorly, and leaves superior acromioclavicular ligaments and trapezius insertion undisturbed.

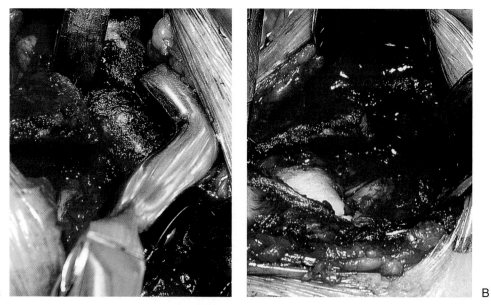

Figure 18-19. A: If the entire distal clavicle is to be resected, a rib cutter may be used to remove it in its entirety. **B:** At the conclusion of the distal clavicle excision, exposure is increased off the retracted supraspinatus tendon. The acromial facet of the acromioclavicular joint should be checked for any residual irregularities.

derlying tendon. However, with a full-thickness tear of the rotator cuff, the bursa may be quite thick, and the difference between the torn edge of the tendon and subacromial bursa may be less clear. Rotating the arm internally exposes the posterior portion of the rotator cuff, and it is here that the interval between bursa and tendon is usually easiest to identify. By placing a blunt clamp between the bursa and tendons, the bursa can be isolated and removed (Fig. 18-20).

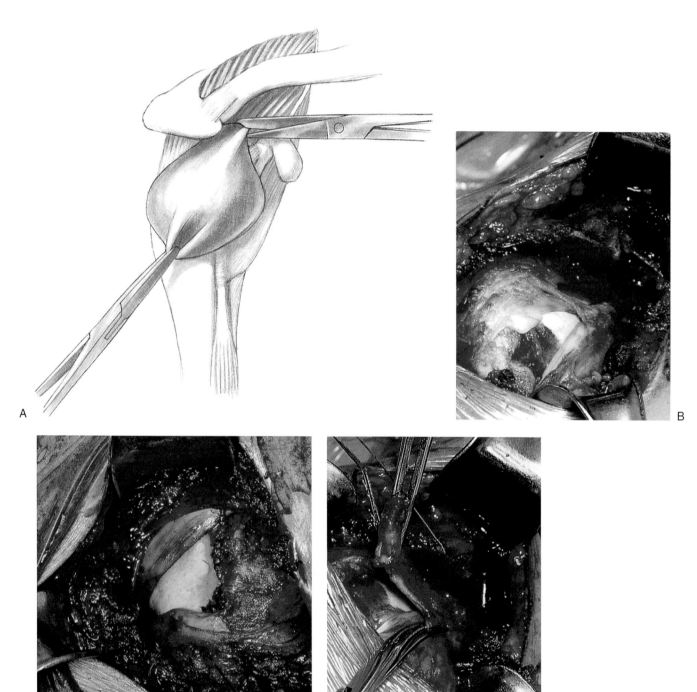

Figure 18-20. A: The thickened adherent subacromial bursa is separated from the torn cuff tissue and removed. **B:** The cuff edge is identified; it is often difficult to distinguish it from thickened subacromial bursa. **C:** Full-thickness rotator cuff tear with a mildly flattened biceps tendon. **D:** Gentle internal and external rotation is helpful in distinguishing the rotator cuff tissue, which can be seen to rotate with the extremity, from the thickened adherent bursa, which is less mobile. Only the abnormal bursal tissue is excised.

At this point, in the presence of a full-thickness tear, the rotator cuff repair commences. With small tears of the rotator cuff, elaborate methods of mobilization and tissue coverage are usually not necessary. It is helpful to identify precisely the rotator cuff anatomy, the shape of the tendon tear, the tendons that are involved and how much they have retracted, and to determine whether there is any deep surface or intratendinous extension of the tendon tear. If an intratendinous split is present, it may be closed prior to commencing the repair of the full-thickness portion (Fig. 18-21). The typical small rotator cuff tear involves the supraspinatus, torn from its attachment on the greater tuberosity. When the supraspinatus retracts posteriorly, it often is scarred to the base of the coracoid process and tethered by the coracohumeral ligament, preventing mobilization. Occasionally a small portion of the supraspinatus may be attached to the coracohumeral ligament in this area. If it is difficult to precisely identify which tendons are involved and to what degree, the biceps tendon can be identified at the rotator interval, between the supraspinatus and the subscapularis; this interval can be opened by incising the fibrous tissue between the supraspinatus and the subscapularis to the base of the coracoid process. Thus, with the rotator interval opened, all the tendon superior (posterior) to the coracoid process is supraspinatus, while all the tendon anterior (inferior) to the coracoid process is subscapularis. Several stay sutures are then placed through the edge of the supraspinatus and the supraspinatus is lifted. While its underside is inspected, intratendinous or deep surface extension of the tendon tear can be identified. Occasionally, deep surface tearing of the rotator cuff can occur in such a way that the deep surface of the supraspinatus is retracted more posteriorly than its superficial surface. It may be fruitful to actually curette this intratendinous component of the tear and repair the deep surface to the superficial surface to prevent further lamellar tearing.

While extensive mobilization is not needed for a small tear, if there is difficulty in mobilizing the supraspinatus it may be because there are adhesions between the deltoid and the cuff in the subdeltoid area, preventing advancement of the tendon. Mobilization can be

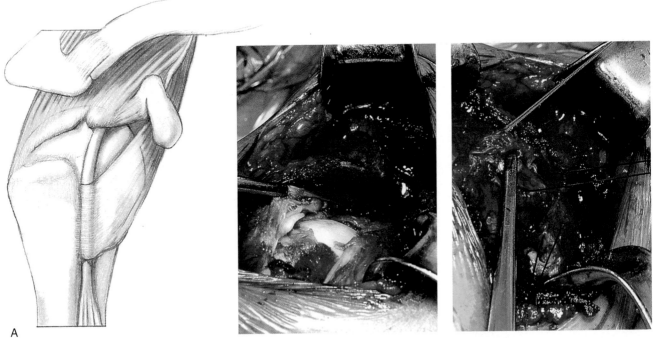

A   B, C

Figure 18-21. A: The torn rotator cuff is identified. The supraspinatus is commonly pulled posteriorly by its attached muscle and inferiorly by adjacent infraspinatus. A tightened coracohumeral ligament may prevent mobilization and advancement of retracted supraspinatus. **B:** The torn leading edge of supraspinatus is identified, lifted up, and any deep surface tearing or intratendinous tearing of the tendon is identified. **C:** If an intratendinous split is present, it is closed before commencing repair of the main tendon tear. Stay sutures are seen in the leading edge of the torn supraspinatus, and can be used to help mobilize the tendon.

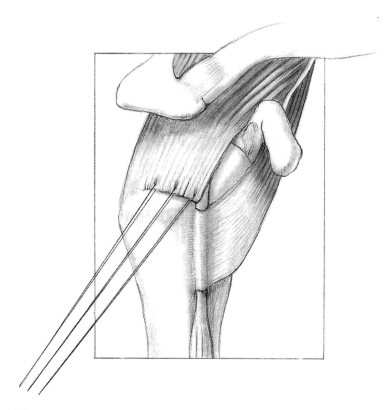

Figure 18-24. The mobilized rotator cuff with its stay sutures is tested for mobility and ease of advancement to the area of the exposed trough.

Drill holes are made at the greater tuberosity with a ⅛-in. drill bit. Likewise, matching drill holes are made in the trough that has been created (Fig. 18-25). In general, the number of drill holes will be determined by the size of the tendon tear and the number of sutures required. The sutures are spaced approximately ½-in. apart and it is quite typical for an isolated supraspinatus tear to require approximately three interrupted sutures. When the

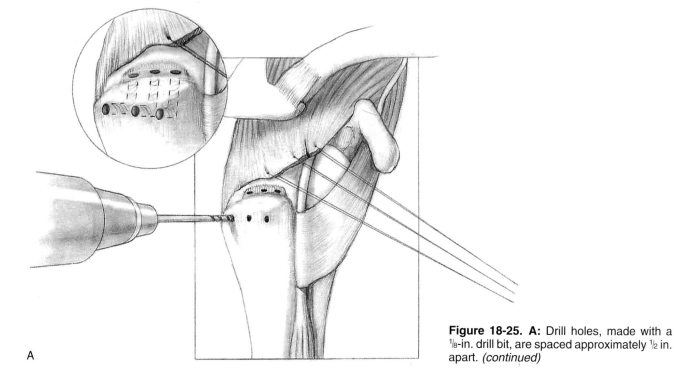

Figure 18-25. A: Drill holes, made with a ⅛-in. drill bit, are spaced approximately ½ in. apart. *(continued)*

A

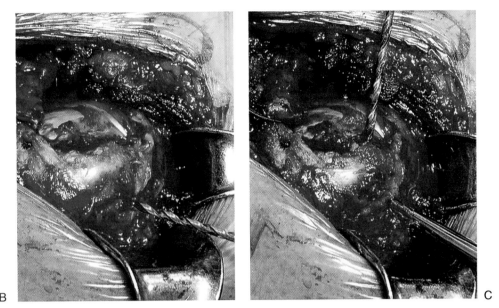

B   C

Figure 18-25. *Continued.* **B:** The drill hole is made in the greater tuberosity, leaving enough cortical bone for an adequate bridge between tuberosity drill hole and prepared trough. **C:** The drill holes in tuberosity and trough are made at 90-degree angles to one another and to the bone, insuring satisfactory bone in the osteopenic patient.

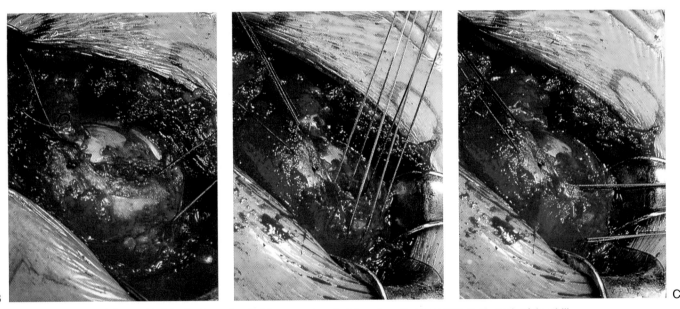

A, B   C

Figure 18-26. **A:** A no. 1 or thicker nonabsorbable suture is passed through each of the drill holes. **B:** A small rotator cuff tear typically uses two to three nonabsorbable sutures, each through its own drill hole. **C:** The previously passed nonabsorbable sutures are tested for anchoring strength, and the mobilized rotator cuff is advanced to its position of insertion.

drill holes have been made, they can be deepened with a small curette. While the holes are usually in continuity with one another at this point, a towel clip or some other grasping clamp can be used to complete the communication between the hole in the tuberosity and the hole in the bony trough. A no. 1 or thicker nonabsorbable suture is then passed through each one of the drill holes (Fig. 18-26). These sutures are passed in a figure-eight fashion through the torn edge of the rotator cuff (Fig. 18-27). Using the stay sutures to take tension off the repair and to advance the rotator cuff into the trough and bone, the cuff is advanced into the bony trough and the nonabsorbable sutures are tied, completing the anatomic repair. If the rotator interval has been opened for exposure or mobilization, this can be closed with a nonabsorbable suture as well (Fig. 18-28).

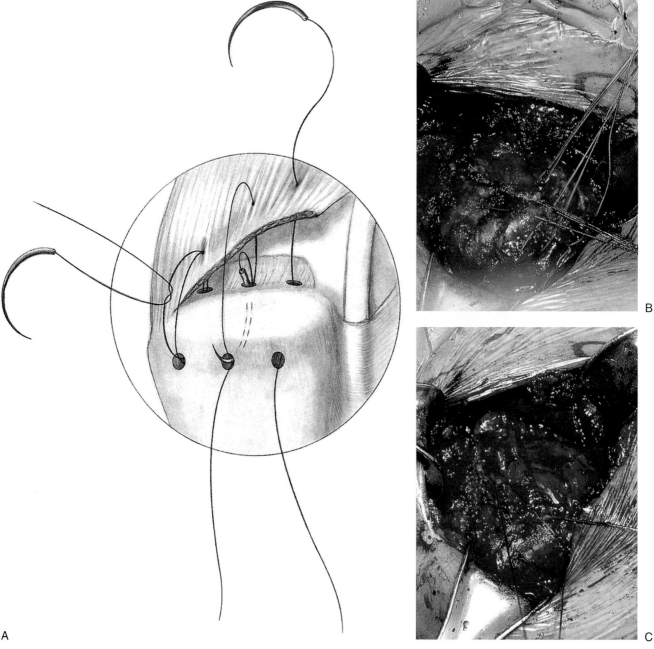

A

B

C

Figure 18-27. A: The nonabsorbable sutures are passed in a figure-eight fashion through the torn edge of the rotator cuff. **B:** The stay sutures may be pulled and used to take tension off the repair during the tying of the knots. **C:** If the sutures in either bone or tendon are loose or insecure, they should be repassed and retied.

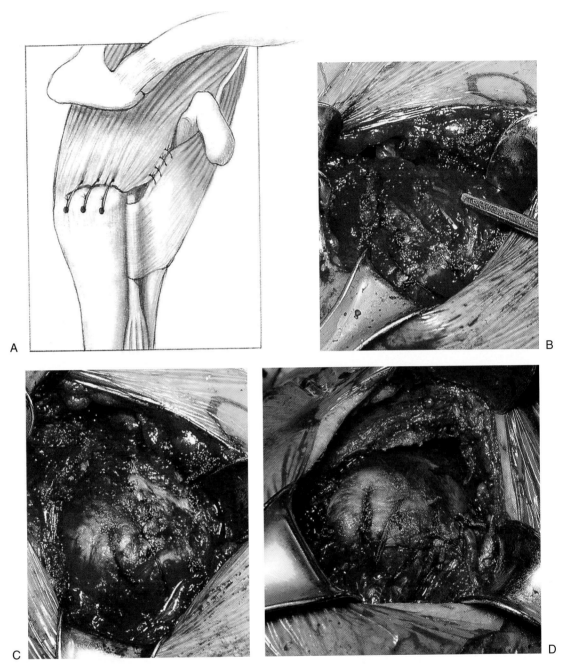

Figure 18-28. A: When the supraspinatus is secured to its greater tuberosity attachment, the rotator interval area may be closed, joining the free edge of the subscapularis to the free edge of supraspinatus. **B:** A clamp points to the superior leading edge of subscapularis, the marker for the rotator interval closure. **C:** The rotator cuff repair completed with nonabsorbable suture. **D:** The completed cuff repair with nonabsorbable suture.

A "mini"-open approach, through a deltoid split, is ideal for use of suture anchors (which may also be used in place of, or in addition to, bone tunnels in open repair). One or more anchors are inserted, and each limb is passed through the mobilized tendon (Fig. 18-29A–D). If a lamellar split has occurred, both suture limbs may be passed through both superior and inferior leaves of the cuff (see Fig. 18-29E).

While the knots for the rotator cuff repair may be tied with the arm in some abduction, taking the tension off the cuff repair, the tension in the sutures should be set with the arm at the side. Any tendon repair that can be repaired only with the arm in full abduction is likely to fail when the arm is permitted to return to the side. In the patient in whom one of

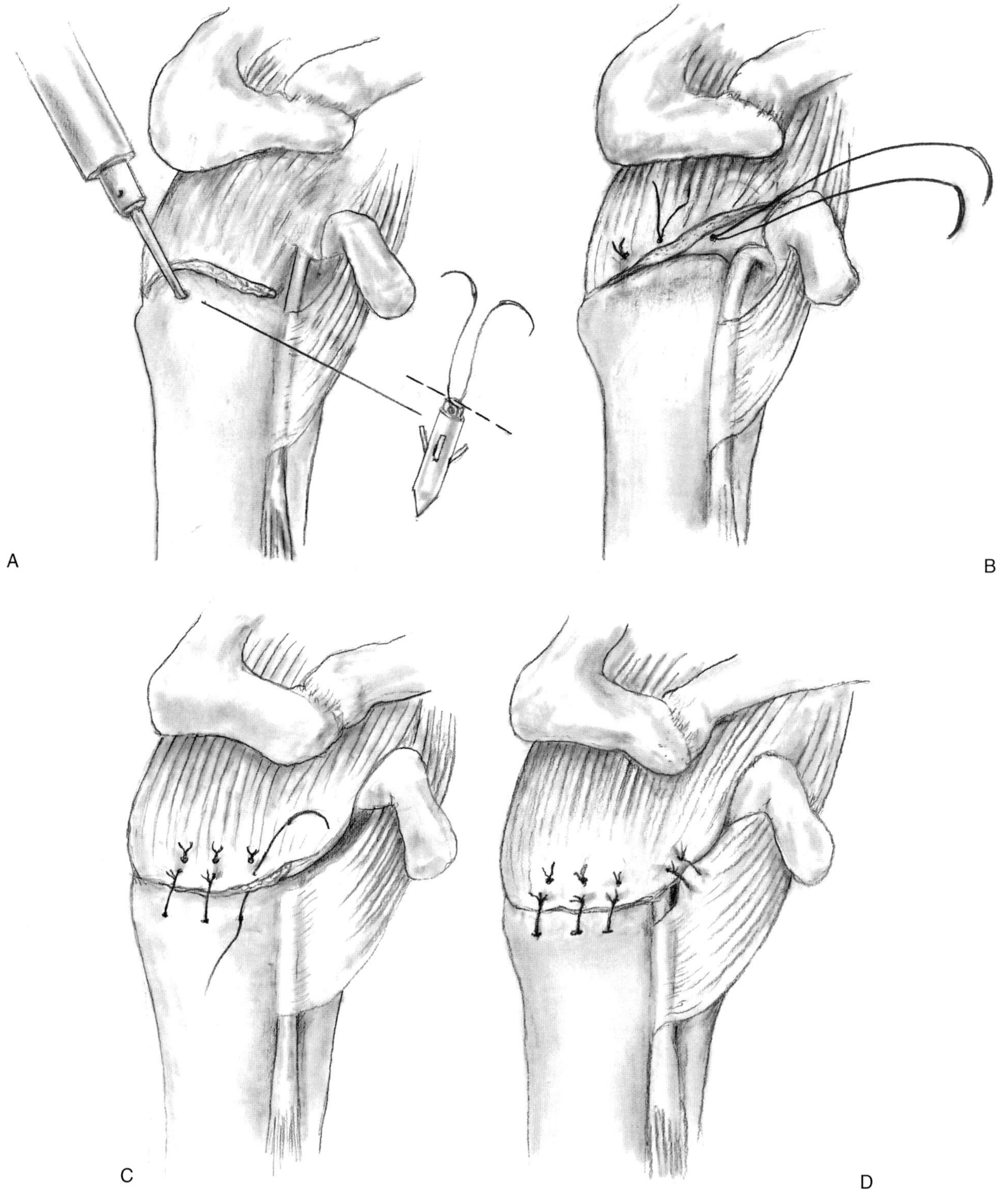

A

B

C

D

Figure 18-29. A: Suture anchors are inserted in the area of decorticated greater tuberosity. **B:** Anchors are spaced 1 cm apart (as with bone tunnels). **C:** With a lamellar split, the limbs of suture can be passed through the top and bottom "leaves" of split tendon. **D:** Bone tunnels can be used in combination with anchors. A more medial row of anchors is augmented by more lateral bone tunnels. This adds to tendon–bone surface contact. *(continued)*

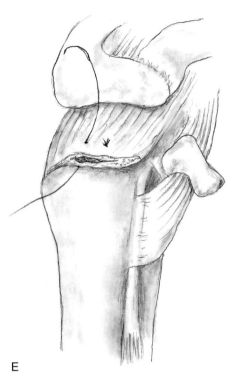

E

Figure 18-29. *Continued.* **E:** The completed double-row repair.

the torn tendons is the subscapularis, there is often medial dislocation of the biceps tendon. If this occurs, the biceps tendon should be replaced in its groove, any associated osteophytes in the bicipital groove removed, and the biceps tendon tenodesed in its groove and incorporated into the supraspinatus and subscapularis repair.

Once the cuff has been sutured, the arm is brought into forward elevation and external rotation, and the adequacy of the decompression and the tension on the sutures are assessed (Fig. 18-30). The wound is then copiously irrigated. If the deltoid has been detached, it must then be meticulously repaired with nonabsorbable suture. I find it helpful to take the

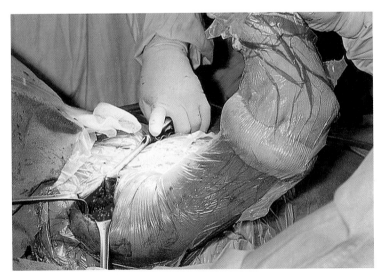

Figure 18-30. Before deltoid closure, the arm is tested in external rotation and forward elevation. Tension and security of cuff repair are examined, and the safe early postoperative range of motion is planned.

corner of the deltoid that has been detached, beginning at the AC joint, and reattach this first, using the superior AC joint capsule and the deep and superficial fasciae of the deltoid in the first stitch. Then from medial to lateral, the anterior deltoid is reattached to the point of its division and to the trapezius insertion with nonabsorbable sutures (Fig. 18-31). It is critical that a secure deltoid repair be obtained. Although it is usually not difficult to repair the deltoid to the point of its division, if there is any question about the security of the deltoid, it may be reattached through a drill hole in the anterior acromion. The skin and subcutaneous tissue are closed with a cosmetic subcuticular closure (Fig. 18-32).

In the patient who does not have a full-thickness rotator cuff tear, following completion of the acromioplasty and inspection of the AC joint, the rotator cuff is manually and visually inspected. If there is an area of significant thinning that is palpable, a tenotomy can be made in the tendon in the area of maximal pathology, in line with the fibers of the cuff tendon. Sutures can be placed on either side of this tenotomy, the tendon then separated, and

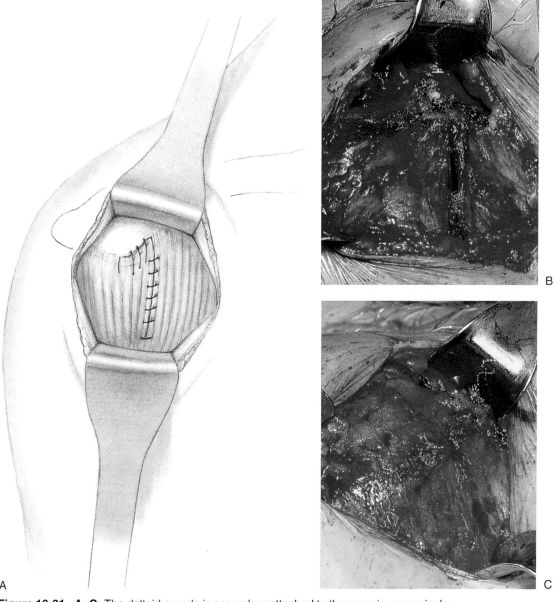

A

B

C

Figure 18-31. A–C: The deltoid muscle is securely reattached to the superior acromioclavicular joint capsule and to the point of its division from the anterior acromion, and the deltoid split is closed.

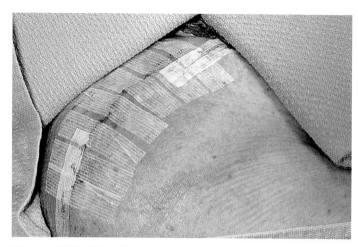

Figure 18-32. The skin is closed with an absorbable subcuticular running stitch.

the deep surface of the tendon inspected. If there is extensive deep-surface or intratendinous tearing, the partially torn area can be resected and the tenotomy closed side to side.

POSTOPERATIVE MANAGEMENT

The postoperative management is decided at the time of the surgical repair of the tendons and must be individualized. Among the factors that need to be taken into consideration are the quality of the tissue of the tendon repair and the sense of security about the sutures holding it, the amount of tension on these sutures with motion, the size of the tendon tear, whether there are associated deltoid problems, and whether there has been prior surgery. Additionally, the level of patient understanding of the nature and goals of the rehabilitation plays a role in the progression of the postoperative program.

I keep a patient either in an abduction brace at approximately 45 degrees or in a postoperative sling (Fig. 18-33). The advantage of sling immobilization is that the sling can be removed for showering, dressing, and initiating postoperative exercises. The advantage of the abduction brace is that active motion is less likely to be initiated by the patient, and protection of the repair is more complete. I try, whenever possible, to use a postoperative sling rather than an abduction brace because of convenience to the patient. However, I use a postoperative abduction brace if the tendon tear is very large, if it is a reoperation for previous failed cuff surgery, or if the patient is not reliable and is likely to use the arm actively. Regardless of the type of protective used, early passive motion begins within the first 24 hours of surgery. The initial physical therapy, while the patient is in bed, is guided by the therapist and consists of supine passive forward flexion and supine passive external rotation with the arm at the side. It is critical that the therapist obtains the patient's confidence and gets the patient to relax enough so that these exercises can be performed safely and confidently. If the patient is in an abduction brace, then the therapist elevates the arm from the brace and lowers it only to the brace. In addition, while the arm is in the abduction brace, it can be externally and internally rotated.

The patient who has a small rotator cuff tear and who is able to cooperate and participate in the rehabilitation is taught an assistive exercise program. When the patient is steady on his or her feet postoperatively, he or she is taught circular Codman exercises, bending over 90 degrees at the waist and rotating the arm in clockwise and counterclockwise directions. The patient is also taught standing forward flexion with a pulley, using the nonoperative arm to motor and raise the operated arm. It must be emphasized to the patient that this is not done using the operated arm actively: All of the power is supplied by the unoperated arm. In addition, the patient is taught assistive external rotation, using a stick, cane, golf

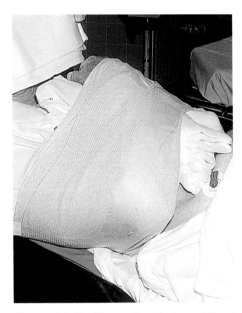

Figure 18-33. The patient is immobilized intraoperatively in a sling and elastic wrap or other support. Pads between the forearm and chest wall keep the arm in slight external or neutral rotation, taking tension off the repair and maintaining the arm in a good position for initiating early postoperative external rotation.

club, or other object. With a pillow under the operated elbow, the elbow is flexed 90 degrees and the unoperated arm moves the operated arm into external rotation.

The patient is kept on this assistive exercise program for 6 weeks and is encouraged to do these exercises five times a day for brief periods of 10 or 15 minutes. At 3 weeks postoperatively, the patient adds extension and internal rotation up behind the back to this assistive program. Before discharge, the decision is made whether a formal physical therapy program will be necessary for the patient. This decision is based on the amount of difficulty the patient is having performing the exercises and how well the patient understands the prohibition of active movement.

The timing for initiation of active movement of the arm and strengthening exercises also depends on the size of the tear and the quality of tissue. In general, at 6 to 8 weeks postoperatively the patient may begin light active use of the arm and some submaximal isometric exercises for both internal and external rotations, and for anterior and middle deltoid strength. Between 10 and 12 weeks postoperatively, unrestricted active use of the unweighted arm may be begun and light resistance is begun with elastic Theraband for anterior deltoid and for internal and external rotation strength. With the larger tears, delay in active use of the arm and resistance exercises may be as long as 3 to 4 months from surgery. Weights are ordinarily not used within the first 3 to 4 months after surgery.

Following open surgical treatment for impingement syndrome, whether or not a small full-thickness tear has been repaired, I ordinarily expect the early postoperative course to be painful for the patient. In addition to the initial soreness from the incision and the extensive soft-tissue dissection, there is ordinarily a painful pulling because of tightness when range-of-motion exercises are being performed. External rotation stretching appears to be the most difficult for the patient. This second type of discomfort ordinarily lasts until the range of motion approaches normal. The third type of discomfort is more variable and is generally thought to be a fatigue aching that exists until the strength of the deltoid and rotator cuff returns to normal. In addition, the patient can commonly experience a weather ache for at least 1 to 2 years from the time of surgery.

When active motion is permitted and initiated, the patient typically has quite a bit of weakness in the deltoid and rotator cuff. The surgeon should not expect that the strength will improve rapidly; the expectation that strength will improve slowly should be communicated to the physical therapist and patient. Therapists may be frustrated and have unrealistic expectations about the rapidity of progress following rotator cuff surgery. I tell patients and therapists that I expect the strength and the movement in the arm to improve over the year following surgery, and I expect the length of rehabilitation to last approximately 1 year from the time of surgery. By 1 year following repair of most small tears, I expect approximately 95% of patients either to be pain-free or to have no more than an occasional ache. I expect the range of motion to be essentially full in forward flexion, external rotation, and internal rotation, and I expect the strength of the arm above shoulder level to be progressing monthly. With a typical 1-cm, full-thickness tear of the rotator cuff, I would expect active and passive motion to be equal at approximately 9 to 12 months from the time of surgery. A smaller percentage of patients may have some residual stiffness in the arm and may have more aching with use of the arm.

My expectations for patients' recovery from very large full-thickness tears are quite different. While the pain relief is usually as good, the return of strength is highly variable and very much depends on the size of the tear, the associated muscle atrophy, and the progress of the rehabilitation. I am careful to tell a patient preoperatively that the return of strength for a massive tear of the rotator cuff is highly unpredictable.

I tell patients that in the early postoperative period, they will feel a tightness and stiffness and have difficulty with their rehabilitation. I tell them that at the end of 3 months, after they have been doing range-of-motion exercises and are just starting to begin strengthening exercises, the pain they have will be noticeably different and less severe than the pain they had before the surgery. They still may not be able to sleep on the involved side, but the pain is often described by patients as a muscle soreness or a "getting better" type of pain. However, at 3 months postoperatively, they are still noticeably weak. At 6 months postoperatively, range of motion should be almost normal passively, perhaps with some end-range stiffness in internal and external rotations. Strength should be improving by this point, and patients will usually have active movement above shoulder level, although the active movement and endurance is often not full by this time. I tell patients at 6 months postoperatively that they probably will have weather ache and fatigue ache following exercise periods. I pay particular attention to tell patients that there is often a slump at about 3 to 4 months postoperatively. Patients have a tremendous letdown at this point, after investing a lot of time, energy, and discomfort in the operation and the early postoperative period, and often they can get quite depressed because there seems to be quite a long way to go. Patients may be frustrated by the inability to see daily improvement, and they need much encouragement to press on. I record the range of motion and strength of patients at each office visit, so that at 3-month intervals they can see that clear progress has been made.

COMPLICATIONS

The most common intraoperative complications are:

Injury to the Terminal Branches of the Axillary Nerve. The axillary nerve fibers course within the deep fascia of the deltoid, approximately 5 cm from the deltoid origin. Splitting or division of the deltoid muscle more than 5 cm from the deltoid origin has the potential to injure the terminal branches of the axillary nerve. This is usually not recognized intraoperatively. If this occurs, deltoid muscle atrophy is seen in that portion of the muscle. I believe there is nothing to do about this complication, except to recognize that it may well affect the ultimate strength of the arm. To avoid this complication, avoid splitting the deltoid more than 5 cm distal to the deltoid origin. A stay suture in the deltoid fascia helps prevent distal splitting during retraction of the deltoid.

Excessive Removal of Acromion. This may be a too-generous amount of acromion removed in an AP direction, leading to shortening of the acromion and difficulty reattaching the anterior deltoid muscle to remaining bone, or it may be extension of the acromioplasty to include the lateral acromion, which may make it difficult or impossible to reattach the middle deltoid fibers. The middle deltoid origin is more muscular than tendinous (unlike the anterior deltoid), and detaching the middle deltoid and removing the lateral acromion can create a very difficult situation in which the middle deltoid retracts and scars to the surface of the rotator cuff, and it is difficult to reattach. In my opinion, a near-complete or radical acromionectomy should never be performed, because this permanently weakens the deltoid origin and can lead to pain, scarring, and an unsightly cosmetic appearance of the shoulder. As the impingement is on the anteroinferior surface of the acromion, it is not necessary to disturb the lateral acromion at all.

Excessive or Protruding Residual Acromion. Another common technical error during the acromioplasty is to angle the cut in such a way as to leave residual medial overhang of the acromion adjacent to the AC joint or to leave lateral inferior protrusion of the acromion adjacent to the anterolateral corner. The way to avoid this is to make sure that the acromioplasty extends from the anterolateral corner to the anteromedial corner of the acromion and that the undersurface of the acromion is completely flat.

Fracture of the Acromion. Angling the osteotome superiorly can fracture through the top of the acromion during the acromioplasty. If this is recognized intraoperatively, the acromion can be fixed with a tension-band technique. Fracture is avoided by angling the osteotome in such a way that it emerges from the inferior cortex of the acromion. If one palpates the superior aspect of the acromion, as the osteotome is directed, the potential for this complication is minimized.

Postoperative Deltoid Avulsion. In the postoperative period, if the deltoid muscle has been detached, the deltoid repair can be pulled off or avulsed by premature active use of the arm or by initiating the strengthening program too soon following surgery. If the deltoid avulses from the anterior acromion in the early postoperative period, I ordinarily leave this alone and continue with the rehabilitation. Although there may be some local tenderness over the prominent anterior acromion not covered by deltoid, it is rare that this small avulsion of the deltoid produces symptoms if an otherwise adequate decompression and cuff repair have been performed.

Retear of the Rotator Cuff. This ordinarily occurs because of inadequate protection postoperatively and beginning active exercises or resistive exercises too early in the postoperative period, and is often related to tissue quality. I believe a certain percentage, perhaps as many as 10% to 15%, of cuff repairs may retear in the postoperative period. If an adequate decompression has been performed and early rehabilitation has eliminated the stiffness, it is unusual for failure of a tendon repair alone to be painful enough to warrant reoperating. Most residual pain is due to inadequate acromioplasty, failure to address pathology in the AC joint, or inadequate rehabilitation with residual stiffness. If retear is recognized in the early postoperative period, I usually continue to press on with the passive and strengthening exercises at the appropriate times and do not recommend immediate re-repair, as pain relief will usually be good despite retear. However, there is one situation that may make me intervene earlier if a cuff retears. If the patient is progressing smoothly with the rehabilitation and has achieved good strength and active motion, and then suffers trauma following which there is dramatic weakness likely to be unacceptable to the patient, early re-repair may be warranted.

Stiffness. This is perhaps the most common complication following cuff surgery. It usually results from tentativeness on the part of the surgeon, therapist, and patient regarding early postoperative motion or lack of clear understanding about the critical nature of early postoperative range-of-motion exercises. If the patient comes to the office with a stiff shoulder in the postoperative period after anterior acromioplasty or rotator cuff repair, I generally have a long discussion about the critical need for postoperative rehabilitation, and I encourage redoubling of the efforts at restoring range of motion in forward flexion, external rotation, and internal rotation. If the patient has not been in a formal outpatient therapy program, one is initiated. Ordinarily, if the efforts of the therapist and the patient are redoubled, the stiffness will gradually be eliminated over time. While the temptation may be great to do a manipulation under anesthesia for postoperative stiffness, I do not manipulate a postoperative shoulder under anesthesia for fear of disrupting the cuff repair or deltoid repair. I believe that the complication of postoperative stiffness is avoidable by beginning early range-of-motion exercises within the first 24 hours of surgery and by emphasizing to the patient the critical need to continue an aggressive rehabilitation program for 6 months to 1 year from the time of surgery.

RECOMMENDED READING

1. Blaine, T.A., Freehill, M.Q., Bigliani, L.U.: Technique of open rotator cuff repair. *Instr Course Lecture (United States)* 50: 43–52, 2001.
2. Burkhart, S.S.: Biomechanics of rotator cuff repair: converting the ritual to a science. *Instr Course Lecture (United States)* 47: 43–50, 1998.
3. Cofield, R.H.: Current concepts review: rotator cuff disease of the shoulder. *J Bone Joint Surg Am* 67: 974–979, 1985.
4. Cofield, R.H., Parvizi, J., Hoffmeyer, P.J., et al.: Surgical repair of chronic rotator cuff tears: a prospective long-term study. *J Bone Joint Surg Am* 83: 71–77, 2001.
5. Craig, E.V.: Open decompression as a treatment of shoulder impingement. *Oper Tech Sports Med* April, 1994.
6. Gerber, C., Fuchs, B., Hodler, J.: The results of repair of massive tears of the rotator cuff. *J Bone Joint Surg Am* 82: 505–515, 2000.
7. Grondel, R.J., Savoie, F.H., Field, L.D.: Rotator cuff repairs in patients 62 years of age or older. *J Shoulder Elbow Surg Am* 10: 97–99, 2001.
8. Hawkins, R.J., Morin, W.D., Bonutti, P.M.: Surgical treatment of full-thickness rotator cuff tears in patients 40 years of age or younger. *J Shoulder Elbow Surg Am* 8: 259–265, 1999.
9. Matsen, F.A. III, Arntz, C.T.: Rotator cuff tendon failure. In: Rockwood, C.A.Jr., Matsen, F.A., III, eds.: *The shoulder.* Philadelphia: WB Saunders, 1990.
10. Neer, C.S. II: Anterior acromioplasty for the chronic impingement syndrome in the shoulder: a preliminary report. *J Bone Joint Surg Am* 54: 41–50, 1972.
11. Neer, C.S. II: Impingement lesions. *Clin Orthop* 173: 70–77, 1983.
12. Warner, J.J.: Management of massive irreparable rotator cuff tears: the role of tendon transfer. *Instr Course Lecture (United States)* 50: 63–71, 2001.
13. Yamaguchi, K.: Mini-open rotator cuff repair: an updated perspective. *Instr Course Lecture (United States)* 50: 53–61, 2001.

19

Repair of Massive Rotator Cuff Tears

John J. Brems

INDICATIONS/CONTRAINDICATIONS

Tears of the rotator cuff are common and result from the unique anatomy and physiology of the shoulder. A combination of vascular and mechanical factors is responsible for this common clinical condition. Although physicians may debate the sequence of events leading up to a rotator cuff tear, impingement of the soft tissues within the confines of the subacromial space appears to be the final common pathway. Whether the initial events occur within the tendon (intrinsic) or from mechanical abrasion from without (extrinsic), the net result is failure of the cuff tendons. The pathophysiology is most likely a spectrum involving mechanical, physiologic, and vascular factors.

Often, rotator cuff tears remain small and are easily treated. When a small rotator cuff tear remains untreated, it may become larger over time. For a variety of reasons, a patient may wish to manage the cuff tear nonoperatively, but careful follow-up evaluations of clinical strength are important to ensure that the cuff tear size is not increasing. It is difficult to predict those patients in whom the cuff tear may increase, but generally, the more active the patient, the more likely the cuff tear will increase in size. Occasionally, the patient with a documented cuff tear may achieve pain relief with a physical therapy program consisting of stretching and strengthening.

Although the primary indication for surgical intervention is pain, some patients are absolutely incapacitated by the weakness associated with a massive cuff tear. In these patients, surgical treatment may be indicated despite little pain.

The contraindications for surgical repair of massive cuff tears include active infection of the glenohumeral joint, often associated with a prior attempt at surgical repair of the rotator cuff; a Charcot shoulder, which may include not only destructive changes of the joint but also severely deficient soft tissue; and failed prior surgical treatment with associated

J. J. Brems, M.D.: Section of Shoulder Surgery, Department of Orthopaedic Surgery, Cleveland Clinic Foundation, Cleveland, Ohio.

deltoid insufficiency. In addition, some patients with failed prior surgery may have had a radical acromionectomy. The devastating combination of cuff loss and resection of the bony origin of the deltoid muscle makes the results of repeat rotator cuff surgery disappointing. In these patients, an alternative form of surgical treatment, such as shoulder arthrodesis, might be considered.

The procedure is relatively contraindicated for the patient who has no pain and is only moderately bothered by the amount of weakness associated with the tendon tear or for the patient who is either unable or unwilling to protect the postoperative repair and cooperate with the critical postoperative rehabilitation program.

In those patients who have a massive cuff tear and arthritis of the glenohumeral joint, repair of the tendons alone is often inadequate to relieve pain, and the tendon repair probably should be combined with shoulder arthroplasty.

PREOPERATIVE PLANNING

The patient with a massive tear of the rotator cuff often has characteristic findings on physical examination. There is atrophy of muscle in the supraspinatus and infraspinatus fossae. There may be a fullness of the shoulder suggestive of fluid underneath the deltoid, which represents fluid leaking out of the cuff tear (Fig. 19-1). There is often an associated tear of the long head of the biceps with the characteristic physical finding of a retracted biceps muscle belly. Palpation of the shoulder may reveal tenderness at the acromioclavicular (AC) joint. There may be crepitus perceived and palpated underneath the deltoid muscle when the arm is passively rotated while in abduction. Hard grinding or crepitation that is deeper may indicate glenohumeral arthritis. The patient may demonstrate surprisingly good passive range of motion. However, the hallmark of the physical examination is weakness of the rotator cuff muscles. While this may be evident in the inability of the patient to actively elevate the arm, pain often impedes active elevation. A more predictable clinical test is for weakness of external rotation. With the patient's arms at the side, both arms can be tested for external rotation strength; the patient with a massive rotator cuff tear often has dramatic inability to maintain external rotation against resistance. In the largest cuff tears, the patient cannot even maintain the arm in position when it is passively placed in external rotation (lag sign).

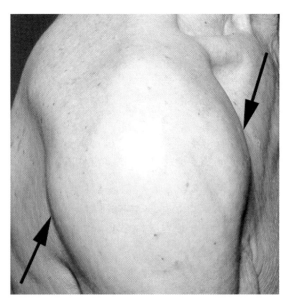

Figure 19-1. This patient has a massive rotator cuff tear. The arrows demonstrate the fullness seen with a "fluid sign."

On plain radiographs, there may be a decrease in the distance between the acromion and the humerus, rounding of the greater tuberosity from impingement against the acromion or a spur, cystic changes or sclerosis in the area of the greater tuberosity, and associated spur formation on the acromion or inferior surface of the AC joint. In the most massive cuff tears of long-standing duration, there are often arthritic changes of the glenohumeral joint. While there is often little doubt about the diagnosis on plain radiographic and physical examination, imaging studies such as magnetic resonance imaging (MRI), ultrasonography, or arthrography clarify the diagnosis. Additionally, an MRI scan has the advantage of demonstrating the precise location, extent, degree of atrophy, and fatty replacement of the torn tissues. Unfortunately, no diagnostic modality is capable of informing the surgeon of the quality and tensile properties of the tissues to be repaired. This additional information may be useful to the patient to help predict the expected outcome of surgical intervention.

SURGERY

Whenever possible, cuff repairs are performed under a combination of regional interscalene block anesthesia and general techniques. The interscalene block provides for preemptive analgesia and prolonged postoperative analgesia. Typical block agents provide 8 to 12 hours of anesthesia after the completion of the procedure. Reports in the anesthesia literature support the concept that if the brain does not perceive the "pain" production during the procedure and for several hours later, the biochemical mediators of pain are much diminished by the time the block agent is no longer effective. Total narcotic use following surgery has also been remarkably lessened. Unfortunately, those agents that provide prolonged analgesia do not provide predictable muscle relaxation; hence, general anesthesia is also used. However, because the brain perceives no pain, the depth of anesthesia is remarkably light, and the patient awakens rapidly, free from pain. Interscalene block anesthesia offers the advantage of less blood loss and is well tolerated by patients with few complications. The prolonged analgesia also provides an opportunity for the surgeon to move the arm following the repair thus allowing the patient to witness the goals and limits of his or her therapy.

If one accepts the premise that subacromial impingement leads to cuff tears, then one must agree that an anterior acromioplasty is a crucial step in the surgical procedure. Some surgeons believe that the acromion is not related to the cause of the cuff tear and believe that the changes in acromial morphology are themselves caused by the impingement process that initiates within the muscle tendon. Regardless of the cause, it remains important to ensure adequate decompression within the subacromial space bounded by the humerus and acromion at the completion of the cuff repair. It is also important to reconstruct the coracoacromial (CA) ligament at the time of deltoid closure. It is increasingly apparent that the CA ligament is an important structure to maintain anterior superior stability especially in the face of a potentially incompetent rotator cuff.

The surgeon must address the AC joint and specifically the lateral clavicle because it is frequently involved in the degenerative process. On the other hand, it is important to correlate clinical findings of pain and tenderness at the AC joint and not merely excise the clavicle because it is hypertrophic on an imaging study. If pain is present at the AC joint during clinical assessment, it should be addressed at the time of surgery. Although there are different methods of dealing with AC joint arthrosis, in the face of massive cuff tears, it is especially important to protect the deltoid. Accordingly, only an inferior resection of the lateral clavicle should be performed. Resection of the lateral clavicle (Mumford) results in potentially significant weakness of the anteromedial deltoid. The combination of a now weakened deltoid in the face of a precarious rotator cuff can result in severe functional disability.

After the acromioplasty and AC joint arthroplasty, the rotator cuff is methodically inspected by internally rotating the arm and examining the posterior cuff muscles then gradually rotating the arm into external rotation while examining the supraspinatus, bicipital tendon, and subscapularis. As often as necessary (predictably 100% of the time), the cuff tendons are repaired to bone. The supraspinatus nearly always tears at its insertion on the greater tuberosity and it must be repaired to that area of the humerus. At the completion of the repair, there should be at most minimal tension along the bone–tendon suture line. Ideally there should be no tension evident at the repair site with the elbow at the patient's side. A massive cuff tear that results in very significant retraction of the muscle and tendon may require an abduction brace for 6 weeks to minimize tension on the repair while it heals. Abduction braces and pillows must be used with caution and recognition that at most they can temporarily relieve tension on the repair. The elbow must still reach the side at the time of cuff closure. If the cuff repair is possible only with the arm abducted and would retear if the elbow were brought to the side, an abduction brace is not appropriate. The brace cannot substitute for cuff tissue, it will tear again as soon as the brace or pillow is removed, even 6 weeks later.

The long head of the biceps tendon is examined at the time of surgery if the cuff tear anatomy permits. If it is frayed and involved in a tenosynovitic process, soft-tissue tenodesis or tenolysis is performed. Although tenolysis is certainly easy, it may leave a disturbing cosmetic deformity and should be discussed with the patient preoperatively. Soft-tissue tenodesis to the transverse humeral ligament or pectoralis insertion is a simple task and avoids the cosmetic event. In either case, there is no significant functional loss to the patient. Neither tenolysis nor tenodesis should be performed unless objective tendonopathy is present. Many investigators believe that the long head of the biceps serves an important role in glenohumeral superior stability, especially in the face of a massive cuff tear.

Technique

The patient is placed in a beach-chair position and the arm is draped to maintain a sterile field (Fig. 19-2). After prepping and draping, the surface anatomy is palpated. A skin marker may be used to outline the pertinent surface features including the clavicle, AC joint, coracoid, and anterior and posterior acromion (Fig. 19-3). The location of the skin incision is variable and depends on surgeon preference. I prefer to make a line from the tip of the coracoid process to a point 1 cm inferior to the midpoint of the lateral acromial length. Besides allowing the incision to be extended posterior, the incision lies in Langer lines and results in a very fine and subtle scar. Incision length is typically 8 to 10 cm (Fig. 19-4).

The incision is carried down to the investing fascia of the deltoid, which is tissue-paper–thin. A self-retaining retractor is placed to hold the skin edges widely open and skin flaps are developed superiorly and inferiorly (Fig. 19-5).

The superior skin flap is developed over the body of the AC joint and the distal skin flap is developed to expose approximately 5 cm of deltoid beginning at the deltoid origin from the anterolateral corner of the acromion (Fig. 19-6).

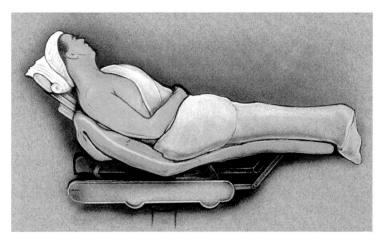

Figure 19-2. The patient is placed in a semi-seated position. This facilitates extension of the arm during mobilization of the superior and posterior cuff tissue.

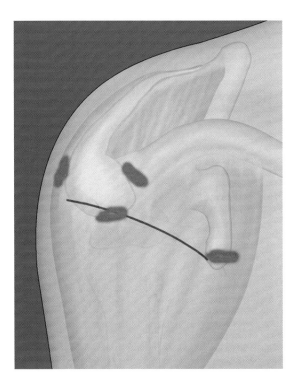

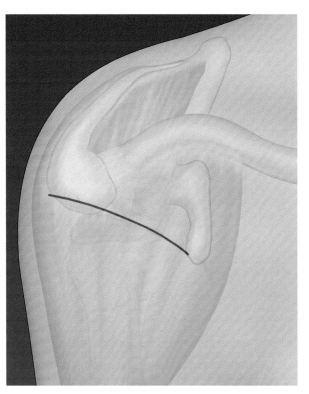

Figure 19-3. The red marks demonstrate the important surface anatomy landmarks. These include the coracoid process, the acromioclavicular joint, and the anterior and posterior corners of the acromion.

Figure 19-4. The skin incision is determined by drawing a line from the tip of the coracoid process to a point off the lateral edge of the acromion.

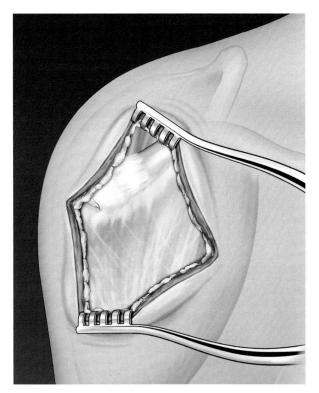

Figure 19-5. After making superior and inferior skin flaps, a self-retaining retractor is used to expose the underlying superficial deltoid fascia.

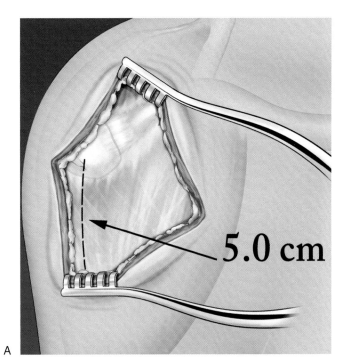

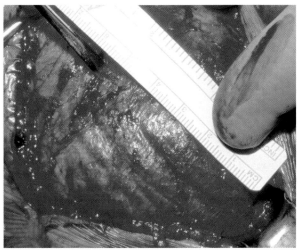

A

B

Figure 19-6. A,B: The deltoid is opened in a line parallel to its fiber orientation. This begins at the anterolateral corner of the acromion and extends not more than 5 cm.

The technique of deltoid opening requires careful planning. The anterior border of the clavicle is palpated, and a marker is used to establish a line across the anterior acromion at the same level as the anterior border of the clavicle. Most often, the acromion extends some distance anterior to the anterior border at the clavicle and represents ossification of the acromial attachment of the CA ligament. When biplanar osteotomy is performed, the anterior acromion will not extend anterior to the anterior border of the clavicle. With a marker, a line is drawn across the anterior border of the clavicle, across the acromion, and down the deltoid parallel with its muscle fibers (Fig. 19-7). A raphe is usually present and represents an anatomic division between the anterior and middle deltoid muscle fibers. Initially, blunt dissectors are used to separate the muscle fibers parallel to their orientation beginning at the anterolateral corner of the acromion and extending the muscle splitting incision inferiorly for about 4 cm (Fig. 19-8). A suture is placed 5 cm from the anterolateral corner of the acromion to prevent the muscle from splitting further and causing injury to branches of the axillary nerve. Over the superior acromion, a cautery needle is used rather than a scalpel because of increased vascularity (Fig. 19-9). The acromial branch of the thoracoacromial trunk lies along the anterior border of the CA ligament (Fig. 19-10). The deltoid muscle sleeve is maintained as one unit and dissected across the anterior acromion medially to the level of the AC joint. If an inferior claviculoplasty is anticipated, the dissection of the deltoid muscle sleeve should proceed medial to the AC joint. Care should be taken to keep the CA ligament on the deep surface of the deltoid so it can be repaired at the time of deltoid closure. When there is ossification of the CA ligament, the dissection should allow maximal preservation of the soft portion of the ligament. Previous techniques have recommended resection of the ligament but newer understanding of physiology and the potential for late superior instability suggests that this ligament is not vestigial and should be protected and repaired when feasible.

A Cobb-type elevator is used to free the undersurface of the acromion from the dense, adherent bursal tissue and periosteum. A blunt retractor is placed behind the posterior corner of the acromion to lever the humeral head inferiorly (Fig. 19-11). With the anterior acromion exposed, a biplanar acromial osteotomy is performed (Fig. 19-12). The surgeon controls the osteotome with both hands while the assistant maneuvers the mallet (Fig. 19-13). This diminishes the risk of potential acromial fracture. A power saw should be used

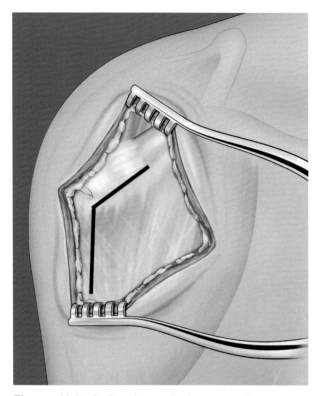

Figure 19-7. A line is marked across the anterior acromion in a line parallel to the anterior border of the clavicle.

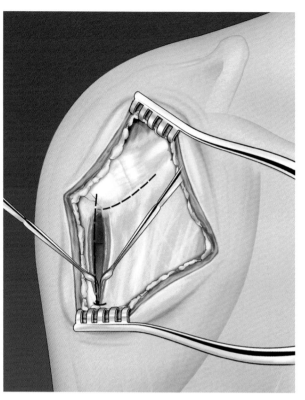

Figure 19-8. Blunt dissectors are used to open the deltoid muscle parallel to its fibers.

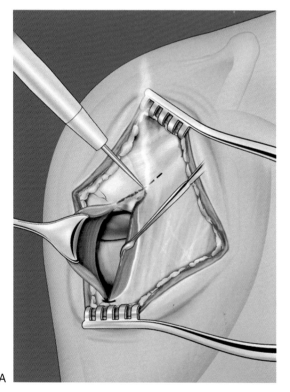

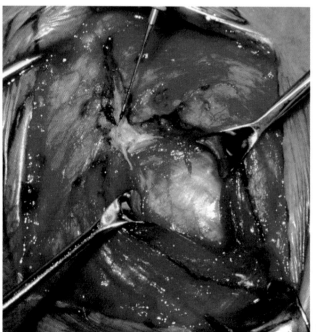

A

B

Figure 19-9. A,B: A needle-tip Bovie is used to remove the superior deltoid from the anterior acromion.

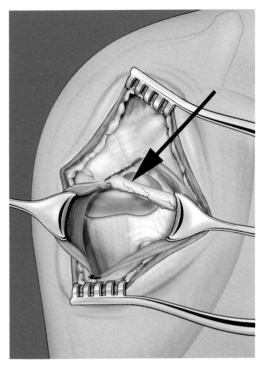

Figure 19-10. The acromial branch of the thoracoacromial trunk lies along the anterior border of the coracoacromial ligament. In the normal dissection, the ligament is kept attached to the deep surface of the deltoid so it can be reapproximated at the time of deltoid closure.

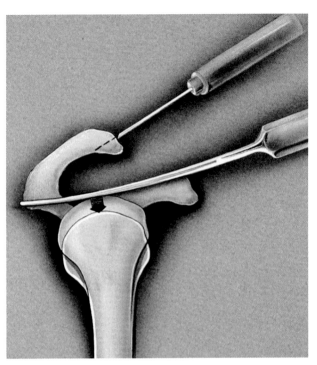

Figure 19-11. A blunt retractor is used to lever the humeral head inferiorly, which facilitates access to the anterior-inferior acromion.

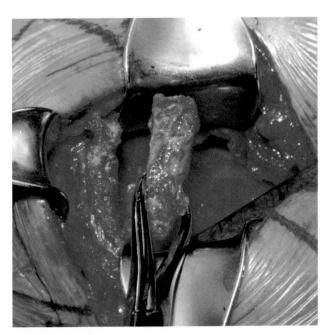

Figure 19-12. Only a small portion of the anterior acromion is removed. Care is taken not to fracture the body of the acromion.

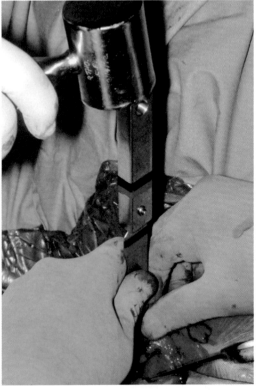

Figure 19-13. A two-handed technique, where the surgeon keeps two hands on the osteotome, provides maximal safety during the acromioplasty.

only with extreme care and with the knowledge that the potential for injury to the lateral deltoid origin is high. For the saw blade to cut the lateral edge of the bone, the "overtravel" of the blade injures the deltoid muscle origin. At the completion of the acromioplasty, the anterior portion of the acromion should not extend anterior to the anterior border of the clavicle. In addition, the undersurface of the acromion should not extend inferior to the clavicle at the AC joint. Only a small amount of cortical bone is removed with the osteotome, typically less than 1.0 cm from anterior to posterior. Most of the bone is removed with a small rasp as the undersurface of the acromion and clavicle are "sculpted" with the rasp (Fig. 19-14).

In the face of a massive cuff tear with supraspinatus retraction, an inferior claviculoplasty will allow improved exposure to the retracted tissue. It is imperative not to disrupt the deltoid muscle origin when removing the inferior clavicle.

A blunt finger is placed in the subacromial space and gentle but persuasive effort is used to free up the bursal adhesions (Fig. 19-15). These adhesions may be quite thick and tenacious but they must be methodically released and excised to permit mobilization of the cuff tissue. A combination of blunt and sharp dissection may be required. The tissue superiorly over the supraspinatus is particularly vascular and vigorous bleeding may be encountered. Anteriorly, the bursa becomes intimately involved with the deep fascia of the deltoid and must be sharply dissected taking care to protect deltoid muscle tissue. It has been my practice to remove as much bursa as possible. I have not done any bursal repairs and do not believe that they are an important aspect of rotator cuff surgery. It is much more important to be certain that bursa is not inadvertently incorporated into the cuff repair. Once the bursa has been thoroughly débrided, the rotator cuff status is fully ascertained.

Typically, the rotator cuff tear initiates at the impingement zone of the greater tuberosity at the point of supraspinatus insertion just posterior to the bicipital groove (Fig. 19-16). As the tear becomes larger, it generally extends posteriorly to involve the infraspinatus before it moves more anteriorly to involve the long head of the biceps and subscapularis tendon. However all combinations of muscle involvement have been documented.

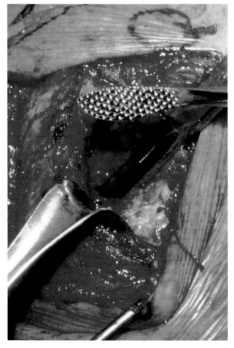

Figure 19-14. Once the osteotome has removed the inferior cortical bone, the inferior acromion is shaped and smoothed with a rasp.

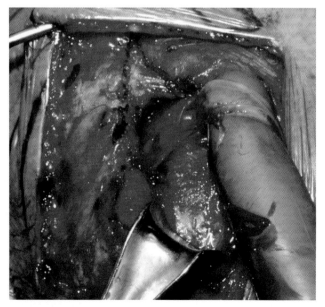

Figure 19-15. A finger is placed within the subacromial space and the adhesions are freed globally about the shoulder.

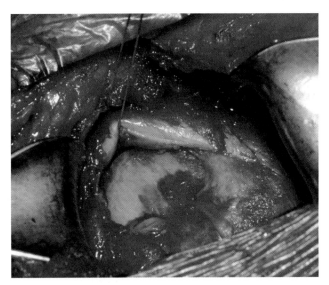

Figure 19-16. The classic rotator cuff tear begins at the greater tuberosity, just posterior to the bicipital groove.

There is much debate and little consensus regarding the definition of a massive cuff tear. Despite the lack of agreement, a body of experts defines a massive tear not by size, but by involvement of more than one tendon. Hence a tear of the supraspinatus with retraction of 4.0 cm may not be defined as massive if the pathology is isolated to a single muscle whereas a combined tear of the supraspinatus and infraspinatus with retraction of 1.5 cm would fit the definition of massive.

In the management of all rotator cuff tears, mobilization of the remaining muscle–tendon units is critical and time-consuming. The process of mobilization must be methodical, anatomic, and thorough. As the tissue is mobilized, sutures should be placed in the tendon edges to avoid the crushing that occurs with clamps. Furthermore, the suture provides a means of testing the tensile strength and quality of the mobilized tissue. If the suture pulls out of the tissue in the fashion of a "cheese-cutting wire," the surgeon knows the tissue quality may preclude a satisfactory repair. The individual muscle–tendon units are first mobilized on their outer bursal surface. Blunt dissectors are placed between the deltoid and cuff tissues posteriorly and superiorly to free adhesions that may be present medially. The bursal surface of the subscapularis must be mobilized with gentle finger dissection under direct vision because the musculocutaneous and axillary nerves lie on its anterior surface, not far from the joint surface.

Mobilization proceeds intraarticularly by passing a no. 15 scalpel blade around the outer aspect of the labrum posteriorly and superiorly. In these portions of the shoulder, the capsule, although adherent to the overlying cuff tissue, is thin and easily released. A Cobb elevator is placed in this interval and the cuff tendons are released from the neck of the glenoid. Great care must be taken not to migrate too medially near the scapular spine because the suprascapular nerve in the spinoglenoid notch is only 1.0 cm from the articular surface. Anteriorly, the capsule and subscapularis tendon are much more intimately related. They too must be separated intraarticularly to allow lateralization of the tendon. Even though the capsular ligaments have been transected, I have never seen a case of resultant clinical instability.

The anterior border of the supraspinatus and the superior border of the subscapularis can be adherent to the base of the coracoid process. With both sharp and blunt dissection, these two tendons must be released from the coracoid. The brachial plexus lies perilously close to the medial side of the coracoid and care must be taken to keep all instruments no more medial than the medial aspect of the bony coracoid.

The coracohumeral ligament is transected close to the base of the coracoid process. This ligament predictably contains a bleeder and hemostasis is easily maintained with simple cautery. As the tendon edges are sequentially mobilized, traction sutures are placed every several centimeters along the tendon edges (Fig. 19-17).

Occasionally the rotator cuff tear is so large that even with maximal soft-tissue mobilization, the tendon edges are not able to reach their anatomic insertion site. In this situation, the tendon edges may be attached to the humerus at a point somewhat medial and cephalad to their normal anatomic insertion sites (Fig. 19-18). In the worst-case situations, the insertion point has been made well into the articular surface with little resultant loss of active elevation. It is important to note that the tendon edges must be adjacent to the greater tuberosity or humeral insertion site with the elbow down by the side. As noted above, if the tendon edges can only reach the bone with the arm held in abduction, then use of an abduction brace or pillow will not result in satisfactory outcome. The brace can only be used to protect a repair, not substitute for a repair.

In massive rotator cuff tears, the long head of the biceps tendon is usually absent and, therefore, not available as a source of graft material. If the long head of the biceps is present but attenuated, a portion of the tendon may be used to reinforce the rotator cuff repair. If it is present and hypertrophied, it should be protected because it is likely involved in the physiologic activity of shoulder function at this time. It may be functioning as a humeral head depressor, and if this structure is sacrificed, a patient with a large cuff tear who did have some active elevation of the arm prior to surgery will be left with very poor elevation, if not complete loss of active use of that extremity.

Sometimes the tendons of a massive cuff tear can be thoroughly mobilized yet not mobilized enough to reach the greater tuberosity. It is then important to try to reestablish force vectors, although a watertight surgical repair may not be possible. Rarely the superior portion of the subscapularis can be transferred to a more superior position so it can better function as a dynamic stabilizer.

Once the tendon edges have been mobilized, they are sutured to the humerus itself. The tendon edges are advanced as much as possible toward their anatomic insertion point on the greater tuberosity with the elbow at the side. To keep the elbow at the side, the insertion point may have to be in the articular segment by as much as 1.0 cm. A rongeur or burr is used to decorticate the bone and to fashion a shallow trough of bleeding bone. The bony

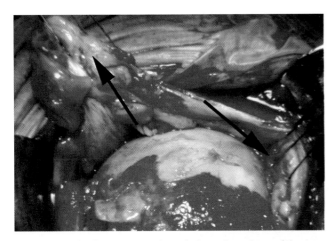

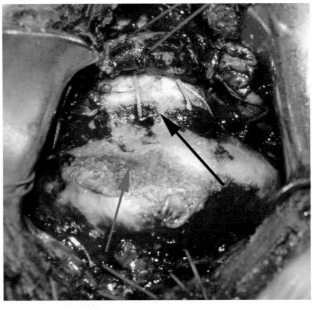

Figure 19-17. Sutures are placed along the edges of the torn tendon. They avoid the problem of crushing the tissue with clamps and provide some ability to determine the tensile strength of the tendon tissue.

Figure 19-18. When the tendon length does not permit repair at the greater tuberosity, the point of reattachment may be moved up to a centimeter into the articular segment as shown by the black arrow. The red arrow points to the anatomic insertion point.

trough is made to allow a vascular surface on the bone coapt against the cuff tendon edges (Fig. 19-19). Multiple holes are made along the trough and through the distal bone to create bone suture tunnels. There are a number of commercially available devices to create these bone tunnels. Except for the smallest tears where there is little retraction and little tension, I prefer not to use bone anchors and believe that bone tunnels provide superior fixation. The vast array of anchors certainly provide ease of use, however, the tendon repair does not permit the cuff edges to lie adjacent to the bone; only the deepest surface of the tendon heals to the bone surface. Furthermore, the extensive "anchor pull-out tests" have all been done on dead bone and never account for the tuberosity osteopenia, which is necessarily present *in vivo* in the presence of long-standing cuff tears. Nonabsorbable suture material of sufficient tensile strength is passed through the tendon using one of two techniques. When the tendon edge is thick, healthy, and robust, a horizontal mattress suture technique is used (Fig. 19-20). If the tendon edges are of poorer quality tissue, a modified Mason-Allen–type suture technique is preferred (Fig. 19-21). After thorough irrigation of the wound, the arm is held abducted while the sutures are tied. The central-most sutures should be tied first, working toward the periphery of the tear last. The arm is slowly brought back down to the side. If the elbow can reach the side but tension appears evident at the suture line, an abduction brace or pillow may be considered. If the elbow cannot be brought down, using a brace will not solve the problem; the repair should be advanced more cranially on the humerus.

A material, now approved by the Food and Drug Administration, is useful in the augmentation of a repair when tissue quality is marginal. Restore (DePuy, Warsaw, IN) is a porcine product, an orthobiologic tissue composed of pig small-intestine submucosa, which has been shown to be of value in the augmentation of poor cuff tissue. However, it is not a

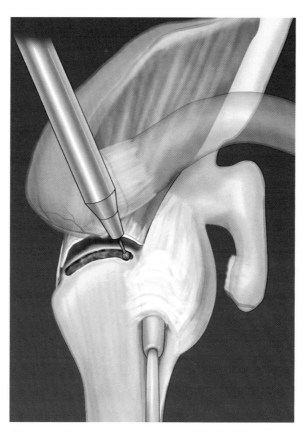

Figure 19-19. A bleeding trough is made in the bone at the point of tendon insertion.

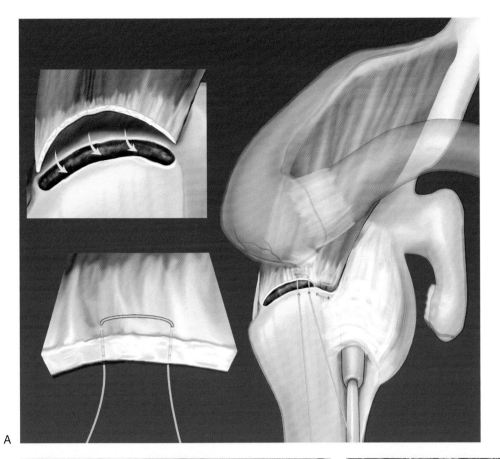

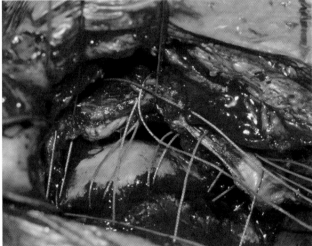

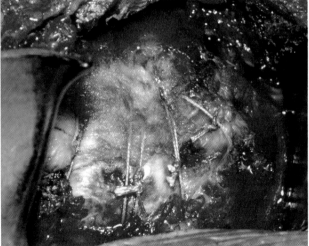

Figure 19-20. A–C: When the tendon to be repaired is thick and robust, a horizontal mattress suture technique is preferred.

substitute for cuff tendon. For a functional rotator cuff, there must be muscle activity; merely filling in the gap of a retracted and inactive muscle will not result in improved active use of the limb. It is of potentially great value in reconstructing massive rotator cuff tears where tissue is present but of poor tensile strength and quality.

If there is a hopelessly massive rotator cuff tear without any evidence of remaining cuff material, the technique that Rockwood has described consisting of joint débridement,

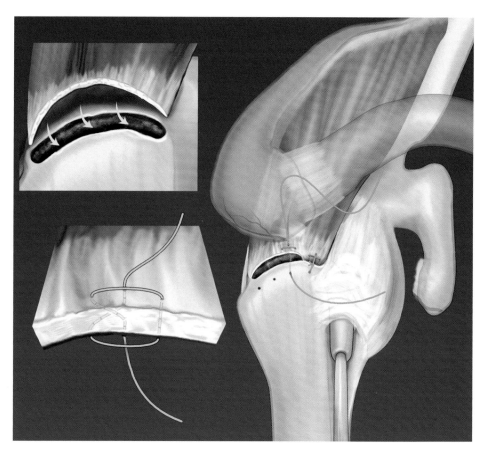

Figure 19-21. When the cuff tissue is of poor quality and of poor tensile strength, a Mason-Allen–type suture is preferred.

acromioplasty, and clean out of the rotator cuff has had very good success. Although functional improvement is minimal and functional deficits persist, shoulder débridement of irreparable massive cuff tears has provided rather significant relief of pain in a high percentage of patients.

At the completion of the cuff repair, the subacromial space is again thoroughly irrigated to remove all blood clot, bone, and soft-tissue debris. The deltoid repair is of critical importance for good functional outcome. The deltoid sleeve is repaired using figure-eight sutures, with the suture being placed through the bone of the acromion on the superior portion of the repair (Fig. 19-22). Usually the needle of the suture is strong enough to pass through the anterior acromion without a drill because the inferior cortex has been removed during the acromioplasty. The superior cortex is usually quite thin, hence the passage of the suture is done with ease. Once the anterior deltoid is securely fixed to the anterior acromion, the intramuscular deltoid split is repaired in a side-to-side fashion with sutures of choice (Fig. 19-23). The subcutaneous tissue is again irrigated to remove fat, blood clot, and debris. In 20 years of experience, I have never placed sutures in the subcutaneous tissue and find no need to do so. The skin is reapproximated using a running subcuticular absorbable suture (Fig. 19-24). Steri-Strips (3M Worldwide, St. Paul, MN) are applied followed by a sterile dressing of choice.

Prior to dressing application, the cognitive patient watches as the arm is placed through a full range of motion. The ability to witness range of motion of their shoulder while anesthetized results in patients having more accelerated progress in physical therapy than those patients who did not have such an opportunity.

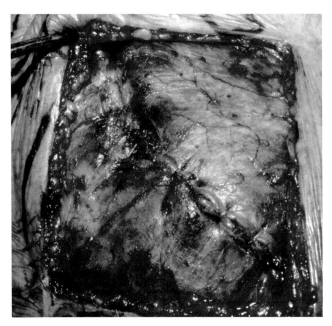

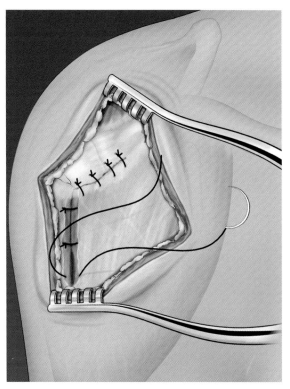

Figure 19-22. The deltoid repair is critical and requires transacromial repair of the deltoid origin.

Figure 19-23. The deltoid intramuscular split is repaired in a side-to-side fashion.

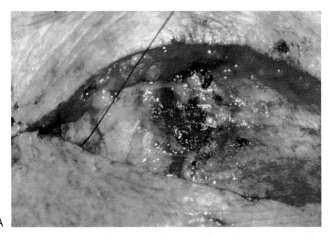

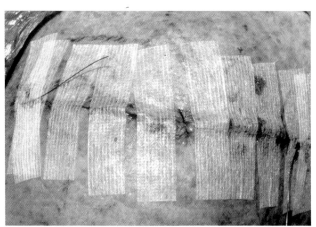

A

B

Figure 19-24. A,B: The skin is closed with a running subcuticular stitch followed by Steri-Strips (3M Worldwide, St. Paul, MN).

POSTOPERATIVE MANAGEMENT

The crux of postoperative management is protection of the repaired tendon and deltoid muscle. Adequate postoperative support such as a sling or abduction pillow or brace may be commonly used. Often, the choice of postoperative protection depends on the type of patient, the adequacy of the soft tissue, the tension on the tendon and sutures, the quality of the deltoid repair, whether an associated procedure to fix an unfused acromial epiphysis was performed, whether the procedure was a revision, or even individual patient preference. While a postoperative sling is more convenient and comfortable than an abduction brace, the surgeon should decide the safest way to protect the repair at the time of cuff repair. The value of preoperative discussion with the patient cannot be overemphasized. Explicit instructions are given to patient and caregiver before the procedure. The patient must demonstrate an understanding of the difference between active and passive motion before undergoing cuff repair. Patients rarely, if ever, become more compliant after a procedure than they were before the surgery. Having repaired hundreds of large cuff tears in the last 20 years, fewer than 10 ever wore an abduction pillow or brace, and even fewer wore slings after the first postoperative day.

Whatever the postoperative immobilization, the rehabilitation commences immediately following the surgery, if not the same day, then certainly within the first 24 hours. Early passive motion to prevent adhesions and postoperative stiffness must be balanced by the need to protect the surgical repair. It really amounts to the patient comprehending the fact that only strict passive motion is allowed, in fact encouraged. Prolonged immobilization without early range of motion exercises often leads to a stiff and painful arm. Active range of motion or passive motion outside the limits of the repair (usually external rotation) has the potential to disrupt the repair. Again, patient education and demonstration of the exercises and limits by the surgeon is a critical concept to maximize benefit and minimize risk of surgical failure. A therapy prescription on a piece of paper to a therapist is really a prescription for failure. There are no routines in the postoperative management of rotator cuff repairs.

Within 24 hours, the physical therapist begins supine passive forward elevation and supine passive external rotation of the arm. The patient and caregiver are instructed in the technique before surgery so the program is somewhat easier to accomplish after the procedure. Exercises of this type are performed two or three times daily for a brief time, typically no longer than 4 to 5 minutes per session. Analgesics and heat application are recommended one half hour before the anticipated exercise session. Forward-bending pendulum exercises (Codman) in the shower are also encouraged before the more formal exercise session. Once the skin suture is removed at 10 to 14 days, the passive internal rotation stretching exercises commence. The use of a pulley has been a tortuous one for me. After several patients had their pulley collapse during their exercise, I have not encouraged its use until the cuff has healed, usually 12 weeks for a massive tear. Furthermore, maintaining strict passivity of the surgical arm is most difficult in using a pulley. There is the inevitable eccentric loading of the cuff and deltoid during the descent phase, which certainly places the repairs of both muscles at risk. Each surgeon must feel comfortable with his or her choice of postoperative protocols as there is clearly no correct "one." The concepts of early passive motion and active motion later should provide the framework for individual choice.

Active exercises are not permitted until the tendon repair is safely healed. It should be remembered that the surgical approach does not shorten or alter the time it takes for the tendon to heal to the bone. Arthroscopic repairs do not heal faster than open repairs and time to actively use the arm is not to be shortened just because a certain technique was used. Light active use of the arm is usually permitted at 12 weeks after surgery when isometric exercises for internal and external rotation and for the deltoid are also begun. Resistive exercises such as the use of Theraband and even light weights are not permitted for at least 3 months postoperatively and may even be delayed for 4 months, depending on the size of the tear and quality of the repair. When a satisfactory range of motion has been achieved and the early strengthening exercises have begun, the patient begins to use the arm more actively. Active use of the arm should preclude sudden deceleration or sudden impact type activities, such as manually starting a lawnmower. In the case of some massive tears, the cuff muscles are so atrophic that even 3 months after surgery, the patient is unable to raise his or her arm against gravity. Patients should be examined to determine if they elevate their arm while supine. Because of the shortened lever arm and diminished effect of gravity, most patients can actively elevate to the limits of their passive motion while supine. In this case, supine active exercises should be performed by having the patient elevate the arm in sets of ten twice daily. When the patient can do so comfortably with no weight in the hand, incremental weights of no more than 0.5 lb should be placed in the hand. This technique allows very gradual strengthening of the cuff and deltoid and recognizes the fact that even the lightest arm probably weighs close to 10 lb. Nearly always, when a patient can lift 8 to 10 lb with the operative arm while supine, upon standing, with no weight in the hand, the arm is easily actively lifted over the head. At this point, the patient begins the routine Theraband and free-weight–strengthening program.

RESULTS

Most reports of the surgical results of massive rotator cuff tears emphasize that pain relief is usually excellent. The patient often experiences three types of postoperative pain. In the early period, there is a soreness from the surgical dissection. As physical therapy is initiated, there is often a sense of tightness or pain as the exercises are performed. Later, when the patient is asked to participate in an active exercise program to rebuild muscle power, there is often an aching that occurs in the muscle being strengthened. Thus, pain in the postoperative period is common and should not frighten the patient or therapist. However, the patient often describes the pain with therapy during the postoperative period as being very different from the preoperative tendon-tear pain. This can be used as a source of encouragement for the patient that the surgical repair has solved the original problem and the new pain is normal during the recovery period. Ultimately, the patient should expect either complete or near-complete pain relief, although there may be weather ache following surgery and there may be a mild ache with overzealous or strenuous use of the arm.

Unfortunately, the return of strength and active use of the arm is much less predictable. Often the patient expects, as the exercise program is begun, to be able to raise the arm above shoulder level, and there is frustration by the tremendous weakness in the arm as the months of rehabilitation progress. The patient should be told that the return to strength depends on the size of the tear, the quality of the soft tissue, whether the repair holds up over time, whether the deltoid muscle is also weak, and whether the recommended rehabilitation program is being followed. It is often 9 months to a year before the arm gets as strong as it is going to be after repair of a massive tear. Ultimately, the patient can expect good use of the arm below shoulder level for rotation inward and outward. Use of the arm above shoulder level is highly variable and ranges from full active use of the arm above shoulder level to an arm that can be used but fatigues easily above shoulder level. In addition, some patients may never reach the ability to use the arm above the level of their shoulder and they should be made aware of that possibility before the surgery. Careful preoperative discussion with patients about realistic expectations of what can and cannot be controlled with repair of massive cuff tears will minimize patient frustration and early expectations following surgery.

The physician's expectations should be much the same as the patient's expectations. It is important to communicate with the physical therapist, who may also be frustrated by the slow progress in muscle strength. The physician should expect that the rehabilitation will be lengthy, that the gains in active motion are unpredictable but should continue over several months to years, and that the relief of pain should be very predictable.

COMPLICATIONS

The most common complications of rotator cuff surgery include the following:

Failure of Repair. Often, surgical failure of the cuff repair is preventable. It can be minimized by achieving maximal mobilization of the cuff tendons, using nonabsorbable sutures through adequate bone tunnels, using suture techniques that account for tissue quality, using nonabsorbable sutures, and repairing the tissue with the elbow at the side under minimal tension. Preventing failure of the repair also depends on a compliant patient who has been given the opportunity to demonstrate the difference between active and passive motion prior to surgery. Certainly, inappropriate early active use of the limb will most certainly result in early disruption. The most common patient contributions to surgical failure are use of weights or other resistive exercises too early, or removing the brace or abduction pillow before being instructed by the physician. There are other medical conditions that are likely associated with surgical failure, such as uncontrollable Parkinson disease, muscle spasms, and other neurologic diseases. Systemic oral steroids for rheumatologic diseases and organ transplant protection adversely affect cross-linking of the collagen fibril and result in poor tensile qualities, leading to high risk of failure.

Glenohumeral Instability. Occasionally the patient who had a massive rotator cuff tear will come to the office complaining of uncontrollable anterosuperior glenohumeral instability as the arm attempts to be elevated. This probably results from the disabling combination of cuff retear, incompetent CA ligament, and extensive mobilization of capsular ligaments. Repair of the CA arch in all patients with cuff surgery cannot be overemphasized. Fortunately, this instability is often painless, although frustrating to the patient. There is no satisfactory treatment for this condition. Despite surgeons' attempts to reconstruct the CA arch with soft-tissue grafts and bone grafts, results have been universally disappointing.

Deltoid Avulsion. The combination of massive tear of the rotator cuff and late deltoid avulsion or failure can be disastrous. This complication is preventable. Intraoperatively, if the deltoid is detached, it must be securely reattached to the bony acromion with nonabsorbable sutures. Care must be taken to only remove the anterior deltoid, as the middle deltoid is often very muscular in its origin and may be very difficult reattach. When the AC joint is clinically symptomatic, only an undersurface claviculoplasty, which protects and preserves the deltoid origin, should be considered. In the presence of massive cuff tears, there are few indications for a Mumford-type lateral clavicular resection. The risk to the deltoid is too great and patients achieve the same level of pain relief with an inferior claviculoplasty. If the deltoid does avulse in the postoperative period, often it will not be painful but attention to its early repair may make the difference in the ultimate ability of the patient to elevate the arm. I have seen many patients with massive cuff tears lift their arm if they have a functioning deltoid, but I have never seen a patient lift his or her arm with a normal cuff and an absent deltoid.

Inadequate Acromioplasty. An anterior acromioplasty is thought by most surgeons to be a critical adjunct to rotator cuff repair for control of pain and prevention of further tearing. If the anterior acromioplasty does not extend completely from the most anteromedial to anterolateral portion of the acromion, residual acromial overhang or spurring can contribute to continued extrinsic impingement and surgical failure of the tendon repair. In addition, overly generous acromioplasty, with excision of the lateral acromion, or more than the anterior underside of the acromion, can make deltoid repair impossible and can permanently weaken the shoulder. There is very little surgical salvage of a radical acromionectomy. The best way to avoid this problem is to make certain that only the anteroinferior surface of acromion is removed at the time of surgery. As discussed previously, use of a two-handed technique and a flexible, thin osteotome provides a great margin of safety during this step of the procedure.

Continued Acromioclavicular Joint Pain. AC arthritis is a frequent companion to massive rotator cuff tears. Failure to recognize this joint as contributory to the pain complex of cuff disease can result in continued pain following cuff repair and lead to an overall surgical failure. The AC joint must be carefully evaluated preoperatively; if there are clinical signs of tenderness with palpation, pain with cross-chest adduction, and pain with reaching the opposite axilla, inferior claviculoplasty should be part of the cuff repair surgical procedure. Conversely, the MRI seems to document AC joint pathology in nearly every scan; do not excise the AC joint merely because there are changes on the MRI. Clinical correlation is necessary in this pathologic environment.

Postoperative Stiffness. Postoperative stiffness usually results from failure to initiate passive range of motion within safe ranges in the early postoperative period. At the time of cuff repair, the surgeon, while observing the repair, should place the shoulder through a range of motion to determine the safe limits. Most commonly, the limiting motion is external rotation, especially in the face of a massive cuff tear and repair. By using long-acting anesthetic agents, the physician can show the patient the limits on the motion while the patient remains free from pain. These limits to motion must also be conveyed to the therapist or care provider. This initiation of early passive motion will minimize the chance of stiffness. If a stiff shoulder presents postoperatively, efforts should be redoubled at restoring passive motion by a combination of passive and assistive exercises. Manipulation under anesthesia should be avoided because this may disrupt the surgical repair.

RECOMMENDED READING

1. Cofield, R.H., Parvizi, J., Hoffmeyer, P.J., et al.: Surgical repair of chronic rotator cuff tears: a prospective long term study. *J Bone Joint Surg* 83A: 71–77, 2001.
2. Davidson, P.A., Rivenburgh, D.W.: Rotator cuff repair tension as a determinant of functional outcome. *J Shoulder Elbow Surg* 9: 502–506, 2000.
3. Dejardin, L.M., Arnoczky, S.P., Ewers, B.J., et al.: Tissue-engineered rotator cuff tendon using porcine small intestine submucosa: histologic and mechanical evaluation in dogs. *Am J Sports Med* 29: 175–184, 2001.
4. Gartsman, G.M.: Massive, irreparable tears of the rotator cuff: results of operative debridement and subacromial decompression. *J Bone Joint Surg Am* 79: 715–721, 1997.
5. Gartsman, G.M., Brinker, M.R., Khan, M.: Early effectiveness of arthroscopic repair for full-thickness tears of the rotator cuff: an outcome analysis. *J Bone Joint Surg Am* 80: 33—40, 1998.
6. Gerber, C., Schneeberger A.G., Perren, S.M., et al.: Experimental rotator cuff repair: a preliminary study. *J Bone Joint Surg Am* 81: 1281–1290, 1999.
7. Gill, T.J., McIrvin, E., Mair, S.D., et al.: Results of biceps tenotomy for treatment of pathology of the long head of the biceps brachii. *J Shoulder Elbow Surg* 10: 247–249, 2001.
8. Hollinshead, R.M., Mohtadi, N.G., Vande Guchte, R.A., et al.: Two 6-year follow up studies of large and massive rotator cuff tears: comparison of outcome measures. *J Shoulder Elbow Surg* 9: 373–381, 2000.
9. Iannotti, J.P.: Full-thickness rotator cuff tears: factors affecting surgical outcome. *J Am Acad Orth Surg* 2: 87–95, 1994.
10. Karas, S.E., Gianchello, T.L.: Subscapularis transfer for reconstruction of massive tears of the rotator cuff. *J Bone Joint Surg Am* 78: 239–245, 1996.
11. Norwood, L.A., Barrack, R., Jacobson, K.E.: Clinical presentation of complete tears of the rotator cuff. *J Bone Joint Surg Am* 71: 499–505, 1989.
12. Rokito, A.S., Cuomo, F., Gallagher, M.A., et al.: Long-term functional outcome of repair of large and massive chronic tears of the rotator cuff. *J Bone Joint Surg Am* 81: 991–997, 1999.
13. Worland, R.L., Arredondo, J., Angles, F., et al.: Repair of massive rotator cuff tears in patients older than 70 years. *J Shoulder Elbow Surg* 8: 26–30, 1999.

20

Latissimus Dorsi Transfers in Rotator Cuff Reconstruction

Thomas F. Holovacs, Norman Espinosa, and Christian Gerber

INDICATIONS/CONTRAINDICATIONS

While there is no universally accepted definition of a "massive rotator cuff tear," we refer to this term if the tear involves disinsertion of no less than two complete tendons (4,11). This is a more anatomic definition than documenting the dimensions of a defect. It should be understood, however, that not only the size of the tendon defect but also the quality of the musculotendinous tissue is an important variable for reparability

Three distinct patterns of massive rotator cuff tears are recognized: posterosuperior, anterosuperior, and global configurations. Posterosuperior rotator cuff tears are the most common type and involve the supraspinatus and infraspinatus (and frequently, the teres minor) tendons.

Although most rotator cuff tears can be repaired successfully, the overall size of the musculotendinous defect, fatty infiltration of the rotator cuff muscles, static superior subluxation of the humeral head, and poor quality tendon/bone may prevent successful repair. In such cases, alternative reconstructive surgical techniques are considered (6).

Historically, the management of irreparable massive rotator cuff tears encompasses a wide range of surgical solutions including: open/arthroscopic débridement, local tendon transposition (upper subscapularis, teres minor, teres major), extrinsic tendon transfer (trapezius), tendon autografts and allografts, synthetic graft material, and deltoid flap reconstruction.

Latissimus dorsi tendon transfer, as described in 1988 by Gerber et al. (6), is our preferred method for the management of the pain and functional deficit caused by irreparable,

T. F. Holovacs, M.D.: Department of Orthopaedic Surgery, Harvard University Medical School; and Harvard Shoulder Service, Massachusetts General Hospital, Boston, Massachusetts.

N. Espinosa, M.D.: Department of Orthopaedic Surgery, University of Zurich, Balgrist University Hospital, Zurich, Switzerland.

C. Gerber, M.D.: Department of Orthopaedics, University of Zurich, and Balgrist University Hospital, Zurich, Switzerland.

massive, posterosuperior rotator cuff tears in individuals with high functional demands. By replacing an irrecoverable musculotendinous cuff unit with healthy extrinsic substitute, this technique alleviates pain and improves function by restoring active external rotation to the glenohumeral joint (1,3,5,6,9).

Indications

The main indication for latissimus dorsi tendon transfer is an irreparable, massive, posterosuperior rotator cuff tear in a patient with intolerable shoulder pain and subjectively unacceptable dysfunction (1,3,5,6,9). Most important is the potential to restore functional active external rotation.

Prior to surgical intervention, it is possible to predict those patients in whom direct, primary repair of a rotator cuff tear is likely to fail (10). Profound weakness of external rotation (both in abduction and adduction), external rotation "lag sign" of more than 30 degrees, superior migration of the humeral head with acromiohumeral distance less than 7 mm, long duration of tendon tear, and computed tomography (CT) or magnetic resonance imaging (MRI) evidence of grade 2 (or worse) fatty replacement of the rotator cuff muscles are all harbingers of unsuccessful rotator cuff repair. This constellation of findings, however, in a patient with shoulder pain and dysfunction highlights the precise indications for latissimus dorsi transfer.

A positive external rotation lag sign provides valuable insight into the specific anatomic areas of the rotator cuff tear. A patient with active external rotation lag with the arm at the side has a massive rotator cuff tear involving the supraspinatus and infraspinatus tendons. Active external rotation lag in abduction signifies extension of the tear into the teres minor. This loss of external rotation can successfully be addressed with latissimus dorsi transfer.

While combined loss of active external rotation and elevation may be an indication for latissimus transfer in a young, active patient, isolated loss of elevation cannot consistently be recovered.

Patients with static superior subluxation of the humeral head with an acromiohumeral distance of less than 7 mm fare just as well after latissimus transfer as those without superior humeral head subluxation.

The optimal indication for this procedure is a patient with a painful shoulder, preserved anterior elevation, and negative "lift-off" sign but with positive "external rotation lag" and "horn-blower" signs.

Contraindications

The mere presence of a massive rotator cuff tear does not necessarily indicate the need for rotator cuff reconstruction with latissimus dorsi transfer. Some patients with massive cuff tears experience minimal pain and maintain good overall shoulder function. Reconstructive surgery in such patients is unnecessary.

Patients with anterosuperior rotator cuff tears, which involve the subscapularis such that the lift-off test is positive, are not good candidates for latissimus dorsi transfers (3,5,6).

Prior failed attempts at primary rotator cuff repair are not necessarily contraindications to subsequent latissimus transfers but as documented by Warner and Parsons (12), salvage reconstruction of failed prior rotator cuff repairs yields more limited gains in satisfaction and function than primary latissimus dorsi transfers. Other relative contraindications include deltoid dysfunction and shoulder stiffness (3,5,6,10,12).

PREOPERATIVE PLANNING

History

The history and physical examination are the diagnostic cornerstones of the massive, irreparable, posterosuperior rotator cuff tear.

Clues to the size of the tendon(s) tear and the quality of the tendon tissue can be expected from the history given by the patient (10). Atraumatic and insidious onset of pain and loss of function over the course of months or years suggest poor tendon quality as well as atrophy and fatty infiltration of the supraspinatus and infraspinatus muscle bellies.

Often the chief complaint is fatigue, especially when using the arm with the shoulder abducted. A frequent scenario is problems when dining because the patient cannot maintain external rotation with the arm at the side. Inability to maintain external rotation forces the patient to compensate by abducting the shoulder, which in turn, encroaches on the adjacent person at the table.

Physical Examination

We begin the physical examination of the shoulder with inspection of the ipsilateral and contralateral shoulders for signs of prior trauma/surgery, atrophy, and deformity. Deformity consistent with static anterosuperior subluxation is an indicator of anterosuperior rotator cuff tear, a contraindication for latissimus dorsi transfer. Furthermore, deltoid defects should be examined closely and interpreted correctly, because they may constitute contraindications for this procedure. Atrophy of the spinati musculature is often readily apparent in patients with long-standing massive rotator cuff tears but is more commonly an indicator that rotator cuff repair is not possible. Spinati atrophy does not constitute a contraindication for latissimus transfer.

Next, we passively assess and document range of motion in elevation, abduction, and internal and external rotation. In our experience, the shoulder must be passively supple for latissimus transfer to be successful. Conversely, loss of passive range of motion constitutes a contraindication for this procedure. The only exception is diminished internal rotation of three to four vertebral levels compared with that of the contralateral side. Internal rotation loss of such a minor degree should not affect successful outcome.

Next, active range of motion is assessed using a goniometer with the patient seated. We document active elevation in the scapular plane and abduction and internal and external rotation at the side and in abduction. Loss of active elevation over 90 degrees is a contraindication to latissimus transfer if it is clearly associated with anterosuperior dynamic subluxation of the humeral head.

A critical physical examination finding is discrepancy between passive and active motion arcs. The external rotation lag sign is highly suggestive of a massive rotator cuff tear with grade 3 fatty infiltration of the infraspinatus. Such a rotator cuff tear is irreparable and amenable to latissimus dorsi transfer. Note that in the presence of subscapularis insufficiency (i.e., positive lift-off test), external rotation lag sign may, in fact be due to testing the shoulder in hyper-external rotation and not because of infraspinatus weakness. In such a situation with subscapularis insufficiency, latissimus dorsi transfer is contraindicated.

Several physical examination findings are specific for massive, posterosuperior rotator cuff tears. In addition to the previously described external rotation lag sign, the horn-blower sign is pathognomonic for a massive rotator cuff tear involving the supraspinatus, infraspinatus, and teres minor (3,6).

After full documentation of active and passive range of motion, formally assess rotator cuff strength. Whereas for purely clinical purposes, manual muscle testing may be acceptable, instrumented strength measurement is mandatory for scientific purposes. Strength in abduction, "empty can" elevation, and internal and external rotation with the arm in adduction and abduction are documented. The lift-off and "belly press" tests for subscapularis competence should be performed. The lift-off must be negative or exhibit only a trace amount of internal rotation lag to consider latissimus dorsi transfer. If passive internal rotation is limited, the belly press test should be used to assess subscapularis function.

Pain can interfere with the accurate assessment of range of motion and strength testing. Specifically, if the patient cannot elevate the arm above the head and it is unclear whether this is due to pain or a structurally based functional compromise, we perform a subacromial impingement test by injecting 15 mL of 1% lidocaine into the subacromial space prior to examining the patient. This intervention will alleviate pain and identify whether the patient is able to actively elevate the arm or at least to maintain the arm above the head if it is lifted into this position.

Imaging Studies

Imaging studies provide important information in the diagnosis and appropriate management of irreparable, massive posterosuperior rotator cuff tears. Our standard plain radiography protocol includes a true anteroposterior (AP) of the shoulder, an axillary view, and supraspinatus outlet views (11).

In the context of massive rotator cuff tears, the true AP of the shoulder is best to demonstrate superior migration of the humeral head and to measure the acromiohumeral distance (ACHD). The normal ACHD averages 10.5 mm. Patients with rotator cuff tears have an average ACHD of 8.2 mm. A value of 7 mm or less suggests an irreparable tear of the infraspinatus and is a strong indicator to consider a latissimus dorsi transfer rather than repair if the clinical findings are compatible with such a procedure.

The axillary radiograph is obtained specifically to demonstrate the presence of an os acromiale, which is more prevalent in the rotator cuff tear population.

As described previously, muscle quality is at least as important as cuff defect size when deciding between an attempt at primary rotator cuff repair or latissimus dorsi transfer. In this context, CT scanning has proven to be an invaluable tool (7). More recently, CT has been gradually superseded by MRI, which in our institution is currently the standard for assessment of muscle quality (2). We perform MRI scans on all patients clinically suspected of having a massive rotator cuff tear. The benefit of MRI is not in the diagnosis of the tear itself but rather, in providing critical information about the degree of muscle atrophy and fatty infiltration in the supraspinatus and infraspinatus muscle bellies. Because several authors have demonstrated that chronic muscle infiltration does not recover after surgical repair, advanced fatty infiltration constitutes an important hallmark for irreparability (5). We document the degree of fatty replacement according to the grading system proposed by Goutallier et al.. (7) and adapted for MRI by Fuchs et al. (2). For our purposes, the oblique sagittal images are the most useful in this regard. We indicate on the MRI requisition the specific reason for obtaining the study (i.e., evaluation of rotator cuff muscle quality) and insist that the imaging sequences include the entire scapula up to its medial border.

SURGERY

Anesthesia/Analgesia Management

Complete intraoperative and perioperative analgesia/anesthesia is critical to the overall success of latissimus dorsi transfers for massive, posterosuperior rotator cuff tears. Because there are two operative fields that are extensive in overall size, general endotracheal anesthesia is required. However, to provide postoperative relief of pain, an anesthesiologist familiar with regional anesthesia, specifically interscalene block and catheterization, evaluates all of our patients preoperatively.

Preoperatively, the anesthesiologist prepares for an interscalene block by placing an indwelling interscalene catheter using electrostimulation technique. During the operative procedure, however, general endotracheal anesthesia is used. Postoperatively, careful neurologic examination of the upper extremity is performed. If the patient's neurologic examination is normal, the interscalene block is activated in order to provide optimal postoperative pain control.

Patient Positioning and Draping

We perform latissimus dorsi transfer for reconstruction of massive, posterosuperior rotator cuff tears in the lateral decubitus position with the trunk elevated into a slight beach-chair

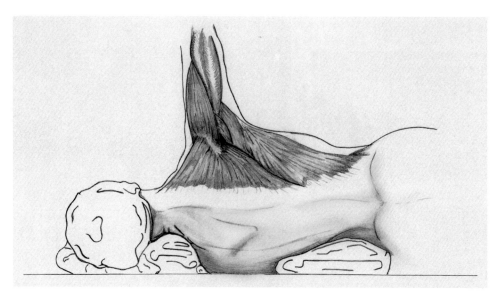

Figure 20-1. Lateral decubitus position. (Copyright Christian Gerber, M.D., University of Zurich.)

position (Fig. 20-1). The patient is positioned as far laterally on the operating table as possible to facilitate optimal positioning for the surgeon. A full-length beanbag is used to support the entire body. An axillary roll is placed beneath the contralateral side and all bony prominences are padded. We mold/contour the full-length beanbag so that it cradles the entire torso in a stable position, ensuring that the beanbag does not encroach on the posterior surgical field.

This procedure requires two separate surgical approaches, anterosuperior and posteroinferior. Therefore, we prepare the entire upper extremity and hemi-torso in a sterile fashion such that the ipsilateral neck, back, chest, and upper extremity will be in the operative field after draping.

The surgeon and the first assistant stand behind the patient during the procedure. Across the operative field, the second assistant stands in front of the patient and maintains the position of the arm and shoulder during the procedure.

Antibiotic prophylaxis with 2 g of Kefazolin is administered intravenously during draping.

Technique

After prepping and draping, the arm is placed at the side and the bony landmarks of the shoulder are palpated and outlined, including; the acromion, acromioclavicular joint, clavicle, and coracoid process. Next, the desired lines of incision for both the rotator cuff exposure and the latissimus dorsi harvest are marked. For the anterosuperior exposure, we draw a straight line over the lateral one third of the acromion parallel to Langer lines. It begins at the posterolateral edge of the acromion and extends anteriorly to 2 to 3 cm lateral to the coracoid process (Fig. 20-2). For the posteroinferior exposure, we draw a line following the anterior border of the latissimus dorsi (or the posterior axillary fold), which curves anteriorly to the anterior inner third of the humerus about 4 cm proximal to the axillary fold (Fig. 20-3). Prior to incising the skin, we use impermeable, bacteriocide-impregnated drapes to cover all exposed skin.

Anterosuperior Exposure. With a no. 10 scalpel blade, the skin is incised over the lateral third of the acromion parallel to Langer lines. Using sharp dissection technique, the skin flaps are elevated around the incision in all directions, just superficial to the deltoid fascia. The skin flaps are retracted medially and laterally with 2-0 nylon sutures (Fig. 20-4).

We split the deltoid muscle in line with its fibers between the anterior and middle del-

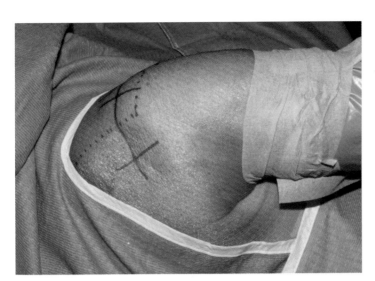

Figure 20-2. Anterosuperior exposure. Line of incision is parallel to Langer lines over the lateral one third of the acromion beginning at the posterolateral edge of the acromion and extending anteriorly to 2 to 3 cm lateral to the coracoid process. (Copyright Christian Gerber, M.D., University of Zurich.)

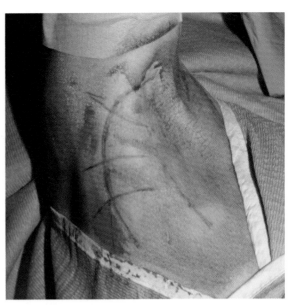

Figure 20-3. Posteroinferior exposure. The line of incision follows the anterior border of the latissimus dorsi and curves anteriorly 4 cm proximal to the axillary fold ending at the inner third of the humerus. (Copyright Christian Gerber, M.D., University of Zurich.)

toid for a distance of 5 cm. With a sharp, straight ½-in. osteotome, the middle deltoid is elevated by removing a thin (1 mm) wafer of bone off the superolateral acromion (Fig. 20-5). An anterior acromioplasty is not routinely performed. If a large spur clearly encroaches on the cuff, this spur is trimmed using a rongeur. In all cases, we preserve the anterior deltoid and the coracoacromial arch.

Using no. 3 Ethibond (Ethicon, Inc., Somerville, NJ), three to four traction sutures are placed through the deltoid muscle and around the shaved wafer of lateral acromion. Gently

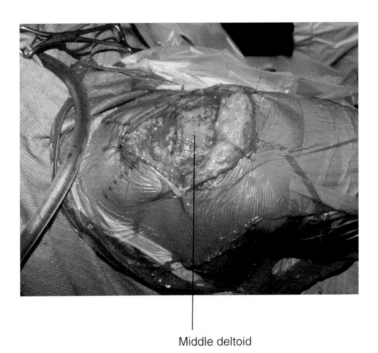

Middle deltoid

Figure 20-4. Deltoid exposure with skin flaps retracted. (Copyright Christian Gerber, M.D., University of Zurich.)

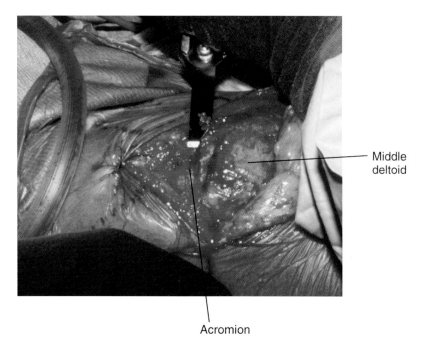

Middle
deltoid

Acromion

Figure 20-5. Middle deltoid detachment. Sharp, straight ½-in. osteotome is used to elevate the middle deltoid by removing a thin (1 mm) wafer of bone from superolateral acromion. (Copyright Christian Gerber, M.D., University of Zurich.)

pulling on these traction sutures allows more complete visualization of the underlying subacromial bursa, retracted rotator cuff, and proximal humerus (Fig. 20-6). Furthermore, these sutures will be the definitive transosseous fixation for deltoid repair at the conclusion of the procedure. We resect the subacromial bursa and identify the edges of the rotator cuff.

Placing a subacromial spreader facilitates visualization of the subacromial space and rotator cuff. Gently grasping the tendon edge with forceps and using a combination of Metzenbaum scissors and long-handled no. 15 scalpel, the retracted rotator cuff tendons are mobilized by releasing the coracohumeral ligament, extraarticular adhesions above the rotator cuff, and intraarticular release in the plane between the superior labrum and the inferior surface of the cuff. When performing the extraarticular lysis of adhesions, we avoid iatrogenic damage to the suprascapular nerve by not releasing more than 1.8 cm medial to the glenoid. If still in place, the tendon of the long biceps is routinely released from its insertion at the supraglenoid tubercle and tenodesed in the bicipital groove

Next, we place three to four no. 3 Ethibond sutures in a modified Mason-Allen configuration into the lateral edge of the rotator cuff from anterior to posterior. These sutures can be used as "traction sutures" to assist in rotator cuff mobilization. Furthermore, they will be the definitive fixation for the cuff after latissimus dorsi harvest.

The greater tuberosity is prepared by abrading its surface with a rongeur. We place a saline-moistened gauze pad into the wound and proceed with latissimus dorsi tendon harvest.

Posteroinferior Exposure. With the second assistant holding the arm in a position of 90 degrees of abduction and internal rotation, the skin is incised with a no. 10 scalpel blade along the previously drawn line (Fig. 20-7). Using sharp dissection, the skin flaps are elevated around the incision in all directions, just superficial to the fascia. The skin flaps are retracted with 2-0 nylon sutures.

The posterior deltoid, long head of the triceps, teres major, and latissimus dorsi muscles are identified (Fig. 20-8). We dissect the anterior border of the latissimus dorsi free from the chest wall fascia, beginning at the level of the muscle belly and proceeding in a superior direction. As the dissection proceeds toward the latissimus insertion, the second assistant maximally internally rotates the shoulder to facilitate exposure of the tendinous insertion. Approaching

(text continues on page 370)

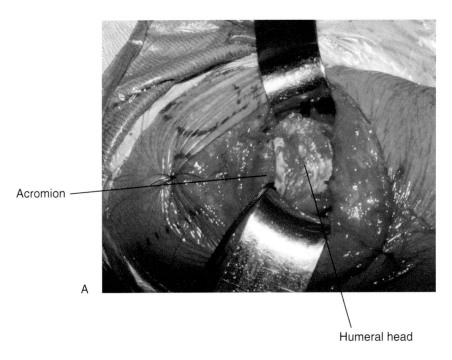

Acromion

Humeral head

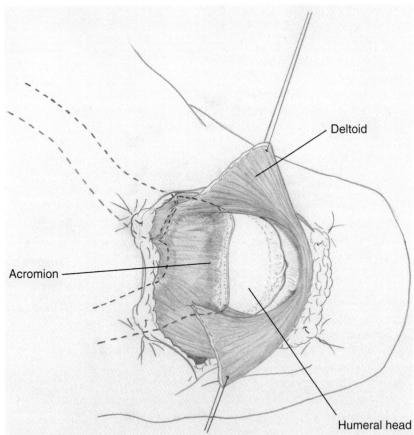

Deltoid

Acromion

Humeral head

Figure 20-6. A,B: Middle deltoid detachment exposing underlying humeral head and remaining rotator cuff. (Copyright Christian Gerber, M.D., University of Zurich.)

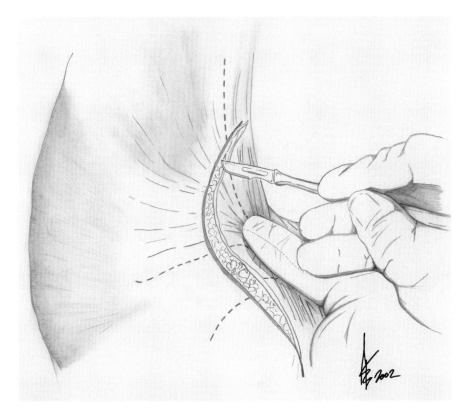

Figure 20-7. Posteroinferior incision. (Copyright Christian Gerber, M.D., University of Zurich.)

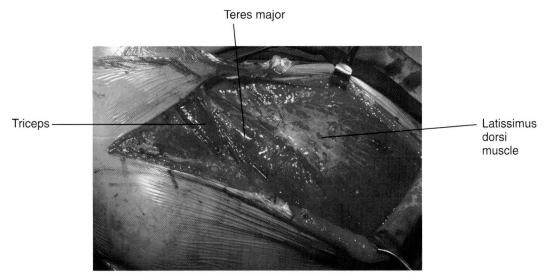

Figure 20-8. Latissimus dorsi exposure. The posterior deltoid, triceps, teres major, and latissimus dorsi muscles are identified. (Copyright Christian Gerber, M.D., University of Zurich.)

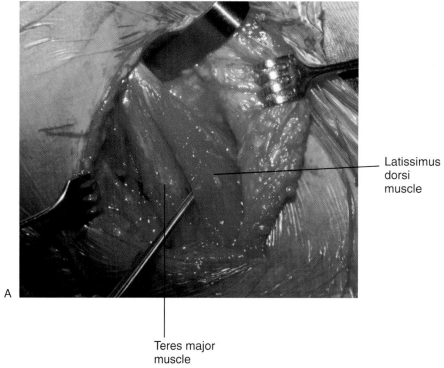

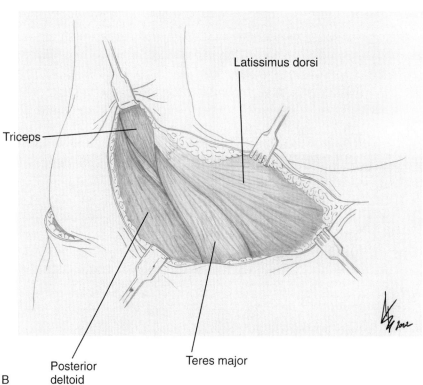

Figure 20-9. A,B: Teres major and latissimus dorsi identification. The tendons of the latissimus dorsi and teres major are closely superimposed atop one another. (Copyright Christian Gerber, M.D., University of Zurich.)

their insertions, the tendons of the latissimus dorsi and teres major are closely superimposed atop one another with the latissimus dorsi being anterior (superficial) to the teres major (Fig. 20-9). The teres major is often muscular to the insertion at the humerus whereas the tendon of the latissimus is long and flat (Fig. 20-10). We believe that the key to dissection is to release the thin latissimus tendon from the humerus with a long-handled no. 15 scalpel or Met-

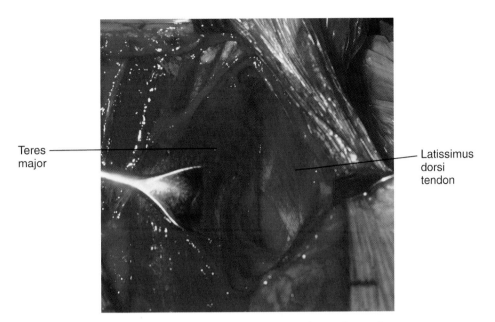

Teres major

Latissimus dorsi tendon

Figure 20-10. Latissimus dorsi tendon. Long, flat tendon is visible from its anterior surface. (Copyright Christian Gerber, M.D., University of Zurich.)

zenbaum scissors before dissecting the interval between the latissimus and teres major (Fig. 20-11). After releasing the tendon, dissection of the interval is greatly facilitated (Fig. 20-12). The two muscle bellies of the latissimus and teres major are often difficult to distinguish. If the surgeon fails to identify the interval properly, he or she is forced to go very proximally or distally to anatomically separate the muscle bellies. Note that the radial nerve crosses over the humerus immediately distal to the latissimus insertion and that the circumflex vessels and axillary nerve are immediately proximal to the latissimus dorsi tendon.

Using no. 3 Ethibond, two sutures are placed through the end of the latissimus dorsi tendon using a Krackow-type stitch to maintain tension on the muscle as the dissection is completed in a retrograde direction toward its origin (Fig. 20-13). The neurovascular pedicle enters the latissimus from its deep surface (anteriorly) and is usually identified when it enters the muscle approximately 10 cm distal to the musculotendinous junction (measured with the muscle under tension) (Fig. 20-14). Identification of the neurovascular pedicle is not mandatory. The anterior aspect of the latissimus is usually under more tension than the posterior aspect. Therefore, the anterior aspect of the muscle–tendon unit must be especially mobilized so that the tendon can easily reach the superolateral aspect of the greater tuberosity.

The edge of the posterior deltoid is identified and, using blunt dissection, we develop the space between the deltoid and teres minor so that it communicates freely with the previously performed anterosuperior exposure. We ensure that there is adequate space under the deltoid for tendon passage and easy excursion. The shoulder is placed in 45 degrees of abduction and 30 degrees of external rotation. From the anterosuperior incision, we use a long, curved clamp to pull the latissimus dorsi tendon and sutures under the posterior deltoid and acromion into the anterosuperior exposure (Figs. 20-14 to 20-16).

Anterosuperior Exposure. We confirm that the latissimus dorsi tendon and muscle are sufficiently mobilized to reach the greater tuberosity (Fig. 20-17). Often slight external rotation may facilitate reinsertion. The humeral head may or may not be fully covered with the tendon. However, it should be remembered that the goal of this tendon transfer is not simply biologic coverage of the humeral head but rather, restoration of active external rotation. Using the previously placed Mason-Allen sutures in the retracted tendons of the rotator cuff, we suture the remaining cuff to a bony trough near the greater tuberosity or to the medial border of the transferred latissimus dorsi tendon. Finally, the two sutures in the end of latissimus dorsi are passed transosseously through the lesser tuberosity with the knot tied over the subscapularis (Fig. 20-18).

(text continues on page 379)

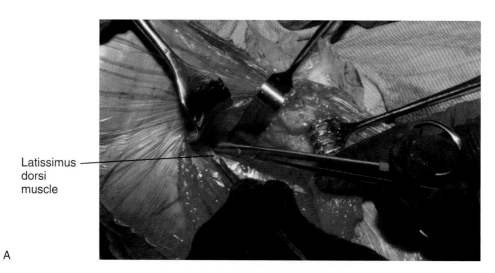

Latissimus
dorsi
muscle

A

Latissimus dorsi
tendon

Teres
major

B

Figure 20-11. A–C: Latissimus dorsi harvest. Release of the latissimus dorsi tendon from its humeral insertion with sharp dissection technique; either long Metzenbaum scissors or no. 15 scalpel blade. (Copyright Christian Gerber, M.D., University of Zurich.) *(continued)*

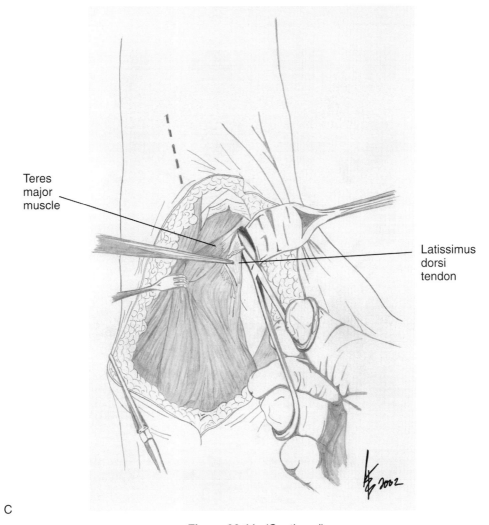

Teres major muscle

Latissimus dorsi tendon

C

Figure 20-11. *(Continued)*

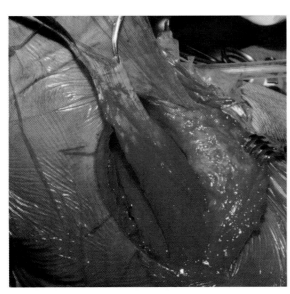

Figure 20-12. Fully released latissimus dorsi tendon. (Copyright Christian Gerber, M.D., University of Zurich.)

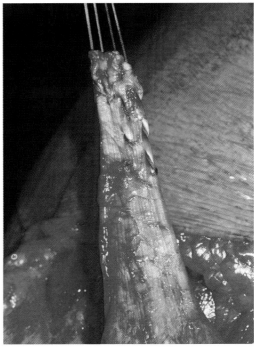

Figure 20-13. Latissimus dorsi tendon with Krackow sutures in end. (Copyright Christian Gerber, M.D., University of Zurich.)

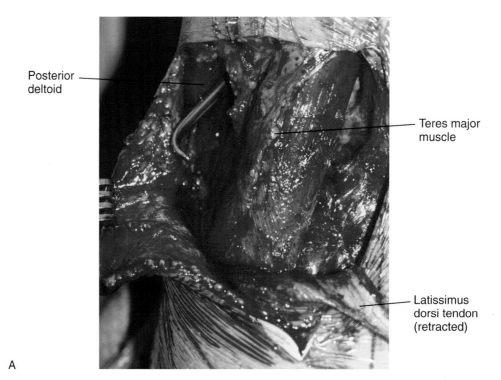

Posterior
deltoid

Teres major
muscle

Latissimus
dorsi tendon
(retracted)

A

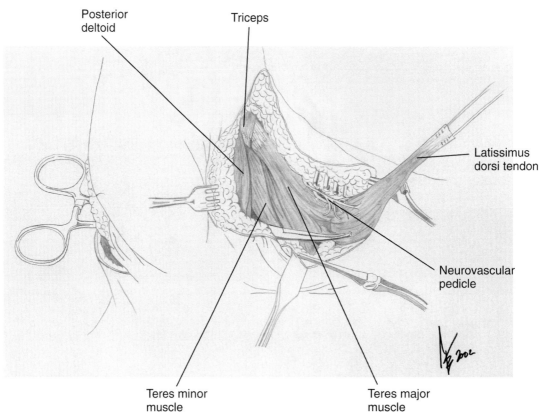

Posterior
deltoid

Triceps

Latissimus
dorsi tendon

Neurovascular
pedicle

Teres minor
muscle

Teres major
muscle

B

Figure 20-14. A,B: Long, curved clamp reaching from anterosuperior incision. Viewed from posteroinferior exposure, the neurovascular pedicle is visible. (Copyright Christian Gerber, M.D., University of Zurich.)

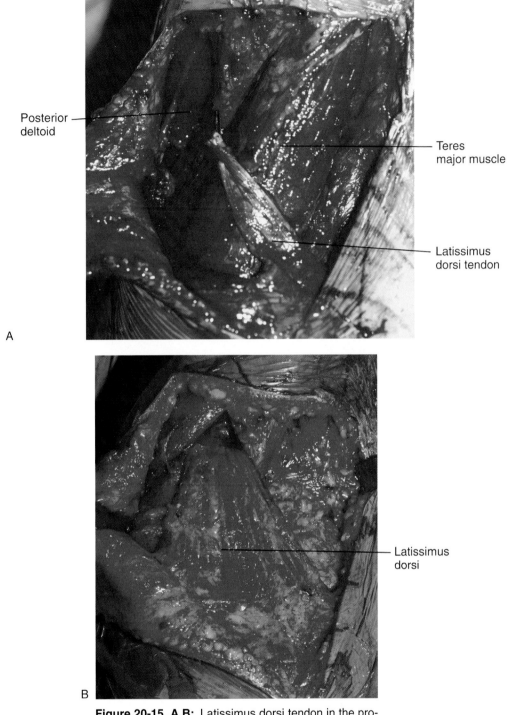

Figure 20-15. A,B: Latissimus dorsi tendon in the process of being pulled up into the anterosuperior exposure. Viewed from posteroinferior exposure, the latissimus dorsi tendon is passed between the posterior deltoid and teres minor. (Copyright Christian Gerber, M.D., University of Zurich.)

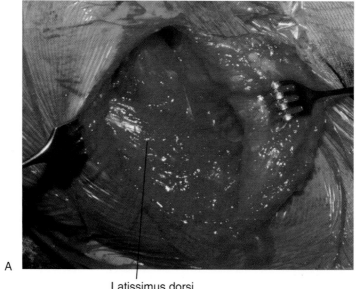

A

Latissimus dorsi

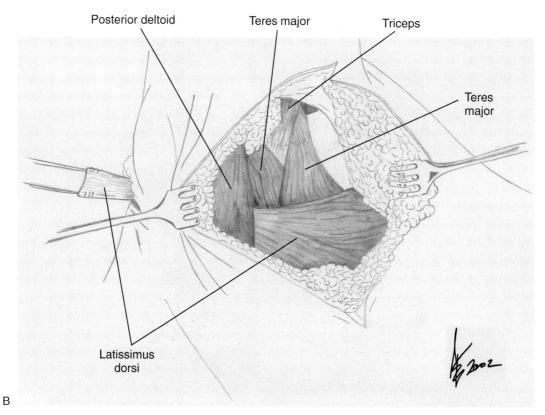

B

Figure 20-16. A,B: Latissimus dorsi tendon pulled completely up into the anterosuperior exposure. Viewed from posteroinferior exposure. (Copyright Christian Gerber, M.D., University of Zurich.)

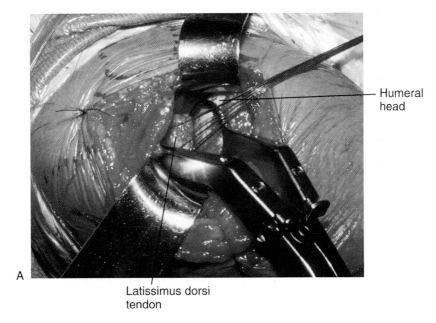

A

B

Humeral
head

Latissimus dorsi
tendon

Latissimus
dorsi tendon

Figure 20-17. A,B: Latissimus dorsi tendon being pulled up over
the humeral head. Viewed from the anterosuperior exposure, the
transferred latissimus dorsi tendon is sufficiently mobilized to
reach the greater tuberosity. (Copyright Christian Gerber, M.D.,
University of Zurich.)

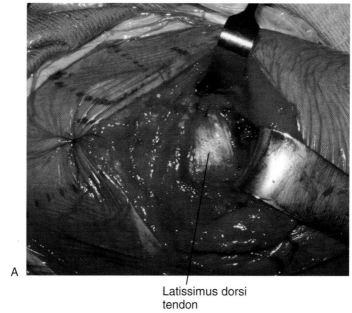

A

Latissimus dorsi
tendon

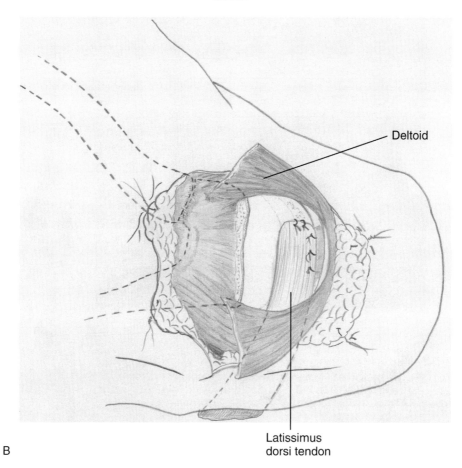

Deltoid

Latissimus
dorsi tendon

B

Figure 20-18. A–C: Latissimus dorsi tendon sutured over the humeral head to the upper
subscapularis tendon. (Copyright Christian Gerber, M.D., University of Zurich.) *(continued)*

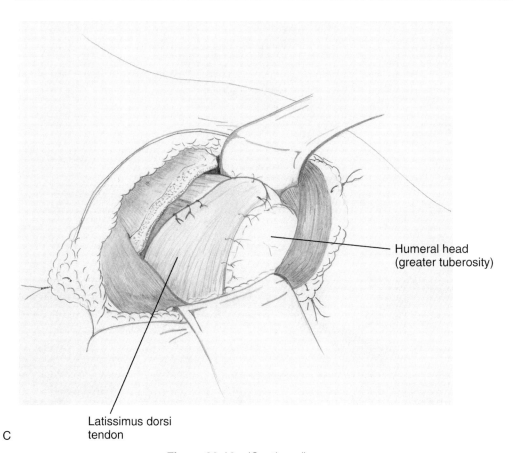

C

Figure 20-18. *(Continued)*

Both wounds are irrigated. Two drains are placed in the inferior wound and one drain is placed in the superior wound. The deltoid split is reapproximated with a running 0 monofilament suture. Using the previously placed no. 3 Ethibond sutures, the deltoid is anatomically reattached transosseously to the lateral acromion (Fig. 20-19).

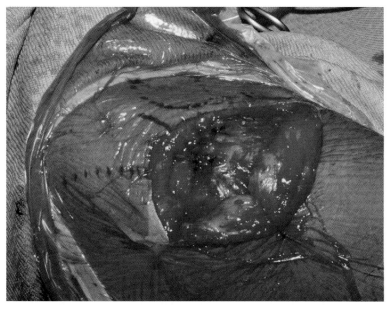

Figure 20-19. Deltoid repair. (Copyright Christian Gerber, M.D., University of Zurich.)

The dermal edges are reapproximated with 4-0 absorbable monofilament. The skin edges are reapproximated with a running, nonabsorbable 4-0 monofilament. Sterile dressings are applied.

In the operating room, an abduction brace is applied (in 45 degrees of abduction and external rotation), which will be worn continuously for 6 weeks.

POSTOPERATIVE MANAGEMENT

Postoperative analgesia in the form of the interscalene catheter and oral pain medicines are provided. The suction drains are removed on postoperative day 2 and the sutures are removed on postoperative day 4. Interscalene anesthesia is stopped after 48 hours.

The abduction brace applied in the operating room maintains the affected extremity in 45 degrees of abduction and external rotation. The patient is instructed to wear the abduction brace continuously for 6 weeks.

Rehabilitation

With the shoulder abducted and externally rotated 45 degrees, the tendon transfer heals in an environment free from tissue tension. During this period a formal physical therapy program is instituted.

During the first 6 weeks postoperatively, the patient remains in the abduction brace but a therapist passively performs gentle abduction and external rotation going into full elevation of the abducted arm. Adduction and forceful internal rotation are forbidden. Passive motion is important to prevent postoperative glenohumeral stiffness and prevent latissimus dorsi tendon adherence to surrounding soft tissues. "Innervation exercises" are initiated immediately to maintain deltoid and latissimus dorsi muscle tone.

After 6 weeks, the abduction brace is removed and the patient is instructed to perform gentle activities of daily living. Physical therapy continues with gentle mobilization maneuvers.

At 3 months postoperatively, active strengthening of the rotator cuff and tendon transfer is begun. Internal rotation, extension, and adduction of the upper extremity are the normal activities for the latissimus dorsi. In its transferred position, however, it must act as an external rotator. Therefore, muscle reeducation is critical for this transfer to function successfully.

Specifically, with a therapist assisting, the shoulder is positioned in the midrange of abduction. The patient is instructed to actively adduct the arm. The latissimus can be palpated during this maneuver and contraction can be easily felt. As it contracts, the therapist gently guides the shoulder into flexion, all the while "coaching" the patient to maintain latissimus contraction. With time, the patient will be able to maintain latissimus contraction to facilitate flexion. Upon mastery of flexion, the same process is used to teach the patient to use the latissimus dorsi for external rotation.

We inform the patient preoperatively and emphasize postoperatively that it may take 12 months for complete retraining of the transferred latissimus dorsi.

RESULTS

Gerber et al. originally reported good-excellent short-term results in four patients after latissimus dorsi transfer (6). Subsequently, Gerber et al. (3) reviewed the results of the first 16 patients an average of 33 months after latissimus dorsi transfer. Subjectively, eight patients reported excellent results, five reported good results, two reported fair, and one reported a poor result. Pain relief at rest was satisfactory in 94% and in 81% with exertion. The average increase in flexion was 51 degrees. External rotation improved an average of 13 degrees. At 65 months postoperatively, pain relief at rest was unchanged but had fallen to 75% with exertion. Results were excellent if the subscapularis was functionally intact and unsatisfactory if in addition to the posterosuperior tear, there was also a subscapularis tear. Miniaci and MacLeod (9) reported results in 17, Aoki et al. (1) in 12, and Warner (10) in six patients; all authors confirmed that provided the indications correspond to those outlined above, this procedure can be performed without significant risk and leads to the results as described by the present authors.

COMPLICATIONS

Complications after latissimus dorsi transfer are relatively rare. In more than 60 procedures, we have observed one infection. Postoperative axillary nerve palsy was observed twice; this resolved fully within 2 months. Pain in the posterolateral scar was observed with the original skin incision, which extended into the axilla. This has led to the modified skin incision described in this chapter, with which we have not observed this complication.

Detachment of the deltoid is a devastating complication after latissimus dorsi transfer (8). This has occurred once in our experience. However, we only detach the lateral deltoid with a thin bone wafer as described above and take utmost care to securely reattach the deltoid and to protect this repair postoperatively with the splint.

Other authors have reported avulsion of the latissimus tendon from its transferred position (10). However, we do not have a documented case of this complication using the surgical technique above. Therefore, we have not found fascia lata augmentation to be necessary. Modifications of mobilization and reinsertion, however, need to be tested for stability of reinsertion.

Persistence of pseudoparalysis (i.e., the inability to elevate the arm above the horizontal) is a potential complication in the chronic long-standing case. Development of pseudoparalysis in a patient who preoperatively could elevate the arm above the horizontal has been observed in four cases. Two were associated with subscapularis tear during a period of time when we were unaware that subscapularis rupture is a contraindication for the procedure. Two further cases were due to deltoid disinsertion one of them with additional temporary axillary nerve palsy. After recovery of the axillary nerve palsy, pseudoparalysis resolved.

ACKNOWLEDGMENT

This chapter was written with support from Resortho Foundation Zurich.

RECOMMENDED READING

1. Aoki, M., Okamura, K., Fukushima, S., et al.: Transfer of latissimus dorsi for irreparable rotator-cuff tears. *J Bone Joint Surg Am* 78: 761–766, 1996.
2. Fuchs, B., Weishaupt, D., Zanetti, M., et al.: Fatty degeneration of the muscles of the rotator cuff: assessment by computed tomography versus magnetic resonance imaging. *J Shoulder Elbow Surg* 8.6: 599–605, 1999.
3. Gerber, C.: Latissimus dorsi transfer for the treatment of irreparable tears of the rotator cuff. *Clinical Orthopaedics and Related Research* 275: 152–160, 1992.
4. Gerber, C.: Massive rotator cuff tears. In: Ianotti, J., Williams, G., Jr., eds.: *Disorders of the shoulder: diagnosis and management.* Philadelphia: Lippincott Williams & Wilkins, 57–92, 1999.
5. Gerber, C., Hersche, O.: Tendon transfers for the treatment of irreparable rotator cuff defects. *Orthop Clin N Am* 28: 195–203, 1997.
6. Gerber, C., Vinh, T.S., Hertel, G.R., et al.: Latissimus dorsi transfer for the treatment of massive tears of the rotator cuff: a preliminary report. *Clin Orthop* 232: 51–61, 1988.
7. Goutallier, D., Bernageau, J.,Patte, D.: L'évaluation par le scanner de las trophicité des muscles des coiffes des rotateurs ayant une rupture tendineuse. *Revue de Chirurgie Orthopedique* 75: 126–127, 1989.
8. Groh, G., Simoni, M.,Rolla, P., et al.: Loss of the deltoid after shoulder operations: an operative disaster. *J Shoulder Elbow Surg* 3: 243–253, 1994.
9. Miniaci, A., MacLeod, M.: Transfer of the latissimus dorsi muscle after failed repair of a massive tear of the rotator cuff. *J Bone Joint Surg Am* 81: 1120–1127, 1999.
10. Warner, J.J.P.: Management of massive irreparable rotator cuff tears: the role of tendon transfer. *J Bone Joint Surg Am* 82: 877–887, 2000.
11. Warner, J.J.P., Gerber, C.: Massive tears of the postero-superior rotator cuff. In: Warner, J.J.P., Ianotti, J., Gerber, C., eds.: *Complex and revision problems in shoulder surgery.* Philadelphia: Lippincott–Raven Publishers, 177, 1997.
12. Warner, J.J.P., Parsons, M. IV: Latissimus dorsi tendon transfer: a comparative analysis of primary and salvage reconstruction of massive, irreparable rotator cuff tears. *J Shoulder Elbow Surg* 10(6); 514–521, 1999.

PART IV

Trauma

21

Open Reduction and Internal Fixation of Fractures and Nonunions of the Clavicle

Peter Kloen and David L. Helfet

INDICATIONS/CONTRAINDICATIONS

Clavicular fractures have been estimated to comprise about 44% of all shoulder girdle injuries. Most of these fractures involve the mid shaft, and most of these heal with nonoperative treatment. Relatively few indications exist for operative treatment of acute clavicular fractures. Among these are open fractures that need irrigation and débridement followed by stable internal fixation; significantly displaced fractures that compromise the underlying neurovascular structures; impending skin penetration by the fracture ends; and the polytrauma patient requiring stabilization of all fractures, to allow early mobilization (7,11). Two other scenarios that have been considered indications for open reduction and internal fixation of acute clavicle fractures are the type II distal clavicle fracture and the floating shoulder. Some recent literature has questioned these last two indications for clavicle open reduction and internal fixation (3,10). The unusual medial clavicular fracture can, rarely, lead to airway and esophageal compromise when the displacement of the clavicle is posteriorly and obviously needs to be reduced and stabilized (4). Relative indications would be severe pain affecting use of the extremity, function for a throwing or similar athlete, and very occasionally, cosmesis.

The second and much larger group of patients that are candidates for operative intervention are those patients who present with a painful clavicular nonunion. The incidence of mid-shaft clavicular nonunions is relatively low (ranging from 0.9% to 4%), but when it occurs, often results in significant discomfort and deformity for these patients. Nonunion rates for lateral clavicle fractures are reportedly higher (22% to 30%) (9,10). Several known factors predispose to the development of a clavicular nonunion: open fracture, segmental

P. Kloen, M.D., Ph.D.: Division of Orthopaedic Trauma, Department of Orthopaedic Surgery, Academic Medical Center, Amsterdam, The Netherlands.

D. L. Helfet, M.D.: Department of Orthopaedic Surgery, Weill Medical College of Cornell University; and Orthopaedic Trauma Service, Hospital for Special Surgery, New York, New York.

comminution, displacement, initial shortening greater than 2 cm, insufficient length of immobilization, operative treatment, and refracture. The pain complaints can vary from a mild ache during overhead activities to severe and disabling resting pain. Neurovascular symptoms can manifest themselves from mild dysesthesias or paresthesias to a full-blown thoracic outlet syndrome with a decreased peripheral pulse and/or venous congestion.

Once patient and physician are convinced that the nonunion is the source of the symptoms, there are essentially no contraindications to surgery other than compromised medical conditions that may place the patient at risk for anesthesia. Aesthetic reasons are a relative contraindication given the unpredictability of the unsightly bump and/or scar formation.

Many techniques have been suggested for the surgical treatment of fractures and nonunions of the clavicle, including pins and wires, intramedullary fixation, plates and screws, (partial) claviculectomy, and external fixation (1,2,5). Most of these pertain to the surgery of fractures and nonunions in the middle third, given the relative scarcity of medial and lateral clavicular fractures. Proponents of intramedullary pin fixation have reported high union rates, but also have stated that hardware removal was often necessary. Proponents of plate fixation question the adequacy but especially the rotational stability of pin fixation. Traditionally, for all internal fixation groups, the hardware is often prominent and painful and needs to be removed.

The senior author has modified the standard clavicle plating technique for mid-shaft clavicle fractures and nonunions to minimize the complications and secondary surgeries previously reported (6). This modified technique positions the reconstruction plate on the anteroinferior border of the clavicle. There are many advantages for this. First, the lateral fragment is lifted up to the medial fragment and supported like a shelf rather than being suspended from cephalad by screws. Second, the length of the screws when aiming obliquely from anteroinferior to superoposterior is longer thus providing more holding power. Third, there is no risk of plunging with the drill or screws because they are aimed away from the neurovascular structures beneath the clavicle. Fourth, the hardware is not prominent or painful, essentially omitting the need for hardware removal.

PREOPERATIVE PLANNING

Given the subcutaneous position of the clavicle, patients presenting with a clavicular fracture or a painful clavicular nonunion do generally not require extensive diagnostic evaluation. The proximal (medial) fragment is relatively more prominent, given the downward pull by the arm of the distal (lateral) fragment. The fracture or nonunion is most likely associated with excess painful mobility and/or crepitus, and the defect can easily be palpated. Occasionally the nonunion is not associated with pain and in these latter instances, a conservative approach should be discussed with the patient. More difficult is the diagnosis of medial and lateral clavicular fractures and nonunions, because these may mimic ligamentous injuries and/or dislocations. Swelling and ecchymosis can obscure subtle deformities.

A careful and detailed neurovascular examination is needed to document any preexisting deficits in the peripheral pulses or brachial plexus. This should include a comparison between left and right, because the extensive collateral circulation of the shoulder might obscure a vascular deficit. Although an associated pneumothorax or hemothorax is rare in these injuries, you should be aware of its possibility; therefore, a complete evaluation should include auscultation for equal breath sounds.

Plain radiographs generally outline the type and location of the mid-shaft fracture or nonunion (Fig. 21-1). In addition to a standard anteroposterior view from the clavicle that visualizes the sternoclavicular and acromioclavicular (AC) joints, a 45-degree cephalad view is helpful. In the former view, the upper lung fields should be evaluated to rule out a pneumothorax. The latter view eliminates the underlying thoracic structures. In case of doubt, a computed tomography (CT) scan can confirm the presence and nature of the nonunion. CT scanning will also allow better evaluation of medial- and lateral-third (especially intraarticular) fracture/dislocations of the clavicle. The medial clavicular injuries are especially difficult to outline on plain radiographs given the overlapping ribs, sternum, and mediastinum.

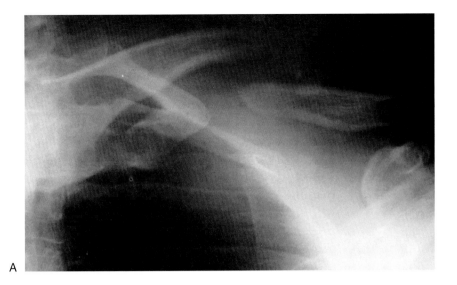

A

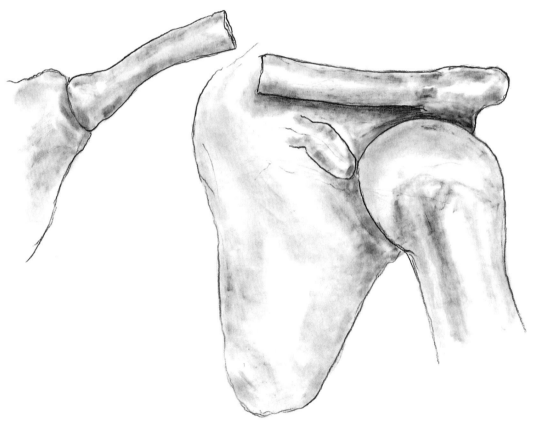

B

Figure 21-1. Anteroposterior radiograph **(A)** and schematic depiction **(B)** of displacement of a midclavicular fracture or nonunion. The proximal fragment is pulled superiorly by the attached muscle.

SURGERY

The patient is placed on the operating room table in a beach-chair position with the aid of a beanbag. Another option is to secure the head to a Mayfield headrest rather than the standard broad headpiece of an operating table. The entire arm of the involved upper extremity should be draped free. The head of the patient should be turned away from the side of the

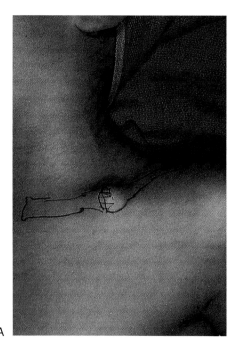

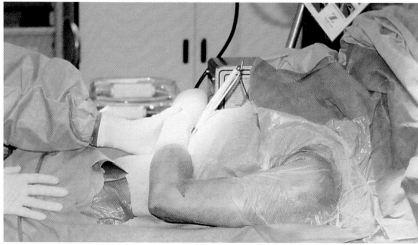

B

A

Figure 21-2. **A:** Clavicle neck and shoulder girdle are prepped and draped free. Location of midclavicular nonunion is outlined on skin. **B:** The patient is positioned supine, the arm draped free, and the iliac crest prepped and draped for the bone graft.

clavicle that is to be operated on. Most often general endotracheal anesthesia is used, although we have successfully performed the procedure with a combination of an interscalene block and spinal anesthesia for the iliac crest bone graft harvest in one patient. To facilitate draping and to expand the operative field, the endotracheal tube is positioned out the opposite corner of the mouth. A rolled up towel is placed between the scapulae to make the clavicle more prominent. If you are planning to use iliac crest bone graft, you should preferably harvest it from the same side (Fig. 21-2).

Mid-shaft Fractures and Nonunions

The incision runs parallel to Langer lines along the inferior border of the clavicle overlying the fracture or nonunion (Fig. 21-3). The dissection is carried down to bone followed by careful subperiosteal dissection (Fig. 21-4). This should be done with caution, taking

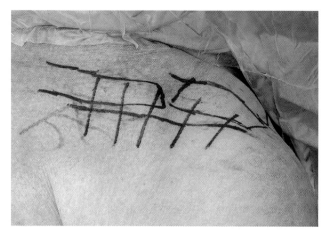

Figure 21-3. Skin incision for anteroinferior plating for midshaft clavicle fractures or nonunions—left shoulder outlined.

care to avoid any potential damage to the anterior divisions of the brachial plexus and the subclavian vessels. In case of a nonunion, there is often a significant amount of intervening soft tissue and scar with displacement of the bony ends. In these instances, it is much safer to proceed with the dissection from known to unknown territory. Using a soft-tissue dissector, the soft tissues are gently pried off the anteroinferior aspect of the bony ends to expose the nonunion site (Fig. 21-5). Since we prefer to position the plate on the anteroinferior aspect of the clavicle, there is no need to do an extensive subperiosteal dissection on the superior surface and edges. Tissue cultures are obtained and antibiotics can now be given.

In case of an atrophic nonunion, remove all intervening tissue using a combination of scalpel and rongeur. If a sclerotic end cap is present on either side of the clavicular nonunion, drilling multiple holes with a small drill can reopen the medullary canal (Fig. 21-6). This only needs to be done over a short distance, just enough to restore bleeding from both ends. We generally do not resect the sclerotic ends because this would necessitate placement of an intercalary graft. In case a defect is present, the decision whether to shorten the clavicle or to place an intercalary graft needs to be made. Some authors have warned against shortening of the clavicle because this could lead to narrowing of the neurovascular space, creating a thoracic outlet syndrome and ipsilateral glenohumeral and/or scapulothoracic dysfunction. However, there are no clear guidelines as to what amount of shortening can be accepted. Obviously, the placement of an intercalary graft mandates two healing sites as opposed to an end-to-end apposition (Fig. 21-7).

In case of a hypertrophic nonunion, the excess callus prevents easy contouring of the plate and places the neurovascular structures at risk of impingement or compression. Therefore, one should remove excess inferior callus to allow apposition of the plate to avoid the compromise of the underlying neurovascular structures. Position small, blunt Hohmann retractors around the bony fragments. Next, you can reduce the nonunion using standard reduction clamps. In case of an oblique fracture or nonunion with relatively little translation and/or displacement (Figs 21-1 and 21-4C), this is relatively straightforward. However, in case of posterior displacement of the lateral fragment, this can be quite cumbersome. Thus in the latter case, it might be helpful to grasp the lateral fragment with a pointed reduction clamp and gently tease it forward, carefully freeing it up from the surrounding muscles. If there is relatively little shortening such as seen in an atrophic nonunion (Fig. 21-8A), the lateral fragment can be pulled medially to meet the medial fragment. A straight 3.5-mm reconstruction plate is contoured to fit the curve of the anteroinferior aspect (rather than the subcutaneous superior aspect) of the clavicle. The use of plate benders and twisters and the design of the 3.5-mm pelvic reconstruction plates greatly facilitate the plate contouring. First, the plate is transfixed to the lateral fragment with one or two screws. To facilitate placement of the screws, grasp the lateral fragment with a reduction clamp and rotate it upward so that the anteroinferior aspect faces more anteriorly. There is no need to keep the nonunion reduced with a clamp at this time. Once the plate is attached to the lateral fragment, reduce the fragment to the medial fragment. A 3.5-mm cortical lag screw is then placed across the nonunion side through the plate by overdrilling the proximal cortex with a 3.5-mm drill and the distal cortex with a 2.5-mm drill bit. Subsequently, place additional 3.5-mm cortical screws for a minimum of three bicortical screws on either side of the nonunion/fracture. This means that we usually use a seven- or eight-hole, 3.5-mm pelvic reconstruction plate (Figs. 21-8B–E and 21-9). Although autogenous cancellous bone graft remains the gold standard, we recently started using demineralized bone matrix with admixed allograft (Grafton DBM Crunch; Osteotech, Eatontown, NJ), which obviates a second incision for iliac crest harvesting. Occasionally, in case of excessive shortening, a tricortical graft is needed to replace the missing bone and restore length. To estimate the needed graft length, measure the distance from the sternal notch to the contralateral acromioclavicular joint. Ideally, you should do this on a preoperative radiograph comparing the involved side with the contralateral healthy side, but you can estimate reasonably well by palpating through the drapes. To harvest the graft, make an incision centered over the anterior iliac crest and expose bone subperiosteally. Use an oscillating saw or osteotome, take the tricortical iliac bone graft. The medial and lateral aspects are fashioned

(text continues on page 396)

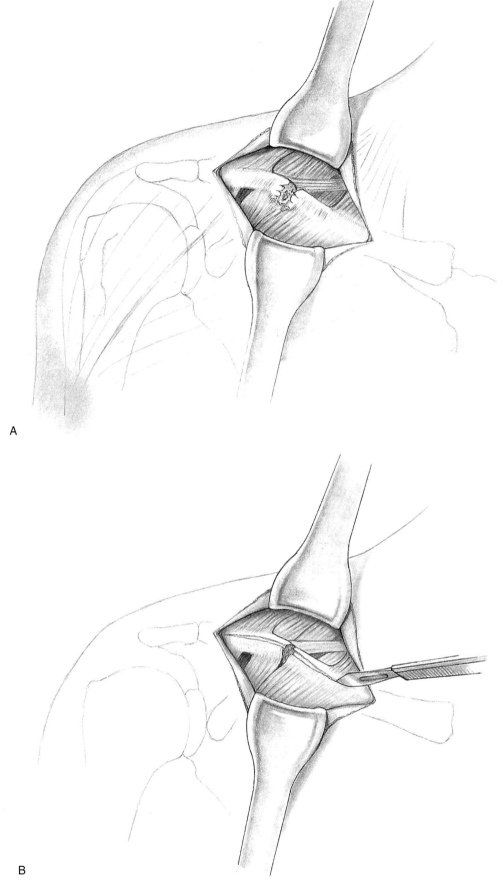

A

B

Figure 21-4. **A:** A horizontal skin incision is made, the flaps are undermined, exposing the trapezius and deltoid fascia at the fracture or nonunion site. **B:** An incision is made in the deltoid–trapezius fasciae, and sutures are placed in the fascial ends for later reattachment. *(continued)*

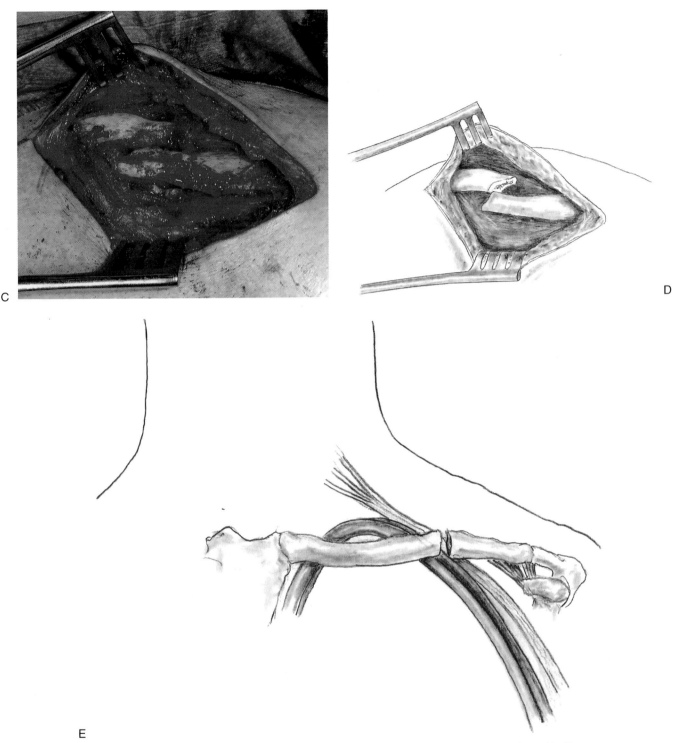

Figure 21-4. *Continued.* **C,D:** Intraoperative view after exposure of the nonunion with displaced fragments. **E:** Proximity of neurovascular structures mandate proceeding with caution, particularly posterior to exposed clavicle.

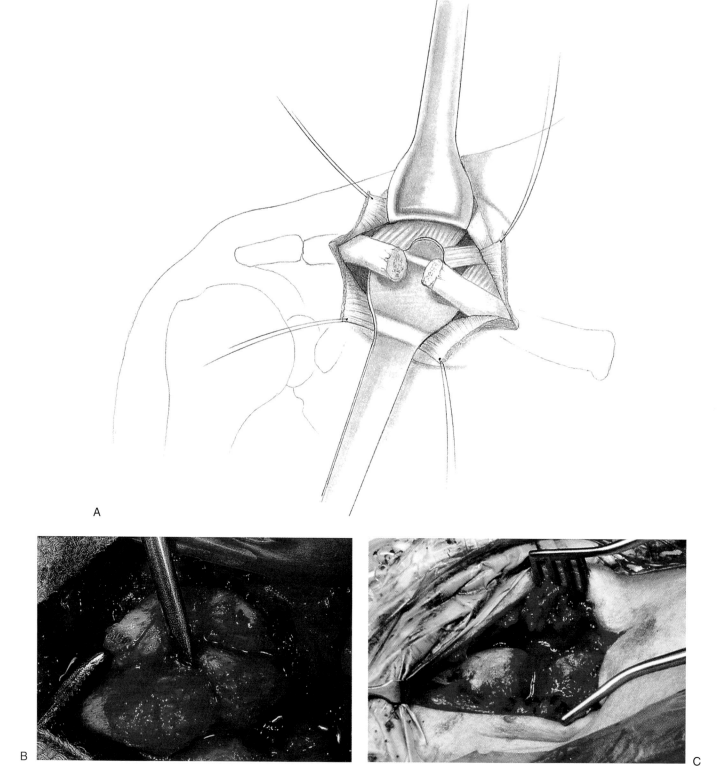

A

B

C

Figure 21-5. A: During exposure of the nonunion, blunt retractors should be placed around the clavicle to protect the vital structures. This is particularly true with the hypertrophic nonunion, in which calluses are often directly adjacent to the subclavian vein. **B:** Intraoperative photograph of nonunion. **C:** Operating room photograph of nonunion exposed. *(continued)*

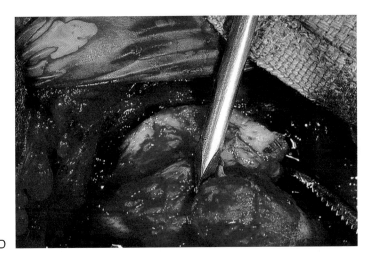

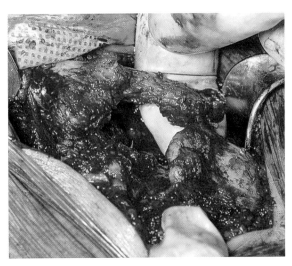

D

Figure 21-5. *Continued.* **D:** The fibrous tissue is removed from the nonunion sites between the clavicular ends and excess bony buildup is removed so the clavicle more closely resembles the normal anatomy.

Figure 21-6. Intraoperative sclerotic nonunion. If a sclerotic end cap is present on either side of the clavicular nonunion, drilling multiple holes with a small drill can reopen the medullary canal.

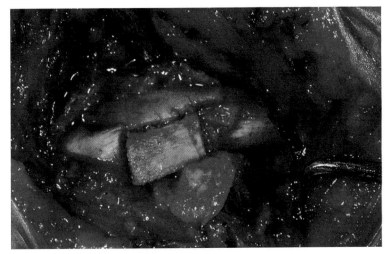

Figure 21-7. An intercalary bone graft may be inserted if a significant defect is present. However, the placement of an intercalary graft requires the healing of two separate sites as opposed to end-to-end apposition.

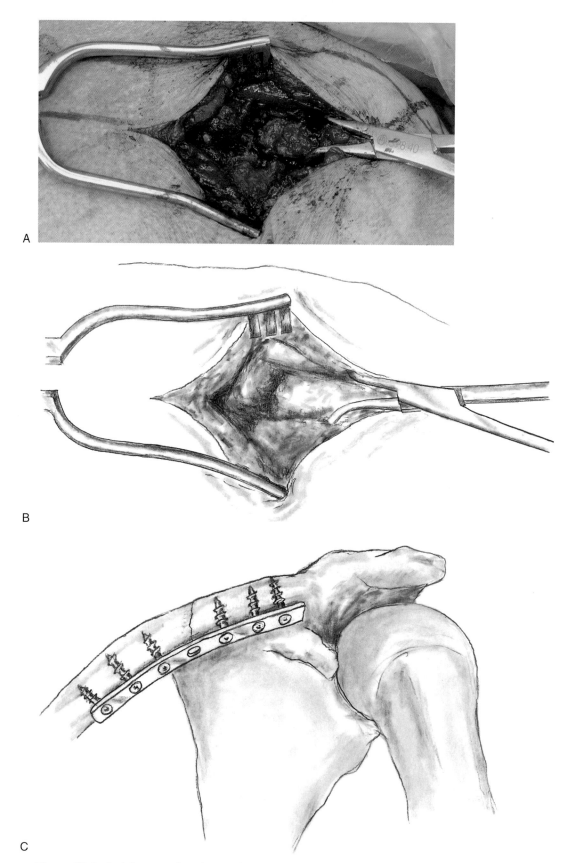

Figure 21-8. A: Intraoperative picture of an atrophic nonunion, showing posterior displacement of the lateral fragment and some shortening, which is corrected by pulling the lateral fragment forward and medially using a bone clamp. **B:** An inferior plate gives apposition of the fracture fragments, good internal fixation, and usually avoids the necessity for later plate removal. **C:** A seven- or eight-hole 3.5-mm pelvic reconstruction plate is usual. A hole is left unfilled with a screw if the screw hole traverses the area of the fracture line. *(continued)*

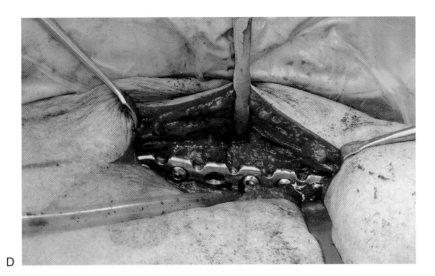

D

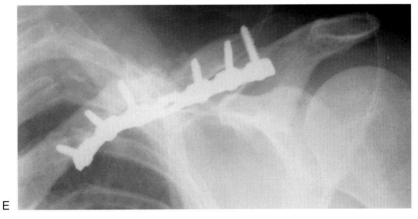

E

Figure 21-8. *Continued.* **D:** After plating, the nonunion with 3.5-mm pelvic reconstruction plate. **E:** Immediate postoperative radiograph showing reduction of the fracture with central screw hole left empty.

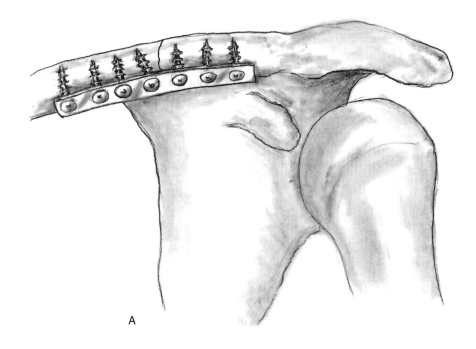

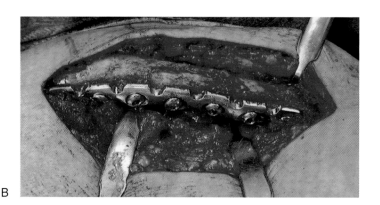

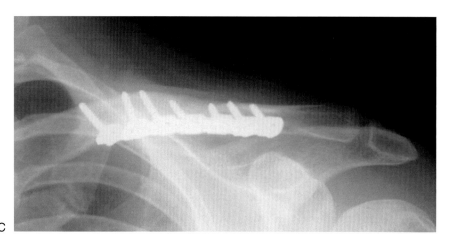

Figure 21-9. A,B: Seven-hole plate with good purchase of four screws on one side of the fracture site and three on the other. With this plating using a seven-hole, 3.5-mm reconstruction plate, there is a lag screw across the oblique nonunion. **C:** Radiograph obtained 1 year after surgery showing excellent healing of the nonunion.

into pegs and plugged into the medullary canals on either side. Depending on the preferred position of the plate (in our case, the anteroinferior aspect) the superior cortical part of the graft is placed opposite the plate to improve the biomechanical strength of the construct. Place at least one screw through the plate and the tricortical graft to secure it in place. Place additional cancellous graft around the nonunion to promote healing.

Assess the stability at the time of surgery to ensure there is no residual micromotion. Also, test the upper extremity/shoulder for a gentle but full range of motion to ensure no neurovascular compromise with position. Radiographs can be obtained at the same time. Finally, after meticulous hemostasis, drains are placed in the wounds, skin is closed using 3-0 monofilament sutures, and Steri-Strips (3M Worldwide, St. Paul, MN) are applied. Drains are usually removed on postoperative day one.

Lateral Clavicular Fractures and Nonunions

In displaced extraarticular fractures of the outer clavicle, the distal fragment retains its normal relationship with the adjacent acromion. As with AC dislocations, loss of the clavicular strength creates the appearance of a shoulder girdle "sag." This also makes the proximal fragment appear to be relatively superiorly displaced. In fact, distal clavicular fractures and nonunions can be confused with high-degree AC separation because of the proximity of the AC joint. These distal clavicle fractures have been classified on the basis of the relationship of the injury to the conoid and trapezoid ligaments. In type IIA fractures, the conoid and trapezoid ligaments are attached to the distal fragment, and the fracture line has a certain obliquity. In type IIB fractures, the trapezoid is attached to the distal fragment, but the fracture is between it and the conoid ligament. In this case, the conoid ligament is ruptured, and the fracture line usually appears to be more vertical than that seen in type IIA (Fig. 21-10).

(text continues on page 400)

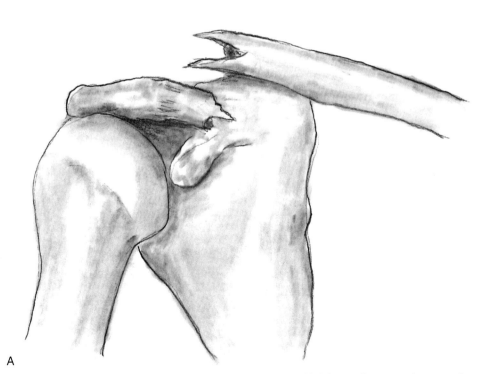

A

Figure 21-10. A: Drawing of a distal clavicle fracture with injury adjacent to the acromioclavicular joint. Proximal fragments may appear superiorly displaced, often confusing the fracture with a high-degree acromioclavicular separation. *(continued)*

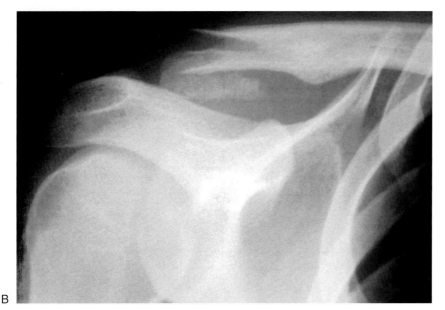

Figure 21-10. *Continued.* **B:** Excellent healing was shown on a radiograph taken 3 months after fixing the fracture with a mini T-plate. **C:** Type IIA fracture with conoid and trapezoid ligaments attached ligament to the distal fragment. The fracture line is oblique. **D:** Diagram of a type IIB fracture with the trapezoid ligament attached to the distal fragment. The fracture occurs between the trapezoid and conoid ligaments. The fracture may appear more vertical than that seen in type IIA.

B

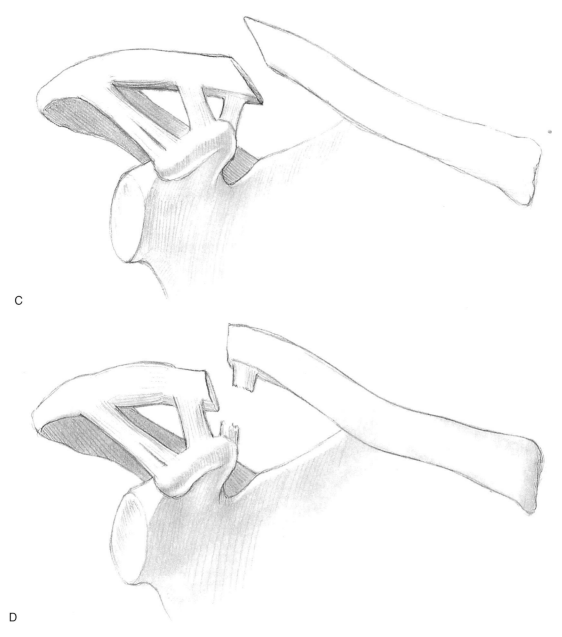

C

D

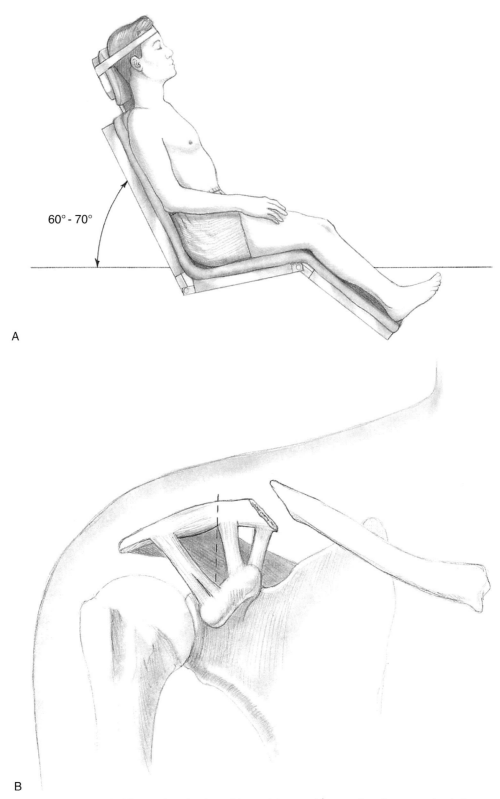

A

B

Figure 21-11. A: The patient is placed in a sitting position so that the upper body is approximately 60 to 70 degrees from the horizontal. *(continued)*

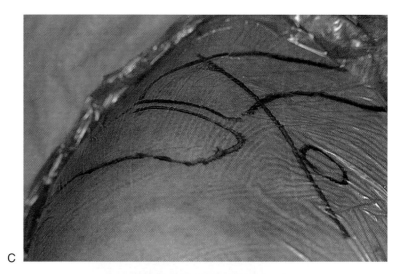

Figure 21-11. *Continued.* **B–D:** The vertical incision allows adequate exposure and results in a more aesthetically pleasing scar. The incision begins at the posterior margin of the clavicle, between the acromioclavicular joint and the fracture fragment, and extends to a point at the superior lateral tip of the coracoid process.

Make a vertical incision (saber cut) between the AC joint and the fracture (Fig. 21-11). Skin flaps are easily raised, if necessary, to increase the surgical exposure. The fracture or nonunion can now be identified and using sharp dissection, the bone ends are exposed (Fig. 21-12). A soft-tissue elevator is needed to complete the dissection subperiosteally (Fig. 21-13). The distal fragment is generally small. Make sure not to compromise any soft-tissue attachments, especially the ligaments. The fracture is temporarily reduced with a small bone-reduction clamp (Fig. 21-14). Depending on the size of the fragment, various techniques are available. In case of a large fragment, we have used a small fragment T-plate (Fig. 21-15).

Other options are the use of a cerclage wire (usually more for oblique lateral clavicle fracture patterns) (Fig 21-16) or intramedullary fixation using a Knowles pin (DePuy, War-

(text continues on page 406)

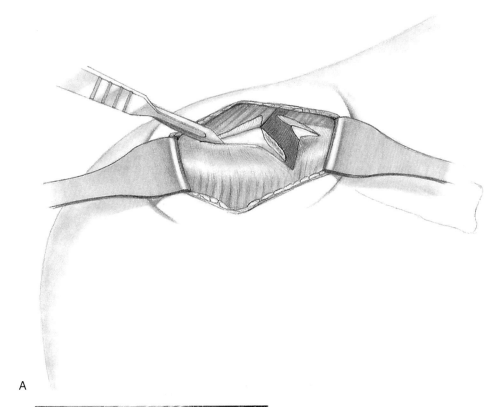

A

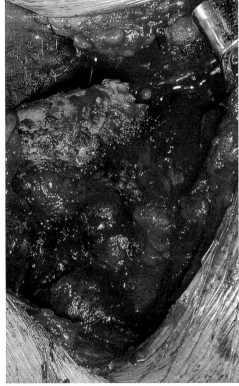

B

Figure 21-12. A,B: Deltoid trapezius fascia is incised transversely far enough to permit mobilization and reduction of the fragments.

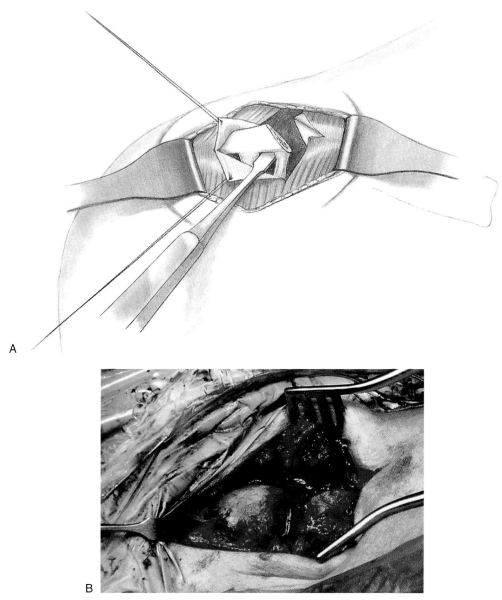

Figure 21-13. A,B: The fracture ends are exposed subperiosteally. A knife is used to begin the dissection plane, which is then continued carefully with a small periosteal elevator. *(continued)*

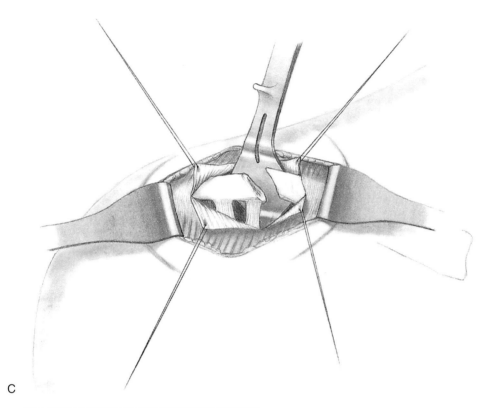

C

D

Figure 21-13. *Continued.* **C,D:** The fracture is exposed circumferentially to allow fragment mobilization, and retractors such as Bennett retractors are placed in the subperiosteal interval. Before insertion of Bennett retractors, the fracture is exposed. Care is taken not to compromise any soft-tissue attachments, particularly the coracoclavicular ligaments.

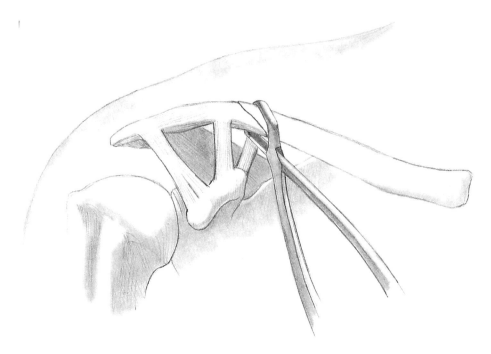

Figure 21-14. The fracture fragments, once mobilized, are reduced and held with a small bone-reduction clamp, with care taken to avoid crushing or comminuting the fracture fragments.

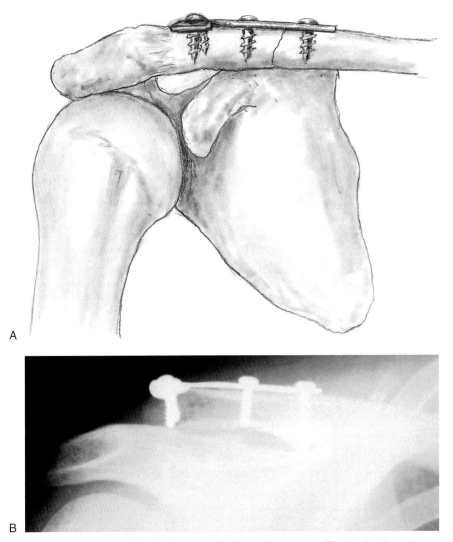

A

B

Figure 21-15. A,B: In the case of a large fragment, a T-plate is placed.

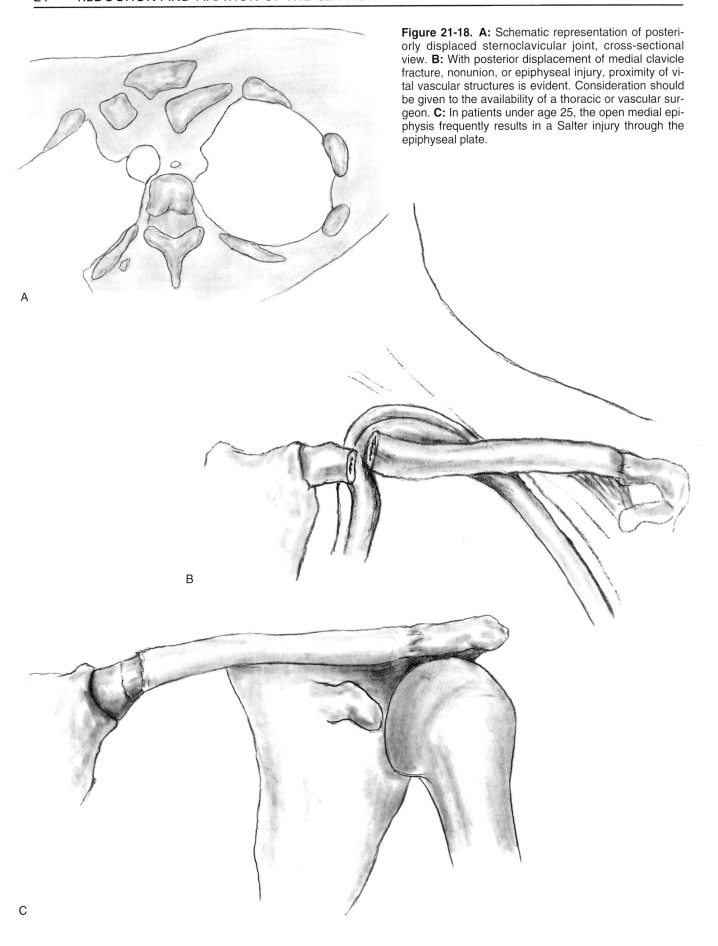

Figure 21-18. A: Schematic representation of posteriorly displaced sternoclavicular joint, cross-sectional view. **B:** With posterior displacement of medial clavicle fracture, nonunion, or epiphyseal injury, proximity of vital vascular structures is evident. Consideration should be given to the availability of a thoracic or vascular surgeon. **C:** In patients under age 25, the open medial epiphysis frequently results in a Salter injury through the epiphyseal plate.

A

B

C

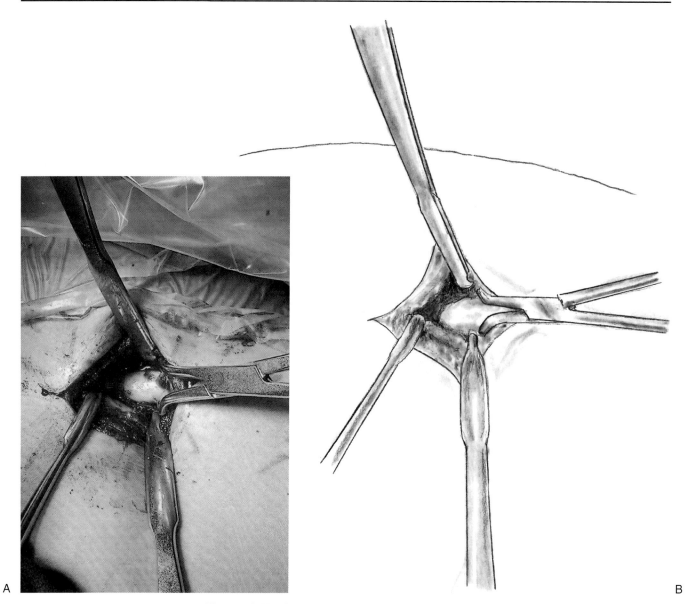

A   B

Figure 21-19. A: Intraoperative open reduction maneuver, pulling forward the lateral clavicle that had buttonholed through the periosteal sleeve. The patient's sternum is to the left of
the picture. **B:** Care must be used in gently maneuvering the fragment into place. One may
have to increase the buttonhole of the posterior capsule and periosteal sleeve to be able to
deliver the displaced fracture anteriorly.

tape or nonabsorbable suture (Ethibond no. 5, Ethicon, Inc.) to secure the clavicle to the underlying first rib or to the manubrium sterni (Fig. 21-20). Whereas others have described
fixing the lateral fragment to the epiphyseal fragment (4), in our experience this medial
fragment is rather small and its mostly cartilaginous structure does not provide adequate
purchase for any type of fixation. We only rarely have used more rigid fixation for medial
sternoclavicular joint fracture–dislocations (Fig. 21-21).

After reduction, with or without stabilization if required, the periosteal sleeve should be
closed. A suction drain is left in place and the skin is closed using a monofilament suture.
The drain is removed on the first postoperative day.

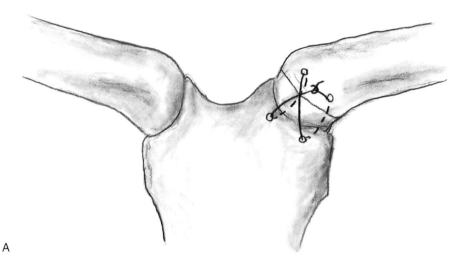

A

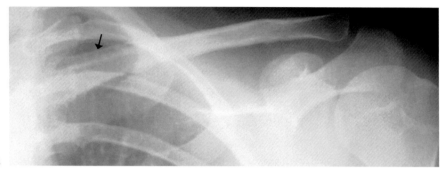

B

Figure 21-20. A: Schematic drawing of the fixation using Ethibond no. 5 suture (Ethicon Inc., Somerville, NJ). Mersilene tape (Ethicon Inc., Somerville, NJ) is an alternative means of fixation. The clavicle is secured to the underlying first rib or to the manubrium sterni. **B:** Radiograph obtained 1 year after surgery shows excellent healing. *Black arrow* points to new bone formation, most likely from within the periosteal sleeve. Patient had returned to athletic activities without restrictions.

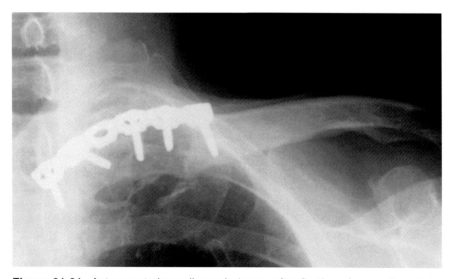

Figure 21-21. Anteroposterior radiograph 1 year after fixation of an acute anterior sternoclavicular fracture dislocation in a 54-year-old man, after it was elected to use the more rigid plate fixation.

POSTOPERATIVE MANAGEMENT

Physical therapy is initiated on the first postoperative day with gentle active and active-assisted Codman and pendulum exercises and the use of gentle overhead pulleys. In addition, elbow flexion/extension range-of-motion exercises without resistance can be initiated. The patient is advised to continue wearing a sling for 10 to 14 days, which is the time of the first postoperative visit. Radiographs are taken at 6-week, 3-month, and 6-month follow-up until crossing trabeculae confirm bony healing. At 3 weeks postoperatively, the patients are started on active and passive range of motion, as tolerated, but no lifting, throwing, or resisted activities until bony healing is confirmed.

RESULTS

We have treated 17 patients with a mid-shaft clavicle nonunion using open reduction and rigid internal fixation with a 3.5-mm reconstruction plate applied to the anteroinferior aspect of the clavicle as described herein. As bone graft we used either autologous iliac crest bone ($n = 13$) or Grafton DBM Crunch ($n = 4$) grafting. All of the nonunions healed, as confirmed both clinically and radiographically. The time to union averaged 3.6 months (range, 2 to 8 months) (6).

COMPLICATIONS

Acute neurovascular injuries are unusual despite the proximity of the brachial plexus and the subclavian vessels. If these do occur, they usually are seen in the more severe injuries of the shoulder girdle including scapular injuries. Compression of the neurovascular structures can be caused at the time of injury, as a result of a displaced fracture or malunion, or even in some rare cases by the hypertrophic callus on the inferior aspect of the clavicle. One of the patients with clavicle nonunion who we treated with anteroinferior plating developed symptoms of a thoracic outlet syndrome secondary to hypertrophic callus that impinged on the neurovascular structure after reduction and plating. This necessitated removal of the callus and revision open reduction and internal fixation during the same hospital stay.

One of the risk factors for developing a nonunion of the clavicular mid shaft is open reduction and internal fixation. Our protocol is to plate the nonunion on the anteroinferior surface as outlined above, regardless of any previous procedure. If a previous incision was slightly more cephalad than our preferred incision, the skin is mobile enough to use this same incision.

Although painful neuromas secondary to injury of the supraclavicular nerves that causes pain and/or dysesthesias on the anterior chest wall have been described, we have not encountered these.

Hardware problems are relatively common. Of these, the most worrisome complication has been the migration of pins, wires, screws, and so forth (8). Not only can this lead to a life-threatening situation, but it also represents failed fixation. Hardware failure is not uncommon, especially in the elderly and those with long-standing nonunions with significant osteopenia. However, the standard plating technique has also been related to nonunions. The failure of standard plate fixation is usually caused by the inadequacy of screw purchase, especially in the distal fragment.

The prominence of the plate, wire, and pin and screw fixation on the superior (subcutaneous) aspect of the clavicle is often uncomfortable and sometimes disabling when wearing a bra or carrying a backpack. This is often a reason for hardware removal, requiring a second operation. Only two patients in our series needed hardware removal because of discomfort. This pertained to the lag screw that was placed outside the plate from superior to inferior (the plate itself did not need removal), illustrating the benefit of the anteroinferior aspect plate and lag screws.

Intraarticular fractures can lead to posttraumatic arthritis. This is more common for the AC than for the sternoclavicular joint. If nonoperative measures fail, the patient might be a candidate for a resection of the medial or lateral aspect. The resection of the medial end of the clavicle should be carefully weighed, because the reconstruction of the sternoclavicular joint is notoriously difficult.

RECOMMENDED READING

1. Boehme, D., Curtis, R.J., DeHaan, J.T., et al.: Nonunion of fractures of the midshaft of the clavicle: treatment with a modified Hagie pin and autogenous bone-grafting. *J Bone Joint Surg Am* 73: 1219–1226, 1991.
2. Boyer, M.I., Axelrod, T.S.: Atrophic nonunion of the clavicle: treatment by compression plate, lag-screw fixation and bone graft. *J Bone Joint Surg Br* 79: 301–303, 1997.
3. Edwards, S.G., Whittle, A.P., Wood, G.W.: Nonoperative treatment of ipsilateral fractures of the scapula and clavicle. *J Bone Joint Surg Am* 82: 774–780, 2000.
4. Goldfarb, C.A., Bassett, G.S., Sullivan, S., et al.: Retrosternal displacement after physeal fracture of the medial clavicle in children. *J Bone Joint Surg Br* 83: 1168–1172, 2001.
5. Jupiter, J.B., Leffert, R.L.: Non-union of the clavicle: associated complications and surgical management. *J Bone Joint Surg Am* 69: 753–760, 1987.
6. Kloen, P., Sorkin, A.T., Rubel, I.F., et al.: Anteroinferior plating of midshaft clavicular nonunions. *J Orthop Trauma* 16:425–430, 2002.
7. Lazarus, M.D.: Fractures of the clavicle. In: Bucholz, R.W., Heckman, J.D., eds.: *Fractures in adults,* 5th ed. Philadelphia: Lippincott Williams & Wilkins, 1041–1078, 2001.
8. Lyons, F.A., Rockwood, C.A.: Current concepts review: migration of pins used in operations on the shoulder. *J Bone Joint Surg Am* 72: 1262–1267, 1990.
9. Neer, C.S.: Fractures of the distal third of the clavicle. *Clin Orthop Rel Res* 58: 43–50, 1968.
10. Nordqvist, A., Petersson, C., Redlund-Johnell, I.: The natural course of lateral clavicle fracture. *Acta Orthop Scan* 64: 87–91, 1993.
11. Ring, D., Jupiter, J.B., Miller, M.E., et al.: Fractures of the clavicle. In: Browner, B.D., Levine, A.M., Jupiter, J.B., et al., eds.: *Skeletal trauma,* 2nd ed. Philadelphia: WB Saunders, 1670–1694, 1992.

22

Operative Treatment of Three-part Proximal Humeral Fractures

Theodore F. Schlegel and Richard J. Hawkins

Displaced three-part proximal humeral fractures remain a challenging problem for the orthopaedic surgeon. Neer's (6) experience with proximal humeral fractures has greatly facilitated a rational guideline for their treatment based on a well-designed classification scheme. Successful treatment relies on the surgeon's ability to make an accurate diagnosis, which requires a thorough understanding of the complex shoulder anatomy coupled with a precise radiographic examination. Appropriate and realistic goals need to be established in all cases. The patient's general medical health, physiologic age, and ability to cooperate with intense and prolonged rehabilitation need to be considered when deciding on treatment.

INDICATIONS/CONTRAINDICATIONS

The primary indications for open reduction and internal fixation (ORIF) of displaced three-part proximal humeral fractures are those occurring in bone of satisfactory quality that permits rigid internal fixation and in young active patients who can tolerate the lengthy postoperative rehabilitation program. Alternatively, in patients who are elderly or infirm with poor bone quality or extensive comminution of the proximal humeral fragments, or in those whom secure internal fixation is likely to be tenuous, consideration might be given for nonoperative treatment or primary prosthetic arthroplasty.

While a number of methods of internal fixation have been described for proximal humeral fractures, we have found that most patients are quite satisfactorily treated with ORIF and tension-band wiring. This method is not technically demanding and in addition to the bone fixation, the tendinous insertion of the rotator cuff is incorporated into the repair.

T. F. Schlegel, M.D.: Englewood, Colorado.

R. J. Hawkins, M.D.: Department of Orthopaedics, University of Colorado, Denver; and Steadman Hawkins Clinic, Vail, Colorado.

The proximal humerus consists of four well-defined parts, which include the humeral head, the lesser and greater tuberosities, and the proximal humeral shaft. There exists a well-defined relationship between those parts, with the neck-shaft inclination angle measuring an average of 145 degrees in relationship to the shaft and retroverted on average 30 degrees. The proximal humerus develops from three distinct ossification centers, including one for the humeral head and one each for the lesser and greater tuberosities. The humeral head ossification center usually appears between the fourth and six months of life. The ossification center of the greater tuberosity arises during the third year of life and the lesser tuberosities fuse together by the fifth year of life, and, in turn, fuse with the humeral head during the seventh year of life. Usually by the age of 19, the head and shaft have fused together. The fusion of the ossification centers creates a weakened area in the construct, known as the epiphyseal scar, making these regions of the proximal humerus susceptible to fracture.

The rotator cuff and shoulder girdle muscles create forces on the proximal humerus as a result of their inherent pull. This balance is disrupted when one or several of the parts of the proximal humerus are fractured. Understanding these deforming forces will facilitate treatment.

The pectoralis major and deltoid are most influential on the shaft, or the distal fracture segment. The pectoralis major inserts along the lateral lip of the proximal bicipital groove, having the greatest effect on the humeral shaft, displacing it anterior and medial. The deltoid, with its more distal insertion on the humeral shaft, is a less deforming force on the distal fracture segment.

The proximal fragments, consisting of the articular head segment as well as the lesser and greater tuberosities, are most influenced by the rotator cuff musculature. Three of the four rotator cuff muscles, including the supraspinatus, infraspinatus, and teres minor, insert onto the greater tuberosity, creating an outward rotational force on the humeral head. The outward rotational force is opposed by the subscapularis muscle, which inserts on the lesser tuberosity, producing an inward rotational force on the head. In the uninjured state, a dynamic balance of these two forces exists. When there is a disruption of these forces, as in the case of a fracture of one of the tuberosity segments, a predictable rotatory deformity of the head occurs.

If the greater tuberosity is fractured, the attached cuff muscles will tend to pull the tuberosity superiorly and posteriorly into an externally rotated position, while the humeral head tends to rotate medially, secondary to the unopposed pull of the subscapularis. In cases in which the lesser tuberosity is fractured, the subscapularis will pull the detached tuberosity medially, while the humeral head will rotate posteriorly and externally as a result of the unopposed pull by the supraspinatus, infraspinatus, and teres minor. Understanding the deformities created by the shoulder girdle and rotator cuff muscles will assist in the classification and treatment of these fractures.

Disruption of the arterial blood supply to the proximal humerus from trauma or surgical intervention can result in avascular necrosis of the humeral head. There are three main arterial contributions to the proximal humerus. The major arterial contribution to the humeral head segment is the superior humeral circumflex artery (Fig. 22-1). This usually lies anterior to the humeral shaft, traveling medial to lateral to anastomose with the posterior humeral circumflex. During its course, it gives off an anterolateral ascending branch. This ascending branch runs parallel to the lateral aspect of the long head of the biceps tendon and enters the humeral head where the proximal end of the intertrabecular groove meets the greater tuberosity. The terminal portion of this vessel, the arcuate artery, is interosseous in nature and perfuses the entire epiphysis. If this vessel is injured, only an anastomosis distal to the lesion can compensate for the resulting loss of blood supply.

Less significant blood supply to the humeral head is delivered by a branch of the posterior humeral circumflex artery and the small vessels entering through the rotator cuff insertions. The posterior humeral circumflex artery, which penetrates the posteromedial cortex of the humeral head, is believed to supply only a small portion of the posteroinferior part of the articular surface of the humerus. The vessels that enter the epiphysis via the rotator cuff insertions are also believed to be inconsequential as well as inconsistent in their vascular supply to the humeral head when compared to the arcuate artery.

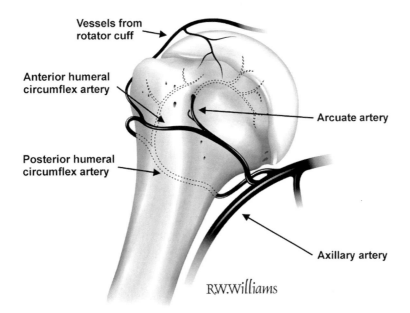

Figure 22-1. Blood supply of the proximal humerus.

Classification

A wide array of classification systems has been proposed. In the past, they have been based on the anatomic level of location of the fracture, mechanism of injury, amount of contact by fracture fragments, degree of displacement, and vascular status of the articular segments. These systems have failed in their ability to provide a functional classification system with an inability to reproduce diagnosis and treat these complex injuries.

Codman (1) was the first to propose that fractures of the proximal humerus occurred in four parts: the greater tuberosity, the lesser tuberosity, the head, and the shaft. He appreciated that the fracture lines followed the old healed epiphyseal plates, delineating the tuberosities and anatomic head from the diaphysis. This was a significant advancement in the understanding of the proximal humeral fractures and their treatment.

In 1970, Neer (5,6) described a classification based on the displacement of these four segments. Later, he eliminated numbered groups and detailed the application of the simplified version, referring only to the segments involved. A segment is considered to be displaced if it is separated from its neighboring segment by more than 1 cm or angulated more than 45 degrees. The fracture pattern refers to the number of displaced parts (segments: two-part, three-part, or four-part). Comminution in a number of fracture fragments or lines is irrelevant unless they fit into a previously described classification. Unfortunately, Neer's system does not consider all the various subpatterns that affect treatment, but it is the accepted standardized classification, at least in North America.

It is important to appreciate that the terminology used to identify proximal humeral fractures denotes first the "pattern of displacement" and second the "key segment" displaced. Thus in the three-part pattern, a displaced tuberosity is always considered the key segment even though a displaced shaft segment is also present (e.g., three-part greater tuberosity displacement). With fracture–dislocations, the fracture pattern is again identified first, but the direction of the dislocation replaces the key segment in the description. A fracture tuberosity segment is always displaced in the direction opposite the dislocation. Therefore, a three-part anterior fracture–dislocation would refer to anterior dislocation of the head and attached lesser tuberosity and posterior displacement of the greater tuberosity. The position of the associated displaced shaft segment is variable.

PREOPERATIVE PLANNING

An accurate diagnosis is essential for the proper treatment of proximal humeral fractures. Three radiographic views are required in any shoulder injury to ensure consistent identification of fracture types (Fig. 22-2). Radiographs of the injured shoulder are taken first, perpendicular to, and second, parallel to, the scapular plane (5). Although fracture fragments may be shifted with any movement of the patient's arm, it is nevertheless important to consider the axillary view in 20 to 40 degrees of abduction essential as a third view, for three reasons. First, it contributes valuable additional information regarding the fracture configuration, since it is oriented at right angles to the two previous views. Second, it is the most reliable means of detecting a locked posterior dislocation with an impression fracture. Third, it provides assessment of the glenoid margins. Each of these views may be obtained with terminal extension and the patient in a standing, sitting, or supine position. These three plain radiographs are sufficient to make an accurate diagnosis. On occasion, computed tomography will be helpful in further defining the magnitude of humeral head defects and assessing glenoid pathologies.

SURGERY

The treatment of displaced three-part proximal humeral fractures is based on proper classification of the fracture type, appreciation of the patient's activity level, and experience of the treating surgeon. Appropriate and realistic goals need to be established. The patient's general medical health, physiologic age, and ability to cooperate with an intense and prolonged rehabilitation should be considered. Based on these features, some patients should not be exposed to operative intervention. It is imperative that there is full appreciation of the fracture pattern, bone quality, and associated injuries when deciding on the method of treatment. Finally, a self-appraisal with regard to knowledge and expertise must be made by the treating surgeon. These complex proximal humeral fractures can challenge even the most experienced shoulder surgeons.

Tension-band Wire Technique

Our preferred method of treatment is based on experience, which was published documenting satisfactory results in a series of 14 patients with three-part proximal humeral fractures (3). The advantages of this method of management include adequate visualization of the fracture fragments, ensuring appropriate reduction with minimal soft-tissue stripping; preservation of the vascular supply to the humeral head; and secure fixation of the fracture fragments, relying on soft tissue and not bone. Complications with this treatment have been

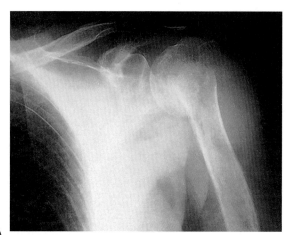

A

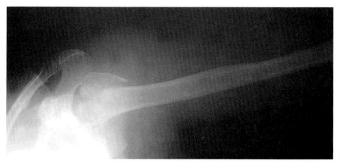

B

Figure 22-2. A,B: Anteroposterior and axillary view radiographs demonstrating a greater tuberosity three-part proximal humeral fracture. Although not shown here, a view parallel to the scapular plane (Y-scapular) radiograph should be obtained to ensure an accurate diagnosis.

reported to be minimal. Avascular necrosis of the humeral head did develop in two patients, only one of whom was symptomatic enough to require revision to hemiarthroplasty. It is unknown if the avascular necrosis was secondary to the initial trauma or a result of surgery. Nevertheless, despite these two cases, the overall complication rate was low and functional results were good.

Tension-band wiring has become the accepted method of treatment for three-part proximal humeral fractures because it allows for reduction and secure enough fixation of the fracture fragments to allow early passive range of motion. It is important to realize that tension-band wiring alone is not satisfactory for two-part shaft displacement fractures. For some reason, the fracture construction is too often unstable, hinging on the tension-band side. This has been our experience and has been recently reported by Koval et al. (4).

Patient Positioning and Preparation

The patient is positioned on the operating room table in a semisitting beach-chair position, intubated, and the head is rotated to the contralateral side. To prevent the patient from sliding down the operating room table, a pillow is placed behind the knees and a seat belt is placed across the patient's thighs. A bladder of a blood pressure cuff may be positioned underneath the ipsilateral scapula and inflated to bring the shoulder into the most advantageous position for surgical approach. A sterile drape is placed across the neck to prevent hair and saliva from contaminating the wound. Intravenous antibiotics are administered to the patient 30 minutes before surgical incision and two doses are given postoperatively. Preoperatively, the patient is instructed to scrub the shoulder and axillary region for a total of 5 minutes with a Hibiclens (AstraZeneca, London, United Kingdom) solution. This allows for the use of a single-step preparation, consisting of a Betadine solution in an alcohol base, to provide antimicrobial properties and to enhance the ability of the drapes to adhere to the patient, maintaining a sterile field. A sterile stockinette allows free manipulation of the arm. A large sterile drape may be applied anteriorly and then wrapped completely and circumferentially to seal off the axilla and to hold the drapes in the appropriate position.

Technique

Bony landmarks are outlined with a surgical marker. An extended deltopectoral approach is used, measuring 12 to 15 cm in length, originating at the anterolateral corner of the acromion, curving toward the coracoid, and ending at the deltoid insertion. The cephalic vein in this case is taken medially so that it is not traumatized during the extensive dissection. If the vein is taken laterally, often excessive tension is placed on the vein, leading to rupture. The insertion of the pectoralis major is partially released for exposure. Abducting the humerus during the procedure aids in relaxing the deltoid. If excessive deltoid tension is present, a transverse division of the anterior 1 cm of the deltoid insertion distally improves exposure and, more important, lessens damage to the deltoid. Blunt dissection is then carried out in the subacromial space to free up any adhesions. A deltoid retractor is placed deep to the deltoid and acromion and superficial to the rotator cuff and humeral head. The coracoacromial ligament may be released superiorly for improved exposure.

The long head of the biceps tendon serves as the key landmark in separating the greater and lesser tuberosity segments, allowing identification of the fracture fragments. Almost all of these fractures involve the greater tuberosity. The fracture pattern is visually confirmed by verifying that the lesser tuberosity remains attached to the humeral head, the displaced greater tuberosity with its attached supraspinatus tendon lies laterally and posteriorly, and there is displacement between the humeral head and shaft. The articular surface of the humeral head is usually directed posteriorly, away from the glenoid fossa, often facing lateral (Fig. 22-3). It is necessary to free the humeral head by blunt dissection and confirm that the head does not have a rare impaction or head-splitting fracture.

A stay suture is placed into the supraspinatus tendon and greater tuberosity, allowing for mobilization of this fragment (Fig. 22-4). This will aid in reduction of the fragment back to

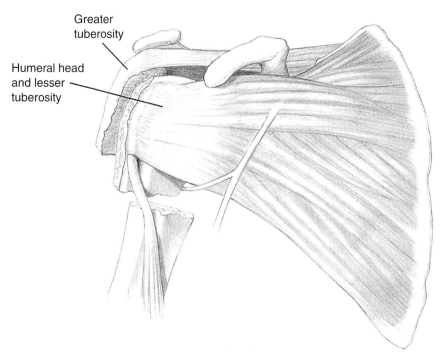

Figure 22-3. A three-part fracture with displaced greater tuberosity and an unimpacted displaced segment of the head.

the bed from which it was avulsed. The humeral head can then be reduced with external rotation of the arm and pushing on the head fragment while rotating it into the glenoid fossa. Simultaneously, the greater tuberosity fragment is brought down to its anatomic position, which assists in holding the head reduced.

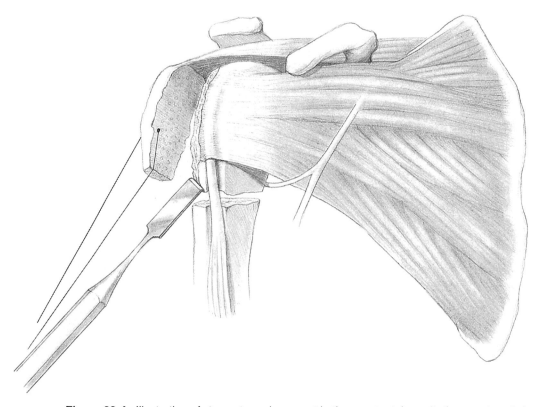

Figure 22-4. Illustration of stay suture placement in the greater tuberosity fragment and elevation of the rotated humeral head fragment.

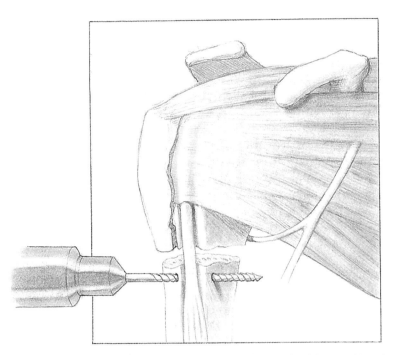

Figure 22-5. Illustration of drill hole placement in the proximal humeral head shaft deep to the bicipital groove for wire placement.

Two sets of drill holes are made perpendicular to the long axis of the shaft through the anterior aspect of the proximal portion of the distal shaft fragment, on each side of the bicipital groove (Fig. 22-5). A 14-gauge, large-bore colpotomy needle (Fig. 22-6), with its stylet in place, is passed through the supraspinatus tendon and its attached greater tuberosity, through the head, and out through the lesser tuberosity and subscapularis tendon (Fig. 22-7). The 18- or 20-gauge wire is then fed from medial to lateral through the first drill hole in the humeral shaft (Fig. 22-8). The needle is then withdrawn to deliver the wire through the above segments. A second wire is passed in a similar manner by placing the colpotomy needle 1 cm above and parallel to the first wire.

The head is then reduced onto the humeral shaft. The free end of the first wire, which lies lateral to the humerus, is then crossed over the fracture site to the medial aspect of the distal fragment segment and passed through the drill hole from medial to lateral (Fig. 22-9).

(text continues on page 422.)

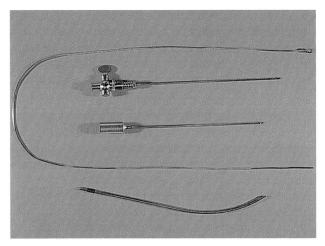

Figure 22-6. Assortment of large needles that can be used to pass cerclage wire; *(top)* medium Verres needle and stylet; *(bottom)* Dingman needle (colpotomy needle not pictured).

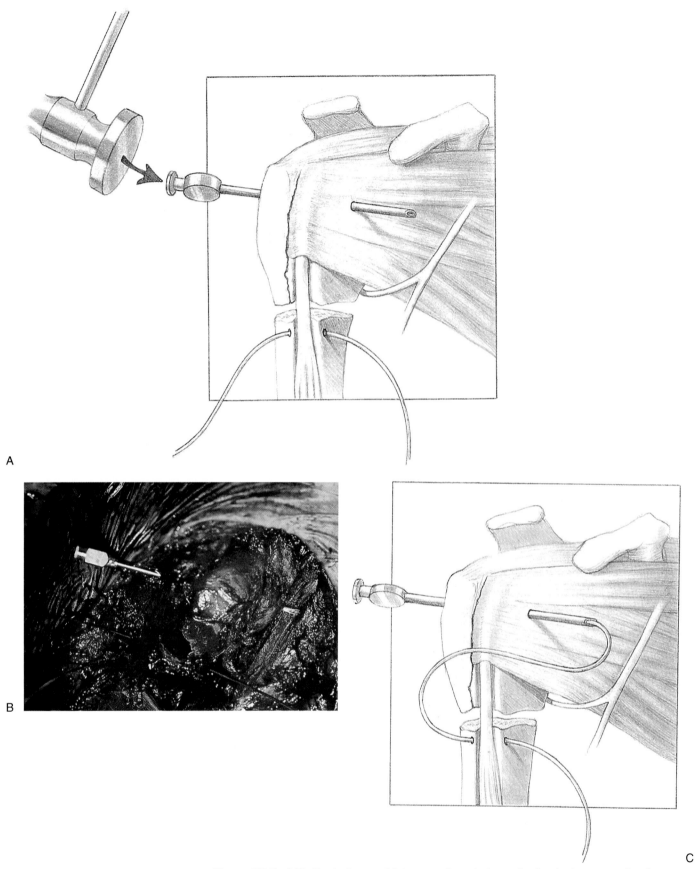

Figure 22-7. A,B: Illustration and intraoperative photograph of colpotomy needle placement through the reduced greater tuberosity and humeral head and attached lesser tuberosity fragment. Note incorporation of the rotator cuff and subscapularis tendons. **C:** Illustration of wire passage through colpotomy needle in figure-eight fashion.

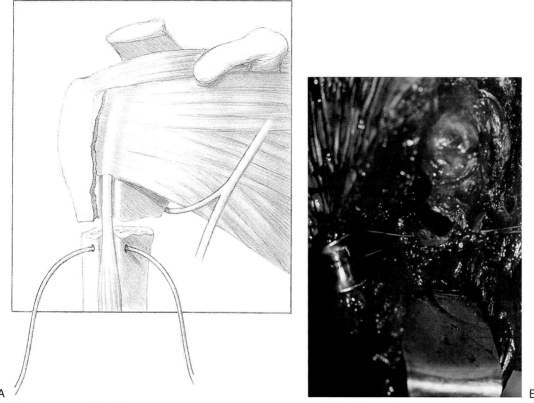

A

B

Figure 22-8. A,B: Illustration and intraoperative photograph showing placement of two twenty-gauge wires deep to the bicipital groove in the humeral shaft.

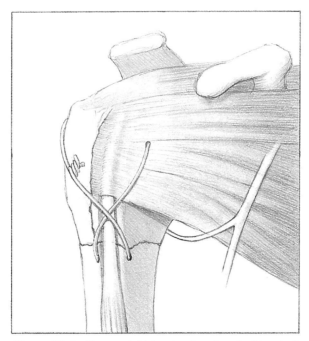

Figure 22-9. Figure-eight tension-band and wiring technique before placement of second wire.

The second wire is passed in an identical fashion through the remaining holes. With the fracture reduced, the wires are secured using a wire tightener (Fig. 22-10). The result is a figure-eight pattern with tension-band wiring of the fracture (Fig. 22-11).

Crossing the wires over the site of the fracture brings the segments of the head and shaft together and compresses the segments of the head and greater tuberosity, thus converting the three-part pattern to a stable one-piece unit. Occasionally, in more stable constructs, one

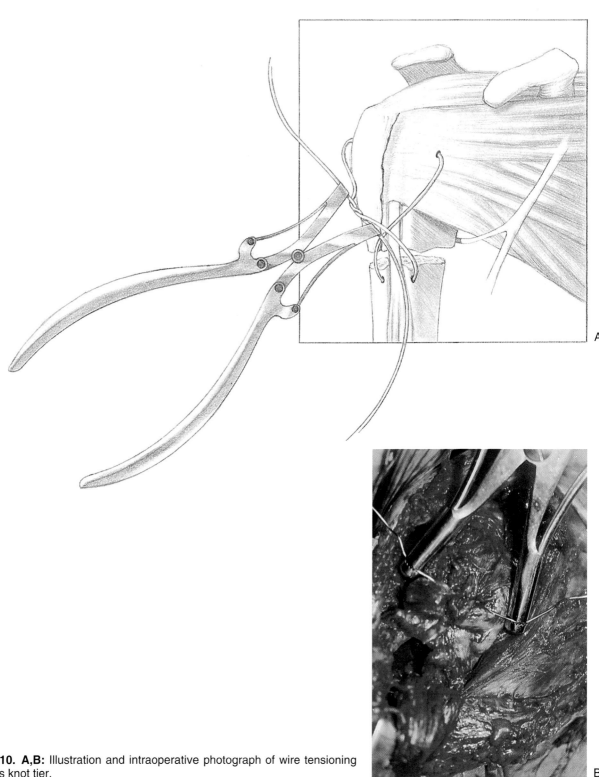

A

B

Figure 22-10. A,B: Illustration and intraoperative photograph of wire tensioning using Harris knot tier.

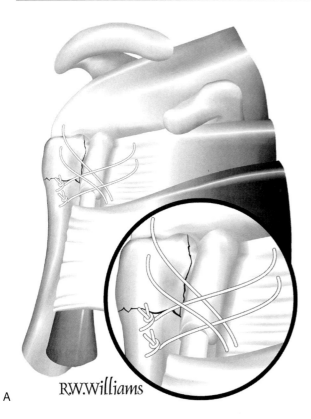

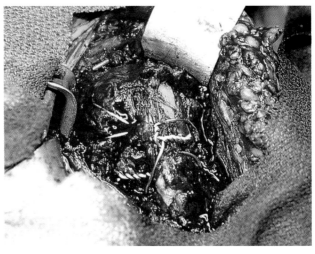

B

A   R.W.Williams

Figure 22-11. A,B: Illustration and intraoperative photograph of final construct with both figure-eight wires in place. Note large rent between subscapularis and supraspinatus tendons.

wire is sufficient. Strong nonabsorbable suture such as a no. 5 could be used, but in our experience it does not cinch down as effectively and does not provide as much stability as wire. The rent between the supraspinatus and subscapularis tendons is then repaired, and the shoulder is carefully moved through a range of motion to confirm the stability of the fracture. Before closure, it is imperative to confirm that the humeral head is reduced within the glenoid.

POSTOPERATIVE MANAGEMENT

Usually, secure fixation of the fracture fragments is obtained and passive range of motion can begin immediately. If, as rarely occurs, the bone is found to be excessively osteoporotic or the rotator cuff is of poor quality, thereby making the fixation tenuous, the patient may be left relatively immobilized in a sling until secure, usually for 3 weeks.

Rehabilitation

Progression of the rehabilitation program must be individualized to optimize the recovery of the shoulder function. The surgeon and physical therapist must convey to the patient a clear understanding of what is expected for short- and long-term goals. The postoperative management program has three well-defined phases: phase I consists of passive or assisted range of motion; phase II is active range of motion with terminal stretching; phase III is a resisted program with ongoing active motion and terminal stretching.

Phase I begins on day 1, especially with the aid of an interscalene block for early pain control, and continues for 6 weeks. It is essential to confirm that the fracture fragments move in unison, signifying fracture stability. This phase may rarely need to be delayed for up to 4 weeks in some cases if the fixation is not rigid. This phase consists of passive forward elevation, and external and internal rotation of the involved shoulder with the assistance of the contralateral extremity. Assisted exercises begin in the supine position with early emphasis on elevation and external rotation. Pendulum exercises are used as a warm up after a few days. Several days later, those exercises are performed sitting or standing. Toward the end of this initial 6-week phase, isometric strengthening may be added. These exercises are performed by applying gentle resistance to inward and outward rotation when the arm is at the side and the elbow is flexed to 90 degrees. Similar exercises are performed for flexion and extension. These activities need to be monitored carefully by the physician and the physical therapist. They are taught to the patient and the patient's spouse so that they can be carried out at home.

Phase II, commencing at 6 weeks, consists of active range of motion exercises with terminal stretching, beginning once early union has been achieved, confirmed clinically and radiographically. When commencing phase II, resumption of the supine position permits concentration on forward elevation and is often advisable when starting the second phase of the program, at least for a few days until the patient is strong enough to elevate in the upright position. Full active range of motion in all planes is sought during this phase.

Phase III, resisted strengthening, begins 10 weeks after surgery when union is assured and adequate range of motion has been obtained. The challenge to achieve normal shoulder function is met with greater resistance during the strengthening exercises and ongoing terminal stretching program. Maximal recovery is rarely achieved before the first postoperative year. All too frequently, the exercise program is abandoned too early which does not allow the patient to reach full recovery potential.

COMPLICATIONS

There have been many reported complications following closed and open treatment of displaced three-part humeral fractures. These can be thought of as nonspecific or specific to the fracture pattern. Infection, neurovascular injury, malunion/nonunion, hardware failure, joint stiffness, and heterotopic ossification can result after the treatment of any proximal humeral fracture. Avascular necrosis, on the other hand, is more likely to occur in four-part displaced proximal humeral fractures and rarely with three-part fractures (6).

Avascular Necrosis

Although the three-part fracture by definition has one tuberosity remaining to give the humeral head blood supply, late avascular necrosis may occur. This most frequently occurs when the lesser tuberosity remains with the humeral head. This potential complication can be minimized by careful patient selection. If doubt exists about adequacy of bone, adequacy of soft-tissue attachment to residual humeral head or tuberosity structures, or failure to obtain secure internal fixation, the surgeon should proceed directly to a primary prosthetic arthroplasty. Should late collapse of the humeral head from avascular necrosis occur, the degree of symptoms may not warrant further surgical intervention. However, should the patient develop symptomatic avascular necrosis following a complex fracture of the proximal humerus, total shoulder replacement rather than hemiarthroplasty is probably the wisest choice.

Infection

Infection is rare with ORIF of displaced three-part proximal humeral fractures. Fortunately, the proximal humerus has adequate soft-tissue coverage with good vascular supply to the tissues, decreasing the risk of infection. However, infection is still possible and it is for this reason that care should be taken to maintain sterility, administer prophylactic antibiotics, and minimize excessive soft-tissue dissection. Obtaining hemostasis at the time of closure and appropriately draining the wound are important to prevent hematoma formation, which increases the risk for infection.

Neurovascular Injuries

Neurovascular injuries have been well documented following displaced proximal three-part humeral fractures. Stableforth (8) reported a 5% incidence of axillary artery compromise and a 6.2% incidence of brachial plexus injuries. Vascular injury most often is associated with penetrating or violent blunt trauma caused by the initial injury, but also occurs after ORIF (2). If a vascular disruption occurs, the lesion is usually found at the junction of the anterior humeral circumflex and axillary artery. The diagnosis is often difficult to make, because peripheral pulses may be normal as a result of collateral circulation. Paresthesias may be a helpful clinical sign. Since early diagnosis and repair are crucial to the outcome, angiography and exploration should be performed immediately when a vascular injury is suspected.

The axillary nerve is susceptible to injury following fractures and their surgical treatment. The axillary nerve provides motor supply to the deltoid and teres major with sensory distribution over the lateral aspect of the upper arm. Sensation over the lateral deltoid region is not a reliable means of determining if there is an axillary nerve injury. A more reliable means of testing the axillary nerve is palpating all three leaves of the deltoid muscle for contraction. Due to pain in an acute fracture, this is often difficult to accurately assess. Electromyelography should be performed if a nerve injury is suspected. This study should be obtained no earlier than 3 weeks after the injury when the results are most accurate, both for documentation and as a baseline for subsequent comparisons of recovery. Most of these injuries are secondary to a neuropraxia and improve with time. If a complete axillary nerve injury does not improve within a 3- to 6-month period, surgical exploration may be considered.

Malunion

True malunion is unusual with this tension-band technique, because the tuberosities are carefully reapproximated to each other and one tuberosity remains attached to the humeral head, thus minimizing the likelihood that the humeral head position will be a problem. Mild degrees of abnormal angulation of the humeral head relative to the shaft may also occur. These are ordinarily not functionally a problem.

A greater degree of malunion of the proximal humerus can cause significant functional limitations, however. In the case in which the greater tuberosity heals in a superior or medial position, the space beneath the subacromial arch will be limited and impingement will occur when the arm is abducted. This problem can be corrected with a salvage surgical procedure, which requires an osteotomy of the greater tuberosity and mobilization of the rotator cuff. This is often difficult because the anatomy is quite distorted and there is often excessive scarring.

Nonunion

With secure internal fixation by this tension-band method, nonunion is rarely seen. Alternate forms of fixation have been associated with a higher incidence of nonunion; this may be related to the extensive dissection required for other internal fixation devices, or it may be related to poor-quality bone inadequately supporting plates and screws. The possibility of nonunion is minimized by careful attention to intraoperative technique, making certain the fracture is well reduced, carefully controlling the direction and degree of arm movement in the early postoperative rehabilitation period. Should nonunion occur, a second operation of internal fixation and bone grafting or prosthetic arthroplasty is usually required.

Stiffness

Postoperative stiffness is not uncommon after the surgical treatment of this complex fracture. Factors contributing to its development include extensive soft-tissue trauma, delay in surgical intervention, necessary protection of comminuted bone fragments, and inability to aggressively institute active and passive motion until satisfactory early healing has occurred. Early passive range-of-motion exercises within safe ranges, careful monitoring of the postoperative rehabilitation, and careful patient selection minimize the likelihood of the development of stiffness.

Heterotopic Ossification

Heterotopic ossification appears to be related to both forceful attempts at closed reduction and delay in open reduction beyond one week for fracture–dislocations. Inadequate irrigation to wash out bony fragments following ORIF may also increase the risk. Exercises to maintain range of motion should be the mainstay of treatment. After 1 year, if a negative bone scan indicates quiescence, excision of the heterotropic bone with soft-tissue releases may be considered.

Wire Breakage and Hardware Complications

Although wire breakage can occur, particularly if the fracture fails to unite, it is not a common complication. Nevertheless, wire breakage has caused some surgeons to recommend very heavy nonabsorbable suture in this tension-band technique. This seems to be a sensible way to avoid this potential complication without compromising the fixation or result.

RECOMMENDED READING

1. Codman, H.A. *The shoulder.* Boston: Thomas Todd, 1934.
2. Hagg, O., Lundberg, B.: Aspects of prognostic factors of comminuted and dislocated proximal humeral fractures. In: Bateman, J.E., Welsh, R.P., eds.: *Surgery of the shoulder.* Philadelphia: B.C. Decker, 1984.
3. Hawkins, R.J., Bell, R.H., Gurr, K.: The three-part fracture of the proximal part of the humerus: operative treatment. *J Bone Joint Surg Am* 68: 1410, 1986.
4. Koval, K.J, Sanders, R., Zuckerman, J.D., et al.: Modified tension band wiring of displaced surgical neck fractures of the humerus. *J Shoulder Elbow Surg* March/April, 1993.
5. Neer, C.S. II. Displaced proximal humeral fractures, I: classification and evaluation. *J Bone Joint Surg Am* 52: 1077, 1970.
6. Neer, C.S. II: Displaced proximal humeral fractures, II: treatment of three-part and four-part displacement. *J Bone Joint Surg Am* 52: 1090, 1970.
7. Paavolainen, P., Bjorkonheim, J.M., Slads, P., et al.: Operative treatment of severe proximal humeral fractures. *Acta Orthop Scand* 54: 374, 1983.
8. Stableforth, P.G.: Four-part fractures of the neck of the humerus. *J Bone Joint Surg Br* 66: 104, 1954.
9. Sturzenegger, M., Fornaro, E., Jakob, R.P.: Results of surgical treatment of multi-fragmented fractures of the humeral head. *Arch Orthop Trauma Surg* 100: 249, 1982.
10. Tanner, M.W., Cofield, R.H.: Prosthetic arthroplasty for fracture and fracture-dislocations of the proximal humerus. *Clin Orthop* 1979: 116, 1983.

23

Proximal Humeral Arthroplasty for Acute Fractures

Gregory N. Lervick and Louis U. Bigliani

INDICATIONS/CONTRAINDICATIONS

Humeral head replacement (HHR) is a useful surgical technique for many acute displaced fractures of the proximal humerus (Fig. 23-1). The indications for the use of a prosthesis are four-part fractures and fracture dislocations; head-splitting fractures; impression fractures involving over 40% of the articular surface; and selected three-part fractures in older patients with osteoporotic bone (1,7). Most severely displaced proximal humeral fractures occur in the older population, particularly in women. Other treatment options include closed reduction, open reduction–internal fixation, head excision, and fusion. Recently, there has been some enthusiasm for percutaneous fixation of valgus-impacted three- and four-part fractures. This may be considered if the fragments remain in reasonable apposition and the medial periosteal sleeve is intact. These forms of treatment have yielded a high percentage of unsatisfactory results in most series, however (2,4).

The contraindications for this procedure are active soft-tissue infection, chronic osteomyelitis, and paralysis of the rotator cuff muscles. Deltoid paralysis is not a contraindication: Adequate yet compromised function can be achieved in such a shoulder.

PREOPERATIVE PLANNING

A detailed history and physical examination are essential, although an adequate clinical evaluation of the injured limb may be difficult because of pain and swelling. It is important

G. N. Lervick, M.D.: Department of Orthopaedics, Park Nicollet Clinic/Methodist Hospital, St. Louis Park, Minnesota.

L. U. Bigliani, M.D.: Department of Orthopaedic Surgery, Columbia University Center for Shoulder, Elbow and Sports Medicine; and Orthopaedic Surgery Service, Columbia-Presbyterian Medical Center, New York, New York.

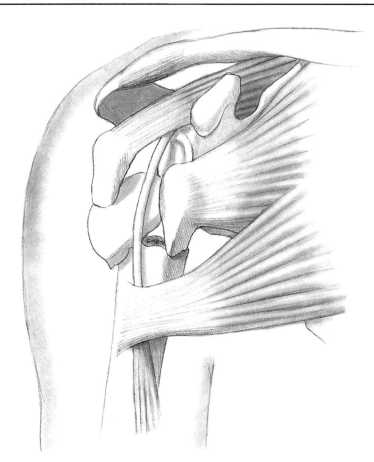

Figure 23-1. A four-part fracture of the proximal humerus. The humeral head is free-floating and displaced from both tuberosities and the shaft. The lesser tuberosity fragment is pulled medially by the subscapularis, the greater tuberosity fragment is pulled posteriorly and superiorly by the supraspinatus and infraspinatus, and the shaft fragment is pulled medially by the pectoralis major.

to establish if the patient has lost consciousness or has had a seizure. Assess the neurovascular status with a high index of suspicion for injuries to the axillary nerve and artery. We treat any injury to the axillary artery as a limb-threatening emergency, evaluate with urgent arteriography, and obtain a vascular surgery consultation. Injuries to the brachial plexus or peripheral nerves can initially be treated conservatively. Electromyographic analysis should be planned 3 to 4 weeks after injury to help clarify the extent of the injury. Do not delay definitive management of the fracture because of a suspected neurologic deficiency. Most injuries are neuropraxias and will resolve over time. If there is no improvement in the neurologic status in the first 3 months after injury, consider further evaluation. Operative exploration with neurolysis and/or nerve grafting may be beneficial, and should be performed in the first 3 to 6 months after injury.

We clearly delineate the fracture pattern on preoperative radiographs. In most cases, this can be done with a standard trauma series (Fig. 23-2). This includes a true anteroposterior (AP) view of the scapula (taken 30 to 40 degrees oblique to the coronal plane of the body), a transscapular lateral or Y view, and an axillary lateral view. The axillary view is taken by abducting the arm 20 to 30 degrees and placing the tube in the axilla with the radiographic plate above the shoulder; there is no need to fully abduct the arm. Often the surgeon must position the arm because of pain. Alternatively, obtain a Velpeau axillary view with the patient remaining in the sling and leaning back over the plate and the tube directed downward. If displacement cannot be determined, or if the anatomy of the articular surface of the humeral head or the glenoid is not clearly defined, obtain a computed tomography scan to

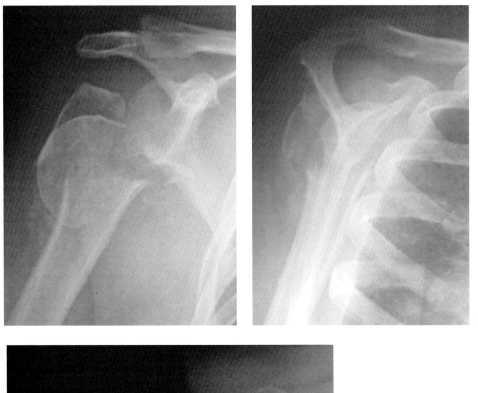

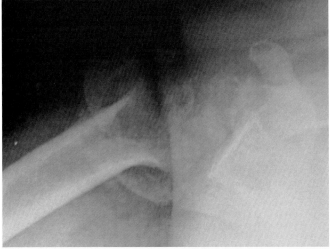

Figure 23-2. A: Anteroposterior radiograph of a four-part fracture. **B:** Lateral view in the scapular plane. **C:** Axillary lateral view.

assist with the diagnosis. Use of a preoperative scanogram of the involved and uninvolved arms often helps establish the proper length of the prosthesis relative to the remaining humeral shaft. In addition, consider obtaining standard radiographs of the contralateral shoulder and using them for preoperative templating.

SURGERY

Patient Positioning

Proper patient positioning is the first step to a successful procedure and its importance cannot be overemphasized. The goal is to have access to the superior, inferior, medial, and lateral aspects of the shoulder. This is achieved by having the involved shoulder elevated from

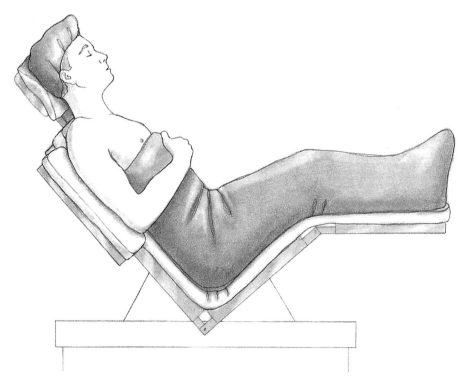

Figure 23-3. Place the patient in a modified beach-chair position with the back flexed approximately 30 to 40 degrees and the lateral border of the scapula and thorax at the edge of the table.

the table and properly supported. We prefer interscalene regional block anesthesia, as it provides excellent muscle relaxation and facilitates exposure. Bring the patient to the edge of the table such that the arm is free, but the lateral border of the scapula and thorax remain supported (Fig. 23-3). Place two small towels under the medial border of the scapula so that the shoulder is elevated off the edge of the table. Remove the top portion of the operating table, and secure the head on a well-padded headrest with the cervical spine in neutral position. Next, place the operating table in a modified beach-chair position by first flexing the table maximally, and then raising the back while slightly lowering the foot of the bed. Elevate the back of the operating table so that the patient sits up at an angle of approximately 30 to 40 degrees. Alternatively, use an operating table designed specifically for shoulder surgery, with an elevated back support and removable lateral portion that leaves the shoulder girdle exposed. Either method will allow adequate superior access to the shoulder. Use a small armboard at the level of the humeral shaft to support the elbow and forearm during the surgery. The armboard may need to be shifted either superiorly or inferiorly to allow enough arm extension for preparation of the shaft. Apply surgical draping to allow exposure to the mid clavicle and axilla, so that the arm is draped free and can be moved throughout the surgery.

Technique

Approach. Use a long deltopectoral approach starting just below the clavicle and extending over the lateral aspect of the coracoid to the deltoid insertion on the humeral shaft (Fig. 23-4). Place large Gelpi retractors in the superficial subcutaneous layer to provide exposure. Identify the cephalic vein in the deltopectoral interval and retract it laterally with the deltoid. There are fewer tributary veins on the medial side than on the lateral side, so retracting the vein laterally generally minimizes bleeding. There is often a large crossover vein superiorly that should be cauterized prior to gaining full superior exposure. It is im-

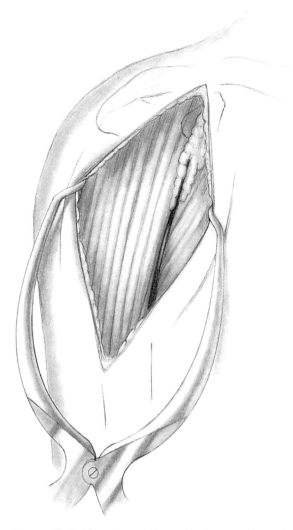

Figure 23-4. Use a long deltopectoral approach starting just below the clavicle and extending over the lateral aspect of the coracoid to the deltoid insertion on the humeral shaft.

portant to preserve the deltoid origin on the clavicle and acromion and its insertion on the humerus. Partially release the proximal aspect of the lateral pectoralis insertion for about one half of its length, and tag with a retention suture to allow later reattachment (Fig. 23-5). Next, identify the coracoid and strap muscles. The coracoid is a lighthouse to the shoulder; avoid dissection medial to this structure, unless the head is displaced (Fig. 23-6). Place a broad retractor beneath the lateral borders of the strap muscles. Do not divide the coracoid muscles or osteotomize the coracoid process, because they provide a barrier to protect the neurovascular bundle. Resect the leading edge of the anterior portion of the coracoacromial (CA) ligament if necessary to facilitate proximal exposure. However, take care to not remove more than the leading edge, as this may compromise superior stability. Place another retractor underneath the deltoid and retract the muscle laterally. Identify the long head of the biceps brachii (LHB) distally and follow it proximally, as this leads to its glenoid insertion and the center of the shoulder (Fig. 23-7).

Exposure of the Fracture. Once deep retractors have been placed in appropriate position, identify and gently excise the hemorrhagic bursa and clavipectoral fascia. This allows exposure of the fracture site and evacuation of the fracture hematoma. Do not remove any substantial fragments of bone that may help support the prosthesis on the shortened

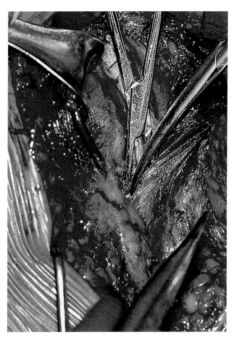

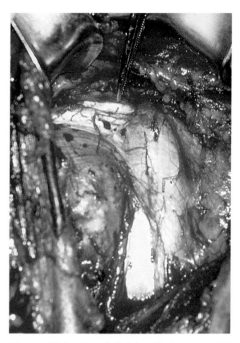

Figure 23-5. We typically detach the superior insertion of the pectoralis major to improve the exposure.

Figure 23-6. Carefully identify the coracoid process, coracoacromial ligament, and conjoined tendon. Define the lateral border of the strap musculature. We often resect the leading edge of the coracoacromial ligament to maximize the proximal exposure. Take care to avoid dissection medial to the strap muscles, as the neurovascular structures are within close proximity.

proximal shaft. The key to recognizing the various components of the fracture is the LHB. As the biceps is followed proximally, the lesser tuberosity is typically on the medial side and the greater tuberosity is on the lateral side (Fig. 23-7). In general, release the soft-tissue attachments between the tuberosity fragments at the rotator interval. The tuberosities are typically fractured in this region of the bicipital groove; opening this interval will allow later mobilization of both tuberosities and allow safe, atraumatic removal of the head (Fig.

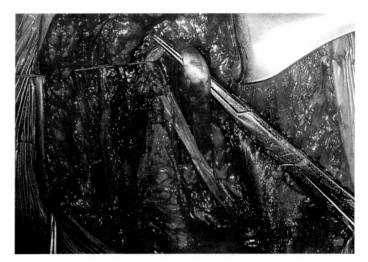

Figure 23-7. Identify the distal portion of the long head of the biceps and follow it proximally. This will help differentiate between the lesser and greater tuberosities and define the rotator interval.

23-8). Use caution when removing the head if it is dislocated anteriorly below the coracoid and under the coracoid muscles, because the neurovascular structures are in close proximity and can be injured by errant dissection. When treatment has been delayed beyond 7 to 10 days, adhesions and early scarring make mobilization even more difficult and potentially dangerous. Perform the dissection carefully in a lateral-to-medial direction and be patient and cautious with head extraction. It is a good idea to have a vascular surgeon available in this situation, given the relative risk of vascular injury.

In rare instances where the head has been dislocated laterally, it may be possible to remove the head and place the prosthesis without disturbing the rotator interval or the soft-tissue attachment between the tuberosities. In this situation, leave the greater and lesser tuberosities together and elevate them as a unit, or "hood." Generally, however, the interval must be opened in the area of the bicipital groove to allow atraumatic removal of the head. In either case, preserve any loose fragments or cancellous bone, including the humeral head, and save them as autogenous graft.

Tuberosity mobilization is critical to adequate reduction and fixation to the shaft. Tag the LHB with a nylon suture and protect it. Begin to mobilize the tuberosities with an elevator and tag with no. 2 nonabsorbable suture. Use swedged-on needles and place them into the tendon proximal to the tuberosity insertion, thereby preserving the integrity of the tuberosity and avoiding further comminution of the fragment. Adequate tuberosity mobilization should be obtained laterally, posteriorly, superiorly, and medially.

We also evaluate the patient for external subacromial impingement. If there is a large subacromial spur in the CA ligament, or if the patient has an impingement configuration of the acromion, it may be worthwhile to perform an anterior acromioplasty. This is not a routine part of the procedure. If an acromioplasty is performed, we recommend a very conservative bony resection, and preservation and repair of the CA ligament to the medial acromion using nonabsorbable nylon sutures. Also, evaluate the patient for a tear in the rotator cuff. Generally, the rotator cuff is intact in this group of patients, unless there is pre-existing cuff disease.

Shaft Preparation and Prosthesis Placement. The proximal shaft of the humerus should be dealt with in a very gentle manner. The bone is often osteoporotic, and there may

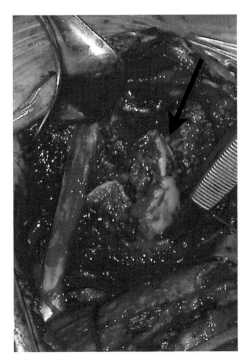

Figure 23-8. The humeral head (*arrow*) is usually a free-floating fragment that can be removed using a metal finger.

be an undisplaced fracture of the shaft, which should be recognized. If there is a shaft component to the fracture, perform fixation before implantation of the prosthesis. This can usually be achieved with cerclage wires and/or heavy nonabsorbable sutures. The addition of the prosthesis and cement usually provides a stable reconstruction with adequate support. Before exposing the shaft, move the armboard either up or down the table to allow the arm to be extended and externally rotated. Lifting the elbow in a distal-to-proximal direction will bring the shaft into the wound. Place medial and lateral Darrach retractors posterior to the shaft for full exposure. Next, prepare the medullary canal with sequential reamers (Fig. 23-9).

It is vitally important to determine proper size and position of the prosthesis. This involves three aspects: retroversion, height, and head size. The current generation of modular prosthetic shoulder implants greatly increases the ability to recreate proximal humeral anatomy. In addition, improved instrumentation allows reproducible version assessment and the ability to trial numerous head sizes and offsets that will maximize motion, stability, and tuberosity repair.

Version may be assessed with use of an intramedullary alignment system equipped with an outrigger that references the forearm (Fig. 23-10). Remember that normal proximal humeral anatomy is variable. We generally position the implant in approximately 25 to 30 degrees of retroversion. The only exception to this rule would be a chronic posterior fracture dislocation, in which case we may choose less retroversion. Other techniques to assess version include positioning of the fins of the prosthesis relative to the distal aspect of the

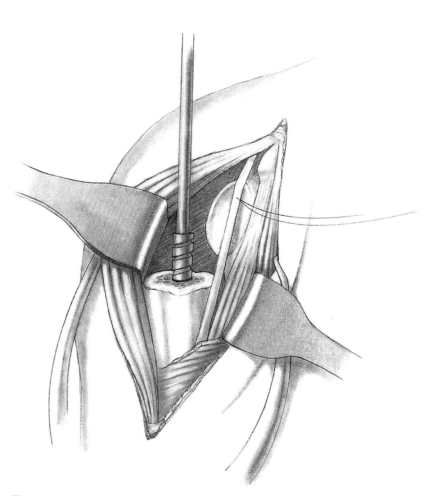

Figure 23-9. Prepare the medullary canal with sequential handheld reamers prior to cement fixation.

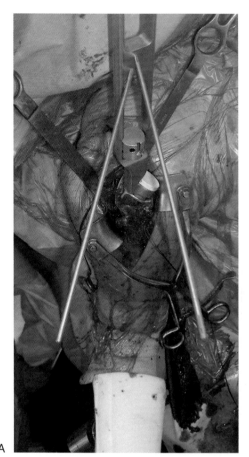

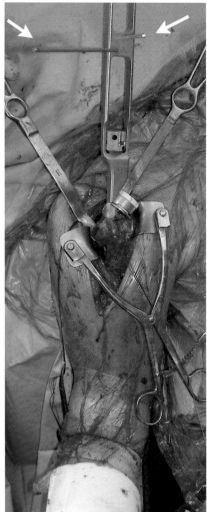

A   B

Figure 23-10. A,B: The use of an instrumentation system with an outrigger (*arrows*) that references the forearm is helpful in assessing retroversion of the component. With the arm in neutral rotation, the humeral head should face the glenoid.

bicipital groove, and palpating and referencing the epicondylar axis of the elbow (Fig. 23-11). Perform the final assessment of version later, when the trial head has been placed and the prosthesis is reduced. Once reduced, the prosthesis should be stable both anteriorly and posteriorly. If the prosthesis subluxates or dislocates posteriorly, there likely is too much retroversion, and this should be decreased. Alternatively, if the prosthesis is unstable anteriorly, this suggests the retroversion is inadequate, and it should be increased. Correct version of the prosthesis will maximize glenohumeral stability, and allow for adequate internal and external rotation of the arm.

Next, assess the height of the prosthesis and size of the head. Seat the trial stem within the canal. Do not seat the collar of the prosthesis so deeply that it is placed against the remaining proximal shaft, because this will usually decrease the length of the humerus and shorten the myofascial sleeve, compromising the mechanical advantage of the deltoid. In general, elevate the collar above the proximal shaft to a position that will allow space for both the greater and the lesser tuberosities to be placed below the level of the head. When the greater tuberosity is reduced, its proximal portion should clear the head and overlap the proximal shaft by only a few millimeters. Use a trial stem with an interference fit to assist

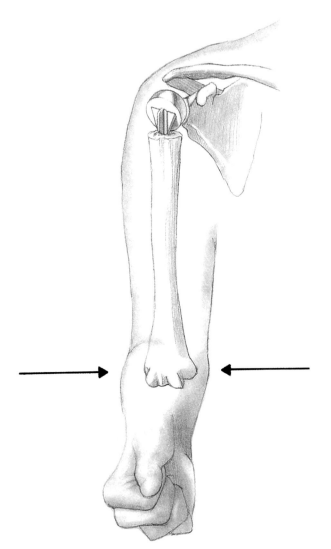

Figure 23-11. Alternatively, palpate the distal humeral epicondyles with the thumb and forefinger. Depending on the implant being used, the fins of the prosthesis can be oriented with reference to the bicipital groove. In fractures, the distal portion of the groove may still be visualized.

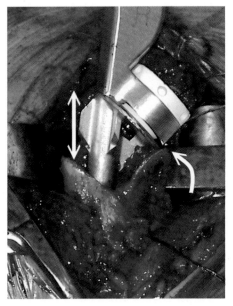

Figure 23-12. Place the trial in the canal in an anatomic position. If the medial neck (*curved arrow*) is intact, it can be used as a reference to the inferior collar of the prosthetic trial. The lateral fins are typically exposed in the region of the displaced greater tuberosity (*straight arrow*). If necessary, a sponge can be placed within the humeral canal to elevate the trial to this anatomic position.

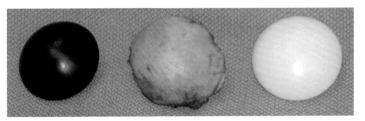

Figure 23-13. Compare the resected humeral head to a prosthetic trial to help determine appropriate sizing.

in maintaining the elevated position of the component when trial reduction is performed. Alternatively, place a sponge in the canal to keep the component elevated (Fig. 23-12).

Next, select and place a trial head. Head selection may be facilitated by templating radiographs of the uninvolved contralateral shoulder and/or by using the head that was removed for comparison (Fig. 23-13). We err toward undersizing the head, because overstuffing the joint increases the likelihood of postoperative stiffness. In general, men require a larger head size and women, a smaller head size. We use a system that provides either standard (concentric) or offset heads in four different radii of curvature that maximize anatomic reproduction and stability.

Now, mobilize the tuberosities out of the way and reduce the trial component. Use the tagging sutures to reduce the tuberosities around the prosthesis (Fig. 23-14A). The tension on the biceps tendon, if it has been preserved, can act as a guide to the proper tension of the entire myofascial sleeve. If the prosthesis is inserted so deeply that the LHB is very slack in its anatomic position, then the prosthesis has likely been placed too deep within the medullary canal. If the LHB is excessively taut, this suggests the prosthesis is too proud. Assess the position of the reduced tuberosities. The tuberosities should be below the head such that subacromial impingement is avoided, and tuberosity to shaft apposition is guaranteed (Fig. 23-14B). Occasionally, the use of intraoperative fluoroscopy is helpful to confirm appropriate position. Perform AP translation and push–pull assessments to confirm stability of the implant. We prefer approximately 50% translation of the head on the glenoid in both anterior-to-posterior and superior-to-inferior directions. Finally, assess the stability of the implant with the arm at the side in 40 to 50 degrees of internal and external rotation. If the prosthesis remains stable, the retroversion is generally appropriate. Prior to removal of the trial prosthesis, measure the distance from the lateral shaft to the lateral aspect of the collar. This will allow reproduction of appropriate height when the actual component is implanted.

Prepare the proximal humerus with drill holes to allow tuberosity fixation with nonabsorbable nylon sutures. We generally drill three or four holes in the area just distal to the tuberosities and bicipital groove (Fig. 23-15A). Pass no. 2 and no. 5 heavy nonabsorbable

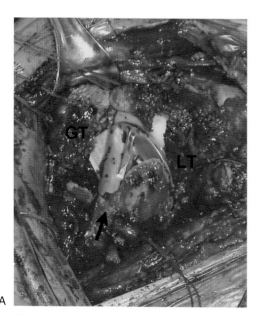
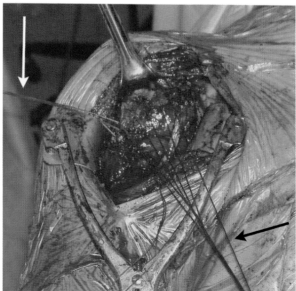

A   B

Figure 23-14. A: After placing the humeral trial, mobilize the tuberosities with the tagging sutures and attempt a trial reduction to the humeral shaft (*arrow*). **B:** The tuberosities should reduce to themselves and the shaft without undue tension. When properly reduced, the tuberosities are located beneath the humeral head and in direct contact with the shaft. The tagging sutures from the lesser tuberosity (*white arrow*) are pulled laterally, and the sutures from the greater tuberosity (*black arrow*) are pulled medially.

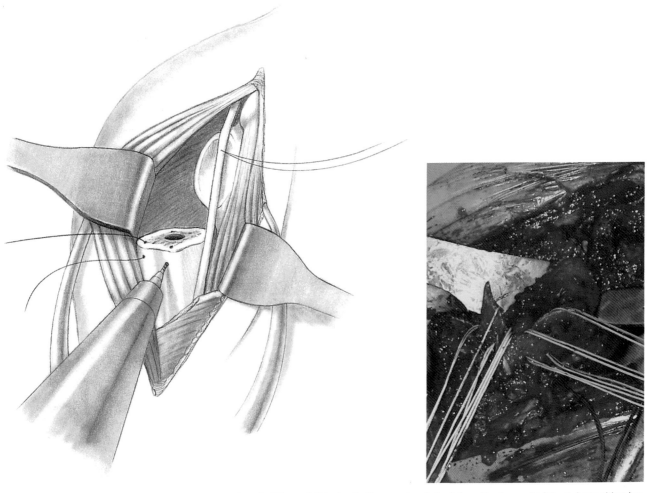

A

B

Figure 23-15. A: Place drill holes in the proximal shaft for attachment of the tuberosities before cementing in the prosthesis. We place two or three holes lateral to the bicipital groove (for the greater tuberosity) and one to two drill holes medial to the groove (for the lesser tuberosity). Pass no. 2 nonabsorbable sutures through the holes from outside the shaft to inside, and tag. **B:** Pass no. 2 and no. 5 nonabsorbable sutures through drill holes both medial and lateral to the bicipital groove. Leave the swedged-on needles on the suture for later passage around the tuberosities through the tendons of the cuff.

nylon sutures with a swedged-on needle through the shaft in an extramedullary to intramedullary direction, and tag them with a clamp (see Fig. 23-15B).

At this stage, turn attention to implantation of the actual prosthesis. In our opinion, cement fixation is required in the setting of a fracture for two reasons. First, there usually is insufficient bone stock to allow adequate press-fit fixation. Second, rotational stability of the implant is lost when the tuberosities are fractured. Therefore, we highly recommend the routine use of cement when performing this operation for acute fractures (Fig. 23-16). However, size the stem close to that of the reamed canal, such that a minimal amount of cement will be required. Place an appropriately sized cement restrictor within the canal, and irrigate the canal to remove excess blood and debris. Inject cement and place the component, using the previous measurements, anatomic landmarks, and instrumentation to assess appropriate height and retroversion. Be careful to remove any excess cement from the proximal canal, because this could prevent tuberosity-to-shaft contact and impede healing. Place the actual head and reduce the prosthesis.

Tuberosity Repair. Tuberosity repair is probably the most important portion of the procedure. Inadequate tuberosity repair is one of the most common and devastating causes of failure. It is far more important to attach the tuberosities to the shaft of the proximal bone

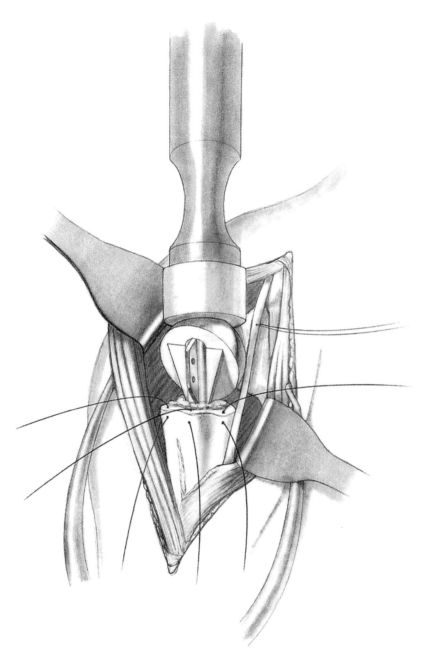

Figure 23-16. Use cement for fixation of the prosthesis within the canal.

than the prosthesis itself (Fig. 23-17). Use the tagging sutures that have been previously placed to mobilize the tuberosities. Place and tag two no. 5 nonabsorbable sutures around the lesser tuberosity, through the lateral fin of the prosthesis, and around the greater tuberosity (Fig. 23-18). Liberally apply cancellous bone as autogenous graft between the tuberosities and shaft and the tuberosities themselves (Fig. 23-19). Reattach the greater tuberosity first, followed by the lesser tuberosity. Use the no. 2 and no. 5 nonabsorbable sutures previously passed through the shaft drill holes, with a total of three to four sutures for the greater tuberosity and two to three for the lesser tuberosity. Then, tie the two sutures placed around the tuberosities and through the fin of the prosthesis. Now, support the arm in a slightly flexed and abducted position. If the LHB has been preserved, reduce it in its groove. Use no. 0 nonabsorbable suture to repair the lateral aspect of the rotator interval

(text continues on page 442)

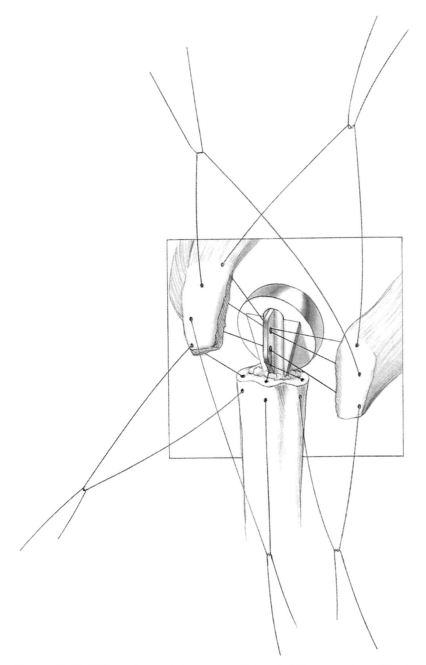

Figure 23-17. Tuberosity repair is an essential part of the procedure. Attach both tuberosities to the shaft and to each other through the fin of the prosthesis. Place bone graft prior to tuberosity fixation.

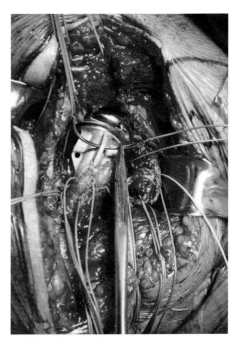

Figure 23-18. A suture can be passed around the lesser tuberosity, through a hole in the fin of the prosthesis, and back around the greater tuberosity. Tie the suture over the tuberosities externally, reducing and securing them to each other.

begin strengthening exercises (6). We obtain radiographs immediately postoperatively, prior to discharge (typically 2 or 3 days after surgery), at 6 weeks, 3 months, and 1 year.

Begin a passive-motion program on the first postoperative day. Base range of motion limitations on the intraoperative assessment of stability following tuberosity repair. Consider the quality of bone, the status of the rotator cuff and deltoid, and the strength of the tuberosity fixation to the shaft. On the first postoperative day, we usually raise the arm in the scapular plane to approximately 80 to 90 degrees to encourage the patient and gain his or her confidence. The therapist then begins gravity-assisted pendulum exercises to allow the patient to warm up. After this, assisted forward elevation and supine external rotation with a stick are performed. After gaining some early motion with the help of a therapist, the patient may lie supine and raise the arm by using the uninvolved contralateral arm. These three exercises are generally done for the first 6 weeks until adequate tuberosity healing has occurred. We do not allow pulley exercises in the first 6 weeks. The goal prior to discharge from the hospital should be approximately 130 degrees of forward elevation in the scapular plane and 30 degrees of external rotation, unless modified by the intraoperative assessment. Take radiographs prior to discharge to ensure that tuberosity displacement has not occurred.

Obtain repeated radiographs at the 6-week follow-up visit (Fig. 23-22). If the tuberosities show evidence of continued healing and no change in alignment, begin active-assisted elevation with a pulley and isometric strengthening exercises for the rotator cuff and deltoid. At 8 to 10 weeks after surgery, add progressive resistive and strengthening exercises. Allow the patient to begin performing activities of daily living (ADLs) such as personal hygiene and eating, as these help build early muscle strength and endurance. Include gentle strengthening as part of a prolonged physical therapy program that is performed on a daily basis. We encourage the patient to continue the daily exercise regimen for at least 6 months, preferably 1 year, to achieve optimal results.

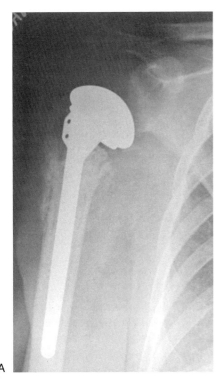

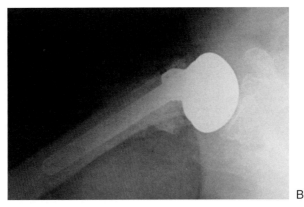

A   B

Figure 23-22. Postoperative anteroposterior **(A)** and axillary lateral **(B)** radiographs demonstrating union of the tuberosities and good positioning of the implant.

RESULTS

Important measures of outcome include pain, range of motion, ability to perform ADLs, complications, and need for further nonsurgical or surgical treatment. Various outcome measurements are used that emphasize certain aspects of outcome more than others; as a result, the reported success rate tends to be variable (5,8–10). At our institution, HHR after acute proximal humerus fracture has been a very successful operation in terms of pain relief. However, outcome with regard to motion and performance of ADLs is somewhat less predictable. It should be remembered that patient satisfaction does not always correlate with functional ability. We counsel patients to expect reliable pain relief after adequate healing of the fracture. The return of range of motion and strength is more difficult to predict and is dependent on many factors, not the least of which is patient motivation. We inform the patient that the rehabilitation process can be prolonged and that slow, continued improvement can be expected for up to 12 to 18 months after the operation.

COMPLICATIONS

Tuberosity Failure

Failure of tuberosity healing is a major factor contributing to poor outcome after HHR (3,12). Complications related to tuberosity fixation include frank nonunion, malunion, tuberosity resorption, and rotator cuff insufficiency, and are usually the result of inadequate fixation at the time of initial surgery. In addition, excessive tuberosity resection and tension overload of the rotator cuff may lead to cuff insufficiency or nonunion or malunion of the tuberosities. There is no clearly accepted radiographic or clinical definition of tuberosity failure, thus resulting in the variable rate reported in the literature. In our opinion, this is the most unfortunate complication following HHR. Most reported cases have extremely limited function and persistent pain, and the results of subsequent treatment have been unpredictable.

Prosthesis Malposition

There are very few reports of component malposition alone as a major reason for clinical failure. However, we have found malposition to be an important factor in poor outcome, and its occurrence may be more frequent than expected (3). The potential malpositions seen clinically are excess anteversion or retroversion, inappropriate prosthetic height, and inappropriate prosthetic humeral head size. It is likely that improper positioning of the humeral component contributes to several more frequently reported complications. These include tuberosity failure, tuberosity malunion, subacromial impingement, rotator cuff insufficiency, and glenohumeral instability. It is important to maintain an awareness of these potential complications and how to avoid them. Templating the contralateral unaffected proximal humerus and use of an intraoperative guide to assess version are both helpful. Strict attention to detail at the time of initial surgery is the best method for avoiding poor component position and/or sizing.

Poor Rehabilitation

Many authors report unsatisfactory results directly related to poor compliance with postoperative rehabilitation. Poor compliance is also associated with increasing patient age and medical comorbidities. It has been shown that physical therapy delayed more than 2 weeks may compromise the ability to regain motion (3,12). We have also seen situations where excessive passive motion, early use of pulleys, or premature active-motion or resistance exercises have resulted in tuberosity failure. Our experience has been that improper or inadequate postoperative therapy contributes to adverse outcome in a significant number of

cases. We therefore emphasize the importance of strict compliance with the postoperative regimen to both the patient and his or her support network (friends and family, when available) during hospitalization. We also strongly recommend direct communication with the patient's outpatient physical and occupational therapists, so that all personnel understand the activity limitations and goals of the rehabilitation program.

Instability

Variable rates of postoperative instability have been reported in most series of hemiarthroplasty for proximal humerus fractures. Definition of the clinical problem is critical in reviewing the true incidence of symptomatic instability. Despite obvious concerns for malpositioning of the humeral component, the occurrence of unidirectional anterior or posterior dislocation is unusual.

The most frequent instability pattern after HHR is likely anterosuperior migration or subluxation of the humeral head. This pattern of proximal migration has been reported by numerous authors and has been shown to adversely affect outcome. In our experience, proximal migration may be associated with rotator cuff insufficiency, failure of tuberosity fixation, improper component position or size, and/or neurologic injury. The affect of anterosuperior migration on functional outcome is dependent on the magnitude of displacement. Small amounts of proximal head displacement are frequently seen and typically do not require surgical revision. However, marked superior migration of the humeral component, in particular when the CA arch is incompetent, severely limits function, and is extremely difficult to treat.

Neurologic Injury

Nerve injury is commonly associated with fractures of the proximal humerus, regardless of whether the injury is treated operatively or nonoperatively. Reported nerve injuries include both isolated peripheral nerve injuries and brachial plexus lesions. They are almost always neuropraxias, with the exception of fractures resulting from penetrating trauma. Since these injuries are reported in both operative and nonoperative series, it can be unclear whether these injuries result from the initial injury or the surgical intervention (3).

Infection

Infection remains a particular concern at the time of initial surgery, as well as in the subacute and late postoperative phases. Infection rates in the literature have been variable following HHR for proximal humerus fracture. As with other major joint arthroplasties, infection most likely results from skin contaminants at the time of original surgery. Theoretically, patients undergoing humeral head arthroplasty for proximal humerus fracture are at risk for postoperative infection for two reasons. First, the patients are often elderly, debilitated, have a poor nutritional state, and multiple medical problems. They not infrequently have other bacterial sources such as the upper respiratory tract and urinary tract. In addition, the acute fracture hematoma and associated soft-tissue injury presents an environment that may be favorable for bacterial growth. The rate of chronic deep infection is quite small, but when it does occur, it frequently requires prosthetic resection or staged revision.

Aseptic Loosening

Symptomatic aseptic loosening is an uncommon complication. Most reported cases have been attributed to cementless fixation of the prosthesis (3). The modest number of aseptically loose implants reported in the literature may also be related to the relative short-term follow up periods of the published series. Aseptic loosening is rare when cement fixation is used for HHR after proximal humerus fracture. We recommend the routine use of cement when performing HHR for acute fractures.

Glenoid Erosion

Glenoid erosion is infrequently cited as a cause of failure following HHR for proximal humeral fractures. It is unclear whether glenoid erosion occurs without the influence of component malposition or instability. More commonly, radiographic changes related to glenoid arthritis are reported. However, most of these patients remain asymptomatic, and relatively few revisions for glenoid erosion have been reported.

Heterotopic Ossification

Ectopic bone formation following fracture of the proximal humerus is a frequent radiographic finding. Neer's (9) initial series noted an association with fracture–dislocation, repeated attempts at reduction, and delayed fracture treatment. Others have demonstrated a relatively frequent occurrence of heterotopic ossification in proximal humerus fractures treated with HHR. The diagnosis can usually be made with standard radiographs. While often noted radiographically, we have found that heterotopic ossification rarely adversely affects outcome or results in reoperation (3).

Tuberosity Prominence/Subacromial Impingement

Prominence of the tuberosities following fracture treatment with HHR has been described. The problem is multifactorial and relates to many of the complications previously discussed, namely failure of tuberosity fixation and/or reduction, inappropriate component height, and the formation of ectopic bone (heterotopic ossification). There have been few published series specifically mentioning impingement syndrome as a complication following HHR. The affect of superior tuberosity displacement on outcome remains somewhat unclear. We have found that impingement often relates to malunion or nonunion of the tuberosities, and therefore strongly recommend excluding failure of tuberosity healing before considering the diagnosis of impingement.

Analysis of Failures

A series of failed hemiarthroplasties for acute proximal humerus fractures has previously been reported from our institution (3). This series of patients represents a large group of patients with unsatisfactory results typically seen in a tertiary care center. A total of 27 patients with 29 shoulders were reviewed, with an average age of 63 years (range, 37 to 79 years). Most patients (79%) were referred from outside institutions. Approximately 75% of the patients in this series had their initial surgery within 15 days of the injury. Overall, 18 patients required revision surgery due to at least one complication.

Analysis of the mode of failure demonstrated the multifactorial nature of the problem. Eighty-three percent of the affected shoulders had more than one complication as the underlying cause of failure. Tuberosity malunion or nonunion was by far the most common complication (15 of 29, 52%). Other contributing factors included improper rehabilitation (41%), neurologic injury (31%), component malposition (31%), and glenoid erosion (24%).

Treatment

Patients presenting with persistent pain or inadequate function following HHR for proximal humerus fracture require a full diagnostic work-up. Obtain a laboratory evaluation including complete blood count, erythrocyte sedimentation rate, and C-reactive protein, and standard radiographs. We consider aspirating the shoulder if the clinical suspicion of infection is high, even if the laboratory values are normal. Patients with identifiable problems on diagnostic imaging or laboratory evaluation will frequently require surgical intervention. Numerous potential treatment options are available to the surgeon depending on the clinical situation. It must be noted, however, that the results of revision surgical treatment have a guarded prognosis.

The treatment of nonunion or malunion of the tuberosities requires mobilization and revision open reduction and internal fixation of the tuberosities, and must be augmented with autogenous or allograft bone graft. If malposition of the component has contributed to the failure of tuberosity healing, limited motion, instability, or glenoid erosion, revision of the humeral component should be performed. Occasionally, tuberosity malunion resulting in impingement alone can be treated successfully with arthroscopic or open acromioplasty and subacromial decompression, with or without tuberoplasty. Arthroscopic treatment with or without manipulation under anesthesia might be considered in the setting of excessive stiffness not explained by improper component size or position, but only if adequate clinical and radiographic healing can be documented.

The treatment of symptomatic instability is complex and depends on many factors including bone quality, component malposition, neurologic injury, and direction or pattern of instability. Component malposition can be corrected with revision. Soft-tissue procedures such as capsular plication, capsular repair, tendon repair, or tendon transfer can be considered when inappropriate component position is ruled out.

In particular, we have found the treatment of severe anterosuperior instability to be challenging. When small to moderate amounts of proximal component migration are seen, we recommend avoiding acromioplasty or decompression of the CA arch. Release of the CA ligament in this setting is potentially disastrous, as it removes the last remaining soft-tissue constraint to superior migration of the humeral head. In situations where anterosuperior instability of the humeral component is severe and the CA arch is compromised, use of an Achilles allograft to reconstruct the CA arch has been described. We have not found static reconstructions of the CA arch to be successful. Dynamic attempts to treat anterosuperior instability include transfer of the pectoralis major tendon and have been performed as an alternative to the static reconstructions. These are salvage situations and it is reasonable to consider these procedures. However, it should be considered as a pain-relieving measure only, since any significant functional benefit, in terms of restoration of motion and strength, has yet to be demonstrated.

The treatment of infection can be problematic. Surgical treatment options include irrigation and débridement with retention of components, one-stage reimplantation, two-stage reimplantation, and resection arthroplasty. Consideration may be given to suppressive antibiotic therapy in patients that are particularly high surgical risk.

The indications for surgical treatment of neurologic dysfunction are unclear. Nerve exploration and grafting has infrequently been described, and its role and effectiveness is uncertain. Tendon or muscle transfers may be helpful in certain situations. However, as a rule, we recommend nonoperative management.

Symptomatic glenoid erosion, as mentioned previously, has not been a significant problem in the short term. A report of HHR converted to total shoulder replacement included a subset of patients who initially had proximal humerus fractures. In that study, improvements in range of motion and pain scores were demonstrated, although functional improvement was more limited (11).

RECOMMENDED READING

1. Bigliani, L.U., Flatow, E.L., Pollock, R.G.: Fractures of the proximal humerus. In: Rockwood, C.A. Jr., Matsen, F.A.I., eds.: *The shoulder,* 3rd ed. Philadelphia: WB Saunders, 337–374, 1998.
2. Cofield, R.H.: Comminuted fractures of the proximal humerus. *Clin Orthop* 230: 49–57, 1988.
3. Compito, C.A., Self, E.B., Bigliani, L.U.: Arthroplasty and acute shoulder trauma: reasons for success and failure. *Clin Orthop* 307: 27–36, 1994.

4. Hawkins, R.J., Angelo, R.L.: Displaced proximal humeral fractures: selecting treatment, avoiding pitfalls. *Orthop Clin N Am* 18: 421–431, 1987.

5. Hawkins, R.J., Switlyk, P.: Acute prosthetic replacement for severe fractures of the proximal humerus. *Clin Orthop* 289: 156–160, 1993.

6. Hughes, M., Neer, C.S. II: Glenohumeral joint replacement and postoperative rehabilitation. *Phys Ther* 55: 850–858, 1975.

7. Levine, W.N., Connor, P.M., Yamaguchi, K., et al.: Humeral head replacement for proximal humeral fractures. *Orthopedics* 21: 68–73, 1998.

8. Moeckel, B.H., Dines, D.M., Warren, R.F., et al.: Modular hemiarthroplasty for fractures of the proximal humerus. *J Bone Joint Surg Am* 74: 884–889, 1992.

9. Neer, C.S. II: Displaced proximal humeral fractures, II: treatment of three- and four-part displacement. *J Bone Joint Surg Am* 52: 1090–1103, 1970.

10. Neer, C.S. II: Recent results and techniques of prosthetic replacement for 4-part proximal humeral fractures. *Orthop Trans* 10: 475, 1986.

11. Sperling, J.W., Cofield, R.H.: Revision total shoulder arthroplasty for the treatment of glenoid arthrosis. *J Bone Joint Surg Am* 80: 860–867, 1998.

12. Tanner, M.W., Cofield, R.H.: Prosthetic arthroplasty for fractures and fracture-dislocations of the proximal humerus. *Clin Orthop* 179: 116–128, 1983.

24

Operative Treatment of Displaced Surgical Neck Fractures of the Proximal Humerus

Charles N. Cornell

INDICATIONS/CONTRAINDICATIONS

Most proximal humeral fractures occur in the elderly, are minimally displaced, and are stable, allowing nonoperative management. However, 15% to 20% of proximal humeral fractures have significant displacement, angulation, malrotation, or tuberosity involvement. Fractures that have 1 cm of displacement, more than 45 degrees of angulation of the humeral head with respect to the shaft, or more than 10 mm of displacement of the tuberosities from their anatomic positions may be candidates for open reduction and internal fixation.

The classification system described by Neer (6) is commonly used and is effective in relating both the severity of the injury and appropriate surgical management. In this system, the four anatomic regions of the proximal humerus are identified, and the involvement of these structures by the fracture is described as one-, two-, three-, or four-part fractures.

One-part fractures are essentially nondisplaced and are amenable to closed treatment. In this classification system, displacement implies that a fragment is shifted by 10 mm or more or is angulated by more than 45 degrees from its normal alignment (greater tuberosity displacement may be an exception and may require reduction if superior displacement of 5 mm or more). Two-part fractures are those with the head and tuberosities intact but separated from the shaft. In three-part fractures, one of the tuberosities, usually the greater, is split off from the head, which is significantly displaced from the shaft. Four-part fractures involve separation of both tuberosities from the head, as well as significant displacement of the head from the shaft.

The classification also describes those injuries associated with dislocation of the head from the glenoid, in addition to the fracture, and identifies these as having a significantly worse prognosis. The greater the number of fragments in a fracture, the greater the risk of

C. N. Cornell, M.D.: Department of Surgery (Orthopaedics), Weill College of Medicine of Cornell University; and Department of Orthopaedic Surgery, Hospital for Special Surgery, New York, New York.

avascular necrosis, with four-part fractures having the highest risk of this complication. For this reason, it is widely accepted that most two- and three-part fractures are candidates for internal fixation, whereas most four-part fractures should be treated with prosthetic replacement. Exceptions to this rule are young patients with good bone stock and valgus-impacted four-part fractures in which surgical repair of the fracture has been followed by predictable success (7).

Most unstable two-, three-, and four-part fractures require surgical management to restore useful shoulder function. Few patients, regardless of age or associated medical conditions, will not benefit from surgical treatment of an unstable proximal humerus fracture. Specific indications for open reduction and internal fixation include open fractures, those that cannot be closed reduced, and fractures in the elderly with poor bone stock not amenable to closed reduction and percutaneous fixation. Young patients with good bone stock, especially those with multiple injuries, are excellent candidates for closed reduction and percutaneous fixation. Specific contraindications to surgery occur in patients with little hope of functional recovery, such as debilitated elderly patients or those with neurologic lesions that preclude useful muscle function. The presence of a severe rotator cuff arthropathy is a relative contraindication to repair and an indication for prosthetic arthroplasty of the humeral head. Four-part fractures with dislocation of the humeral head are associated with nearly a 100% incidence of osteonecrosis and should be selected for hemiarthroplasty.

Most proximal humeral fractures occur in elderly women after slips and falls. The bone of the proximal humerus is osteoporotic and provides for poor fixation when plates or screws are used (4,5). Hawkins et al. (4,5) pointed out that the soft-tissue attachments of the rotator cuff tendons are usually strong in spite of poor adjacent bone quality. They demonstrated that these soft tissues provide excellent sites of fracture fixation when tension-band wiring techniques are used. Furthermore, tension-band wiring does not violate the subacromial space or lead to postoperative impingement and minimizes the stripping and interference with blood supply associated with plates. In younger patients, bone quality is usually superior, allowing excellent fixation with plates and screws. In many cases, fractures in young individuals are the result of high-energy trauma and as such can be severely comminuted in the metaphyseal region. This comminution creates instability that precludes the use of the screw-tension-band technique, as it leads to excessive shortening with loss of deltoid power and inferior subluxation of the humeral head. In such cases, a buttress plate is needed to restore and maintain length. Small fragment plates such as the cloverleaf plate fit the proximal humerus well and provide for multiple screw purchase into the humeral head. These are the ideal plates for these fractures because they avoid the bulk of the large fragment plates and the multiple screw purchase provides more secure fixation. In all cases, a tension-band wire can be used to help neutralize the pull of the rotator cuff, significantly enhancing the security of fixation. In summary, two- and three-part fractures in both young and old patients without significant comminution can be ideally managed with the screw-tension-band technique. Four-part fractures, nonunions, and fractures with metaphyseal comminution are better treated with cloverleaf plate and tension-band wire. In the future, locking small fragment plates will replace the cloverleaf design.

PREOPERATIVE PLANNING

In patients with injuries to the shoulder, a careful history should be taken to document the mechanism of injury as well as the presence of associated injuries. The physical examination should assess the degree of swelling, with a careful search for neurovascular injury. Although vascular injury is rare, axillary artery disruption does occur and is most commonly associated with numbness and paresthesia in the limb and an expanding axillary hematoma. Because the collateral circulation of the upper limb is extensive, the presence of pulses at the wrist does not preclude a significant proximal vascular injury. The axillary and musculocutaneous nerves are the most commonly injured nerves, and their function at the time of presentation must be carefully documented. Radiographs should include a true anteroposterior and transthoracic lateral of the scapula and an axillary lateral of the glenohumeral joint. If significant comminution exists, full-length views of the humerus may be necessary. If there is a question of comminution of the humeral articular fragment, or if the precise location of the tuberosities is unclear, a computed tomography scan may be helpful. The surgeon may wish to obtain a view of the opposite shoulder to act as a guide for restoration of the injured side.

The surgeon should develop a careful preoperative plan and create a surgical tactic. Preoperative planning in these cases consists of a careful analysis of the injury radiographs to determine the number and location of the fracture fragments (Fig. 24-1). A surgical drawing can trace the preoperative location of the humeral head, shaft, and greater and lesser tuberosities. A second drawing is prepared to locate the position of the fragments after open reduction is performed. The position of the screw and tension-band wires is included in this second drawing (Fig. 24-2). The surgical approach to a proximal humeral fracture can be difficult. Swelling, hematoma, and the disruption of the normal soft-tissue and bony landmarks can frustrate even experienced surgeons. I have found that careful preoperative planning helps predict what the anatomy will look like at the time of surgical exposure. Hasty preparation will lead to longer operative time and a much more frustrating learning curve with this technique.

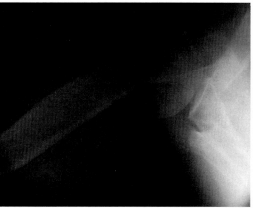

C

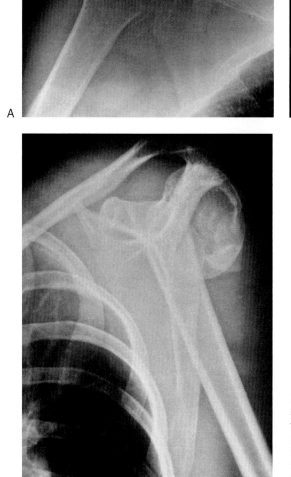

A

B

Figure 24-1. Anteroposterior **(A)**, lateral **(B)**, and axillary **(C)** views of a three-part fracture of the right proximal humerus. (From Cornell, C.N.: Proximal humeral fractures: open reduction internal fixation. In: Wiss, D.A., ed.: *Master techniques of orthopaedic surgery: fractures.* Philadelphia: Lippincott–Raven Publishers, 35–46, 1998.)

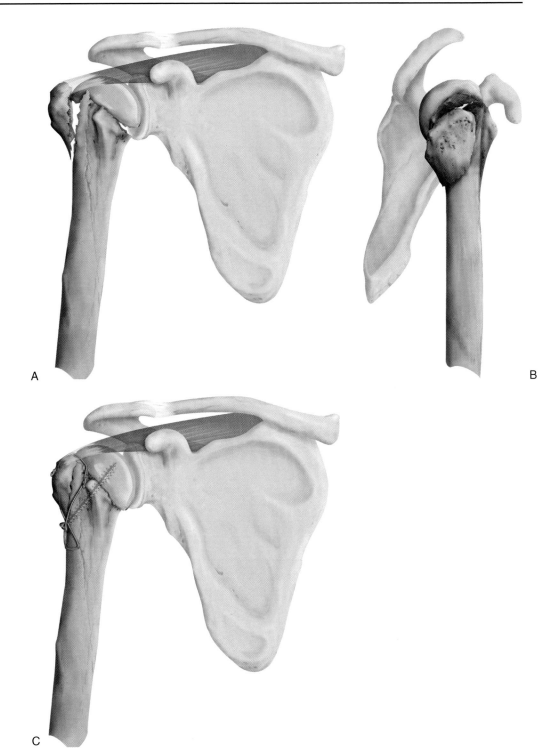

A

B

C

Figure 24-2. A–C: Preoperative drawing of the surgical tactic involves identifying the fracture fragments on the injury radiographs and approximating their position after reduction. The internal fixation also can be diagrammed. (From Cornell, C.N.: Proximal humeral fractures: open reduction internal fixation. In: Wiss, D.A., ed.: *Master techniques of orthopaedic surgery: fractures.* Philadelphia: Lippincott–Raven Publishers, 35–46, 1998.)

SURGERY

Screw-tension Band Wiring

Regional anesthesia is frequently used for this procedure. Interscalene block provides adequate anesthesia during the case and can provide postoperative pain relief if long-acting local anesthetics are used. The surgeon can supplement the block with local anesthetics and epinephrine to ensure adequate cutaneous anesthesia and to retard bleeding from the skin and subcutaneous tissues during the surgical exposure. General anesthesia is reserved for uncooperative patients and for those with severe chronic pulmonary disease. An interscalene block paralyzes the ipsilateral diaphragm, which can lead to respiratory distress in patients with severe preoperative pulmonary compromise.

For use of the image intensifier during the procedure, the patient must be carefully positioned. A radiolucent table and a "beanbag" are helpful. The patient is positioned in the beach-chair position with the head elevated 60 to 75 degrees. The patient is positioned so that the shoulder protrudes off the side of the table, allowing access for the image intensifier. The beanbag is necessary to secure this positioning. The affected arm is draped free with access for an extended deltopectoral incision (Fig. 24-3). An interscapular pad and careful molding of the beanbag are needed to allow manipulation of the arm and shoulder during the procedure.

A deltopectoral incision is made, beginning at the edge of the acromion and extending distally to the level of the deltoid insertion. The cephalic vein is identified and can be sacrificed or, preferably, mobilized and medially retracted. We frequently release the anterior part of the distal deltoid insertion to facilitate retraction of the anterior deltoid thus improving exposure of the proximal humerus and rotator cuff. Failure to do this makes placement of the tension-wire bands extremely difficult. The deltoid tendon is released subperiosteally in line with the long axis of the humerus, after which the shoulder is gently abducted. The clavipectoral fascia is incised, allowing entry into the subacromial space. Aufranc or Howman retractors are placed superiorly and laterally, exposing the humeral head, shaft, and rotator cuff (Fig. 24-4).

A pointed tenaculum clamp is used to grasp the humeral head, providing provisional control of the proximal fragment. The fracture site is débrided of hematoma and soft tissue.

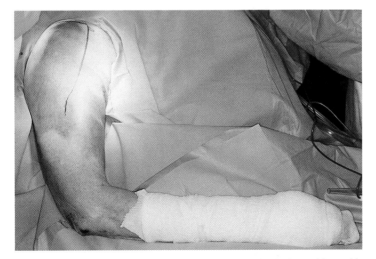

Figure 24-3. The patient is placed in the beach-chair position with the entire extremity draped free. An extended deltopectoral incision is made. (From Cornell, C.N.: Proximal humeral fractures: open reduction internal fixation. In: Wiss, D.A., ed.: *Master techniques of orthopaedic surgery: fractures.* Philadelphia: Lippincott–Raven Publishers, 35–46, 1998.)

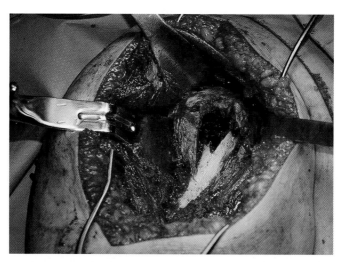

Figure 24-4. After development of the deltopectoral interval, the distal deltoid insertion is released subperiosteally in line with the humerus. After the clavipectoral fascia is opened, retractors can be placed in the subacromial space, exposing the fracture and humeral head. (From Cornell, C.N.: Proximal humeral fractures: open reduction internal fixation. In: Wiss, D.A., ed.: *Master techniques of orthopaedic surgery: fractures.* Philadelphia: Lippincott–Raven Publishers, 35–46, 1998.)

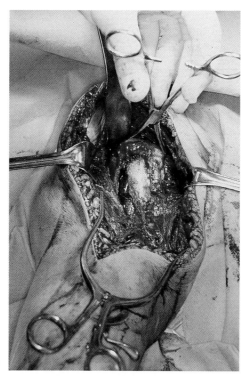

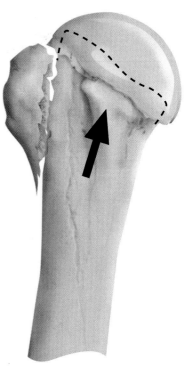

A   B

Figure 24-5. A: The humeral head is grasped with a pointed clamp and reduced to the shaft. **B:** The shaft is impacted into the humeral head. (From Cornell, C.N.: Proximal humeral fractures: open reduction internal fixation. In: Wiss, D.A., ed.: *Master techniques of orthopaedic surgery: fractures.* Philadelphia: Lippincott–Raven Publishers, 35–46, 1998.)

The head and shaft are then impacted, reducing the fracture and creating a stable configuration (Fig. 24-5).

Fracture fixation is achieved by placing a 6.5- or 4.5-mm lag screw from the proximal lateral humeral shaft into the humeral head (Fig. 24-6). The screw size is based on the size of the bone and bone quality. Recently we found that 4.5-mm cortical screws inserted in a lag fashion achieve excellent purchase with little risk of additional comminution of the fragile humeral cortex. The lateral cortex is overdrilled with a 4.5-mm drill, and a countersink is used. If the tuberosities are displaced, they can now be reduced to the head and shaft and fixed with an additional lag screw or heavy suture into the humeral head (Fig. 24-7).

Two 18-gauge wires are then placed through a drill hole in the humeral shaft. The drill hole is placed 3 to 4 cm below the fracture site in intact cortex. A 3.2-mm drill bit is used. The hole is drilled from anterior to posterior. Two wires are then passed from anterior to posterior through this hole. One wire is passed beneath the supraspinatus tendon as a figure-eight tension band. The other wire is passed through the tuberosities, also in figure-eight fashion. A 14-gauge angiocatheter or culposcopy needle can be used as a cannula to facilitate passage of the wires (Fig. 24-8). Two twists for tightening are used in each wire on each side of the shaft. Ideally, the twists are placed at the level of the junction of the head and shaft to achieve maximal tightening of the wires (Fig. 24-9).

Many surgeons may wish to substitute heavy Dacron suture or tape for the stainless-steel wires. I prefer using wire because I believe that its greater stiffness allows it to be more securely tightened. In addition, sharp bone fragments and edges occur at the fracture site, which may lead to fretting and premature breakage of suture materials, which is better resisted by the steel wire.

When completed, the construct is inspected by using the image intensifier. The length of the screws in the humeral head should be verified and shortened if there is a risk of intraarticular protrusion. The position of the fragments and accuracy of the reduction are determined. An idealized construct is illustrated schematically in Fig. 24-10. The stability of the reduction with passive range of motion also should be confirmed.

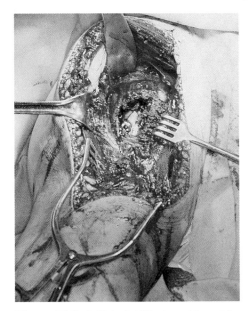

Figure 24-6. Initial stability is achieved by placing a 4.5- or 6.5-mm lag screw from the lateral humeral cortex into the humeral head. (From Cornell, C.N.: Proximal humeral fractures: open reduction internal fixation. In: Wiss, D.A., ed.: *Master techniques of orthopaedic surgery: fractures.* Philadelphia: Lippincott–Raven Publishers, 35–46, 1998.)

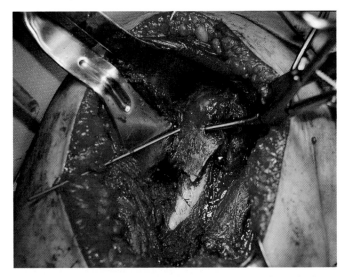

Figure 24-7. In a three-part fracture, the greater tuberosity is reduced to the humeral head and shaft and held with a pointed clamp. A guidewire has been placed in preparation for insertion of a cannulated lag screw. (From Cornell, C.N.: Proximal humeral fractures: open reduction internal fixation. In: Wiss, D.A., ed.: *Master techniques of orthopaedic surgery: fractures.* Philadelphia: Lippincott–Raven Publishers, 35–46, 1998.)

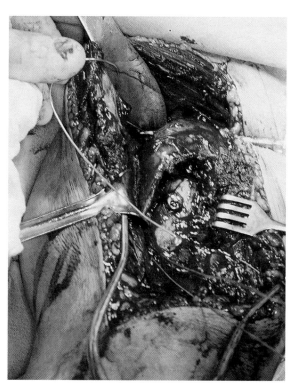

Figure 24-8. A 14-gauge angiocatheter is used as a wire-passing cannula. It is passed beneath the supraspinatus tendon just medial to its insertion on the greater tuberosity. (From Cornell, C.N.: Proximal humeral fractures: open reduction internal fixation. In: Wiss, D.A., ed.: *Master techniques of orthopaedic surgery: fractures.* Philadelphia: Lippincott–Raven Publishers, 35–46, 1998.)

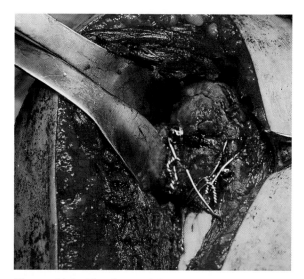

Figure 24-9. The figure-eight wires are passed and tightened by using two twists in each wire. The twists are placed close to the fracture site to achieve maximal tightening. (From Cornell, C.N.: Proximal humeral fractures: open reduction internal fixation. In: Wiss, D.A., ed.: *Master techniques of orthopaedic surgery: fractures.* Philadelphia: Lippincott–Raven Publishers, 35–46, 1998.)

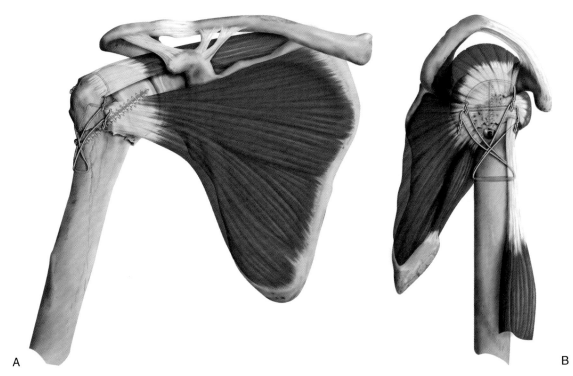

A   B

Figure 24-10. A,B: Anteroposterior and lateral drawings illustrating fracture reduction and placement of internal fixation. (From Cornell, C.N.: Proximal humeral fractures: open reduction internal fixation. In: Wiss, D.A., ed.: *Master techniques of orthopaedic surgery: fractures.* Philadelphia: Lippincott–Raven Publishers, 35–46, 1998.)

The wound is irrigated and then closed over a drain. The deltoid tendon is repaired back to its origin with heavy resorbable suture. The deltopectoral interval is reapproximated with a few resorbable sutures, and the subcutaneous layer is carefully closed. A subcuticular skin closure can be performed for optimal cosmetic healing of the skin.

Plate-tension Band for Four-part Fractures and Those with Comminution

The patient positioning and surgical approach to the four-part or comminuted fracture is identical to that described above. After exposure is achieved and the fracture site is prepared, the tuberosities are reapproximated and reduced to the humeral head. The reduced position can be provisionally maintained by suturing the tuberosities together. Kirschner wires, which are placed proximally to not interfere with plate placement, can stabilize the tuberosities to the articular segment. The cloverleaf plate is trimmed to remove the most superior extension of the plate and it is slightly contoured to fit the proximal humerus. The plate is anatomically positioned to the proximal fragment and fixed with several 4.0-mm fully threaded cancellous screws. The position of the plate on the proximal fragment must be perfect to ensure anatomic reduction of the fracture after the plate is approximated distally to the shaft. After placing enough screws into the humeral head to achieve secure purchase of the proximal segment, the plate is reduced to the shaft and held with a fracture reduction clamp. The image intensifier is then used to determine that an adequate reduction has been achieved and that no screws are protruding into the shoulder joint. The plate is secured to the humeral shaft using at least three 3.5-mm cortical screws. Before securing the plate to the shaft, an 18-gauge stainless-steel wire is placed under the midportion of the plate for use as the tension band. The tension-band wire is placed under the supraspinatus tendon in figure-eight fashion and is tightened with two twists (Fig. 24-11). The wound closure is similar to that for the screw-tension band procedure described above.

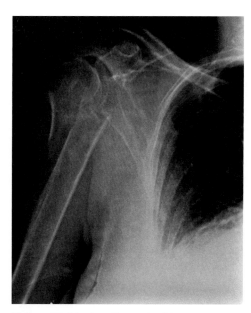

Figure 24-11. A radiograph of two-part proximal humerus fracture in a 63-year-old, right-
hand-dominant woman. (From Cornell, C.N.:
Proximal humeral fractures: open reduction
internal fixation. In: Wiss, D.A., ed.: *Master
techniques of orthopaedic surgery: fractures.*
Philadelphia: Lippincott–Raven Publishers,
35–46, 1998.)

POSTOPERATIVE MANAGEMENT

A sterile dressing is applied, and the arm is immobilized in a sling or shoulder immobilizer.
Gentle, passive pendulum exercises and active elbow exercises are started on the first postoperative day. Passive exercises are performed for the first four postoperative weeks. Active-assisted exercises are initiated at week 3 or 4 and are continued until the sixth postoperative week. Thereafter, active range of motion and strengthening exercises are instituted.
Supervised physical therapy is continued until maximal recovery is achieved, which on average requires 6 months of treatment. In the early postoperative period, patients are seen in
the outpatient department frequently. Patients are asked to return every 2 weeks for the first
6 weeks for examination of the surgical wound and to determine the compliance with the
exercise program. Radiographs are obtained to ensure no loss of fracture stability has occurred. Generally by the sixth postoperative week, adequate fracture healing has occurred
to allow a progressive range-of-motion and muscle-strengthening program. The frequency
of outpatient visits is reduced to monthly or greater. Nearly full passive range of motion
should be recovered by 6 weeks after surgery. Active range of motion, which relies on adequate strength and coordination of the deltoid and rotator cuff, requires prolonged therapy.
The goal for these patients should be overhead function of the arm with 120 degrees or
more of forward flexion and adequate internal and external rotation. Return of the ability
to perform activities of daily living is achieved in nearly all patients. Return to sports that
require throwing or vigorous overhead use of the arm, as in tennis or swimming, is more
difficult to achieve. I tell my patients that recovery from this surgery can be slow and frustrating in the early months. However, I encourage them to be patient and persistent with
their therapy. With a stable, near-anatomic reconstruction, excellent functional results are
usually achieved.

Hawkins et al. (5) reported on treatment of a series of three-part fractures of the proximal humerus with the tension-band technique. Patients averaged 126 degrees of forward elevation, with 8 of 15 patients subjectively scoring their results as functionally good to ex-

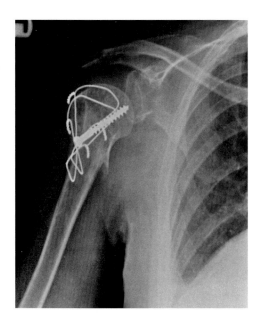

Figure 24-12. Postoperative radiographs after open reduction and internal fixation. (From Cornell, C.N.: Proximal humeral fractures: open reduction internal fixation. In: Wiss, D.A., ed.: *Master techniques of orthopaedic surgery: fractures.* Philadelphia: Lippincott–Raven Publishers, 35–46, 1998.)

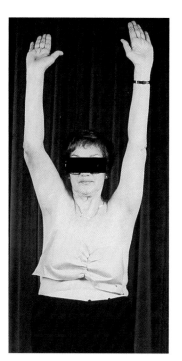

Figure 24-13. A clinical photograph demonstrating the shoulder motion in forward flexion at 1 year after surgery. (From Cornell, C.N.: Proximal humeral fractures: open reduction internal fixation. In: Wiss, D.A., ed.: *Master techniques of orthopaedic surgery: fractures.* Philadelphia: Lippincott–Raven Publishers, 35–46, 1998.)

cellent. All but two patients had excellent pain relief. The two poor results occurred in a patient with a broken tension-band wire and in one patient with osteonecrosis of the humeral head. Both required secondary surgery.

In our own experience with the technique in two- and three-part fractures (3), excellent results were achieved in 10 of 13 patients. Early aggressive range-of-motion exercises led to an average forward flexion of 160 degrees. This technique is ideal for the elderly patient with osteopenic bone. Properly done, the technique offers excellent fracture fixation, allowing early mobilization of the shoulder (Figs. 24-12 and 24-13). In addition, the implants are small, avoiding subacromial impingement or devascularization of the humeral head that has been associated with T-shaped or cloverleaf plates. The incidence of avascular necrosis of the head is reported to be lower using tension banding as compared with plates for three- and four-part fractures (7).

COMPLICATIONS

Injury to the axillary nerve has been reported after this procedure, and care must be taken to avoid injury to the nerve as it courses through the deltoid muscle. Most axillary nerve palsies are neuropraxias and carry a good prognosis for recovery. Electromyography is useful for monitoring the course of recovery, especially in situations in which little return of function is noted by 3 months. Avascular necrosis occurs in approximately 15% to 20% of three-part fractures and between 50% and 75% of four-part fractures (2). Avascular necrosis usually leads to pain and a poor result. Prosthetic replacement of the humeral head or

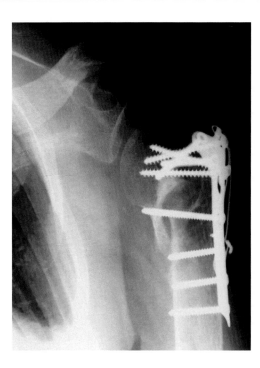

Figure 24-14. Anteroposterior radiograph of a left proximal humerus after repair of a nonunion using the cloverleaf plate and tension band.

total shoulder replacement may be needed as salvage. Breakage of the tension-band wires is reported sporadically and when it occurs, it can cause an impingement syndrome. When this happens, removal of the broken wires should be performed. If excessive comminution of the shaft occurs, excessive shortening above the deltoid insertion occurs, which can lead to pseudosubluxation and prolonged weakness of the rotator cuff. When significant comminution is present, the cloverleaf plate should be used (Fig. 24-14). In the future, locking plates designed for the proximal humerus will be available, providing even better strength of fixation.

Residual shoulder stiffness and loss of shoulder rotation is a frequent complication after any shoulder injury. Perhaps the best defense against this complication is immediate postoperative rehabilitation, which is allowed by these tension-band techniques. When stiffness that limits function occurs, persistent but gentle range of motion is needed. Occasionally, a gentle manipulation under anesthesia may be performed in a patient who tolerates therapy poorly, provided the fracture appears well healed. Pain consistent with rotator cuff impingement is frequently encountered, and subacromial corticosteroid injection will often ease the pain and improve the results of therapy. In our experience, arthroscopic decompression or lysis of adhesions has not been necessary. In most cases, patience and persistence generally provide the best results.

RECOMMENDED READING

1. Bigliani, L.U.: Treatment of two and three part fractures of the proximal humerus. *Instr Course Lect* 38: 231–244, 1989.
2. Brooks, C.H., Revell, W.J., Heatley, F.W.: Vascularity of the humeral head after proximal humeral fracture. *J Bone Joint Surg Br* 75: 132–136, 1993.
3. Cornell, C.N., Levine, D., Pagnani, M.J.: Internal fixation of proximal humerus fractures using the screw-tension band technique. *J Orthop Trauma* 8: 23–27, 1994.
4. Hawkins, R.J, Bell, R.H., Gun, K.: Three part fractures of the proximal part of the humerus. *J Bone Joint Surg Am* 68: 1410–1414, 1986.
5. Hawkins, R.J., Kiefer, G.N.: Internal fixation techniques for proximal humerus fracture. *Clin Orthop* 223: 77–85, 1987.
6. Szyskowitz, R., Seggl, W., Schleifer, P., et al.: Proximal humeral fractures: management and expected results. *Clin Orthop* 292: 13–25, 1993.
7. Young, T.B., Wallace, W.A.: Conservative treatment of fractures and fracture dislocations of the upper limb of the humerus. *J Bone Joint Surg Br* 67: 373–377, 1985.

25

Open Reduction and Internal Fixation of Glenoid Fractures

Thomas P. Goss

INDICATIONS/CONTRAINDICATIONS

Fractures of the scapula comprise approximately 1% of all fractures. Because direct high-energy trauma is generally involved, there is a high incidence (80% to 95%) of associated osseous and soft-tissue injuries, which may be multiple, major, and threaten limb or life. Fractures of the glenoid process account for approximately one third of scapular fractures and include disruptions of the glenoid cavity (the glenoid rim and the glenoid fossa; Fig. 25-1) and disruptions of the glenoid neck (Fig. 25-2). Although more than 90% of glenoid fractures are minimally displaced and can be treated nonoperatively, approximately 10% are significantly displaced and require surgical reconstruction. Fractures of the glenoid rim are managed surgically if the injury causes persistent subluxation of the humeral head or if the reduction is unstable. Instability can be anticipated if the fracture is displaced 10 mm or more and one fourth or more of the glenoid cavity anteriorly or one third or more of the glenoid cavity posteriorly is involved. Surgical indications for glenoid fossa fractures include (a) an articular step-off of 5 mm or more, (b) such severe separation of the fragments that a nonunion is likely, and (c) a fracture pattern that allows displacement of the humeral head out of the center of the glenoid cavity. Surgical treatment of glenoid neck fractures is considered if there is translational displacement of the glenoid fragment 1 cm or more or angular displacement of the fragment 40 degrees or more in either the coronal or sagittal plane (type II fractures) or both. Contraindications include severely comminuted fractures of the glenoid cavity and glenoid fractures in which comminution of the surrounding osseous structures precludes satisfactory fixation.

T. P. Goss, M.D.: Department of Orthopedics, University of Massachusetts Medical School; and University of Massachusetts Memorial Health Care, Worcester, Massachusetts.

Glenoid Rim Fractures

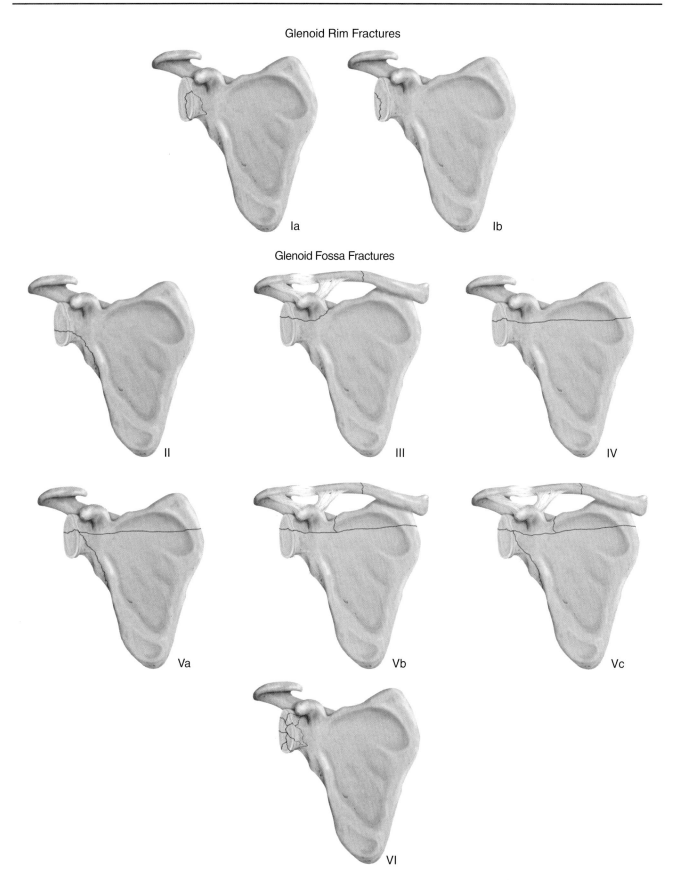

Figure 25-1. Goss-Ideberg classification for fractures of the glenoid cavity. (From Goss, T.P.: Glenoid fractures: open reduction internal fixation. In: Wiss, D.A., ed.: *Master techniques of orthopaedic surgery: fractures.* Philadelphia: Lippincott–Raven Publishers, 1–17, 1998.)

Type I Fractures

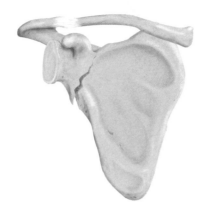

Type II Fractures

Translational Displacement

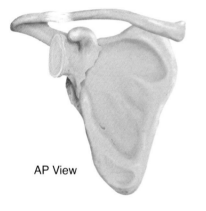

AP View

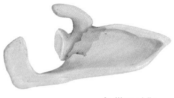

Axillary View

Angulatory Displacement

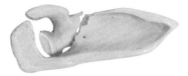

Axillary View

Figure 25-2. Classification for fractures of the glenoid neck. (From Goss, T.P.: Glenoid fractures: open reduction internal fixation. In: Wiss, D.A., ed.: *Master techniques of orthopaedic surgery: fractures.* Philadelphia: Lippincott–Raven Publishers, 1–17, 1998.)

PREOPERATIVE PLANNING

Diagnosis is radiologic and begins with a "scapula trauma series," composed of true anteroposterior and lateral views of the scapula and an axillary projection of the glenohumeral joint. Because of the complex bony anatomy in the area, however, a computed tomography scan is often required to accurately define these injuries and to allow optimal preoperative planning. Three-dimensional scanning can be extremely helpful to the orthopaedist trying to evaluate the most complex fracture patterns. These radiographs should also be reviewed carefully to identify associated fractures of the shoulder girdle including the remainder of the scapula, the clavicle, and the proximal humerus, as well as disruptions of the acromio-clavicular, glenohumeral, sternoclavicular, and scapulothoracic articulations. Abrasions and open wounds involving the superficial soft tissues must be inspected carefully, and surgery may need to be delayed until they are adequately clean. Although vascular injury is quite uncommon, distal pulses should be palpated and if absent or questionable, arteri-ography should be performed. Injury to the brachial plexus also is uncommon, but a thor-ough neurologic examination is necessary to document function of the axillary, musculo-cutaneous, median, radial, and ulnar nerves. Electromyographic (EMG) testing can be performed 3 weeks after injury if a deficit is found or suspected. Scapulothoracic dissocia-tion is a distinct clinical entity that should be considered. It has a very high incidence of neurovascular involvement and is characterized by (a) a history of violent trauma, (b) mas-sive swelling of the shoulder girdle, and (c) posterolateral displacement of the scapula rel-ative to the rib cage.

Should it be determined that surgical management for the glenoid fracture is necessary, a thorough knowledge of the shoulder anatomy is essential. Depending upon the clinical situation, the glenoid process may be approached from three directions or combinations thereof. The specific type and location of the fracture is a prime determinant of the specific surgical approach. Frequently, combined approaches are used.

The anterior approach is used for fractures of the anterior glenoid rim (type Ia; Fig 25-1) and some fractures involving the superior aspect of the glenoid fossa (types III, IV, and Vb). The posterior approach is used at least in part for fractures of the posterior rim (type Ib), most fractures of the glenoid fossa (types II, III, IV, and V), and fractures of the glenoid neck. The superior approach may be used for (a) fractures of the glenoid fossa with a diffi-cult-to-control superior fragment (in conjunction with either a posterior or an anterior ex-posure) (types III, IV, V) and (b) fractures of the glenoid neck with a difficult-to-control glenoid fragment (in conjunction with a posterior exposure). Basic orthopaedic and shoul-der instruments should be available and fixation devices should include Kirschner wires (K-wires), 3.5- and 4.0-mm cannulated compression screws, and 3.5-mm malleable recon-struction plates. K-wires can be used for temporary or definitive fixation of glenoid frag-ments. The latter is the case when significantly displaced fracture fragments are too small to allow more substantial fixation but one must be sure to bend the K-wire at its point of entry to avoid migration. The 3.5-mm malleable reconstruction plates are particularly help-ful in the management of glenoid neck fractures. The 3.5- and 4.0-mm cannulated com-pression screws are especially useful in stabilizing fractures of the glenoid rim and the glenoid fossa. For patients with anterior rim, posterior rim, and type II glenoid cavity frac-tures, the iliac crest should be prepped and draped in case the fragment is comminuted, re-quiring placement of a tricortical graft to restore glenohumeral stability.

SURGERY

Although nerve block techniques are available, in most cases, general anesthesia is advis-able because of (a) the awkward positioning that may be required, (b) the extensive dis-section and manipulation that may be necessary, (c) the prolonged operative time that fre-quently occurs, and (d) the proximity of the patient's head to the work being done. A regional block before the administration of general anesthesia, however, may be used for postoperative pain control.

The shoulder should be prepped and draped widely in case combined approaches or ad-ditional exposures are necessary.

Anterior Approach

The patient is placed on the operating room table in the beach-chair position (Fig. 25-3). Bony landmarks are outlined with a marking pen (Fig. 25-4). An incision is made in Langer's lines, centered over the glenohumeral joint, and running from the superior to the

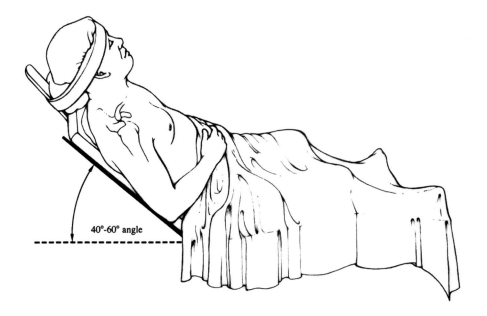

Figure 25-3. The beach-chair position used for anterior approaches to the glenoid process.

40°-60° angle

inferior margin of the humeral head (Fig. 25-5). The deltoid muscle is exposed (Fig. 25-6) and split in the line of its fibers directly over the coracoid process (Fig. 25-7). The conjoined tendon and the pectoralis major muscle are retracted medially, while the deltoid muscle is retracted laterally. The arm is externally rotated onto a sterile arm support or positioner and the subacromial bursa is removed, exposing the subscapularis tendon (Fig. 25-8). (For fractures involving the superior aspect of the glenoid fossa, opening the rotator interval may allow sufficient exposure; Fig. 25-9.) The subscapularis tendon is incised 2.5 cm medial to the medial border of the bicipital groove and along its superior and inferior borders. It is then dissected off the underlying anterior glenohumeral capsule/glenoid neck

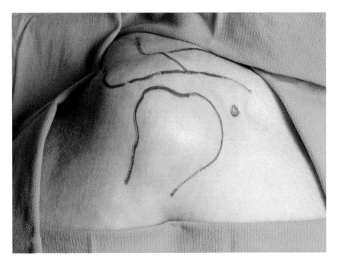

Figure 25-4. The anterior shoulder complex bony landmarks: humerus, acromion, clavicle, coracoid.

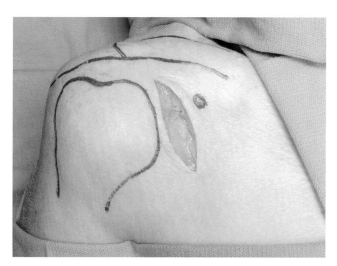

Figure 25-5. The standard anterior incision extending from the superior to the inferior margin of the humeral head, centered over the glenohumeral joint, and in Langer's lines.

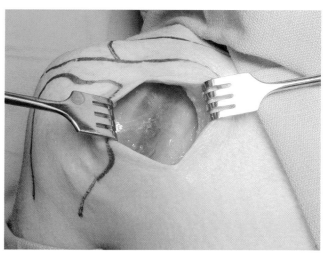

Figure 25-6. Elevation of the superficial soft-tissue flaps to expose the deltoid muscle.

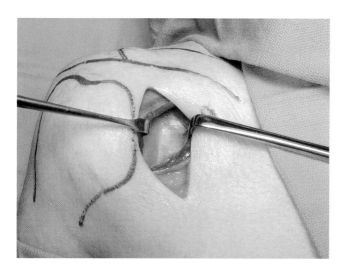

Figure 25-7. The deltoid muscle is split in the line of its fibers directly over the palpable coracoid process and retracted medially and laterally.

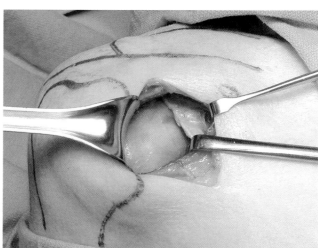

Figure 25-8. The lateral portion of the deltoid is retracted laterally, the medial portion of the deltoid and the underlying conjoined tendon are retracted medially, the arm is externally rotated, and the subacromial bursa is removed allowing visualization of the subscapularis tendon.

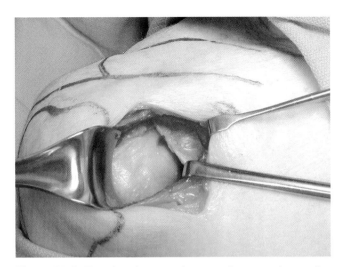

Figure 25-9. Drawing down on the arm allows one to see the rotator interval, which can be incised to gain access to the superior aspect of the glenoid process.

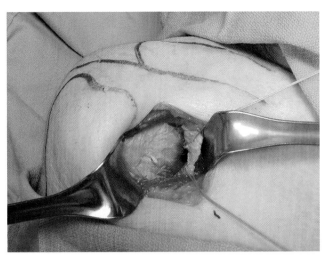

Figure 25-10. The subscapularis tendon is incised vertically 2.5 cm medial to its insertion over the greater tuberosity and along its superior and inferior borders, dissected off the underlying anterior glenohumeral joint capsule, tagged, and turned back medially.

periosteum and turned back medially (Fig. 25-10). The anterior glenohumeral capsule is incised in the same fashion and turned back medially (Fig. 25-11). With a humeral head retractor inserted into the glenohumeral joint (a Fukuda ring retractor is especially useful) and holding the humeral head out of the way, the entire glenoid cavity can be inspected and the surgeon has ready access to the anterior rim (Fig. 25-12). Support of the humerus, slight abduction, and slight external rotation of the humerus aid in relaxing the soft tissue and augment anterior exposure. One must take care to avoid injury to the nearby axillary nerve.

Figure 25-13 is an example of a case that required an anterior approach.

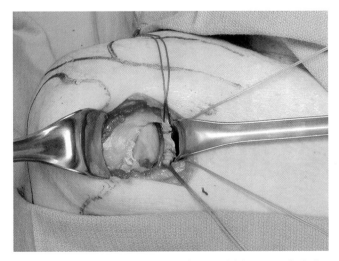

Figure 25-11. The anterior glenohumeral joint capsule is incised similarly to the subscapularis tendon, tagged, and turned back medially.

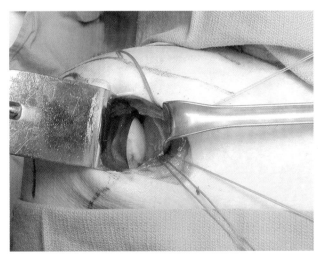

Figure 25-12. With the anterior glenohumeral joint capsule reflected medially and a humeral head retractor in place, ready access is available to the glenoid fossa and the anterior glenoid rim.

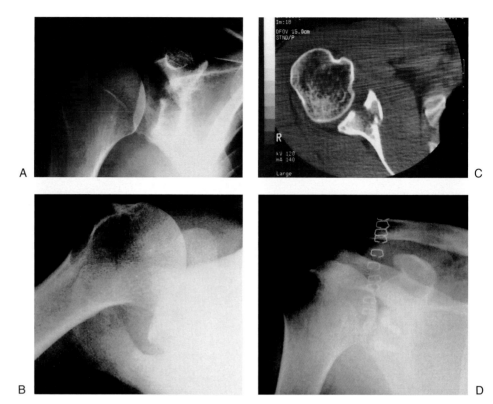

Figure 25-13. Radiographs of a person who sustained a type Ia fracture of the glenoid cavity: **(A)** a preoperative anteroposterior radiograph showing what appears to be a fracture of the anteroinferior glenoid rim; **(B)** a preoperative axillary radiograph showing what appears to be a fracture of the anterior glenoid rim with anterior subluxation of the humeral head; **(C)** an axial computed tomography image showing a severely displaced fracture of the anterior glenoid rim; and **(D)** a postoperative anteroposterior radiograph showing reduction and stabilization of the anteroinferior glenoid rim fragment with two cannulated interfragmentary screws.

Posterior Approach

The patient is placed on the operating room table in the lateral decubitus position—nonoperative side down (a towel roll placed in the axilla), operative side up, and the torso stabilized by a beanbag (Fig. 25-14). The upper extremity and shoulder complex are prepped and draped free; the elbow, forearm, and wrist/hand are encased in a sterile wrap; and a well-padded sterile-draped Mayo stand is prepared to serve as a mobile, adjustable arm rest. Bony landmarks are outlined with a marking pen (Fig. 25-15). An incision is made over the lateral third of the scapular spine, along the posterior aspect of the acromion to its lateral tip and distally in the mid-lateral line for a distance of 2.5 cm (Fig. 25-16). Via sharp and blunt dissection deep to the subcutaneous layer, soft-tissue flaps are developed and retracted, exposing the posterior deltoid muscle (Fig. 25-17). The posterior deltoid is dissected sharply off the scapular spine and acromion and split in the line of its fibers for a distance of not more than 2.5 cm, starting at the lateral tip of the acromion. A blunt retractor such as a Darrach is helpful in identifying the deltoid–infraspinatus interval along the spine of the scapula. The posterior deltoid is bluntly separated off the underlying infraspinatus and teres minor musculotendinous units and retracted down to but not below the inferior margin of the teres minor (Fig. 25-18). The inferior half of the infraspinatus tendon is incised vertically 2 cm posterior to the greater tuberosity, and the infraspinatus/teres minor interval is opened. The infraspinatus can then be dissected off the underlying posterior glenohumeral joint capsule and retracted superiorly (Fig. 25-19). The posterior glenohumeral capsule is incised in the same fashion, separated subperiosteally off the posterior glenoid process, and retracted superiorly (Fig. 25-20). With

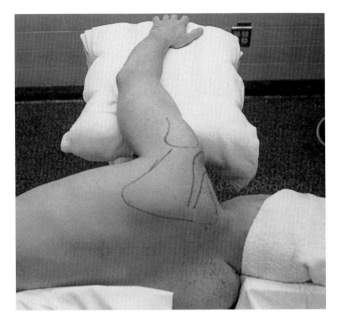

Figure 25-14. The lateral decubitus position used for posterior and posterosuperior approaches to the glenoid process. (From Goss, T.P.: Glenoid fractures: open reduction internal fixation. In: Wiss, D.A., ed.: *Master techniques of orthopaedic surgery: fractures.* Philadelphia: Lippincott–Raven Publishers, 1–17, 1998.)

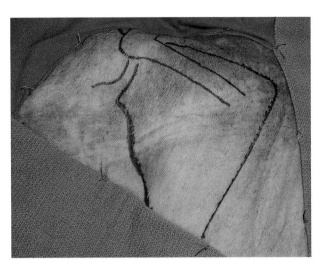

Figure 25-15. The posterior shoulder complex bony landmarks: humeral head, scapular body, scapular spine. (From Goss, T.P.: Glenoid fractures: open reduction internal fixation. In: Wiss, D.A., ed.: *Master techniques of orthopaedic surgery: fractures.* Philadelphia: Lippincott–Raven Publishers, 1–17, 1998.)

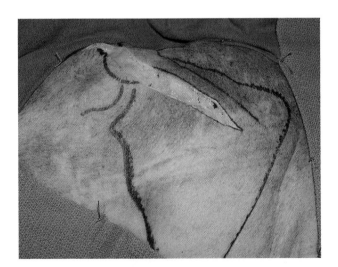

Figure 25-16. The standard posterior incision extending along the inferior margin of the scapular spine and the acromion. At the lateral tip of the acromion, the incision continues in the midlateral line for 2.5 cm. (From Goss, T.P.: Glenoid fractures: open reduction internal fixation. In: Wiss, D.A., ed.: *Master techniques of orthopaedic surgery: fractures.* Philadelphia: Lippincott–Raven Publishers, 1–17, 1998.)

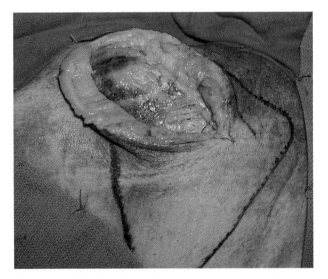

Figure 25-17. Elevation of superficial soft-tissue flaps to expose the origin of the posterior and middle heads of the deltoid muscle. (From Goss, T.P.: Glenoid fractures: open reduction internal fixation. In: Wiss, D.A., ed.: *Master techniques of orthopaedic surgery: fractures.* Philadelphia: Lippincott–Raven Publishers, 1–17, 1998.)

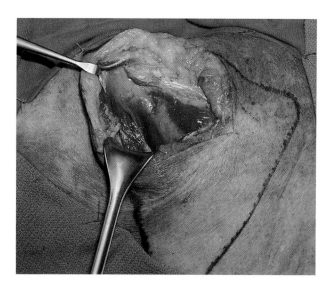

Figure 25-18. The posterior and middle heads of the deltoid muscle have been detached from the scapular spine/posterior acromial process and retracted distally to expose the infraspinatus musculotendinous unit. (From Goss, T.P.: Glenoid fractures: open reduction internal fixation. In: Wiss, D.A., ed.: *Master techniques of orthopaedic surgery: fractures.* Philadelphia: Lippincott–Raven Publishers, 1–17, 1998.)

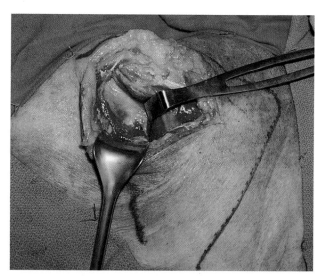

Figure 25-19. The infraspinatus/teres minor interval has been developed, with the infraspinatus retracted superiorly and the teres minor retracted inferiorly to expose the posterior glenohumeral joint capsule (the inferior portion of the infraspinatus insertion has been released). (From Goss, T.P.: Glenoid fractures: open reduction internal fixation. In: Wiss, D.A., ed.: *Master techniques of orthopaedic surgery: fractures.* Philadelphia: Lippincott–Raven Publishers, 1–17, 1998.)

a Fukuda retractor inserted into the joint and holding the humeral head out of the way, behind the anterior glenoid rim, the entire glenoid cavity can be inspected and the surgeon has ready access to the posterior aspect of the glenoid process (Fig. 25-21). The entire infraspinatus tendon/posterior glenohumeral capsule can be detached laterally and superiorly and turned back medially for maximal exposure. With injuries that involve only the posteroinferior or inferior aspect of the glenoid cavity, one may be able to avoid detaching these structures completely— simply developing the infraspinatus/teres minor interval and making a linear incision in the

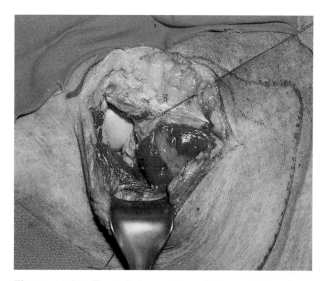

Figure 25-20. The inferior portion of the posterior glenohumeral joint capsule has been incised and reflected medially to expose the humeral head and glenohumeral joint space. (From Goss, T.P.: Glenoid fractures: open reduction internal fixation. In: Wiss, D.A., ed.: *Master techniques of orthopaedic surgery: fractures.* Philadelphia: Lippincott–Raven Publishers, 1–17, 1998.)

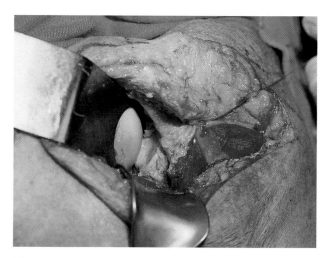

Figure 25-21. With the posterior glenohumeral joint capsule reflected medially and a humeral head retractor in place, ready access is available to the glenoid fossa and the posterior glenoid rim. (From Goss, T.P.: Glenoid fractures: open reduction internal fixation. In: Wiss, D.A., ed.: *Master techniques of orthopaedic surgery: fractures.* Philadelphia: Lippincott–Raven Publishers, 1–17, 1998.)

capsule may allow adequate access. This is the so-called safe interval, safe because the infraspinatus is innervated by the suprascapular nerve from above, and the teres minor is innervated by the axillary nerve from below. The interval between the infraspinatus and teres minor muscles can be developed further, the underlying soft tissues elevated subperiosteally, and the long head of the triceps detached to gain access to the inferior aspect of the glenoid process and lateral border of the scapular body (Fig. 25-22). One must take particular care to protect and avoid injury to the nearby suprascapular and axillary nerves.

Figures 25-23 and 25-24 are examples of cases that required a posterior approach.

Superior Approach

The superior approach can be added to the anterior or the posterior exposure if a displaced difficult-to-control or -stabilize superior glenoid cavity fragment or glenoid process fragment is present (Figs. 27-25 to 25-27). Either incision is extended over the superior aspect of the shoulder. Soft-tissue flaps are developed and retracted, exposing the superior aspect of the distal clavicle, the AC joint, the acromion, and the trapezius muscle. In the interval between the clavicle and the acromion (posteromedial to the acromioclavicular joint), the trapezius muscle and the underlying supraspinatus tendon are split in the line of their fibers bringing one down upon the superior aspect of the glenoid process (the superior glenoid rim is located posterolaterally while the base of the coracoid process is located anteromedially). A 2.0-mm guide wire can then be placed into the superior fragment and used to manipulate it into position while visualizing the reduction via the anterior or posterior exposure. One must take care to protect and avoid injury to the suprascapular nerve and vessels that lie medial to the coracoid process.

Bone Stock and Fixation Techniques

Thick solid bone for internal fixation is at a premium because much of the scapula is paper-thin. Four regions of substantial bone stock are available, however: the glenoid process, the coracoid process, the acromial process/scapular spine, and the lateral border of the scapular body (Fig. 25-28). A variety of fixation devices are available but the most useful are (a) easily contoured 3.5-mm reconstruction plates, (b) 3.5- and 4.0-mm cannulated in-

(text continues on page 474)

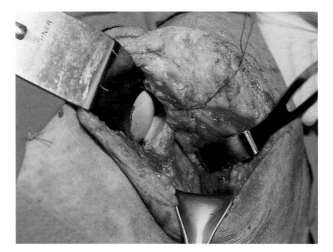

Figure 25-22. With the infraspinatus/teres minor interval developed further, the two musculotendinous units retracted, and the long head of the triceps muscle released, access to the inferior aspect of the glenoid process and the lateral scapular border is available. (From Goss, T.P.: Glenoid fractures: open reduction internal fixation. In: Wiss, D.A., ed.: *Master techniques of orthopaedic surgery: fractures.* Philadelphia: Lippincott–Raven Publishers, 1–17, 1998.)

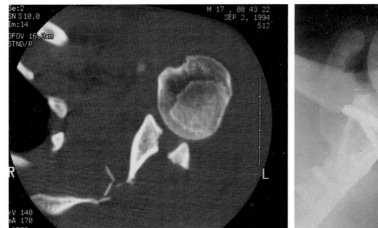
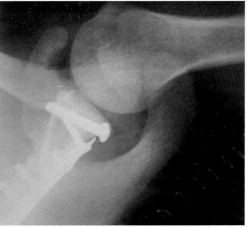

Figure 25-23. A 17-year-old boy had multiple blunt trauma including a left shoulder injury after a motor vehicle collision. Plain radiographs and a computed tomography scan **(A)** showed a severely displaced posterior glenoid rim fragment with a significant articular step-off and posterior subluxation of the humeral head (a type Ib fracture of the glenoid cavity). Five days after injury, he underwent an open reduction and internal fixation via a posterior approach. Fixation was achieved with two interfragmentary cannulated screws and a buttress plate. Articular congruity and glenohumeral stability were restored **(B)**. (From Goss, T.P.: Glenoid fractures: open reduction internal fixation. In: Wiss, D.A., ed.: *Master techniques of orthopaedic surgery: fractures.* Philadelphia: Lippincott–Raven Publishers, 1–17, 1998.)

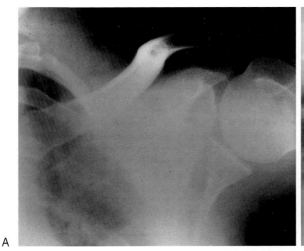
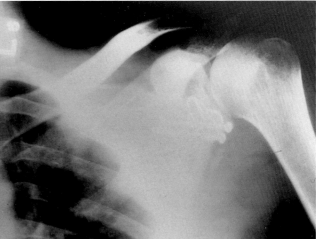

Figure 25-24. A 37-year-old man had blunt trauma to his left shoulder caused by a fall down a flight of stairs. Plain radiographs **(A)** showed a severely displaced inferior glenoid cavity fragment (type II fracture) with a significant articular step-off and inferior subluxation of the humeral head. Two days after the injury, he underwent an open reduction and internal fixation via a posterior approach. Fixation was achieved with two interfragmentary compression screws and a cerclage wire. Articular congruity and glenohumeral stability were restored **(B)**. (From Goss, T.P.: Glenoid fractures: open reduction internal fixation. In: Wiss, D.A., ed.: *Master techniques of orthopaedic surgery: fractures.* Philadelphia: Lippincott–Raven Publishers, 1–17, 1998.)

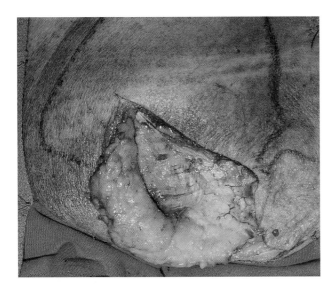

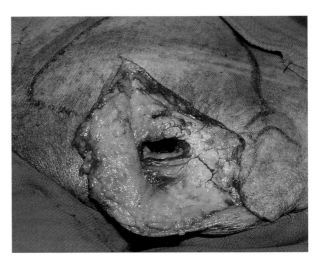

Figure 25-25. This and the next two figures show the superior approach to the glenoid process. The inferior aspect of the scapular body is at the top, the superior angle of the scapula is to the left, and the glenohumeral joint is to the right. The incision is the same as that in Figure 25-16; however, in this case, the superior soft-tissue flap has been developed and reflected, exposing the trapezius muscle (in the center of the figure), which is inserting along the scapular spine and acromial process. (From Goss, T.P.: Glenoid fractures: open reduction internal fixation. In: Wiss, D.A., ed.: *Master techniques of orthopaedic surgery: fractures.* Philadelphia: Lippincott–Raven Publishers, 1–17, 1998.)

Figure 25-26. In the interval between the clavicle and the scapular spine/acromial process, the trapezius has been split in the line of its fibers to expose the underlying supraspinatus muscle. (From Goss, T.P.: Glenoid fractures: open reduction internal fixation. In: Wiss, D.A., ed.: *Master techniques of orthopaedic surgery: fractures.* Philadelphia: Lippincott–Raven Publishers, 1–17, 1998.)

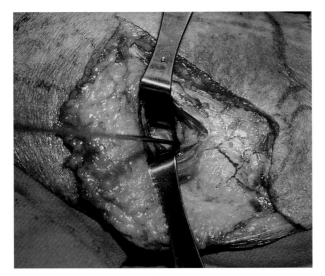

Figure 25-27. In the interval between the clavicle and scapular spine/acromial process, the trapezius muscle and the supraspinatus musculotendinous unit have been split in the line of their fibers and retracted to expose the superior aspect of the glenoid process lateral to the coracoid process. A K-wire has been placed into the glenoid process. If this were a separate fracture fragment, the K-wire could be used to manipulate the fragment into position relative to the remainder of the glenoid process (a posterior exposure is necessary to make sure articular congruity has been restored). The K-wire could then be used to place a cannulated interfragmentary compression screw. (From Goss, T.P.: Glenoid fractures: open reduction internal fixation. In: Wiss, D.A., ed.: *Master techniques of orthopaedic surgery: fractures.* Philadelphia: Lippincott–Raven Publishers, 1–17, 1998.)

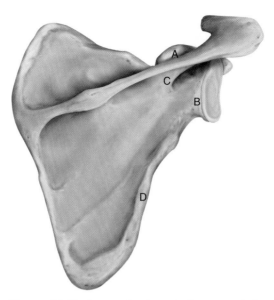

Figure 25-28. Areas of adequate bone stock for internal fixation on the glenoid region of the scapula. **A:** coracoid process; **(B)** glenoid neck; **(C)** acromial process/scapular spine; **(D)** lateral border of the scapula. (From Goss, T.P.: Glenoid fractures: open reduction internal fixation. In: Wiss, D.A., ed.: *Master techniques of orthopaedic surgery: fractures.* Philadelphia: Lippincott–Raven Publishers, 1–17, 1998.)

terfragmentary compression screws, and (c) K-wires (Figs. 25-29 to 25-31). These devices may be used alone or in combination depending upon the clinical situation and taking into account the available bone stock and the surgeon's preference and experience. Obviously, stable rigid internal fixation is desirable but frequently, lesser fixation is all that can be provided and does not preclude an excellent anatomic and functional result. The anterior and posterior exposures should be sufficient for type Ia (anterior rim) and type Ib (posterior rim) fractures, respectively. The glenoid rim fracture is reduced anatomically and fixed in position with two 2.0-mm guide wires. These wires are then used to drill, tap, and finally insert two 4.0-mm cannulated compression screws (the second screw is placed to control rotation). If the rim fragment is comminuted, a tricortical bone graft harvested from the iliac crest is used to reconstruct the margin. The posterior approach is used for type II glenoid cavity fractures and similar fixation is provided. However, the inferior fragment must be well mobilized by dissecting subperiosteally inferiorly and anteriorly; the cannulated screws are placed posteroinferiorly to anterosuperiorly.

Type III fractures are approached either anteriorly or posteriorly with a supplemental superior exposure if necessary. The superior glenoid fragment is reduced as anatomically as possible and stabilized with a cannulated screw passed superiorly to inferiorly. Type IV fractures are usually approached posteriorly, generally with a supplemental superior exposure. The superior glenoscapular fragment is reduced as anatomically as possible relative to the inferior glenoscapular fragment and stabilized with a cannulated screw passed superiorly to inferiorly.

Type V fractures of the glenoid cavity are combinations of the type II, III, and IV injuries and therefore follow the same management principles. Fractures of the glenoid neck are approached posteriorly, supplemented by a superior exposure as necessary (Fig. 25-32). The infraspinatus/teres minor interval is developed, exposing the lateral scapular border. The glenoid fragment is then reduced as anatomically as possible relative to the scapular body and fixed in position with a contoured 3.5-mm reconstruction plate applied along the posterior aspect of the glenoid fragment and the lateral scapular border.

If bleeding is a concern, medium hemovac drains are placed in the wound. Closure of the wound follows routine surgical principles.

(text continues on page 478)

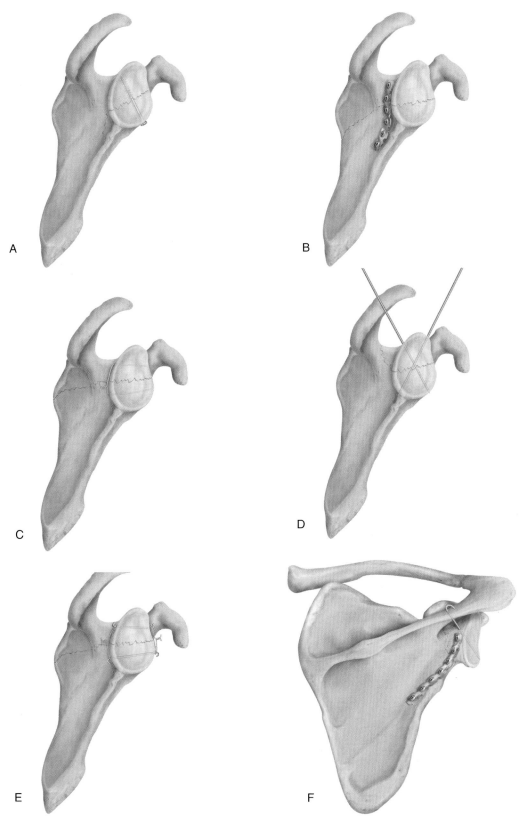

Figure 25-29. Internal fixation techniques for stabilization of glenoid process fractures. **A:** Interfragmentary compression screw. **B:** Reconstruction plate. **C:** Cerclage wire/suture. **D:** K-wires. **E:** Two K-wire-cerclage wire/suture technique. **F:** Reconstruction plate plus K-wire (used for temporary or permanent fixation). (From Goss, T.P.: Glenoid fractures: open reduction internal fixation. In: Wiss, D.A., ed.: *Master techniques of orthopaedic surgery: fractures.* Philadelphia: Lippincott–Raven Publishers, 1–17, 1998.)

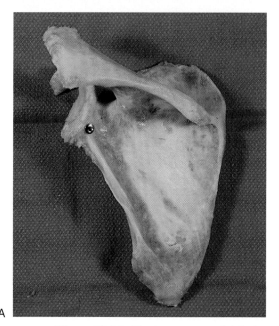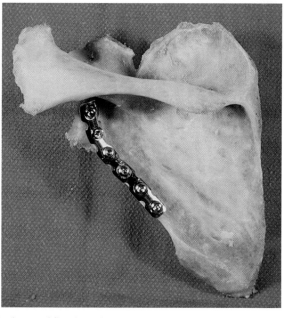

Figure 25-30. The two most useful devices for internal fixation of glenoid process fractures. **A:** A cannulated interfragmentary compression screw. **B:** A 3.5-mm malleable reconstruction plate. (From Goss, T.P.: Glenoid fractures: open reduction internal fixation. In: Wiss, D.A., ed.: *Master techniques of orthopaedic surgery: fractures.* Philadelphia: Lippincott–Raven Publishers, 1–17, 1998.)

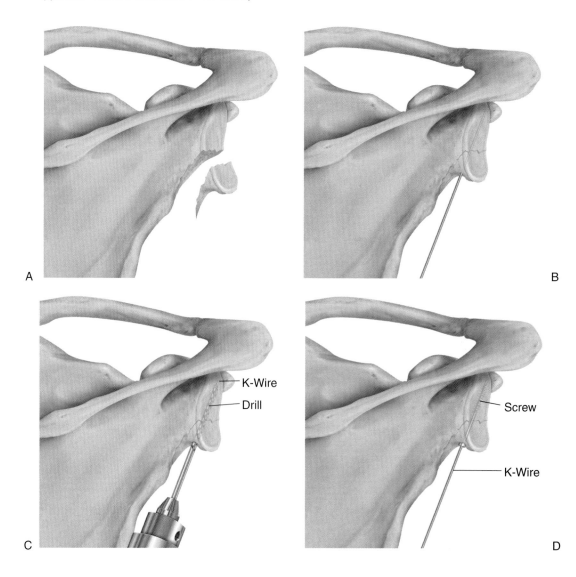

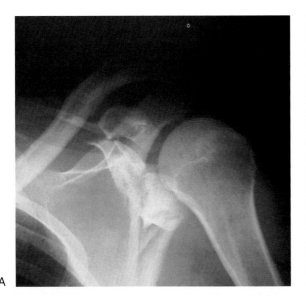

A

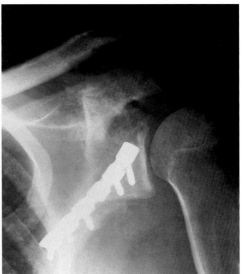

C

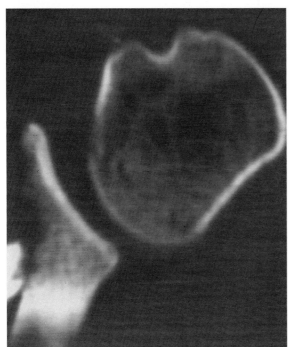

B

Figure 25-32. A 27-year-old man was involved in a motor vehicle collision, sustaining multiple blunt trauma, including an injury to his left shoulder. Plain radiographs **(A)** and a computed tomography scan **(B)** showed a complete fracture of the glenoid neck and a fracture of the coracoid process, resulting in severe angulatory displacement of the glenoid fragment (a type II glenoid neck fracture). Two days after the injury, he underwent an open reduction and internal fixation via a combined posterior/superior approach. **C:** Fixation was achieved with a 3.5-mm reconstruction plate. Anatomic position and stabilization of the glenoid fragment were achieved. (From Goss, T.P.: Glenoid fractures: open reduction internal fixation. In: Wiss, D.A., ed.: *Master techniques of orthopaedic surgery: fractures.* Philadelphia: Lippincott–Raven Publishers, 1–17, 1998.)

Figure 25-31. Reduction and internal fixation of a glenoid fracture by using an interfragmentary cannulated compression screw. **A:** Displaced type II glenoid cavity fracture. **B:** Temporary reduction and fixation of fragment by using a K-wire. **C:** Passage of a cannulated drill using the K-wire as a guide. **D:** Passage of a cannulated compression screw using the K-wire as a guide. (From Goss, T.P.: Glenoid fractures: open reduction internal fixation. In: Wiss, D.A., ed.: *Master techniques of orthopaedic surgery: fractures.* Philadelphia: Lippincott–Raven Publishers, 1–17, 1998.)

POSTOPERATIVE MANAGEMENT

Most patients are discharged to home with their arms immobilized in a sling-and-swathe bandage. Early care after operative treatment of glenoid fractures is dependent on the degree of stability achieved. With stable internal fixation, patients are begun on a program of simple passive range-of-motion exercises, which include dependent circular and pendulum movements and external rotation to but not past neutral during the first 2 weeks after surgery. Assistive or passive exercises permit restoration of motion while protecting muscles that may have been detached or split (deltoid, infraspinatus, subscapularis). Between weeks three and six, further passive stretching exercises in all ranges are initiated. The goal is to achieve 90 degrees of forward flexion by postoperative day 14, 120 degrees by postoperative day 28, and 150 degrees by postoperative day 42; internal rotation to the small of the back by postoperative day 28 and to the high part of the lower back by postoperative day 42; and 0 degrees of external rotation by postoperative day 14, 30 degrees of external rotation by postoperative day 28, and 60 degrees of external rotation by postoperative day 42. The patient sees a therapist two to three times a week and performs a self-directed home exercise program three to four times a day.

During the first 2 weeks, the patient's arm is totally immobilized between physiotherapy sessions. Light use of the arm while sitting is allowed during the third and fourth weeks. Light use of the arm when indoors is permitted during weeks 5 and 6. The patient is seen by the physician at 2-week intervals between weeks 1 and 6. Anteroposterior radiographs in neutral rotation and axillary views of the shoulder are obtained on each occasion to ensure maintenance of the reduction and hardware and correct positioning of the humeral head within the glenoid cavity. Range of motion of the shoulder is documented, and updated physiotherapy instructions are generated accordingly. If fixation is with K-wires, cerclage wires, or isolated screws, the shoulder may need to be immobilized in a sling-and-swathe dressing, an abduction brace, or even overhead olecranon pin traction for 7 to 14 days to allow early healing to occur before beginning any physiotherapy. At 6 weeks, healing is usually complete, protection is discontinued, and functional use of the shoulder is encouraged. As range of motion improves, progressive strengthening exercises are added. The rehabilitation program continues until range of motion and strength are maximized. The patient should limit the use of the arm to light activities through week 12, and heavy, physical athletic activities are prohibited for 4 to 6 months after surgery.

RESULTS

Scapular fractures are uncommon, so few large studies exist. Hardegger et al. (6) reported 79% good-to-excellent results associated with five displaced glenoid neck fractures treated surgically (6.5-year follow-up). Kavanaugh et al. (7) at Mayo Clinic reviewed ten displaced glenoid cavity fractures treated with open reduction and internal fixation (ORIF) and found it to be a "useful and safe technique which can restore excellent function of the shoulder." Until more data are available, it is reasonable to predict a good-to-excellent functional result if (a) surgical management restores normal or near-normal glenoid anatomy/articular congruity/glenohumeral stability, (b) the fixation is secure, and (c) there is a well-structured and intensive rehabilitation program.

COMPLICATIONS

Complications associated with fractures of the glenoid are in four categories (examples of each are provided):

1. Complications associated with injuries to bony and soft-tissue structures in the zone of injury due to the severe traumatic forces involved.

   Although uncommon, injuries to the axillary nerve do occur but usually represent a neurapraxia and have a good prognosis for recovery. EMG testing may be performed 3 weeks after injury or as needed thereafter to monitor recovery. Exploration and repair should be considered between 3 and 6 months after injury if there is no sign of function or if improvement is not satisfactory. Exploration and repair should be performed by 12 months at the latest. Glenohumeral arthrodesis should be considered if the patient fails to recover functional elevation.

Fractures (or late deformity and callus) in the area of the spinoglenoid notch may injure or compress the suprascapular nerve, thus affecting the neuromuscular integrity of the supraspinatus and infraspinatus muscles.

On occasion, fractures of the glenoid neck may be associated with a fracture of the clavicle. This combination of injuries has been called a "floating shoulder" and represents a double disruption of the superior shoulder suspensory complex. Because of instability, the glenoid neck or clavicle fracture can be severely displaced. Gross shoulder instability results and may be felt by the patient as a "shift" of the shoulder girdle. Stabilization of one or both bones is suggested to improve comfort and aid in overall management. Regardless of how the glenoid neck fracture is managed, if unacceptable displacement persists at the clavicular fracture site, ORIF is indicated.

2. Complications associated with the scapular fracture itself.

If ORIF of a glenoid fossa fracture fails to restore satisfactory articular congruity, resulting in symptomatic posttraumatic glenohumeral arthritis, a shoulder arthroplasty may be indicated. In older individuals, a total replacement is the procedure of choice. In younger individuals, a hemiarthroplasty with or without reshaping of the glenoid and biologic resurfacing (with the option to convert to a total shoulder replacement at a later date) may be considered. Arthrodesis is an option in those who must use their shoulders for heavy, manual, physical work.

3. Complications associated with the surgical management.

Superficial infections are managed with local irrigation and débridement, closure over drains, and a short course of appropriate antibiotic therapy. Deep infections must be recognized as early as possible and treated aggressively. The wound is opened surgically, thoroughly débrided and irrigated, and closed over drains. Hardware is maintained if possible and certainly if fixation is firm. Six weeks of appropriate intravenous antibiotic therapy is frequently indicated. Iatrogenic damage to the axillary or suprascapular nerves may also occur, resulting in compromised infraspinatus, supraspinatus, or deltoid function.

4. Complications associated with the postoperative management.

Shoulder joint stiffness may result with either nonoperative or operative treatment. Close follow-up by the physician, dedication on the part of the therapist, and maximal effort by the patient should result in functional shoulder range of motion. Most patients will lose some range of motion; however, 135 degrees or more of forward flexion, internal rotation to the small of the back, and 30 degrees of external rotation should be achieved. If postoperative loss of motion occurs, a closed manipulation under anesthesia is generally unsuccessful because this type of shoulder stiffness is caused by dense posttraumatic and postoperative scarring. An open surgical release may result in even more scarring and loss of motion. Treatment therefore consists of a long-term aggressive stretching program, hoping that the contracted soft tissues will gradually stretch out over time.

RECOMMENDED READING

1. Butters, K.P.: The scapula. In Rockwood, C.A. Jr., Matsen, F.A. II, eds.: *The shoulder.* Vol. 1. Philadelphia: WB Saunders, 335–366, 1990.
2. Goss, T.P.: Fractures of the glenoid cavity. *J Bone Joint Surg Am* 74: 299–305, 1992.
3. Goss, T.P.: Fractures of the glenoid cavity: operative principles and techniques. *Techn Orthop* 8: 199–204, 1994.
4. Goss, T.P.: Fractures of the scapula: diagnosis and treatment. In: Iannotti, J.P., Williams, G.G., eds.: *Disorders of the shoulder: diagnosis and treatment.* Philadelphia: Lippincott Williams & Wilkins, 597–637, 1999.
5. Goss, T.P.: Scapular fractures and dislocations: diagnosis and treatment. *J Am Acad Orthop Surg* 3(l): 22–33, 1995.
6. Hardegger, F.H., Simpson, L.A., Weber, B.G.: The operative treatment of scapular fractures. *J Bone Joint Surg Br* 66: 725–731, 1984.
7. Kavanaugh, B.F., Bradway, J.K., Cofield, R.H.: Open reduction and internal fixation of displaced intraarticular fractures of the glenoid fossa. *J Bone Joint Surg Am* 75: 479–484, 1993.

26

Percutaneous Fixation of Proximal Humeral Fractures

Raymond R. White

INDICATIONS/CONTRAINDICATIONS

Percutaneous fixation of proximal humeral fractures is an excellent example of indirect reduction and minimal stable fixation. This procedure allows rapid healing and return to a normal function. The Neer classification accounts for displacement and angulation and is used to classify proximal humerus fractures (Fig. 26-1). Percutaneous fixation is most commonly used to treat two-part fractures or those involving the surgical neck and the isolated greater tuberosity fracture. However, this technique is also optimal for three-part fractures because it preserves the tenuous blood supply to the head fragment. This technique, therefore, should be considered for physiologically young patients who wish to save their own humeral head and avoid prosthetic replacement. Occasionally percutaneous fixation can be used on four-part fractures. The risk of avascular necrosis associated with this procedure precludes its use in circumstances other than for young patients who want to save the humeral head.

Contraindications for percutaneous fixation are head-splitting fractures; four-part fractures in the elderly; uncooperative patients; pathologic bone; and metaphyseal extension. This technique is not a substitute for prosthetic replacement in the elderly with four-part fractures or fractures in which the humeral head is split and not able to be reconstructed. Patients must be cooperative and not confused. Postoperative patient confusion may lead to loss of fixation and poor results. If adequate fixation is not possible because of osteopenia or pathologic (tumor) bone, another technique should be used. This technique cannot be used in fractures with metaphyseal comminution. These fractures, in which length is an important issue, should be stabilized with plate fixation.

R. R. White, M.D.: Department of Orthopaedics, University of Vermont, Burlington, Vermont; and Orthopaedic Trauma Division, Maine Medical Center, Portland, Maine.

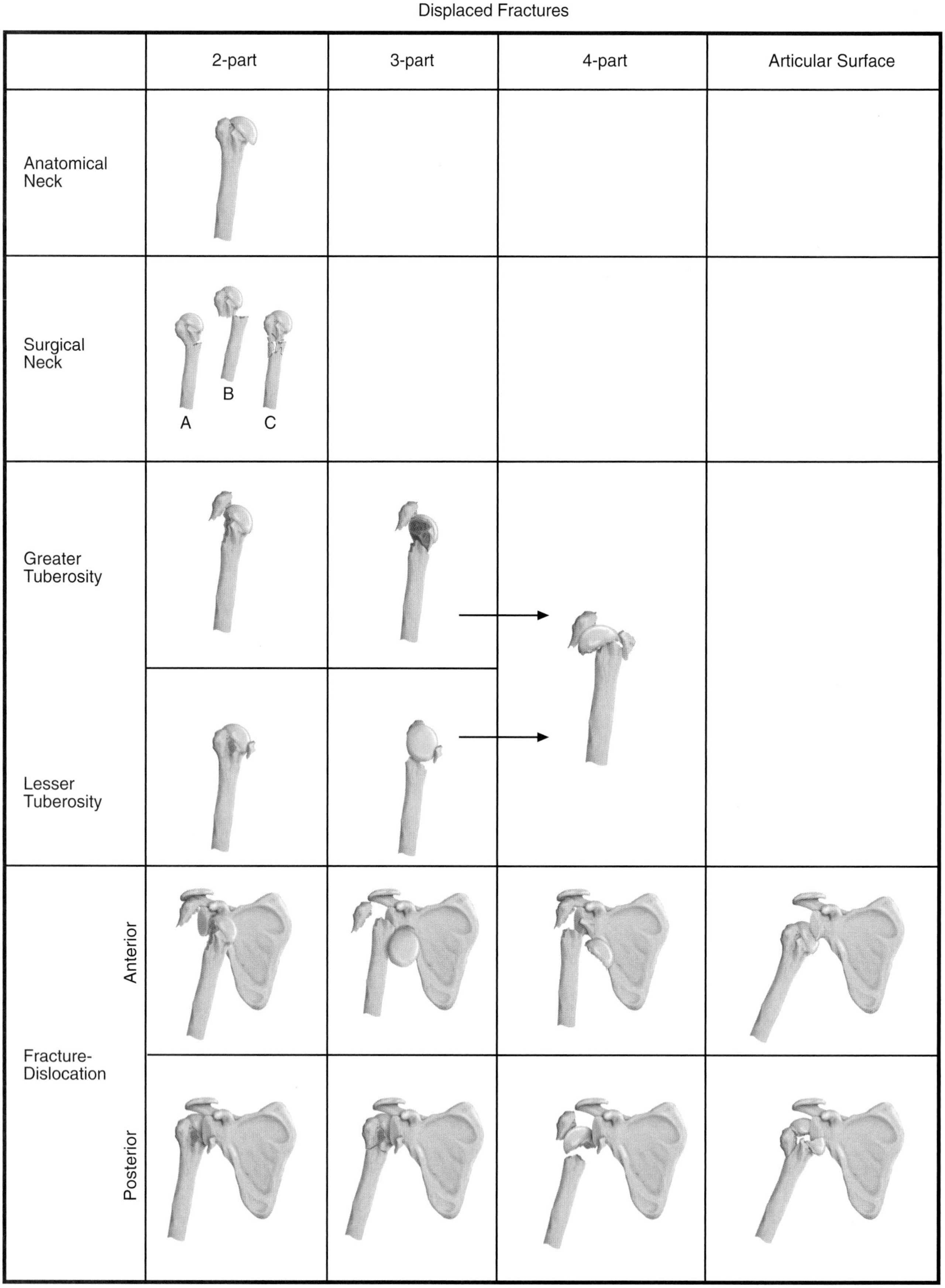

Displaced Fractures

	2-part	3-part	4-part	Articular Surface
Anatomical Neck				
Surgical Neck	A B C			
Greater Tuberosity				
Lesser Tuberosity				
Fracture-Dislocation — Anterior				
Fracture-Dislocation — Posterior				

Figure 26-1. Neer classification of proximal humerus fractures. (From White, R.R.: Proximal humeral fractures: percutaneous fixation. In: Wiss, D.A., ed.: *Master techniques of orthopaedic surgery: fractures.* Philadelphia: Lippincott–Raven Publishers, 19–33, 1998.)

PREOPERATIVE PLANNING

Initially, the patient's limb is evaluated for neurovascular compromise, especially the axillary nerve. Considerable shoulder swelling is not unusual, and ecchymosis often extends into the forearm and chest wall.

Radiographic views include an anteroposterior (AP), scapular Y, and axillary lateral views of the shoulder (Fig. 26-2). A true AP view of the humerus (with the arm in a neutral position) may be useful to determine head impaction. The axillary view is helpful in determining AP angulation and lesser tuberosity displacement. A computed tomography scan is rarely necessary, and magnetic resonance imaging is not helpful in determining head vascularity in the acute phase.

Timing of the surgery is critical only if the head is dislocated. A dislocated humeral head must be relocated as an emergency. Occasionally it is possible to reduce the head dislocation by closed methods, but an open approach is usually required. If the head is not dislocated, surgery can be done on an elective basis, usually 3 to 7 days after injury. If there are no associated medical problems, surgery can be done in an outpatient setting. The patient is placed in a sling-and-swathe shoulder immobilizer until surgery. Pre- and postoperative pain management are the same: The patients are given scheduled acetaminophen (1,000 mg every 6 hours) and ibuprofen (400 mg every 6 hours), with oxycodone (5 to 10 mg every 2 hours) for breakthrough pain.

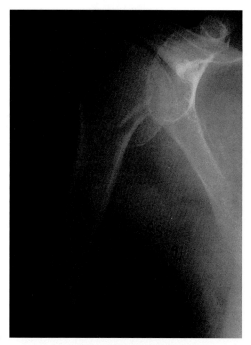

A

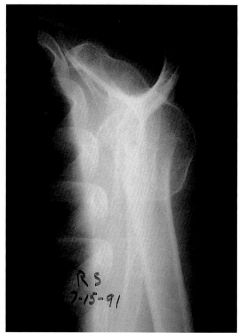

B

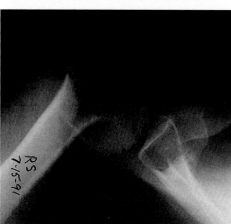

C

Figure 26-2. A: Anteroposterior radiograph. **B:** "Y" radiograph. **C:** Axillary radiograph. (From White, R.R.: Proximal humeral fractures: percutaneous fixation. In: Wiss, D.A., ed.: *Master techniques of orthopaedic surgery: fractures.* Philadelphia: Lippincott–Raven Publishers, 19–33, 1998.)

SURGERY

After the patient is anesthetized, the table is turned 90 degrees, with the anesthesia staff and their equipment on the unaffected side, allowing sufficient room for the surgeon on the affected side. The image intensifier is positioned at the head of the table with the video monitors near the base unit on the affected side (Fig. 26-3A). The C-arm is positioned so the

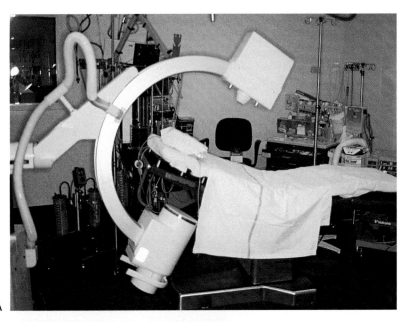

A

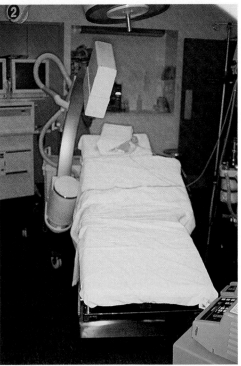

B

Figure 26-3. **A:** The position of the operating room equipment. The table is turned 90 degrees, with the anesthetist and equipment on the unaffected side and the image intensifier at the head of the table. **B:** The C-arm position as seen from the end of the table. Note that the C is tilted to avoid the table's interfering with the image. (From White, R.R.: Proximal humeral fractures: percutaneous fixation. In: Wiss, D.A., ed.: *Master techniques of orthopaedic surgery: fractures.* Philadelphia: Lippincott–Raven Publishers, 19–33, 1998.)

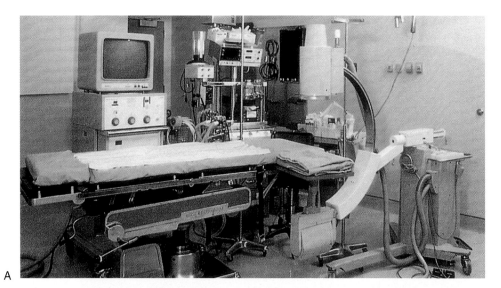

A

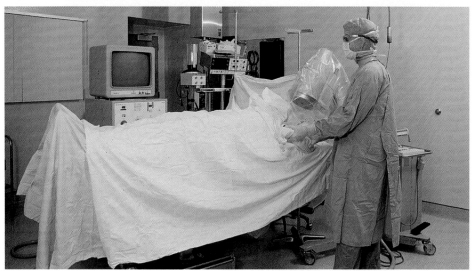

B

Figure 26-4. A: The patient is positioned flat on the operating room table. The patient's head is at the foot of the table. This keeps the table cranks from interfering with the image intensifier. **B:** The axillary view is easy to obtain in this position by swinging the image under the shoulder. (From White, R.R.: Proximal humeral fractures: percutaneous fixation. In: Wiss, D.A., ed.: *Master techniques of orthopaedic surgery: fractures.* Philadelphia: Lippincott–Raven Publishers, 19–33, 1998.)

machine can swing 90 degrees to obtain an axillary view. The "C" should be positioned to swing either under or over, depending on the position of the patient. It is helpful to tilt the upper portion of the "C" medially and the lower portion of the "C" laterally to keep the table from interfering with the image (Fig. 26-3B).

Patients can be positioned in one of two ways. The first is to place the patient flat on a level operating room table with the head at the foot of the table (backward on the table), so the table cranks are not in the way of the x-ray machine (Fig. 26-4A). The patient is then moved laterally on a radiolucent board so the shoulder is over the edge of the table. The advantage of this position is threefold: two-part fractures tend to stay reduced; the image-intensifier sending unit is below the table and farther from the surgeon; and the image swings under the drapes, facilitating an axillary view (Fig. 26-4B).

In the second position, the patient is placed in a beach-chair position (Fig. 26-5A) with the shoulder over the edge of the table. The image intensifier is turned so the sending unit is up and can be swung over the top for the axillary view. This position provides an easy table setup, and if open reduction is necessary, the position is a familiar one. Unfortunately,

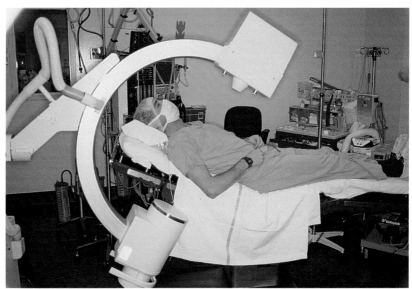

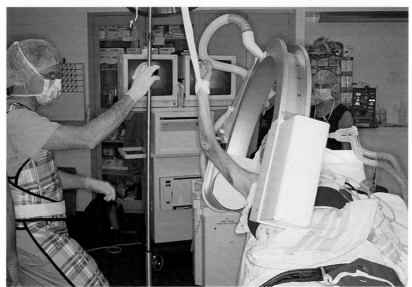

Figure 26-5. A: The beach-chair position is shown. **B:** The image must be swung over the top for the axillary view. (From White, R.R.: Proximal humeral fractures: percutaneous fixation. In: Wiss, D.A., ed.: *Master techniques of orthopaedic surgery: fractures.* Philadelphia: Lippincott–Raven Publishers, 19–33, 1998.)

the C-arm must be swung over the top to obtain an axillary view, and the x-ray unit is closer to the surgeon's head, increasing exposure to the surgeon (see Fig. 26-5B).

Reduction

Head-shaft Reduction. It is imperative that the head be properly reduced onto the shaft. The pectoralis major pulls the shaft medially, anteriorly, and into internal rotation, exerting a deforming force. The supraspinatus, the other major deforming force, abducts the head fragment. Reduction can usually be accomplished by reversing the deforming forces. The reduction maneuver is longitudinal traction, abduction, posterior displacement, and slight external rotation of the shaft fragment relative to the proximal fragment (Fig. 26-6A). When impaction is a major component of the fracture, the shaft fragment may need to be moved posteriorly and outward (while longitudinal traction is applied; Fig. 26-6B).

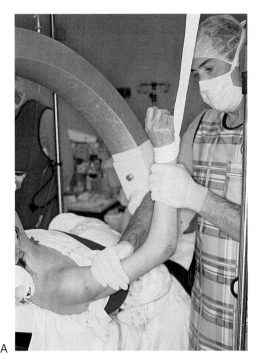

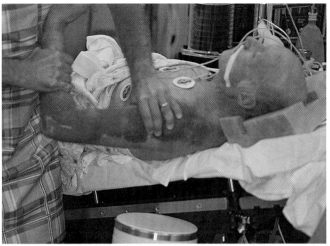

A

B

Figure 26-6. A,B: The maneuver used to reduce two- and three-part fractures. The shaft is distracted and mobilized posteriorly relative to the head fragment. (From White, R.R.: Proximal humeral fractures: percutaneous fixation. In: Wiss, D.A., ed.: *Master techniques of orthopaedic surgery: fractures.* Philadelphia: Lippincott–Raven Publishers, 19–33, 1998.)

This movement can be aided by placing a rolled towel in the axilla to act as a fulcrum. Reduction must be confirmed in both AP and axillary planes by using the image intensifier before fixation.

Once reduction is obtained, it can usually be maintained by holding the arm suspended while prepping and draping is carried out (Fig. 26-7). After draping, the assistant holds the reduction while the surgeon places the fixation.

If an acceptable reduction cannot be obtained or maintained, a small-diameter Schanz pin inserted into the head acts as a joystick. The pin should be placed via the greater

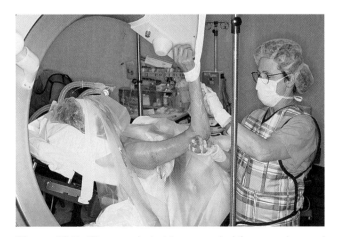

Figure 26-7. The arm is held suspended for prepping and draping. This position usually holds the reduction. (From White, R.R.: Proximal humeral fractures: percutaneous fixation. In: Wiss, D.A., ed.: *Master techniques of orthopaedic surgery: fractures.* Philadelphia: Lippincott–Raven Publishers, 19–33, 1998.)

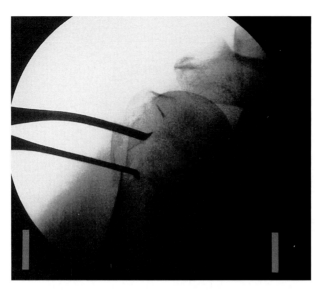

Figure 26-8. The impacted head fragment of this three-part fracture is reduced through a percutaneous incision with a lamina spreader. (From White, R.R.: Proximal humeral fractures: percutaneous fixation. In: Wiss, D.A., ed.: *Master techniques of orthopaedic surgery: fractures.* Philadelphia: Lippincott–Raven Publishers, 19–33, 1998.)

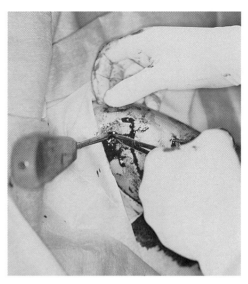

Figure 26-9. The soft tissues are spread with a hemostat when screws and washers are passed through them. (From White, R.R.: Proximal humeral fractures: percutaneous fixation. In: Wiss, D.A., ed.: *Master techniques of orthopaedic surgery: fractures.* Philadelphia: Lippincott–Raven Publishers, 19–33, 1998.)

tuberosity to control the head fragment so the shaft fragment can be reduced to it.

Occasionally, the fracture cannot be reduced closed because of biceps tendon interposition. A limited deltopectoral approach can be used to remove the tendon, permitting fracture reduction. Formal open reduction is occasionally necessary when there is a significant displacement or irreducible impaction. In these cases, fixation can be either percutaneous or internal.

Greater Tuberosity Reduction. Greater tuberosity fractures can be reduced percutaneously. First, rotate the shoulder until the displaced fragment is seen in its greatest profile and displacement. The fragment is usually a little posterior; some internal rotation of the arm will give the best view of displacement. A cannulated screw guide pin is placed via a 1.5-cm deltoid splitting into the center of the fragment. If the displacement is lateral only, the pin can be directed into the humeral head. If the displacement is superior and lateral, the pin should be directed more inferiorly. The cannulated screw (usually with a washer) will push the fragment either medially, or medially and distally when tightened, thereby reducing the fracture.

Three-part Fractures. Three-part fractures in which the head is impacted and the greater tuberosity laterally displaced can also be reduced percutaneously. A 2.0-cm deltoid-splitting incision is made at the level of the fracture (this is localized with the image intensifier). A lamina spreader is introduced into the fracture site, and the head is disimpacted by opening the jaws of the spreader (Fig. 26-8); this tilts the head fragment into position by rotating it around the intact medial soft-tissue structures. The head is then held in place with pins (as described subsequently). The greater tuberosity can then key into place if the head has been tilted into the correct position. It is reduced as described previously, and fixed as noted subsequently (see Fixation).

Fixation

Greater Tuberosity Fractures. In minimally displaced or comminuted tuberosity fractures, a large cannulated cancellous screw (7.0 or 7.3 mm) can be used to obtain both the reduction and the fixation. By using the image intensifier, the arm is rotated until the tuberosity is in greatest profile and displacement. Next, the cannulated screw guide pin is placed through a 1.5-cm incision into the center of the fragment and into the opposite cortex. A screw with a washer is then placed in the standard fashion. As the screw is tightened, the reduction is accomplished. A washer must be used to distribute the force of this powerful screw over a large area to avoid fragmenting the tuberosity. Care must be taken not to entrap the deltoid muscle beneath the washer. A curved hemostat or similar instrument is used to mobilize the muscle as the screw and washer pass through the deltoid (Figs. 26-9 and 26-10).

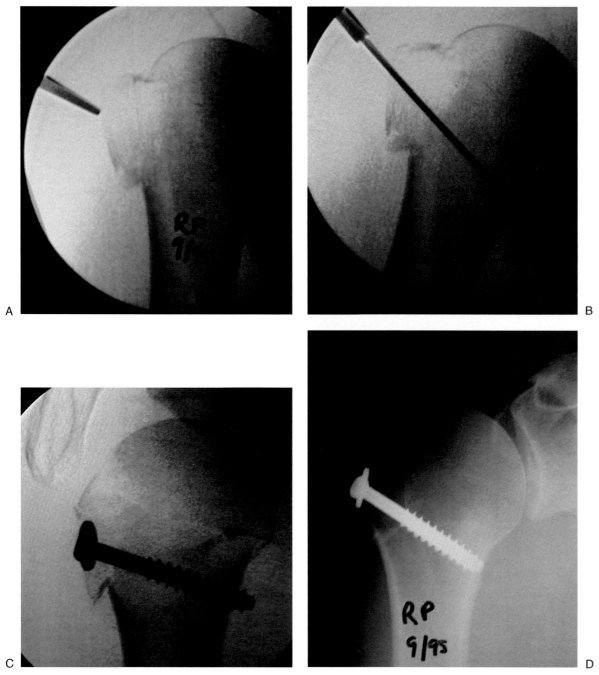

Figure 26-10. **A:** The greater tuberosity is seen on greatest profile, and the starting point is identified with a straight hemostat. **B:** A cannulated screw guide pin is passed through the greater tuberosity and into the medial cortex. **C:** The cannulated screw is placed, and the fracture is reduced by the screw and washer. **D:** Result at follow-up. (From White, R.R.: Proximal humeral fractures: percutaneous fixation. In: Wiss, D.A., ed.: *Master techniques of orthopaedic surgery: fractures.* Philadelphia: Lippincott–Raven Publishers, 19–33, 1998.)

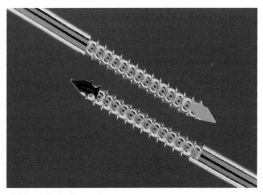

Figure 26-11. Terminally threaded pins used for percutaneous fixation. (From White, R.R.: Proximal humeral fractures: percutaneous fixation. In: Wiss, D.A., ed.: *Master techniques of orthopaedic surgery: fractures.* Philadelphia: Lippincott–Raven Publishers, 19–33, 1998.)

Two-part Fractures. For fixation of a two-part proximal humeral fracture, we use 2.5 × 150-mm terminally threaded pins (Fig. 26-11) to decrease the chance of pin migration. If these are not available, the terminally threaded guide pins can be used with a compression hip screw.

By using the image intensifier, position a pin on the anterior shoulder along the ideal line for placement, and mark the line with a skin marker. This line functions as the anteversion guide pin does in pinning femoral neck or intertrochanteric fractures. Ideally, it should be placed just above the deltoid insertion, but it is usually placed a little higher. Care must be taken to avoid damaging the axillary nerve. Four pins should be placed; they need not be parallel. An attempt should be made to spread the pins in the humeral head. Pin placement should be checked on both views with the image intensifier to be certain that they are contained within the humeral head. After the pins have been placed properly, they are cut off beneath the skin (Fig. 26-12).

Another method of fixation uses cannulated screws. With this method, it is possible to use only one or two cannulated screws because of the limiting factor of the size of the starting point, the lateral humeral shaft. The fixation used most often is two 7.0-mm cannulated cancellous screws oriented vertically along the shaft and into the head.

Three- and Four-part Fractures. In three- and four-part fractures, the head fragment is stabilized in the same way as in two-part fractures. The greater tuberosity fragment is stabilized with a single large cannulated cancellous screw. This screw is directed into the humeral head or into the proximal metaphysis, depending on which way will best reduce the fragment (see the previous section on fixation of greater tuberosity fractures) (Fig. 26-13). The lesser tuberosity is not usually stabilized in four-part fractures.

POSTOPERATIVE MANAGEMENT

The strength of the fixation and the reliability of the patient determine whether the arm is placed in a sling or sling-and-swathe. If the patient is cooperative and excellent fixation was obtained, only a sling is used. If there are any concerns, the swathe also is used. Physical therapy is started 5 to 7 days after surgery. Initial physical therapy consists of gentle pendulum exercises. Active and active-assisted range of motion is started 3 to 4 weeks after surgery, depending on the fixation quality and the healing. The sling protection is discontinued 4 to 6 weeks after surgery, depending on healing. Strengthening begins at this time. Unrestricted activity begins when healing is complete, usually within 6 to 10 weeks.

The pins are removed at 4 to 6 weeks, depending on healing. This is generally done in the office with local anesthesia. Sometimes sedation is necessary; extremely squeamish patients require a light general anesthetic.

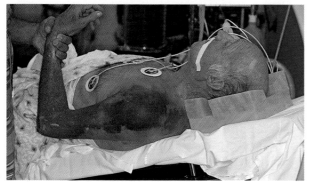

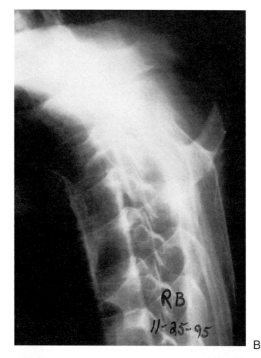

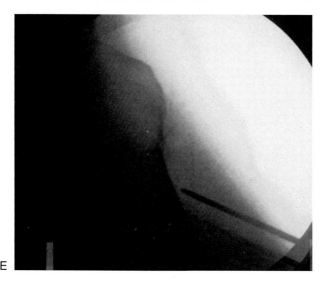

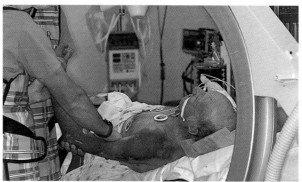

Figure 26-12. A,B: Anteroposterior (AP) and Y-view of a patient. **C:** Supine position of the patient on the table. Note the extensive hematoma as a result of this fracture. **D:** The reduction maneuver. The shaft is mobilized distal, posterior, and lateral relative to the head fragment. **E:** The position of the fragments after reduction and before pinning. This shows a pin placed outside the skin to localize the skin incision. *(continued)*

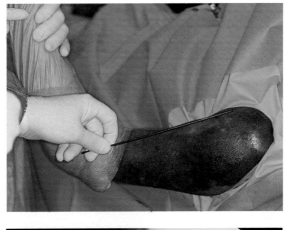

F

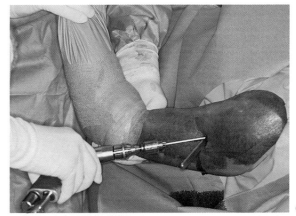

G

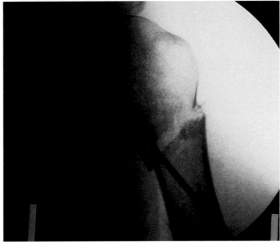

H

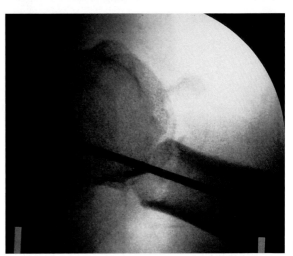

I

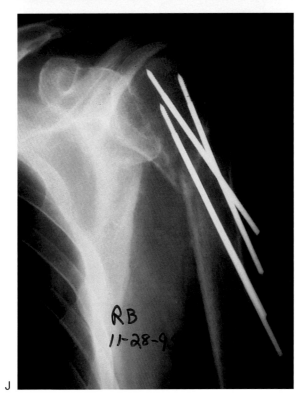

J

Figure 26-12. *Continued.* **F:** A pin is placed on the anterior aspect of the shoulder to estimate the direction in which the pins should be directed. **G:** The first pin is drilled. Note the pin is directed in line with the shaft. This will place the pin in the head fragment. **H,I:** The intraoperative placement of the first pin in the AP and axillary views. **J:** The radiograph at 3 weeks shows the final position, and one pin has slightly backed out. (From White, R.R.: Proximal humeral fractures: percutaneous fixation. In: Wiss, D.A., ed.: *Master techniques of orthopaedic surgery: fractures.* Philadelphia: Lippincott–Raven Publishers, 19–33, 1998.)

COMPLICATIONS

Pin Protrusion or Migration

The most common causes of pin protrusion through the skin are reduction of swelling in the upper area and outward migration of the pins.

In the first type, the surgeon has two choices: (a) remove the pin if healing has progressed and if the remainder of the fixation is adequate to the point that removal of the pin will not jeopardize the fixation; or (b) leave the protruding pin in place, and treat the pin site as if it were an external fixator pin site. I generally choose the latter approach and have done so without further problems.

Migrating pins pose a more serious problem. The first sign of a migrating pin may be a sudden increase in pain, in either the shoulder or the soft tissues. If the pin has migrated outward and still provides fixation, it can be treated as a protruding pin, as noted previously. If it is no longer providing fixation, protruding through the skin, and causing enough irritation to hamper rehabilitation, it is best removed. If a pin should migrate inward and pen-

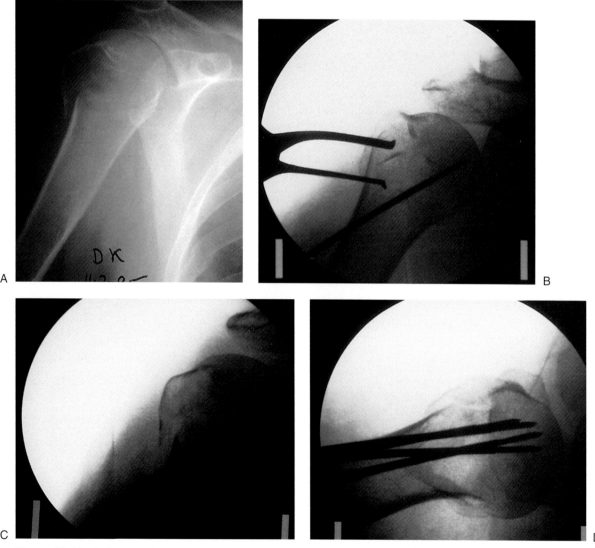

Figure 26-13. A: Impacted three-part fracture. The head fragment is impacted into a valgus position, and the tuberosity fragment is laterally displaced. **B:** The lamina spreader is shown in position. The head has been elevated and the first K-wire is in place. **C,D:** The position of the pins in the anteroposterior and axillary views. The tuberosity is still displaced. *(continued)*

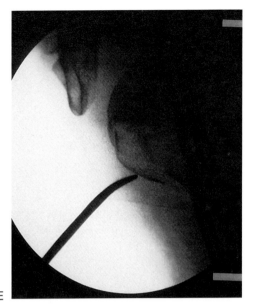
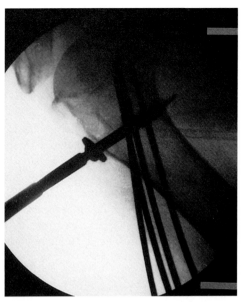

E   F

Figure 26-13. *Continued.* **E:** An instrument is shown localizing the appropriate starting point for the screw. **F:** The final position after the cannulated screw is placed. The tuberosity is reduced. (From White, R.R.: Proximal humeral fractures: percutaneous fixation. In: Wiss, D.A., ed.: *Master techniques of orthopaedic surgery: fractures.* Philadelphia: Lippincott–Raven Publishers, 19–33, 1998.)

etrate the humeral head, it must be removed immediately. These pins are not repositioned because enough healing has taken place that replacement is not necessary.

Loss of Reduction

Loss of reduction is usually associated with fixation failure, either pin or bone failure. Because many patients with proximal humerus fractures are elderly, the problem of poor bone quality is of great concern. In addition, many elderly patients become confused and may be more active than they should be. When a patient becomes confused and requires restraints, the arm should be placed in a sling-and-swathe. A fiberglass cast may be used for the swathe so it cannot be removed by the patient.

RECOMMENDED READING

1. Cornell, C.N., Levine, D., Pagnani, M.J.: Internal fixation of proximal humerus fractures using the screwtension band technique. *J Orthop Trauma* 8: 23–27, 1994.
2. Flatow, E.L., Cuomo, F., Maday, M.G., et al.: Open reduction and internal fixation of two-part displaced fractures of the greater tuberosity of the proximal part of the humerus. *J Bone Joint Surg Am* 73: 1213–1218, 1991.
3. Jaberg, H., Warner, J.J., Jakob, R.P.: Percutaneous stabilization of unstable fractures of the humerus. *J Bone Joint Surg Am* 74: 508–515, 1992.
4. Kocialkowski, A., Wallace, W.A.: Closed percutaneous K-wire stabilization for displaced fractures of the surgical neck of the humerus. *Br J Accident Surg* 21: 209–212, 1990.
5. Koval, K.J., Sanders, R., Zuckerman, J.D., et al.: Modified-tension band wiring of displaced surgical neck fractures of the humerus. *J Shoulder Elbow Surg* 2: 85–92, 1993.
6. Ruedi, T., Schweiberer.: Fractures of the proximal humerus. In: Allgöwer, M., ed.: *Manual of internal fixation,* 3rd ed. New York: Springer-Verlag, 438–441, 1992.

27

Operative Treatment of Tuberosity Fractures, Malunions, and Nonunions

Edward V. Craig

FRACTURES OF THE GREATER TUBEROSITY

INDICATIONS/CONTRAINDICATIONS

Fractures of the greater tuberosity continue to present a challenge for the clinician treating trauma to the shoulder. Because of the small amount of space available to the rotator cuff passing under the coracoacromial arch, small degrees of tuberosity displacement may produce severe functional deficits.

Greater tuberosity fractures occur both in association with and in the absence of anterior glenohumeral dislocations. A greater tuberosity fracture without an associated dislocation may be nondisplaced, minimally displaced, or displaced. When displacement occurs, it is usually posterior or superior. In some instances, "open-book" displacement occurs with opening anteriorly and the fragment "hinged" posteriorly.

A greater tuberosity that fractures in association with an anterior glenohumeral dislocation may produce unique problems for the surgeon. If the associated soft-tissue attachments to the shaft of the humerus and periosteum are disrupted, the rotator cuff attached to the greater tuberosity may displace the greater tuberosity in such a way that when the humeral head is relocated, anatomic restoration of the greater tuberosity may not occur. If the greater tuberosity remains in an anatomic position following relocation, there is little long-term deficit. After a brief period of immobilization, rehabilitation may be begun with range-of-motion exercises, followed by exercises that are more aggressive after the healing of the fracture.

E. V. Craig, M.D.: Department of Orthopaedics, Weill Medical College of Cornell University; and Hospital for Special Surgery, New York, New York.

My indications for operative fixation of an acute greater tuberosity fracture with or without an associated humeral head dislocation are the following:

- Displacement of the greater tuberosity in a superior or posterior direction more than 0.5 to 1 cm (Figs. 27-1 and 27-2).

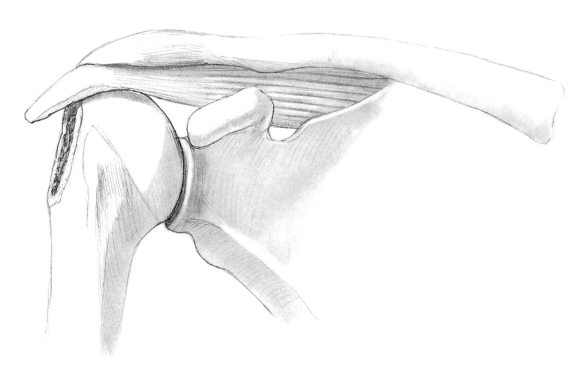

Figure 27-1. Pathologic fracture anatomy. The greater tuberosity segment is pulled superiorly by the supra- and infraspinatus muscles. This fragment displaces into the subacromial space, limiting abduction and forward elevation and producing a mechanical block to elevation of the extremity.

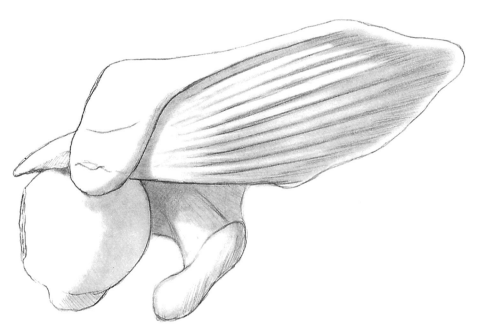

Figure 27-2. In some patients, the large tuberosity fragment is pulled posteriorly, coming to rest behind the humeral head. This fragment may heal to the shaft of the humerus or the posterior glenoid, and it is often associated with contracted external rotators and posterior capsule.

- Displacement of the greater tuberosity 0.3 to 0.5 cm in a superior direction in an over-head athlete or in someone who needs normal, asymptomatic function for overhead use of the arm.
- Irreducible dislocation of the humeral head requiring open reduction.

In general, the only contraindications for acute operative treatment of a greater tuberosity fracture are little or no displacement of the tuberosity segment; displacement that is neither posterior nor anterior, but directly lateral, or hinges open on one side; or if the patient's medical condition precludes surgical intervention.

PREOPERATIVE PLANNING

A patient who has a displaced greater tuberosity fracture, whether or not the humeral head is dislocated, presents with the arm splinted at the side. Any movement of the arm is exquisitely tender and painful. Examination of the extremity usually shows ecchymosis and swelling over the shoulder girdle, and there is often crepitus with gentle rotation of the glenohumeral joint. There is usually point tenderness in the area of the greater tuberosity attachment. If the greater tuberosity fracture is accompanied by an anterior dislocation of the glenohumeral joint, there is, in addition, a fullness in the subcoracoid area. As in any anterior dislocation, there may be a flattening lateral to the acromial process, but the associated fracture of the tuberosity, with its attendant bleeding and swelling, may mask the usual flattened appearance, the result of the empty glenoid that frequently accompanies traumatic anterior dislocations of the shoulder.

I routinely order three radiographs to assess the degree of displacement of the greater tuberosity in an acute fracture: an anteroposterior (AP) view of the glenohumeral joint, which provides information on the degree of superior displacement of the greater tuberosity and identifies the proximity of the greater tuberosity to its donor fracture site; a true lateral view of the scapula, which gives information about the extent of superior and posterior displacement of the greater tuberosity segment and the degree of comminution of the fragment; and an axillary view, which demonstrates the presence or absence of an associated glenohumeral joint dislocation, gives some information on the extent of posterior displacement of the greater tuberosity segment, and may show any associated fracture of the glenoid that accompanies a fracture dislocation. Additionally, I usually order a computed tomography (CT) scan of the involved shoulder. The CT scan shows precisely the location of the greater tuberosity donor site and provides invaluable information about the degree of posterior displacement of the greater tuberosity segment. In addition, accompanying scapula (glenoid) pathology is well seen.

Occasionally, one may identify a greater tuberosity segment that is quite small and appears to be only one of the facets of rotator cuff attachment. This may be accompanied by a more severe soft-tissue injury, such as full-thickness tear of the rotator cuff, consisting of the supraspinatus and all or some of the external rotators. In this instance, the supraspinatus and infraspinatus may be torn at their insertions. Instead of the teres minor tearing, this tendon may avulse the small segment of bone visible radiographically. Thus, the radiographically evident piece of bone represents a much more significant soft-tissue injury. If, following reduction of the humeral head and near-anatomic restoration of the greater tuberosity segment, there is significant weakness, as one might find with a cuff tear, it may be reasonable to consider a magnetic resonance imaging (MRI) scan instead of a CT scan, as this may provide information of associated soft-tissue damage and the extent of bony pathology accompanying the fracture.

SURGERY

The patient is brought to the operating room and placed in a semisitting, beach-chair position. As with most shoulder procedures, the involved extremity is draped free. For an acute fracture, the incision is an anterosuperior one, extending from just lateral to the anterior acromion to just lateral to the coracoid process (Fig. 27-3). The subcutaneous tissue is then sharply divided in line with the skin incision, flaps are developed, and retractors are placed.

With an acute greater tuberosity fracture, under most circumstances, the open reduction and internal fixation can be performed by splitting the deltoid muscle. A vertical split is made in the deltoid muscle at the anterolateral corner or at the acromioclavicular (AC) joint, depending on the location of the greater tuberosity segment (Fig. 27-4). If the displacement is predominantly superior, the deltoid split can be made beginning at the AC joint. If the displacement is predominantly posterior, the fragment is usually easier to retrieve by a more posterior split, beginning at the anterolateral corner of the acromion (Fig. 27-5). In any case, the split in the deltoid does not extend longer than 4 to 5 cm to avoid injury to the terminal branch of the axillary nerve. A stay suture is placed in the deltoid muscle to prevent further splitting during retraction. The fibers of the deltoid are retracted and a blunt instrument is used to free the subdeltoid area of any adhesions and to ensure that free access to the greater tuberosity segment is achieved. Blood, clot, and debris are removed from the subacromial space, and a bursectomy is performed. The donor site from the area of the greater tuberosity adjacent to the bicipital groove is identified and clot is removed from this area as well. For access to the greater tuberosity segment and for ease of mobilization of the segment, several stay sutures are placed at the greater tuberosity–cuff junction (Fig. 27-6). This provides good control of the greater tuberosity fragment. Traction on the sutures enables the tuberosity fragment to be manipulated into its anatomic location, particularly if a little external rotation is applied to the humerus.

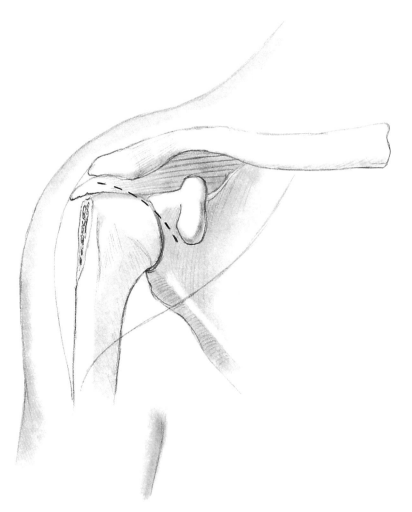

Figure 27-3. The incision for acute fracture internal fixation is an anterosuperior one, extending from just lateral to the anterior acromion to just lateral to the coracoid process.

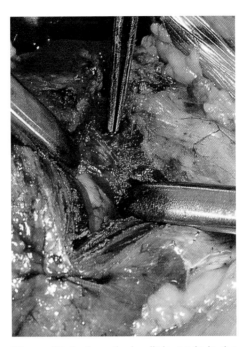

Figure 27-4. A vertical split is made in the deltoid muscle beginning at the acromio-clavicular joint and extending a distance of 5 cm. The distal-most aspect of the deltoid split is marked with a stay suture, protecting the terminal branches of the axillary nerve from injury.

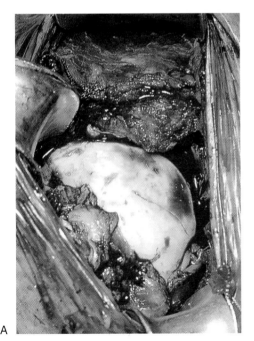

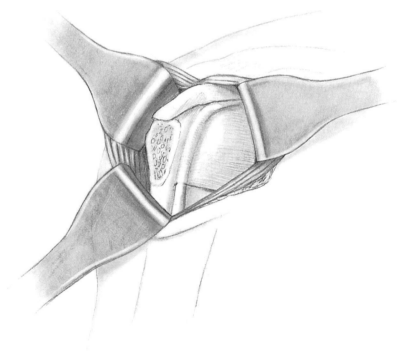

A

B

Figure 27-5. A,B: Intraoperative surgical pathology. The retracted greater tuberosity is displaced by the attached supra- and infraspinatus muscles. There is a split in the rotator interval, exposing the humeral head articular surface prior to cuff and tuberosity fixation.

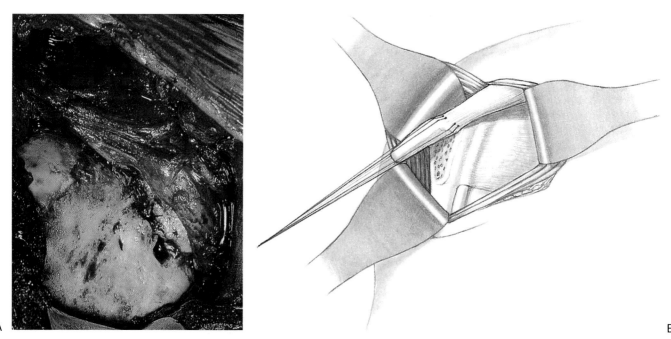

A

B

Figure 27-6. A,B: Stay sutures are placed at the tuberosity cuff juncture for ease of mobilization of the tuberosity fragment. The donor site is prepared by removing clot, fibrous tissue, and debris prior to reattachment of the greater tuberosity fragment.

Many methods of internal fixation have been described for acute fractures of the greater tuberosity. One of these is a screw and washer. The screw may be drilled through the greater tuberosity segment in an inferomedial direction to engage the opposite cortex of the upper metaphysis of the humerus, or it may be drilled horizontally if bone purchase is secure (Fig. 27-7). One or more screws can be used, depending on size, amount of comminution, and bone quality of the greater tuberosity piece.

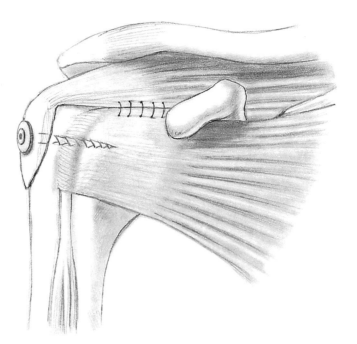

Figure 27-7. For an acute fracture, a screw and washer may be used to fix the fragment to the humeral shaft segment. The rotator interval tear is then closed.

Alternatively, heavy suture (or wire) can be used to secure the greater tuberosity segment to its donor site (Fig. 27-8). If a suture is to be used, no. 5 nonabsorbable suture is strong, secure, and easy to work with. Drill holes are made in the humeral shaft inferior to the donor site, several no. 5 Tevdek sutures are placed through these drill holes, and the sutures emerge from the cancellous donor site. Likewise, drill holes also may be made in the greater tuberosity segment itself.

The rent in the rotator interval between supraspinatus and subscapularis (which invariably accompanies this injury) is repaired. Side-to-side closure of the rotator interval will take tension off the rotator cuff and the greater tuberosity fracture and will help to prevent retraction of the tuberosity piece while preparation is being made for open reduction–internal fixation. The no. 5 Tevdek suture that has been placed through the humeral cortex to emerge from the donor site is then brought through the greater tuberosity fragment from inside out, and the greater tuberosity fragment is anatomically positioned in the proximal humerus and tied with a no. 5 nonabsorbable suture or wire.

If the bone is osteopenic, or if the greater tuberosity piece is fragmented and comminuted, drill holes through the greater tuberosity may not be secure. The no. 5 nonabsorbable suture that has been brought through the drill holes in the humerus may encircle the greater tuberosity by being brought from the inside out at the greater tuberosity–rotator cuff junction.

A word of caution: If the displaced greater tuberosity fracture has occurred as a part of a fracture dislocation, particularly in a young or athletic person, there may be an associated Bankart lesion accompanying the fracture dislocation. While restoration of the greater tuberosity ordinarily will provide stability to the shoulder, if the Bankart lesion is large, consideration should be given to repairing this acutely. Thus, at the time of tuberosity repair, the anterior glenoid should be inspected. This can usually be done prior to reduction of the tuberosity if traction is placed on the arm and the glenoid inspected through the interval between supraspinatus and subscapularis. If the Bankart lesion is to be repaired acutely, prior to reduction of the greater tuberosity segment, the rotator interval tear is extended, a tag suture is placed around the superior edge of subscapularis so this can be retracted, and the glenoid with anterior glenoid rim is inspected through the rent in the rotator interval. Several sutures or suture anchors can then be placed in the Bankart lesion

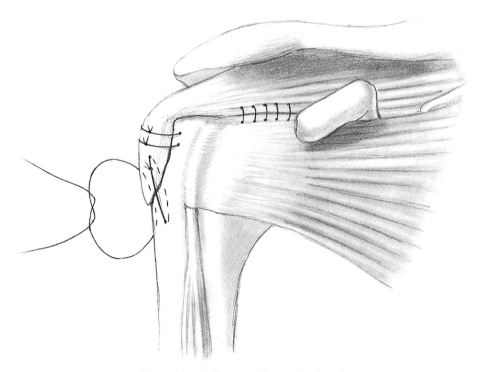

Figure 27-8. Figure-eight tension band.

through this rent in the rotator interval without having to make a separate anterior incision in the subscapularis.

If the patient is older than age 35 and the greater tuberosity is internally fixed, consideration may be given to adding an anterior acromioplasty and coracoacromial ligament excision. Fracture with its attendant trauma in the subacromial space may lead to enough scarring in the subacromial space that late impingement may occur. I ordinarily add an anterior acromioplasty if there is evidence that previous rotator cuff disease existed, if the patient is older than age 35, or if there is an abnormal shape or slope to the acromion.

After secure fixation of the greater tuberosity fragment, the deltoid must be meticulously repaired. In the case of an acute fracture, if the deltoid has been split it is simply closed with nonabsorbable suture. If more extensive exposure has been necessary and a portion of anterior deltoid is detached, it must be secured to the point of its division and to the superior AC joint capsule prior to closure of the deltoid split. The subcutaneous tissue and skin are then closed in layers with absorbable suture. The patient is placed in a canvas sling with an Ace wrap to secure the operated extremity to the chest wall.

POSTOPERATIVE MANAGEMENT

After internal fixation of the fragment, the arm is tested in forward elevation, internal rotation, and external rotation. If there is secure fixation of the greater tuberosity reattachment, early rehabilitation with range-of-motion exercises is begun.

The patient is immobilized in a sling and swathe for the first 24 hours after surgery. At 24 hours, the patient is given a removable sling and begins supine passive forward flexion and supine passive external rotation exercises with the assistance of a therapist. When the patient is steady enough to participate in the exercise program, circular Codman exercises are begun, followed by passive use of the overhead pulley, using the nonoperated arm to motor the operated arm.

At approximately 4 to 6 weeks postoperatively, submaximal isometrics for the deltoid and rotator cuff are begun. When there are radiographic signs of healing of the tuberosity segment to the shaft of the humerus, more resistive exercises are begun, adding an elastic or rubber band for strengthening of the cuff and deltoid. Whether the fragment was initially displaced or not, the rehabilitation can be difficult, frustrating, and lengthy. Return of range of motion and strength may take 1 year or more.

Pain in the early postoperative period is expected because of the fracture and the surgical dissection. As this subsides, there is ordinarily pain while doing exercises, particularly at the end of the range of motion, because of tightness in the glenohumeral joint. Later, after fracture healing, as progressive resistive exercises are being added, muscle fatigue may produce aching, which persists until the strength of the deltoid and rotator cuff are restored to normal. At the end of 1 year following fracture, most patients will have a range of motion within 10 degrees of the maximal forward elevation of the uninvolved side, and external rotation within 10 to 15 degrees of that of the contralateral side, and they will be essentially pain-free (except for weather ache), if anatomic restoration has occurred.

COMPLICATIONS

There are ordinarily few complications following open reduction internal fixation of a greater tuberosity fracture.

Nonunion

If nonunion of the greater tuberosity exists, it may be treated with open reduction internal fixation and iliac crest bone grafting, using either a tension-band technique or a screw-and-washer technique.

Stiffness

As with most surgical procedures on the shoulder, stiffness is best treated by prevention, with a very early range-of-motion program concentrating on forward flexion, external rotation, and internal rotation. If stiffness continues to be a problem following fracture healing, continued aggressive stretching for range of motion, with or without formal physical therapy, is indicated. If at the end of 6 months there is still a significant amount of stiffness of the shoulder, I would consider an open lysis of adhesions with hardware removal if a screw and washer have been utilized. I would under no circumstances do a manipulation under anesthesia because of the fear of refracture of the tuberosity.

MALUNIONS AND NONUNIONS OF THE GREATER TUBEROSITY

INDICATIONS/CONTRAINDICATIONS

Malunions and nonunions of the greater tuberosity occur when a displaced greater tuberosity segment remains, healed or not, in the displaced position, either superiorly or posteriorly. These are extremely difficult problems to treat. While it may be attractive to treat the mechanical problems with subacromial decompression alone, this is usually not successful, and repositioning of the tuberosity segment is usually necessary.

The indications for surgical treatment of a greater tuberosity malunion or nonunion include significant displacement, either superiorly or posteriorly, of the greater tuberosity, and some functional deficit caused either by pain or significant limitation of range of motion.

There are no absolute contraindications to surgical treatment of a symptomatic malunion in a patient who presents with anatomic displacement, pain, or significant limitation of range of motion and who had a functional extremity prior to the injury. If the fragment remains ununited to the shaft, it may be mobilized and fixed to the donor site.

PREOPERATIVE PLANNING

The patient with a greater tuberosity malunion or nonunion may present in a number of ways. There is usually a history of prior trauma, and the patient may or may not have had a previous radiograph. It is interesting that a number of patients have presented following trauma with so-called calcific tendonitis, that is, a calcific deposit in the subacromial space. Further evaluation and analysis in fact reveals that this "calcium" is a displaced tuberosity segment. Thus, a careful history, physical examination, and thorough radiographic analysis are critical.

Physical examination is usually significant for a block to forward elevation if the greater tuberosity is malunited superiorly in the subacromial space, and a block to external rotation if the greater tuberosity is malunited posteriorly behind the humeral head. The classic, although not specific, sign on physical examination is the absence of the ability to externally rotate the humerus with the arm in maximal abduction.

Because the greater tuberosity is in a nonanatomic position, the rotator cuff is also in a nonanatomic position with regard to its musculotendinous length. Thus, there is typically weakness of external rotation. If there is significant posterior malunion of the greater tuberosity, the proximity of the greater tuberosity to the posterior glenoid may cause the humeral head to lever out of the glenoid in external rotation, and the patient may have the sense of recurrent anterior instability (Fig. 27-16C).

The radiographs routinely ordered to evaluate malunion are the same as those ordered for acute fractures of the greater tuberosity: AP, lateral, and axillary views. Because there is frequently a block to external rotation, the AP view is usually with the humerus in internal rotation. In this view, one may see the donor defect and the greater tuberosity clearly displaced from the defect. Superior displacement is usually easily recognizable in the AP view. However, if there is not much superior displacement, the amount of posterior displacement may be confusing and may be difficult to interpret on plain radiograph. A lateral radiograph usually gives a clearer picture of the malunion. The axillary radiograph may show the greater tuberosity healed to the shaft of the humerus. Occasionally the tuberosity itself, if severely retracted, may fail to unite to the humerus and may actually heal to the posterior glenoid.

A CT scan is extremely useful for identifying the precise position of the greater tuberosity relative to its donor defect. If an associated rotator cuff tear is suspected, imaging studies, such as arthrography or MRI, may be added.

SURGERY

The surgical approach and procedure are quite similar to those for acute fractures of the greater tuberosity. If the tuberosity is malunited, the healing of the greater tuberosity to the shaft of the humerus in the displaced position presents extreme challenges for the surgeon. The retracted fixed tuberosity is associated with contracted, shortened capsule and rotator cuff, requiring extensive release and mobilization if an anatomic repositioning is to be obtained.

The patient is positioned in a beach-chair position, and the arm is draped completely free. An anterosuperior approach is used, as when fixing an acute fracture (Fig. 27-9). However, more extensive exposure is needed for mobilization, and it is useful to detach a portion of the anterior deltoid in addition to the usual deltoid split (Fig. 27-10). The deltoid is split beginning at the AC joint and then is detached from the anterior acromion out to the anterolateral edge of the acromion. Because of the extensive disease in the subacromial space, an anterior acromioplasty and excision of the coracoacromial ligament is usually added.

In the subacromial space, the humeral head is usually covered by a thin film of bursa, and because of the displaced greater tuberosity with attached rotator cuff, the usual tendinous coverage of the superior humeral head is not present. The supraspinatus and infraspinatus are attached to the greater tuberosity, and are identified by their positions relative to it (Fig. 27-11).

To reposition the malunited greater tuberosity anatomically, it is necessary to osteotomize the greater tuberosity segment. The donor defect, adjacent to the bicipital groove, from which the greater tuberosity has been fractured, is usually quite sclerotic and should be decorticated so that a bed of bleeding bone can be prepared for advancement of the greater tuberosity segment (Fig. 27-12). To osteotomize the segment, several drill holes are made in the most inferior aspect of the greater tuberosity malunion, and an estimate is made as to where the callus from the fracture begins and where the greater tuberosity piece ends (Fig. 27-13). It is usually best to err on the side of too large a piece of bone. Care must be taken, if the tuberosity is malunited to the posterior shaft of the humerus, to protect the axillary nerve throughout the osteotomy, since the emergence of the osteotomy site may be quite close to the quadrilateral space (Fig. 27-14). A blunt retractor may be placed in the area of the quadrilateral space at the time of the osteotomy of the posteriorly malunited greater tuberosity, so that the tuberosity can be osteotomized safely without risk to the axillary nerve. Once the tuberosity is osteotomized, several heavy nonabsorbable sutures are placed at the juncture of the greater tuberosity and the rotator cuff to better control the cuff and tuberosity segment.

The rotator cuff is usually shortened and the posterior capsule quite tight and contracted. Mobilization of the fragment is impossible without adequate release of the contracted tissue. The greater tuberosity segment is everted, and the superior and posterior glenohumeral joint capsules may be capsulotomized to help effect tuberosity advancement (Fig. 27-15). Any extraarticular adhesions binding the greater tuberosity segment are released and a subdeltoid bursectomy is performed. After careful lysis of adhesions extraarticularly and intraarticularly, with capsulotomy superiorly and posteriorly, the fragment of the greater

(text continues on page 508)

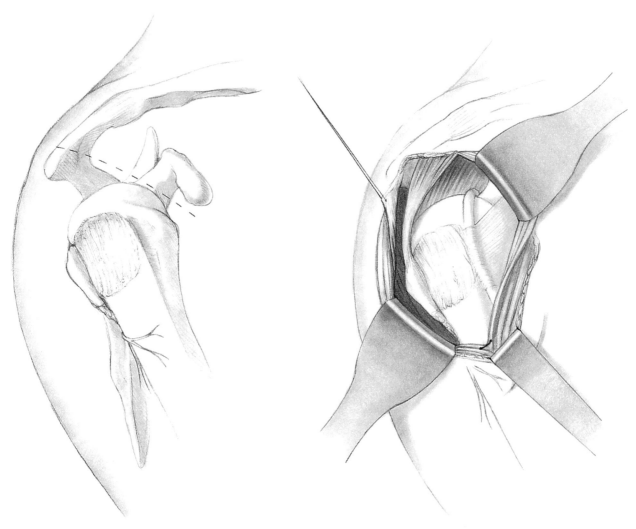

Figure 27-9. In the presence of a malunion or nonunion, a more extensile anterosuperior exposure is necessary. The skin incision is brought over the top of the anterolateral acromion and extends more inferiorly than the incision used in an acute fracture.

Figure 27-10. In addition to the split in the deltoid, it is typical for a portion of anterior deltoid to require detachment, because exposure to, retrieval of, and mobilization of the malunited greater tuberosity segment is more difficult. An anterior acromioplasty is often added to the procedure.

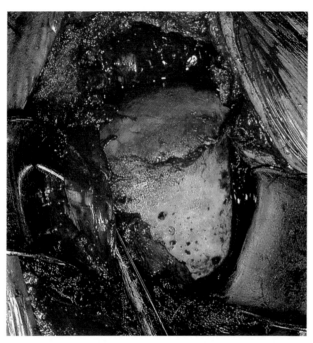

Figure 27-11. The exposed humeral head is identified. The donor site of the tuberosity is often sclerotic. The greater tuberosity is malunited to the posterior shaft of the humerus, and a clamp identifies the attachment site of the supraspinatus; the entire rotator cuff is attached posteriorly.

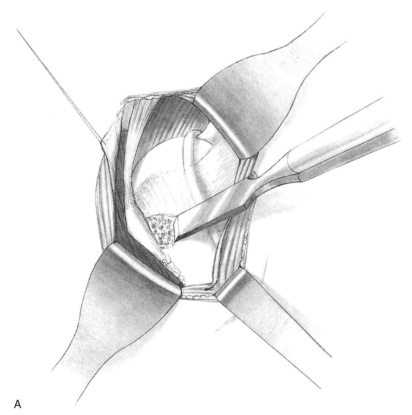

A

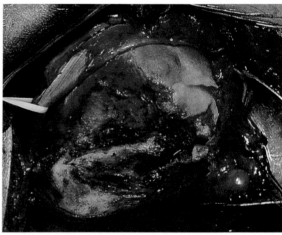

B

Figure 27-12. A,B: The donor defect, adjacent to the bicipital groove, is decorticated so that a bed of bleeding bone can be prepared for better healing of the greater tuberosity segment.

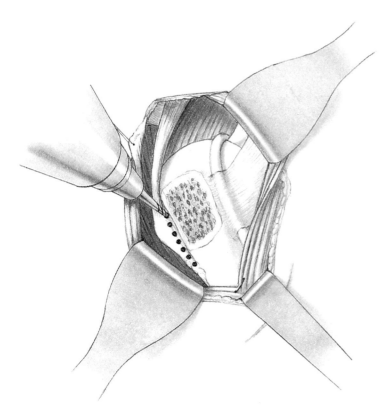

Figure 27-13. Prior to osteotomy of the malunited fragment, drill holes mark the site of osteotomy, so that the cut in the bone can be made precisely, minimizing fracture and fragmentation of the tuberosity piece.

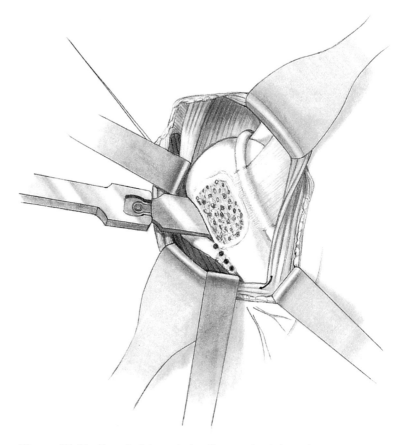

Figure 27-14. Care is taken during the greater tuberosity osteotomy to avoid the axillary nerve as it emerges from the quadralateral space near the site of bone detachment. It is often difficult to distinguish tuberosity segment from fracture callus.

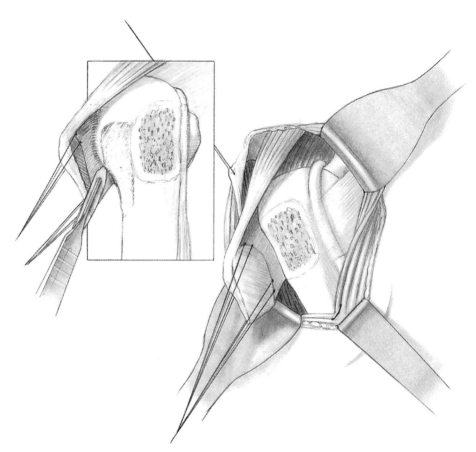

Figure 27-15. Because of the shortened rotator cuff and contracted posterior capsule, eversion of the greater tuberosity segment combined with extensive capsulotomy is usually necessary for mobilization of the fracture fragment.

tuberosity can usually be brought to the point of its origin, although external rotation of the humerus may be necessary. Other techniques of mobilization include interval release, late coracohumeral ligament release, and resection.

As was noted previously, if the greater tuberosity has been fractured in conjunction with an anterior fracture dislocation, there may be an associated Bankart lesion with destabilization of the glenohumeral ligaments. If this Bankart lesion is not addressed, extreme external rotation, often necessary to reposition the greater tuberosity anatomically, may actually result in a redislocation of the humeral head. Before advancing the greater tuberosity to its original place, I routinely examine the anterior glenoid rim through the rent in the rotator interval. If there is a Bankart lesion, it usually can be repaired with an anchor to the glenoid rim through a split in the rotator interval before the bony repair.

At this point, the greater tuberosity segment usually must be contoured to the donor defect. Unlike in an acute fracture setting, the fragment of greater tuberosity may be sclerotic and rounded, and it may contain callus, so that it often does not fit exactly into the area of the defect. However, in a chronic malunion, the bone quality is usually quite good. Iliac bone graft may be added if the greater tuberosity malunion is quite sclerotic, and it is always used in the presence of an ununited fragment. For internal fixation, my preference is to use one or two AO screws and washers for fixation of this fragment to the shaft of the humerus (Fig. 27-16). One or two screws are angled from the greater tuberosity inferomedially to engage the medial cortex of the humerus. Care must be taken to make certain that the screw does not penetrate the articular cartilage of the humeral head. The rotator interval is closed and the range of motion of the shoulder is tested. The security of the fixation and the range of motion of the shoulder are noted. The deltoid is meticulously repaired, and the wound is closed in layers.

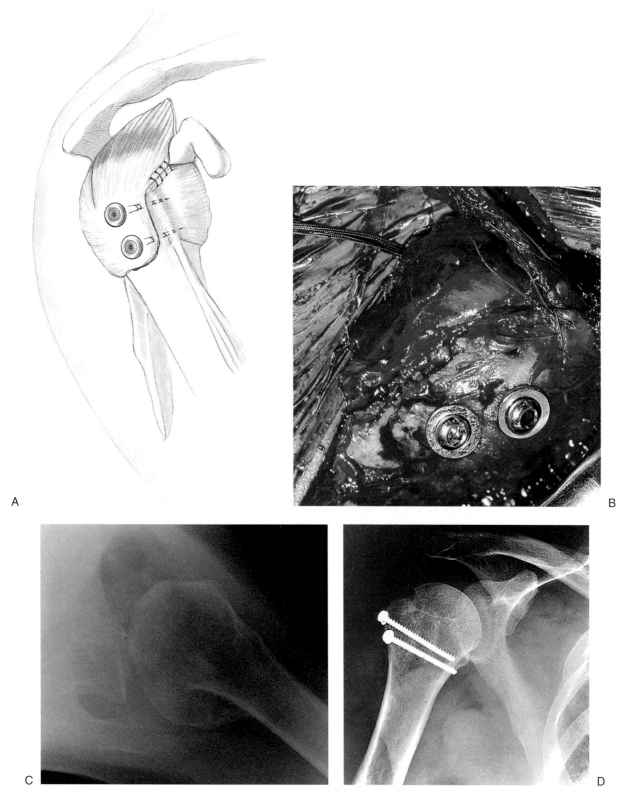

Figure 27-16. A,B: The osteotomized tuberosity segment is secured to the bed of bleeding bone with one or two AO screws, and the rotator interval tear is closed. **C:** An axillary radiograph reveals a posteriorly malunited greater tuberosity segment accompanied by anterior subluxation of the humeral head. **D:** The tuberosity segment after the osteotomy is secured to the humeral shaft with two screws and washers.

In the case of an ununited fragment, the surgical approach is identical. The tuberosity piece is prepared in similar fashion before insertion into the donor defect. Mobilization is usually necessary, and iliac crest bone graft is added at the time of internal fixation.

POSTOPERATIVE MANAGEMENT

The patient is placed in a sling and swathe in the operating room. Radiographs are routinely ordered either the day of or the day after surgery, prior to the beginning of any rehabilitation. If the internal fixation of the ununited or malunited fragment is secure, early postoperative rehabilitation is begun.

On the first postoperative day, passive supine forward flexion and passive supine external rotation are initiated by a physical therapist. The rehabilitation program consists of mobilization of the shoulder while protecting the fragment fixation. The patient who can understand and learn the program is begun on Codman circular exercises, assistive forward elevation with an overhead pulley, and supine external rotation within the first week following surgery. This assisted range-of-motion program is continued until there is radiographic evidence of union of the fragment.

At approximately 6 weeks postoperatively, or when radiographically there is solid union of the fracture fragment, isometric exercises for the rotator cuff and deltoid are begun. At approximately 10 weeks postoperatively, resistive exercises using an elastic band or a light weight may be added for further strengthening of the deltoid and cuff muscles. After this reconstruction, it is not uncommon for the shoulder to remain stiff for a long period and for the return of range of motion to be frustratingly slow. The patients are ordinarily followed at 6-week intervals until radiographically there is secure union of the fragment. The patients are then followed intermittently, depending on how difficultly or smoothly the postoperative rehabilitation program is progressing.

The expectations for the procedure depend on the length of time that the tuberosity was displaced and on the amount of associated rotator cuff dysfunction and damage to the glenohumeral joint, and is predicated on the successful union of the tuberosity fragments.

If there has been long-standing retraction and malunion of the greater tuberosity, some limitation of passive motion is frequently present at the time of reconstruction. In the presence of the fixed shortening of the rotator cuff, permanent weakness of external rotation and elevation above shoulder level may result. However, after osteotomy of the tuberosity and repositioning, and once the greater tuberosity heals to the shaft of the humerus, improved function of the rotator cuff is quite typical.

I tell my patients to expect that at approximately 6 months after surgery, if there has been adequate healing of the tuberosity, approximately two thirds of normal forward elevation will be present. By the end of 1 year, approximately 80% of normal forward elevation and external rotation can be expected. The strength and active movement of the arm, particularly above shoulder level, may be limited, and, again, they depend on healing of the tuberosity and length of time between injury and reconstruction.

COMPLICATIONS

Nonunion

The likelihood of this is increased with comminution, osteopenic bone, inadequate internal fixation, and the introduction of active or resistant exercises too early after repair. Rigid internal fixation and carefully controlled rehabilitation offer the best protection against this complication.

Fixed Anterior Dislocation of the Shoulder

This may occur if an unrecognized and unrepaired Bankart lesion is present, especially if external rotation is needed for greater tuberosity relocation. To avoid this, the anterior glenoid rim should be inspected, and, if a Bankart lesion is present, it should be repaired at the time of reconstruction.

Axillary Nerve Injury

This may occur either to the terminal branches at the time of the deltoid split or to the main branch at the time of the osteotomy emergence into quadrilateral space. The course and the position of the nerve should be understood and recognized, particularly in the presence of old trauma, scar, or malunited bone.

RECOMMENDED READING

1. Bigliani, L.U.: Fractures of the proximal humerus. In: Rockwood, C.A., Jr., Matsen, F.A., eds.: *The shoulder.* Philadelphia: WB Saunders, 278, 1990.
2. Bono, C.M., Renard, R., Levine, R.G., et al.: Effect of displacement of fractures of the greater tuberosity on the mechanics of the shoulder. *J Bone Joint Surg Br* 83: 1056–1062, 2001.
3. Flatow, E.L., Cuomo, F., Maday, M., et al.: Open reduction and internal fixation of 2-part displacement fractures of the greater tuberosity of the proximal part of the humerus. *J Bone Joint Surg Am* 73: 1213–1218, 1991.
4. Neer, C.S.: Displaced proximal humeral fractures, I: classification and evaluation. *J Bone Joint Surg Am* 52: 1077–1089, 1970.
5. Neer, C.S., II: Shoulder reconstruction. In: Rockwood, C.A., Jr., Matsen, F.A., eds.: *The shoulder.* Philadelphia: WB Saunders, 377–380, 1990.
6. McLaughlin, H.L.: Dislocation of the shoulder with tuberosity fracture. *Surg Clin North Am* 43: 1615, 1963.
7. Takase, K., Imakiire A., Burkhead, W.Z., Jr.: Radiographic study of the anatomic relationships of the greater tuberosity. *J Shoulder Elbow Surg* 11: 557–561, 2002.
8. Williams, G.R., Wong, K.L.: Two-part and three-part fractures: open reduction and internal fixation versus closed reduction and percutaneous pinning. *Orthop Clin North Am* 31: 1–21, 2000.

PART V

Arthroplasty and Arthroplasty Alternatives

28

Total Shoulder Replacement with Intact Bone and Soft Tissue

Edward V. Craig

INDICATIONS/CONTRAINDICATIONS

The first humeral head replacement in the United States was implanted for a proximal humeral fracture in 1953. In 1971, a matching polyethylene glenoid component was used as the first total shoulder replacement. Since that time, a variety of designs has been identified for glenohumeral arthroplasty, with most being of the unconstrained variety. Implant designs exist with variable humeral head sizes and stem lengths, with or without modularity, and matched with glenoid components of differing designs. However, all designs have in common the lack of constraint in the prosthetic components, allowing reattachment of the rotator cuff muscles around the implant and thus permitting the shoulder to be rehabilitated for motion and strength without mechanical blocks to motion.

The indications for total shoulder arthroplasty are pain from an incongruous joint associated with glenohumeral arthritis and the attendant loss of function. Stiffness of the shoulder in the absence of pain is only rarely an indication for glenohumeral joint arthroplasty. However, in some arthritic conditions such as ankylosing spondylitis, which may be associated with a stiff elbow and a stiff shoulder, glenohumeral arthroplasty may be considered to improve overall function in the extremity. The single most common indication for total shoulder arthroplasty is pain that is unresponsive to nonoperative treatment such as antiinflammatory medications and rest. In some glenohumeral arthritic conditions, it may be reasonable to consider intraarticular steroid injection prior to a glenohumeral arthroplasty. However, in most patients, pain from loss of the glenohumeral joint space accompanying glenohumeral arthritis is inadequately addressed with intraarticular injections, which provide short-term relief, if any at all. In some cases of early osteoarthritis, arthroscopic débridement of the joint, débridement of osteophytes, or loose body removal (with or without soft-tissue releases to gain increased range of motion) may be considered.

E. V. Craig, M.D.: Department of Orthopaedics, Weill Medical College of Cornell University; and Hospital for Special Surgery, New York, New York.

Glenohumeral arthroplasty is contraindicated in a patient whose symptoms are not sufficiently disabling to warrant an operation, in a patient who has loss or paralysis of both rotator cuff and deltoid, and in a patient with active infection. Loss of the rotator cuff alone or deltoid alone may be handled with soft-tissue procedures and/or muscle transfers and is not necessarily a contraindication for a nonconstrained arthroplasty of the shoulder. In addition, a neuropathic joint is generally considered a contraindication to a glenohumeral joint arthroplasty.

While many types of glenohumeral arthritis have intact bone in rotator cuff, including osteoarthritis, avascular necrosis, capsulorraphy arthropathy, dislocation arthropathy, and some cases of rheumatoid arthritis, the prototype for the prototypic patient undergoing total shoulder replacement with intact soft tissues is the patient with osteoarthritis or osteonecrosis.

PREOPERATIVE PLANNING

The patient who presents with glenohumeral arthritis requiring total shoulder arthroplasty gives a characteristic history. There is usually a several-year history of gradually progressive shoulder pain. Accompanying the shoulder pain is a progressive stiffness and loss of motion, and the patient often experiences a grinding or grating within the shoulder joint that is disturbing and painful.

There are many different causes of glenohumeral joint arthritis, any of which can become sufficiently symptomatic to warrant total shoulder arthroplasty. These include primary osteoarthritis, rheumatoid arthritis, dislocation arthropathy, postcapsulorraphy arthopathy, posttraumatic arthritis, osteonecrosis, cuff tear arthropathy, and septic arthritis. The history and extent of disability are highly individualized and depend on the type of arthritis that is present. Patients with osteonecrosis may have a history of predisposing factors such as oral corticosteroids, alcoholic excess, or collagen vascular disease.

On physical examination, the patient usually has a degree of posterior joint-line tenderness that is different from that of the contralateral shoulder, unless the condition is bilateral. There is usually restricted passive range of motion. Motion of the shoulder in forward elevation, external rotation, and internal rotation is usually painful. This passive restriction of motion is usually accompanied by a sense of deep grinding or grating, typical of an incongruous glenohumeral joint with cartilage loss. The patient with primary osteoarthritis of the shoulder may have some flattening of the anterior shoulder and fullness posteriorly, because asymmetric wear of the glenoid may cause the humeral head to translate posteriorly, producing the so-called pseudosubluxation of primary osteoarthritis. When the strength of the shoulder is tested in a patient with osteoarthritis or avascular necrosis, there is usually not much noticeable weakness of external rotation strength, as the rotator cuff in these conditions is usually normal. However, when the patient is asked to contract the external rotators against resistance, there is a ratcheting-type of grinding from the joint incongruity. Patients with rheumatoid arthritis may have an intact rotator cuff but some weakness on cuff testing due to the myopathy of rheumatoid arthritis, the myopathy associated with clinical steroid therapy, or rotator cuff tearing.

The standard radiographs requested are a true anteroposterior (AP) view of the glenohumeral joint, a scapula lateral view, and an axillary view. The AP provides a view of the extent of glenohumeral joint space narrowing, the position of the tuberosities relative to the humeral head, and the position of the humeral head relative to the acromion. In primary osteoarthritis, characteristic radiographic features include an inferior protruding osteophyte, which is, in fact, a circumferential osteophyte, and sclerosis or cystic changes in the humeral head. A supine axillary view will confirm the presence of narrowing of the joint and will indicate whether the glenoid may be worn asymmetrically. In addition, in primary osteoarthritis there is often a radiographic subluxation of the humeral head posteriorly, because of the excessive posterior wear on the face of the glenoid. However, the true amount of asymmetry of glenoid wear may be difficult to determine by plain axillary view.

If there is a suggestion of significant asymmetric wear, or in conditions where the position of the tuberosities relative to the head may be unclear, a computed tomography scan can be useful to define the precise bony anatomy. With a severe amount of glenoid wear posteriorly, plans may be made for possible intraoperative glenoid bone graft.

Patients with primary osteoarthritis and osteonecrosis usually have an intact rotator cuff. Occasionally, there will be a rotator cuff tear that is small and easily repairable. It is not standard for me to order an arthrogram or a magnetic resonance imaging scan in a patient who has classic radiographic findings of osteoarthritis. If there has been previous trauma, prior surgery, or any other situation in which nerve damage may have occurred, an electromyogram is performed.

SURGERY

Either regional anesthesia with interscalene block or general anesthesia is used for total shoulder replacement arthroplasty.

The patient is positioned in the beach-chair position with the affected arm supported on an armrest that may be moved in and out of the operating field. For work on the humeral head, cuff, and glenoid, the arm is best supported on the armrest. However, for intramedullary insertion of the prosthetic device, hyperextension of the arm off the side of the operating table is usually needed. Alternatively, a beanbag may permit molding with support of the elbow while permitting extension of the humerus for humeral shaft insertion. A towel is placed behind the scapula, the head is secured to the operating table or to a head holder, and the arm is prepped to the level of the hand and wrist. The hand is wrapped in a waterproof bag with an Ace bandage or a sterile stocking to the level of the elbow, which is then secured. The operating field is then draped with a U-drape. The topographic markings are made with a skin marker and Steri-Drape (3M Worldwide, St. Paul, MN) is applied.

The skin incision is deltopectoral, originating at the inferior border of the clavicle, halfway between the acromioclavicular joint and the coracoid process, and extending inferiorly and laterally to the deltoid insertion, ending just lateral to the muscle belly of the biceps (Fig. 28-1). The skin and subcutaneous tissue are divided to the level of the deltoid.

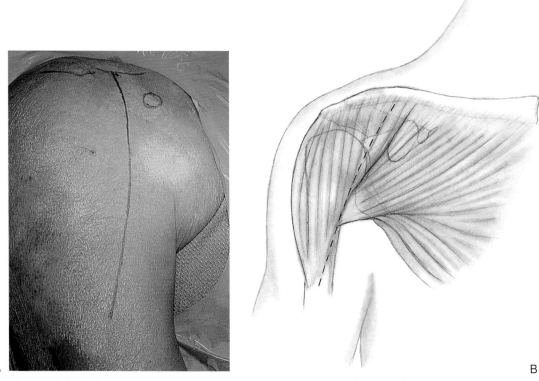

A   B

Figure 28-1. A,B: A long deltopectoral incision is the usual surgical approach for shoulder arthroplasty.

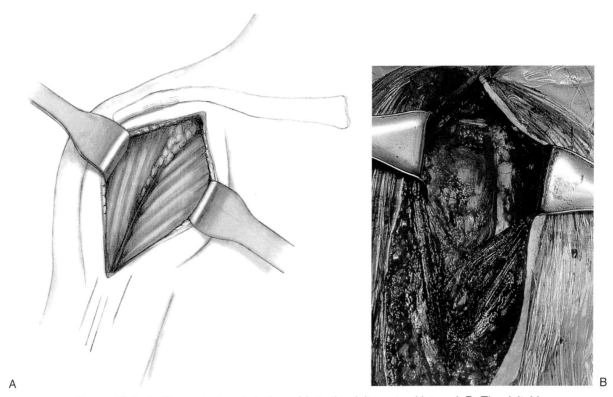

Figure 28-2. A: The cephalic vein is the guide to the deltopectoral interval. **B:** The deltoid and pectoralis are retracted, exposing the conjoined tendon medially and the coracoacromial ligament in the superior aspect of the wound.

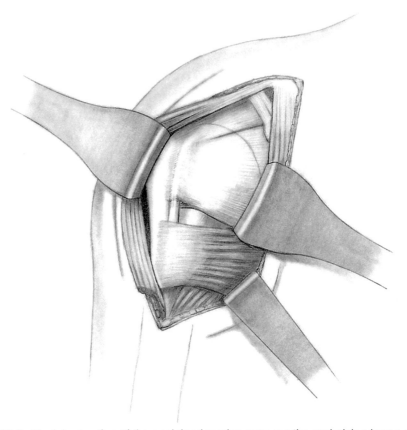

Figure 28-3. Medial retraction of the conjoined tendon exposes the underlying bursa and subscapularis.

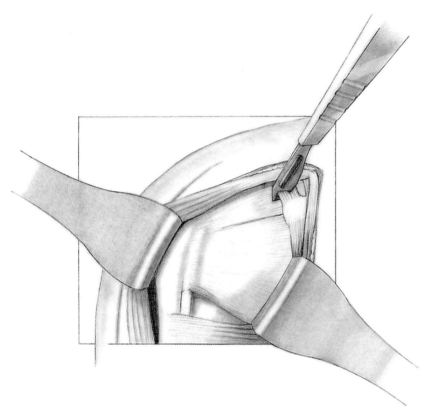

Figure 28-4. The coracoacromial ligament is often excised, and its excision may aid exposure. In those patients with rotator cuff weakness or insufficiency, this ligament is kept undivided, as a superior buttress.

The deltopectoral interval is then identified, usually by the cephalic vein, which has fat overlying it (Fig. 28-2). If there is difficulty identifying the deltopectoral interval, external rotation of the humerus puts the pectoralis under some tension and makes the superior fibers of the pectoralis more easily identifiable. In addition, the interval may be found in the superior aspect of the wound at the level of the coracoid process. Although the cephalic vein may be able to be preserved, it may also be ligated and excised to ensure against intraoperative avulsion. The clavipectoral fascia adjacent to the conjoined tendon is identified and incised up to the level of the coracoacromial ligament. Often there are significant muscle fibers of the brachialis and short head of the biceps, which extend somewhat laterally to the tendinous portion of the conjoined tendon. These should be included with the conjoined tendon and retracted medially; the underlying bursa and subscapularis are then exposed (Fig. 28-3). Electrocauterization can be used to handle the branch of the thoracoacromial trunk, a troublesome bleeder in the superior aspect of the wound. The coracoacromial ligament may also be excised (Fig. 28-4). If necessary for exposure, the upper one fourth of pectoralis tendon may be divided and the deltoid insertion along the lateral aspect of the humerus may be divided or elevated subperiosteally. This release of the deltoid distally makes it less likely that the deltoid muscle will be significantly traumatized during retraction. At this point, the amount of passive external rotation may be tested with the arm at the side. In some patients, internal rotation contracture may severely limit external rotation. In this situation, a Z-lengthening of the subscapularis is necessary to provide external rotation. If, however, passive external rotation is 10 degrees or greater, the lengthening of the subscapularis is not needed. The anterior humeral circumflex vessels are cauterized as the dissection continues.

The subscapularis and anterior capsule are then divided together from the level of the rotator interval to the most inferior border of the subscapularis insertion (Fig. 28-5). These are divided approximately 2 cm from the lesser tuberosity insertion of the subscapularis.

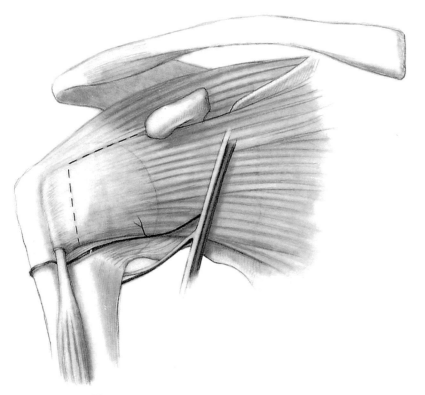

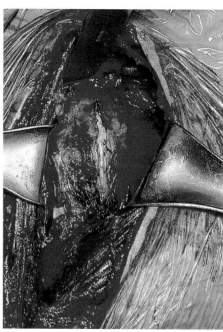

A   B

Figure 28-5. A,B: Subscapularis and capsule are divided in their entirety and the incision may be extended toward the coracoid process, completely opening the rotator interval.

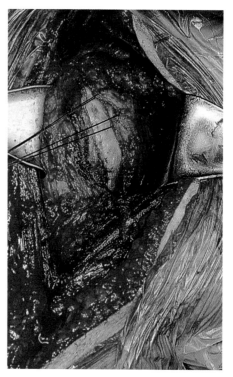

Figure 28-6. The subscapularis is tagged with temporary stay sutures and retracted medially.

Care must be taken when dividing the subscapularis superiorly, so that the biceps tendon in the rotator interval is not inadvertently sectioned. Care must also be taken when dividing the subscapularis inferiorly, so that the axillary nerve is not inadvertently injured. The axillary nerve crosses beneath the subscapularis tendon approximately 3 mm medial to the musculotendinous junction. External rotation of the humerus while the subscapularis is being divided will minimize the likelihood that the axillary nerve will be inadvertently injured. In addition, a blunt retractor beneath the subscapularis also minimizes potential for nerve injury. Care must be taken to divide the capsule as far inferiorly as possible. This not only helps in a tight shoulder to expose the joint for dislocation of the humeral head but also permits adequate humeral retraction posteriorly for glenoid exposure. With the subscapularis divided, the rotator interval is incised medially to the level of the coracoid process, and the subscapularis muscle is tagged with stay sutures and retracted medially (Fig. 28-6). The humeral head is then dislocated by hyperextending and externally rotating the arm. It is often helpful to place a blunt retractor superiorly over the neck of the humerus, under the biceps tendon and supraspinatus and inferiorly under the neck of the humerus, inside the capsule. With dislocation of the humeral head and delivery into the wound, preparation is made for humeral head resection and osteotomy. Marginal osteophytes are removed (Fig. 28-7). Patients with osteoarthritis often have intraarticular loose bodies, which should be removed. In addition, during inferior capsular division, in the presence of a very large inferior osteophyte, the axillary nerve may be quite close to the inferior aspect of the humeral head and osteophyte, and caution should be used while dissecting in this area.

Exactly how the humeral head and neck osteotomy is performed depends on the total shoulder system being used. What follows is a description of the Biomed Atlas Trimodular Shoulder Arthroplasty (an integrated shoulder system). Whatever the shoulder system used, the osteotomy of the head of the humerus consists of only that portion of the head ordinarily covered with articular cartilage. The head is osteotomized in 30 degrees of retroversion, which mimics the normal amount of retroversion of the humerus. In addition, the

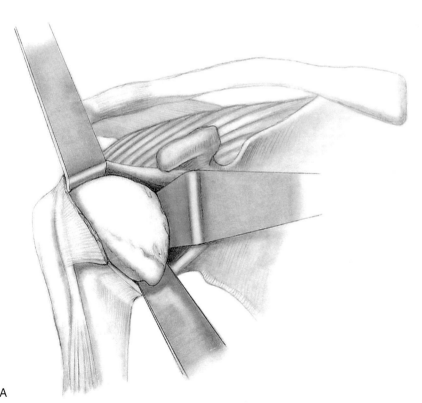

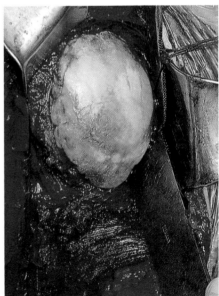

A

B

Figure 28-7. A,B: The humeral head is dislocated, retractors are placed superiorly and inferiorly, and the marginal osteophytes are identified. *(continued)*

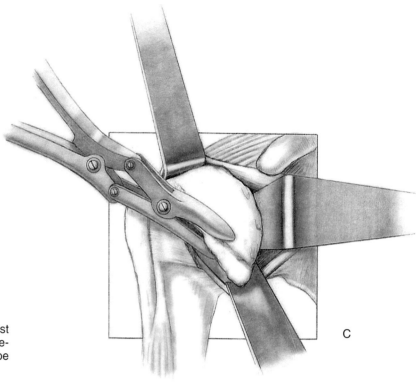

Figure 28-7. *Continued.* **C:** The most prominent marginal osteophytes are removed. Any residual osteophytes can be excised after the trial stem is inserted.

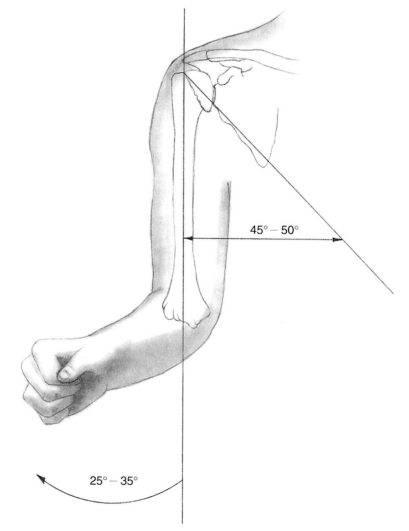

Figure 28-8. The osteotomy is angled approximately 45 to 50 degrees to the shaft of the humerus.

osteotomy is at an angle of approximately 45 to 50 degrees to the shaft of the humerus (Fig. 28-8). If the osteotomy is to be made freehand, a trial prosthesis may be placed against the proximal humerus and the angle of the osteotomy outlined with a cautery (Fig. 28-9). With the elbow bent 90 degrees, the forearm in neutral rotation, the arm externally rotated 35 degrees, and the osteotomy angled directly from anterior to posterior, a retroversion cut of 30 degrees is produced.

Alternatively, a humeral head resection guide may be used. In this system, the resection guide is placed on the intramedullary T-handled reamer. A ¼-in. drill bit is used to make a pilot hole just posterior to the bicipital groove, approximately 1 to 1.5 cm from the greater tuberosity into the medullary canal of the humerus (Fig. 28-10). The sequential T-handled reamers are then used to prepare the humerus to the point at which resistance, or "chatter," is felt in the shaft of the humerus (Fig. 28-11). At this point, the humeral head resection guide is assembled directly onto the T-handled reamer. The humeral head resection guide ensures that the angle relative to the shaft of the humerus will be 45 to 50 degrees (Fig. 28-12). A retroversion guide rod inserted into the resection guide and kept parallel to the forearm ensures the appropriate amount of retroversion for the cut (Fig. 28-13). In this particular system, it is possible to make the cut in 20, 30, or 40 degrees of retroversion. The usual cut for primary osteoarthritis and osteonecrosis will be made in 30 degrees of retroversion. Less retroversion may be needed if there is a possibility of posterior instability of the implant. More retroversion may be needed in some cases of malunion following fracture.

When the humeral head resection guide is lined up appropriately, ⅛-in. drill bits are used to secure it to the shaft of the humerus, and the cutting block is used to make the appropriate angle cut and resect the appropriate amount of humerus (Figs. 28-14 and 28-15). In the Biomed Atlas or Integrated System, a rotator cuff probe inserted under the cuff and fit into

(text continues on page 528)

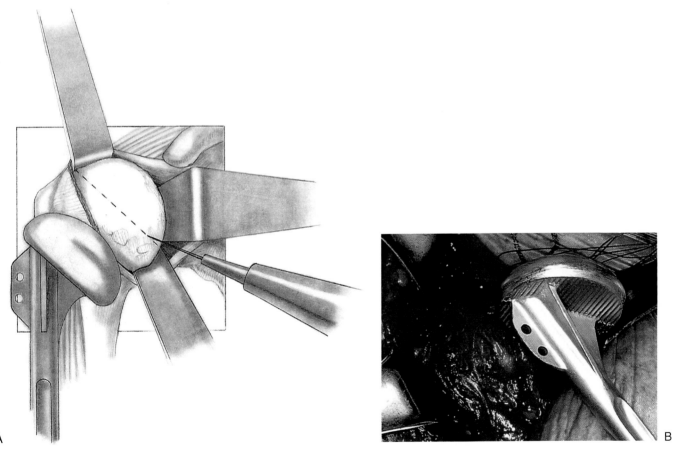

A   B

Figure 28-9. A,B: If the osteotomy is to be made freehand, without a resection guide, a trial prosthesis can be used to identify the osteotomy site.

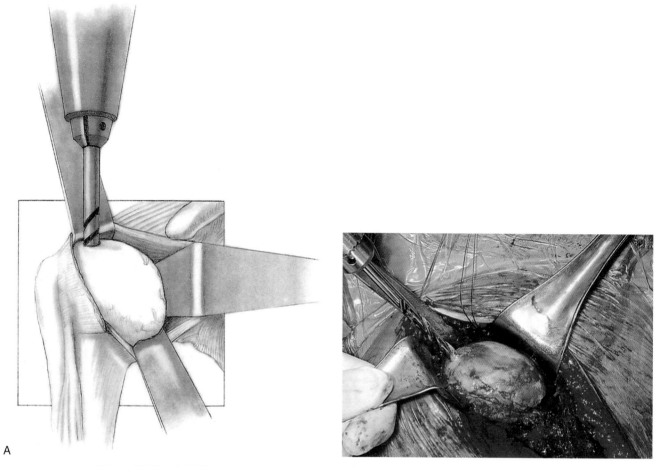

A   B

Figure 28-10. A,B: If a resection guide is used, a $^1/_4$-in. drill bit is used to make the initial intramedullary pilot hole.

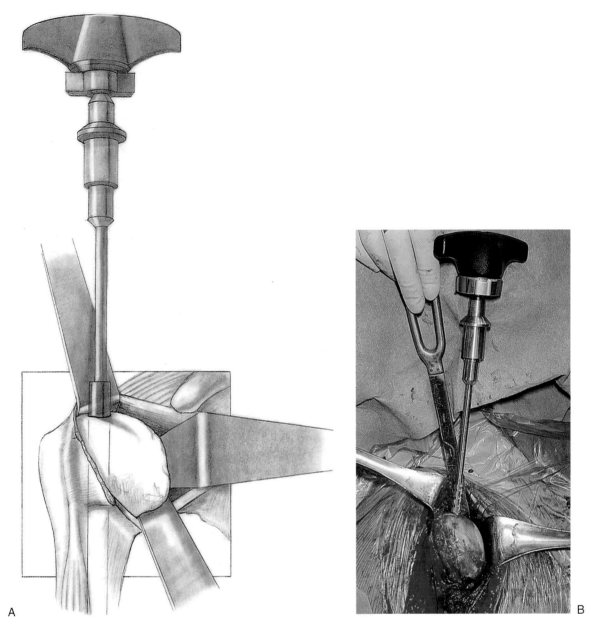

A

B

Figure 28-11. A,B: T-handled reamers sequentially enlarge the intramedullary canal to prepare the humeral shaft.

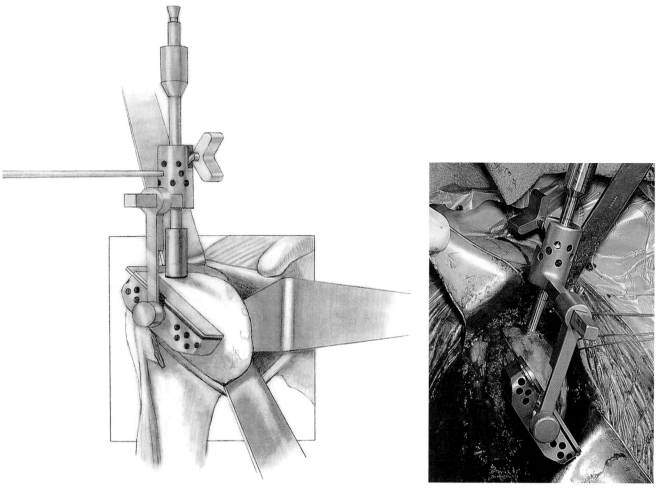

A

B

Figure 28-12. A,B: The humeral head resection guide is assembled directly onto the T-handled reamer. The holes on the cutting jig are for pin placement to secure the cutting jig to the humerus. A flexible rotator cuff probe is placed beneath the supraspinatus and the biceps tendon to insure the proper exit site for the osteotomy cut.

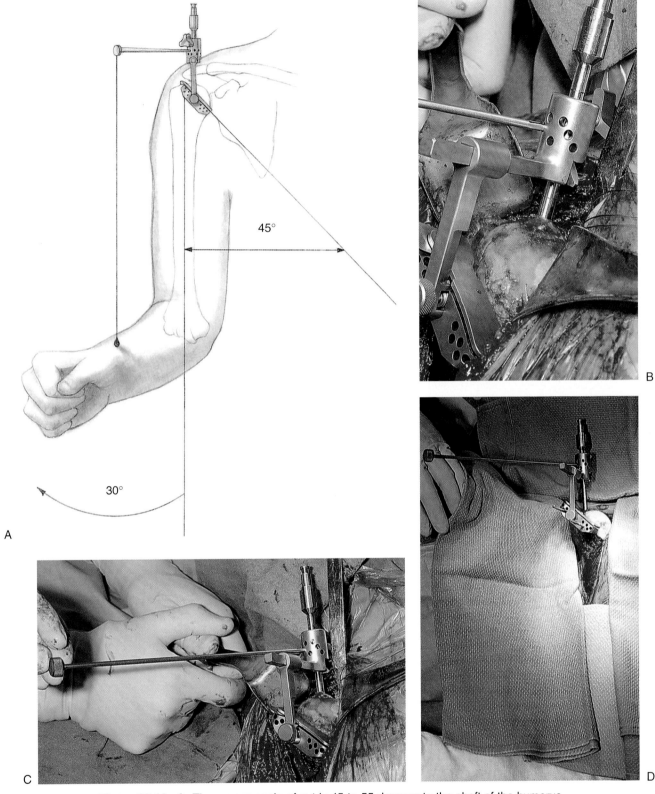

Figure 28-13. A: The proper angle of cut is 45 to 55 degrees to the shaft of the humerus and 25 to 35 degrees of retroversion. To ensure the precise amount of retroversion, the re-section guide uses a version rod, which is aligned precisely parallel to the long axis of the forearm. **B,C:** The version rod is placed in the hole of the resection guide, marked with the precise amount of retroversion desired. **D:** Version rod parallel to the long axis of the forearm.

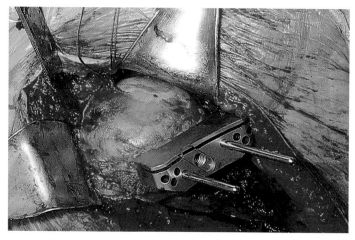

Figure 28-14. When the precise angle of the cut is determined, ¹/₈-in. drill bits secure the cutting block to the shaft of the humerus.

the cutting block assists in determining the precise cut location. The two pitfalls at this part of the procedure are as follows:

Incorrect Amount Resected

If too little humeral head is resected, there will be a ridge of bone remaining inside the joint, leading to tightness of the joint, incomplete seating of the humeral prosthesis, and difficulty in exposing the glenoid for the implantation of the glenoid component. Alternatively, if the resection of the humeral head is too extensive, the egress of the osteotomy may be either into the rotator cuff or even into the greater tuberosity, in which case fracture of the greater

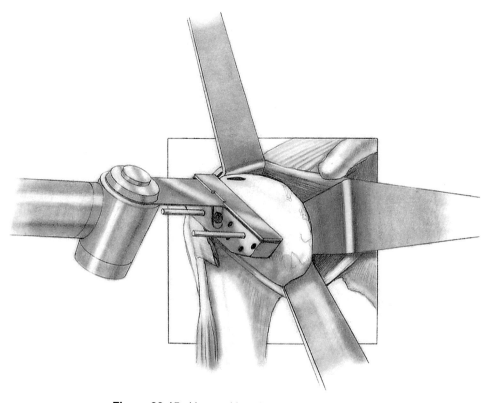

Figure 28-15. Humeral head osteotomy is performed.

tuberosity results. The osteotomy cut should emerge precisely at the position where the rotator cuff inserts on the greater tuberosity (Fig. 28-16). No ridge should be able to be felt between the rotator cuff tendinous and capsular insertion and the free cut of the humeral head.

Inadvertent Sectioning of Biceps Tendon

Care must be taken that during the cutting of the humeral osteotomy, the biceps tendon is protected so that it is not inadvertently sectioned. The resected humeral head is then removed.

Once the osteotomy is complete, a trial humeral stem is inserted and seated fully in the intramedullary canal in the appropriate amount of version (Fig. 28-17). The following guides to the appropriate version of the humerus can be observed when the fin of the prosthesis is placed just posterior (lateral) to the bicipital groove:

- With the elbow at 90 degrees and the arm facing straight ahead, the humeral component should face directly toward the glenoid.
- When looking at the forearm and shoulder from above, the fin of the implant should make an angle of approximately 30 degrees with the transverse axis of the elbow.

With the humeral trial seated securely on the osteotomy cut, any marginal peripheral osteophyte that extends past the humeral trial component may be removed (Fig. 28-18). It is quite common for a peripheral osteophyte to be present both inferiorly and posteriorly in primary osteoarthritis of the shoulder.

The trial humeral component is again removed and the arm is positioned for exposure of the glenoid. The extremity is resting on an armboard or beanbag, with or without rolled sheets to act as bolsters. A glenoid retractor (ring or Fukuda) is placed around the posterior rim of the glenoid, and the proximal humerus is gently retracted (Fig. 28-19). Exposure of

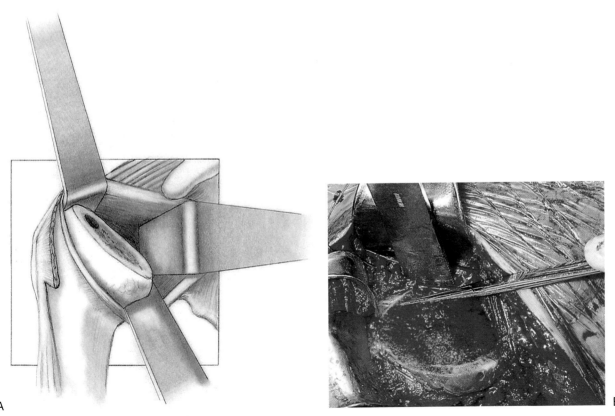

A   B

Figure 28-16. A,B: The osteotomy cut should emerge precisely at the position of rotator cuff insertion on the greater tuberosity.

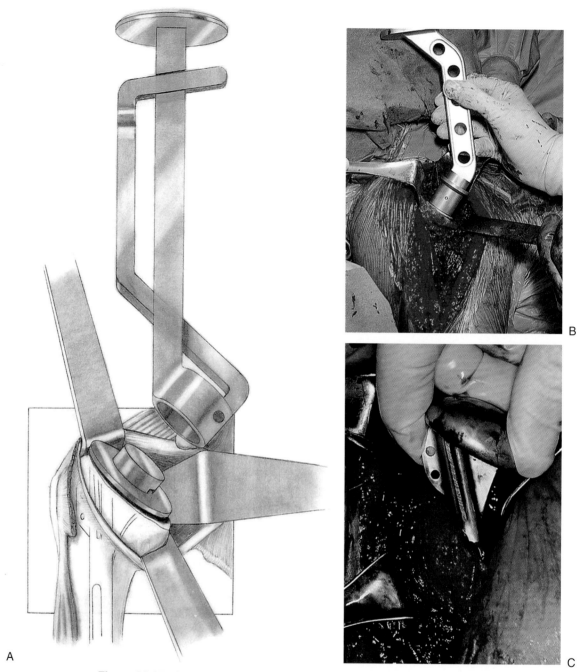

Figure 28-17. A,B: The trial humeral stem is inserted in the appropriate amount of version, and seated securely on the osteotomy resection site. **C:** Alternatively, in the nonmodular system, a fixed-stem humeral trial may be inserted in the proper depth and version.

the glenoid is critical for satisfactory insertion of a glenoid prosthesis. In most instances, whenever glenoid exposure is inadequate or the working space too tight, it is usually because of inadequate soft-tissue release. To expose the glenoid, I make certain that the anterior capsular attachment at the rim of the glenoid is released from superior to inferior, so that the entire neck of the glenoid can be palpated from superior to inferior (Fig. 28-20). This may be facilitated by developing the interval between the subscapularis and capsule. The subscapularis may then be retracted interiorly and the entire capsule released and resected. The axillary nerve should be palpated and consideration given to a blood retractor inferiorly below the capsule to protect the axillary nerve while the capsule is released.

The anterior and posterior glenoid labrums are excised in their entirety and any proliferative synovium is removed as well. Care must be taken when removing the glenoid labrum

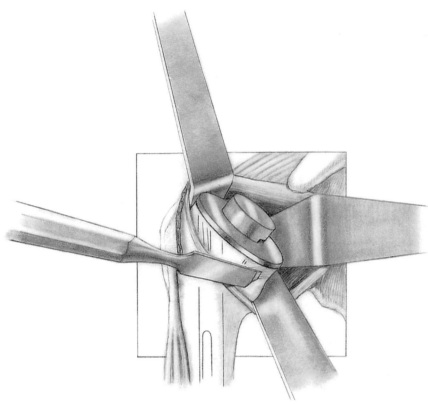

Figure 28-18. With the implant fully seated, any residual protruding osteophyte and excess bone is removed. This minimizes the likelihood that osteophytes will obstruct exposure of the glenoid fossa.

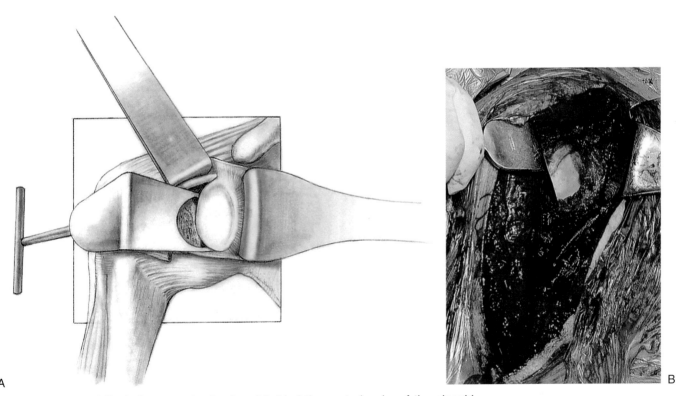

A   B

Figure 28-19. A,B: A ring retractor is placed behind the posterior rim of the glenoid, exposing the glenoid fossa and retracting the humeral shaft.

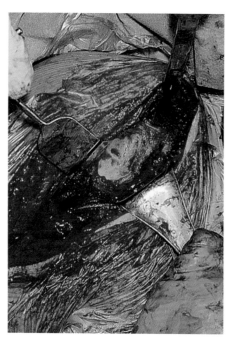

Figure 28-20. The anterior capsular attachment to the glenoid rim is released from superior to inferior, ensuring that the neck of the glenoid can be palpated. This ensures that the slot will be deepened in the normal cancellous anatomic neck of glenoid.

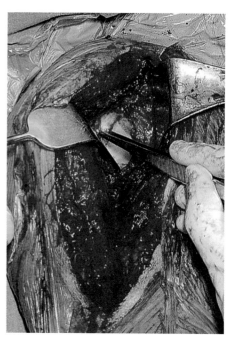

Figure 28-21. Posterior labrum is removed from the biceps insertion to the inferior glenoid. Anterior glenoid labrum may be removed as well.

not to detach the biceps tendon from the supraglenoid tubercle (Fig. 28-21). If necessary, the posterior capsule may be released from superior to inferior as well. Although maintaining the most inferior capsular attachment from humerus to glenoid helps protect the axillary nerve coursing underneath the soft-tissue capsular structure, if need be, a circumfer-

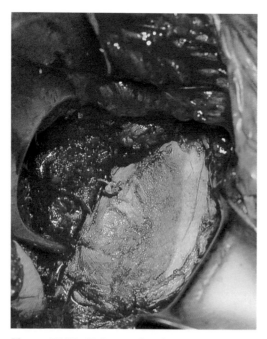

Figure 28-22. Release of anterior and posterior capsule and contracted soft tissue, combined with labral excision, exposes the glenoid face for direct access during glenoid preparation.

ential capsulotomy may be performed so that the humerus can be retracted. A blunt retractor, such as a forked glenoid or Darrach, is placed deep to the subscapularis and anterior capsule, exposing the anterior glenoid rim. A second blunt retractor, such as a Darrach, may be placed beneath the biceps tendon insertion, so that the most superior portion of the glenoid can be exposed.

Occasionally, residual inferior humeral osteophyte will protrude through the ring retractor, interfering with glenoid exposure, preparation, and implantation of the glenoid component. This osteophyte becomes less prominent if the arm is brought into external rotation, but if the inferior aspect of the proximal humeral osteophyte is protruding through the ring retractor and interfering with exposure, it may be trimmed further.

With the face of the glenoid exposed, any residual cartilage may be removed from the face of the glenoid (Fig. 28-22). It is important at this point to judge the wear pattern of the glenoid, to try to decide whether there is indeed osteophyte formation that distorts the exposed face of the glenoid, and to try to identify the center of the glenoid, under which is the cancellous neck. A straight instrument or a gloved finger can palpate the anterior border of the glenoid neck and give the surgeon an idea of the angle of the glenoid neck, so a centering hole can be made. Total shoulder systems use either keel- or pegged-typed glenoid component. Preparation depends on the type of glenoid used. The atlas system component I most frequently use is a keeled glenoid component. For this reason, using a burr, an estimate is made of the approximate middle of the glenoid neck and a small slot from superior to inferior is made in the normal axis of the glenoid fossa (Fig. 28-23). This slot is neither deepened excessively, nor widened, until it is clearly observed that this centering hole and slot are indeed in the cancellous portion of the neck of the glenoid. Excessive posterior or anterior wear of the glenoid, or excessive osteophyte formation, can make the surgeon create a keel for the glenoid, away from the anatomic cancellous center of the glenoid, leading to cortical penetration or fracture of the glenoid during preparation.

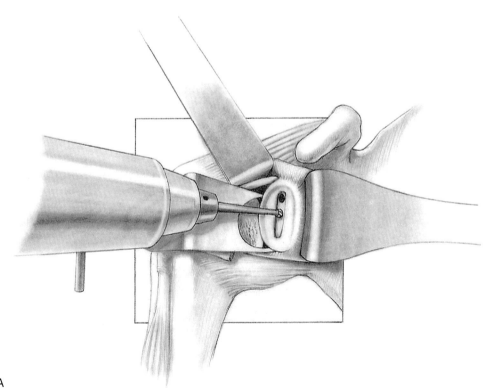

A

Figure 28-23. A–C: In this arthroplasty system, a slot is created from superior to inferior to house the glenoid keel. This slot should be widened only to the normal glenoid component width, but it may be undermined superiorly and inferiorly for better and more secure cement penetration. *(continued)*

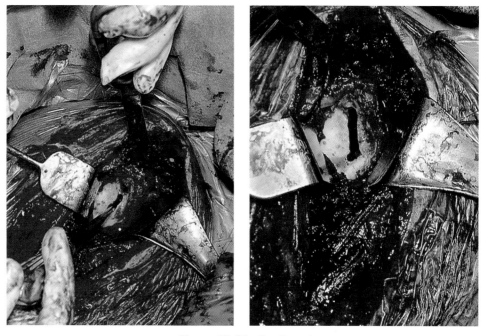

Figure 28-23. *Continued.*

A small curette is then placed in the trial slot that has been created and the direction of the cancellous neck of the glenoid is found. Once this is found, the remaining slot can be deepened in a superior and inferior direction for insertion of the keel of the Atlas glenoid design. Once the superior-to-inferior slot is created, a broach can be used to prepare the neck of the glenoid for receipt of the trial prosthesis (Fig. 28-24). A glenoid-contouring device is used to contour the exposed surface of the glenoid to the exact curvature of the posterior surface of the prosthesis so they match precisely and the prosthesis sits on solid sub-

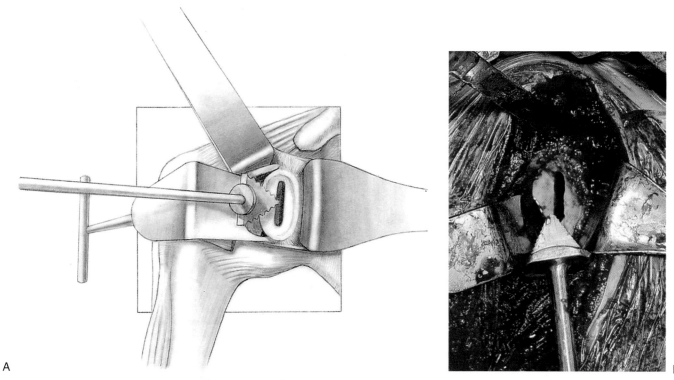

Figure 28-24. A,B: The glenoid broach to deepen the slot for the glenoid keel.

chondral bone (Fig. 28-25). The slot is deepened in the cancellous neck of the glenoid, and then undermined superiorly and inferiorly for further cement purchase. Although there is usually very little distortion of the anatomy in osteonecrosis, it is very common for patients who have primary osteoarthritis of the shoulder to wear the glenoid more posteriorly than anteriorly and thus to have some posterior sloping of the glenoid. If this is not taken into

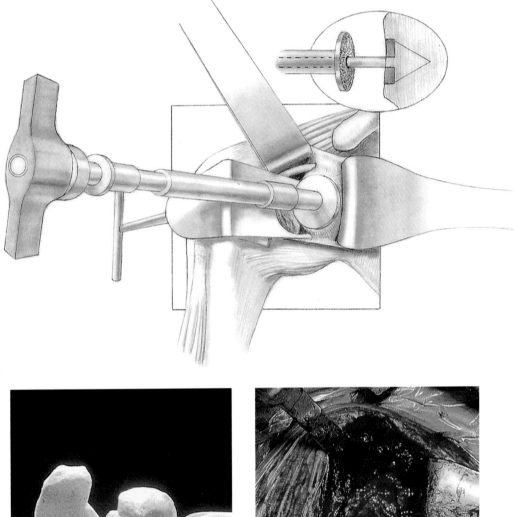

A

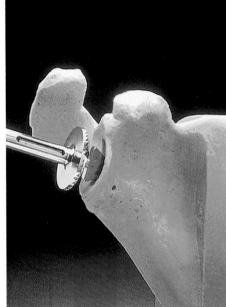

B

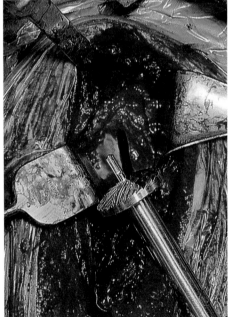

C

Figure 28-25. A–C: The glenoid-contouring device is used to prepare the exposed glenoid face to match precisely the posterior surface of the glenoid prosthesis. The keel attachment to the contouring device ensures contouring of only that amount of glenoid resurfaced by the prosthesis. The contouring device moves back and forth along the exposed extension of the stem–keel instrument.

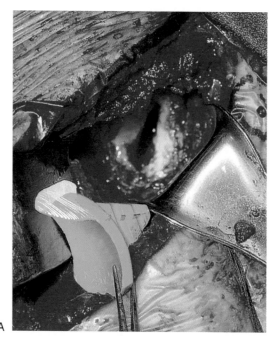
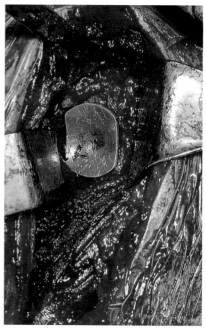

Figure 28-26. A,B: The standard polyethylene glenoid trial component is placed in the prepared glenoid. Alternative sizes with identical curvature and keel depth are available.

consideration, the posterior half of the glenoid component may not seat securely on sub-chondral bone, resulting in a gap between posterior prosthesis and posterior glenoid. Thus, the surgeon has three options if there is excessive wear in the posterior half of the glenoid:

- Burr down the anterior half of the glenoid bone to match the extent of posterior wear.
- Bone graft the posterior glenoid so that the implant seats securely on anterior and posterior bone.
- Use a glenoid component that already takes into account asymmetry of glenoid wear (posterior built-up glenoid).

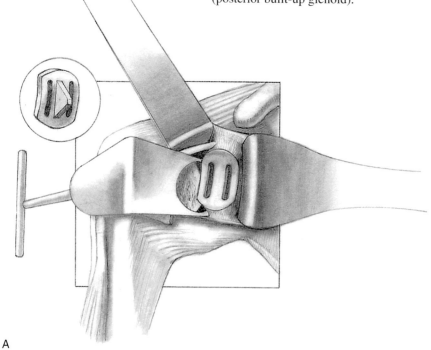
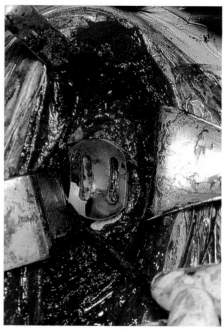

Figure 28-27. A,B: A slotted glenoid trial can be used to make certain that the implant seats securely on both anterior and posterior subchondral bone.

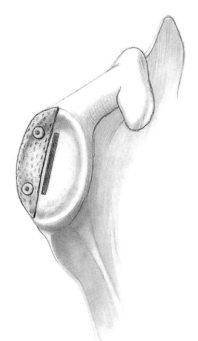

Figure 28-28. With severe asymmetric glenoid wear, a bone graft can be contoured from humeral head to build up the excessively worn posterior glenoid, and is secured to the glenoid bone by internal fixation.

Under most circumstances, the anterior glenoid bone can be burred down and contoured so that the posterior glenoid does not need to be grafted. This is done relatively easily with the glenoid-contouring device, which can asymmetrically burr down the prominent high anterior wall of the glenoid. The glenoid trial component is inserted (Fig. 28-26). A slotted glenoid trial can be used to make certain that both the anterior and posterior halves of the glenoid component seat securely on subchondral bone (Fig. 28-27). The preparation of the glenoid is completed when both anterior and posterior surfaces of the component seat on subchondral bone and there is no excessive rocking or toggle of the component. Three glenoid sizes are available to match the exposed glenoid face. All have the same radius of curvature and the same keel size and depth. All glenoids match all humeral head sizes.

In those unusual circumstances in which it is elected to use bone graft, the resected humeral head can be used, a wedge-shaped piece of corticocancellous bone can be created, and one or two screws can secure the bone graft in the posterior glenoid (Fig. 28-28).

Once the glenoid is contoured to match the posterior face of the implant, several subchondral drill holes are made in the exposed surface of the glenoid (Fig. 28-29). The glenoid face and slot are meticulously dried, using either pulsating lavage or an epinephrine-soaked sponge. Methacrylate is pressurized into the slot of the glenoid, and the polyethylene glenoid component is cemented into place. An ingrowth glenoid or pegged glenoid is available, but I have chosen in most patients to use a polyethylene component (Fig. 28-30). If cortical penetration occurs during glenoid preparation, cancellous graft from the humeral head can be used to pack this defect prior to cementation of the glenoid component.

If the disease process creates where so far medial (in some cases even medial to the coracoid base) that there is not enough bone to support a glenoid component, the surgeon can consider a hemiarthroplasty alone or consider hemiarthroplasty using soft tissue into position, such as a fascia lata or Achilles allograft, to act instead of a polyethylene glenoid component.

Once the glenoid is cemented into place and excess cement is removed, the osteotomy site is again exposed on the humerus (Fig. 28-31). Care must be taken when exposing the proximal humerus so that, as the arm is externally rotated for access to the medullary canal, the greater tuberosity does not lever on the inserted glenoid component. A bone hook applying lateral traction will minimize the likelihood of this happening. The deltoid is re-

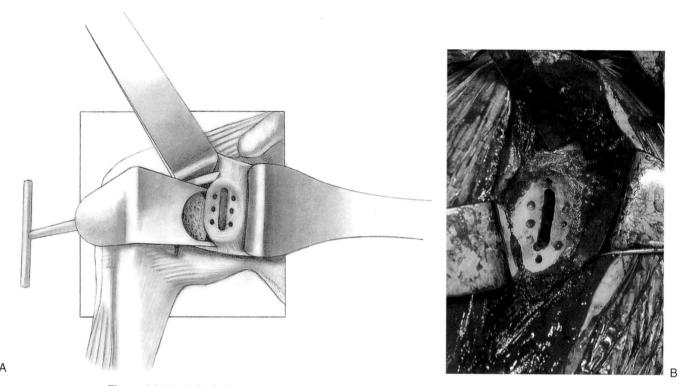

A

B

Figure 28-29. A,B: Subchondral drill holes made in the exposed glenoid for added cement penetration.

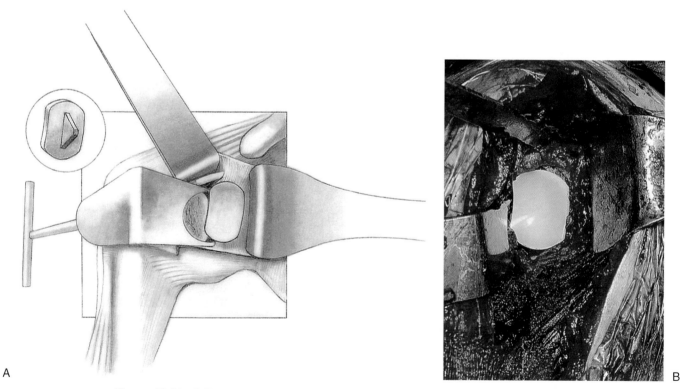

A

B

Figure 28-30. A,B: A standard polyethylene glenoid component is cemented into place.

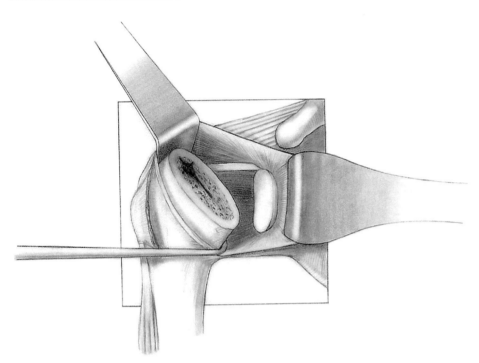

Figure 28-31. With the glenoid implantation completed, the humeral osteotomy site is exposed. Lateral traction with a bone hook during external rotation diminishes the likelihood that the greater tuberosity will impinge and lever on the posterior glenoid component.

tracted out of the way, the humerus is externally rotated and brought into the wound, and slight hyperextension exposes the proximal humerus and its medullary canal. At this point, a trial humeral component is selected. With the Atlas design, several stem thicknesses and lengths are available, and options exist for varied head sizes. In the Neer design, proximal humeral modularity is also available and both proximal and distal humeral components may be sized independently (Fig. 28-32).

In general, the thickest stem that will fit securely into the medullary canal is selected. Likewise, the largest head that will allow closure of the subscapularis around it is selected. I decide on the head size both by the size of the head that has been resected originally and

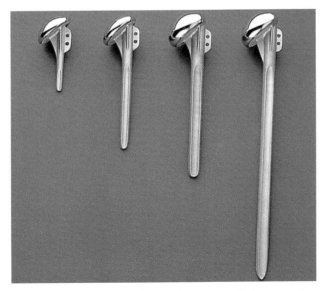

Figure 28-32. The Neer humeral components have varying stem lengths and thicknesses and offer two head sizes.

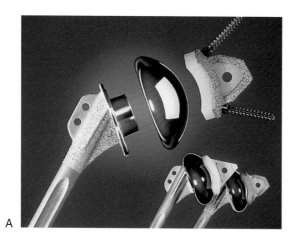
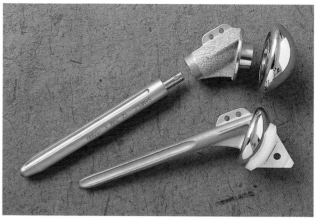

A   B

Figure 28-33. A: Modularity in the Kirschner II-C system offers greater flexibility in head size, stem thickness, stem length, and, thus, intraoperative soft-tissue tensioning. **B:** The proximal humeral modulant adds the ability to independently size the proximal and distal humerus.

by how tight the rotator cuff is after the humeral trial is in place and the shoulder is reduced. In general, a larger head size will allow greater tension in the surrounding soft tissues, and it will potentially permit more power (Fig. 28–33). A smaller head size allows easier closure of the rotator cuff and more play in the glenohumeral joint, and it will avoid overstuffing the joint (Fig. 28-34). With the humeral head reduced, the humerus should be stable in the glenoid yet permit some anterior and posterior translation. In addition, inferior traction should permit the humeral head to translate inferiorly somewhat. The correct position of the humerus is with the top of the humeral head component approximately 3 to 5 mm above the top of the greater tuberosity. Too prominent a greater tuberosity will cause impingement of the tuberosity on the acromion, while too proud a head may concentrate pressure on the superior glenoid once the shoulder is relocated. The humeral component may be cemented into place or may be a press fit, if a secure press fit can be obtained (Figs. 28-35 and 28-36). After this final insertion of the humeral component, the shoulder is again reduced. Stability and motion are again tested (Fig. 28-37). It should be recognized that some laxity will be present under regional or general anesthesia, particularly if extensive

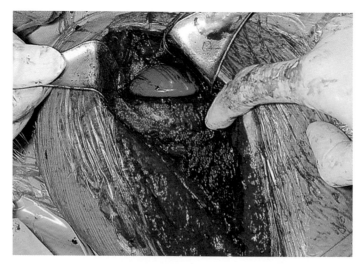

Figure 28-34. The modular head trial may be used to gauge soft-tissue tensioning, prosthetic stability, and ease of rotator cuff closure. Without changing the humeral stem, greater flexibility in soft-tissue tension is possible with a change in head size alone.

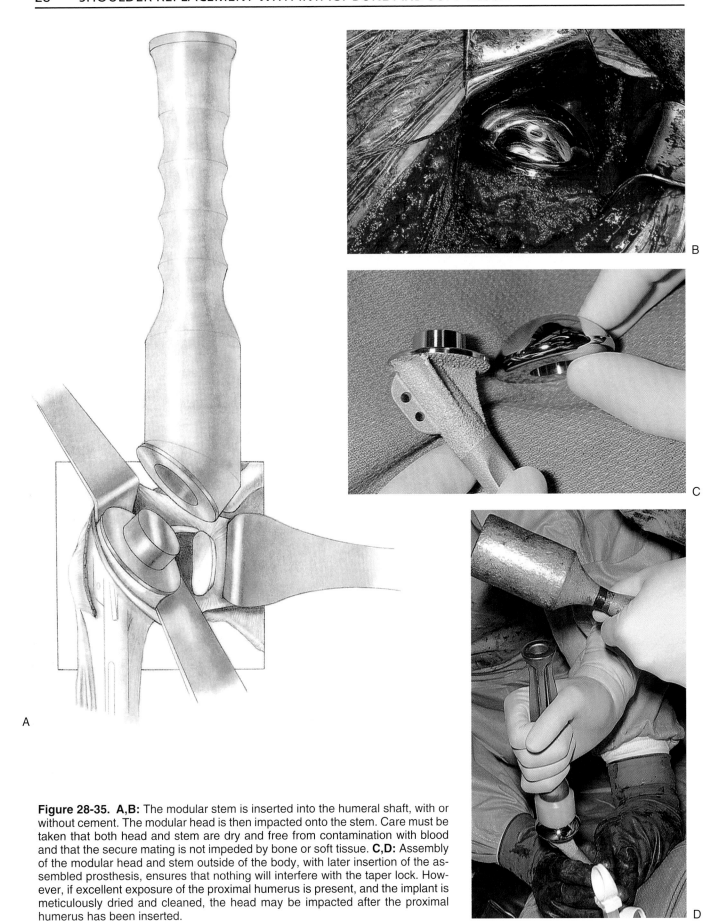

A

B

C

D

Figure 28-35. A,B: The modular stem is inserted into the humeral shaft, with or without cement. The modular head is then impacted onto the stem. Care must be taken that both head and stem are dry and free from contamination with blood and that the secure mating is not impeded by bone or soft tissue. **C,D:** Assembly of the modular head and stem outside of the body, with later insertion of the assembled prosthesis, ensures that nothing will interfere with the taper lock. However, if excellent exposure of the proximal humerus is present, and the implant is meticulously dried and cleaned, the head may be impacted after the proximal humerus has been inserted.

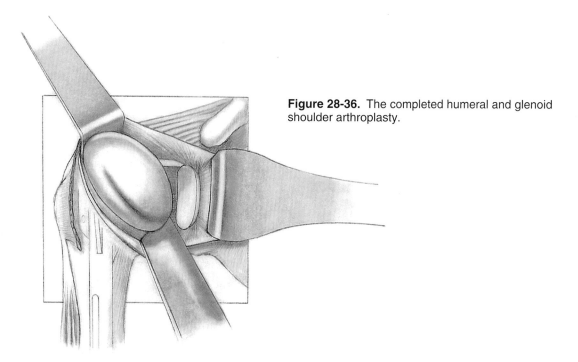

Figure 28-36. The completed humeral and glenoid shoulder arthroplasty.

capsule or resection has occurred. Postoperatively, muscle tone quickly assists in stabilizing the implant. If there is frank posterior dislocation intraoperatively (which may occur because of the asymmetric wear of the glenoid), a number of options exist:

- The larger humeral head may be inserted, thus creating more tension in the capsular tissue.
- The humeral component may be placed in less retroversion.
- The posterior capsule of the shoulder may be directly tightened to create more soft-tissue tension.

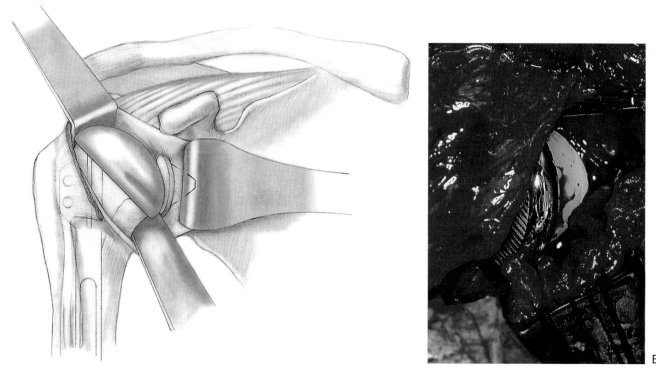

A   B

Figure 28-37. A: The humeral head is reduced, and motion and stability are tested. **B:** With humerus and glenoid in place, the subscapularis is ready to be closed around the completed arthroplasty.

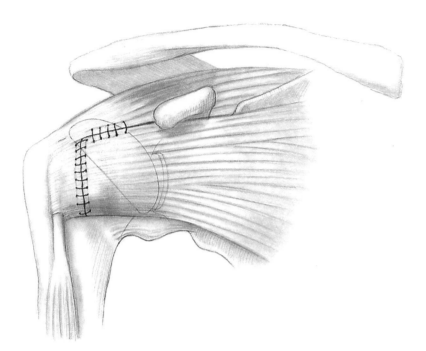

Figure 28-38. The subscapularis is closed to the point of its division and the interval between supraspinatus and subscapularis is sutured.

- The postoperative course may be altered, either with immobilization in some external rotation, or with restriction of postoperative range of motion to avoid the frontal plane.

First, the humerus is implanted because occasionally it is not cemented. Once the humerus is implanted and the shoulder is reduced, the subscapularis is repaired anatomically to the supraspinatus and to the point of its division, making no attempt to close the anterior or posterior capsule (Fig. 28-38). Heavy no. 2 nonabsorbable suture or fiber wire is used for subscapularis closure. Testing the motion in forward friction and external rotation provide information on subscapularis tension and implant stability and can guide both the extent and position of the postoperative range of motion. A Hemovac is placed deep to the deltoid, exiting through a separate stab wound. The deltopectoral interval is closed with absorbable suture. Subcutaneous tissue is closed with absorbable suture and a subcuticular running stitch is made, followed by approximation of the skin with Steri-Strips and the addition of a sterile dressing.

POSTOPERATIVE MANAGEMENT

The patient leaves the operating room with the arm immobilized at the side. Based on the range of motion and stability of the prosthesis, which has been tested intraoperatively, physical therapy begins on the first postoperative day, and radiographs should be obtained in the early postoperative period, particularly prior to initiation of physical therapy, to make certain that the humeral head is located prior to initiation of range of motion. Working with a therapist, the patient begins supine passive forward flexion and supine passive external rotation. When the patient is steady on his or her feet, participation in the postoperative rehabilitation is permitted. The patient is taught circular Codman exercises and an assistive program with a standing overhead pulley, using the unoperated arm to power or move the operated arm. Likewise, the patient begins assistive external rotation with a stick or a cane, using the unoperated arm to bring the operated arm into external rotation. It is emphasized to the patient that the exercises must be performed four to five times a day for brief, 10- to 15-minute sessions.

Since under most circumstances, the only muscle that has been divided at the time of surgery is the subscapularis, this is the only muscle that need be protected in the postoperative period. Therefore, the only motion that is not permitted is active internal rotation of the shoulder. With an otherwise intact rotator cuff, the patient is able at approximately 10 days postoperatively to begin light, gentle isometrics of the external rotators and deltoid. The patient is permitted to use the arm for light activity beginning at approximately 4 weeks postoperatively. At 6 weeks postoperatively, the sling is removed, active internal rotation exercises are begun, and resistive exercises for external rotation and the anterior and middle deltoid are permitted. Unrestricted active use of the arm is begun at 8 weeks postoperatively. At 12 to 16 weeks, if there is residual tightness in forward elevation, internal rotation, or external rotation, this may be addressed by end-range stretching exercises.

After total shoulder arthroplasty for osteoarthritis, it must be emphasized to the patient and the therapist that rehabilitation may take 8 months to 1 year from the time of surgery before the patient achieves maximum improvement in motion, strength, endurance, and activity. I usually tell the patient that the rehabilitation takes quite a long time and that at about 3 months postoperatively most patients are reasonably comfortable, have motion about half normal, but do notice some weakness. At 6 months postoperatively, most patients are pain-free, except for weather ache, and have motion and strength about two thirds of normal. I tell them that they can usually return to sedentary work within 2 to 3 weeks from the time of surgery, but that heavy work is forbidden for 4 months or more and depends greatly on the motion and strength of the shoulder and how they are progressing.

I tell patients to expect the following during the postoperative period: Under normal circumstances, the patients often will wake up from surgery in a great deal of pain. However, they frequently note that the hard type of pain typical of arthritis is gone and that the type of pain they are having, although not inconsequential, is quite different from what they had preoperatively. The patients also notice that when the arm has begun to be moved by the physical therapist during the assistive exercise program, the hard grating and grinding so typical of an arthritic shoulder is no longer there. The patients do have several types of pain postoperatively:

- A soreness from the extensive soft-tissue dissection, which lasts for a few weeks.
- A soreness and stiffness pain while exercises are being performed, which is oftentimes described as a "getting better" type of pain, a muscle soreness rather than an incapacitating type of pain. This usually continues to improve as the range of motion improves and eventually resolves when the range of motion is back to normal.

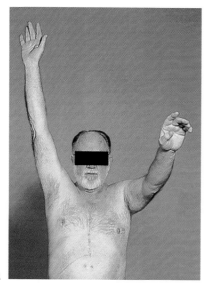
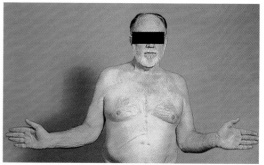

Figure 28-39. A: Examination reveals restricted active and passive forward elevation. **B:** Limited external rotation of left shoulder because of joint incongruity and soft-tissue contracture.

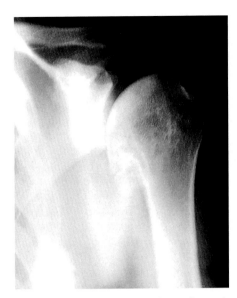

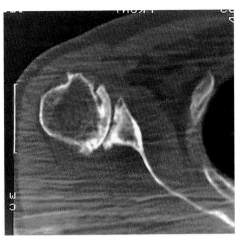

Figure 28-40. Anteroposterior radiograph showing findings consistent with primary osteoarthritis. Humeral head sclerosis and large inferior osteophyte present classic radiographic changes.

Figure 28-41. Computed tomography scan illustrates marginal osteophyte and cystic changes in glenoid and humeral head and shows that the glenoid surface is worn symmetrically on anterior and posterior surfaces. There is adequate bone stock for glenoid component.

- An aching that may be fatigue aching of the deltoid or rotator cuff, which usually lasts until the strength gets back to normal.
- A weather ache, which may last 1 or 2 years, and is related to the surgical treatment rather than to the prosthesis itself.

Nevertheless, it is reasonable to expect that at 1 year postoperatively, approximately 95% of the patients will be pain-free, and the remaining will usually have no more than a weather ache or an occasional ache with excessive activity. Likewise, because the deltoid is ordinarily normal and the rotator cuff is typically normal in primary osteoarthritis, I think it is reasonable to expect that there will not be significant strength limitations (Figs. 28-39 to 28-43).

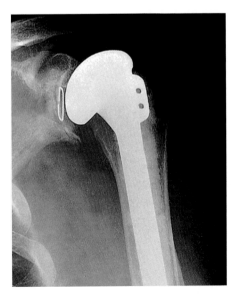

Figure 28-42. Postoperative radiograph showing position of humeral head and glenoid component.

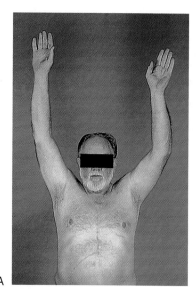
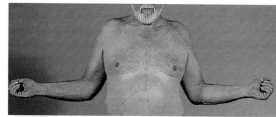
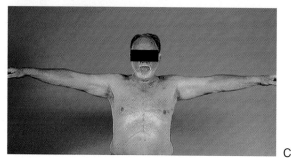

Figure 28-43. A–C: At 6 months postoperatively, after careful rehabilitation, the patient had near-normal forward elevation, external rotation, and abduction.

COMPLICATIONS

The most common complications noted after shoulder arthroplasty are the following:

Shoulder Stiffness

An arthritic shoulder is often very tight to begin with. There may be soft-tissue contracture and subscapularis shortening, and these may be worsened by filling the joint with a prosthetic humerus and glenoid. In general, postoperative stiffness is minimized by making certain that all adhesions are released intraoperatively, any capsular contracture or tightness is dealt with at the time of implantation, any subscapularis shortening is addressed by subscapularis lengthening, and an overly large humeral head component is not put into the shoulder. If postoperative stiffness is a problem in a shoulder in which motion was obtained intraoperatively, this is usually a result of inadequate rehabilitation. The patient needs to be given encouragement to redouble the efforts for restoration of motion and forward flexion, external rotation, and internal rotation. If the patient comes into the office with stiffness postoperatively and it is unexpected, I ask the patient to redouble the efforts and to see a physical therapist for passive stretching exercises.

Posterior Instability of the Humerus

Posterior subluxation and dislocation may occur in primary osteoarthritis from asymmetric wear of the glenoid. Asymmetric wear of the glenoid can lead to the glenoid component being placed in too much retroversion, and the humeral component can slide down the face of the glenoid, subluxating posteriorly. If this posterior instability is recognized intraoperatively, I address it before final prosthetic implantation (see Surgery section). In a patient who presents with late posterior instability that was not recognized initially, the position of the component should be checked radiographically. If rehabilitation of the rotator cuff muscles does not provide some dynamic stability to the shoulder or if the components are malpositioned, prosthetic revision may need to be considered.

Late Anterior Dislocation of the Humeral Head

It has recently been recognized that anterior dislocation of the humerus following a total shoulder arthroplasty may occur. This is usually associated with rupture of the subscapularis repair. If this occurs and is recognized early, the subscapularis can be directly repaired. If, after subsequent subscapularis repair, there is still anterior instability, components may need to be revised, or the anterior structures may need to be augmented with allograft material, such as Achilles tendon material.

Neurovascular or Brachial Plexus Injury

While any one neurologic complication is not common, it is not uncommon to have mild brachial plexus irritation after total shoulder arthroplasty. This usually manifests itself as paresthesia; occasionally frank paralysis may occur. Nerve injury can be avoided by making certain that all nerves are protected adequately, that all soft tissues are released, and that there is no excessive traction placed on the brachial plexus intraoperatively. If a nerve injury is discovered postoperatively, it is usually a neuropraxia, and time is given for this to resolve. If there is no resolution, nerve studies may be used, and if there is question about the integrity of the nerve, it can be explored.

Glenoid Loosening

Although the incidence of clinical loosening following total shoulder replacement is extremely small, and the revision rate is extremely low, the presence of lucent lines is not infrequent radiographically. Those patients who are asymptomatic and present with radiolucent lines in the glenoid need only be followed clinically and radiographically. If the patient comes in with symptomatic painful shoulder after shoulder arthroplasty and glenoid looseness is suspected, the usual evaluation for painful arthroplasty is begun, including cultures and paired isotope scanning, with examination under anesthesia.

RECOMMENDED READING

1. Bigliani, L.U., Bauer, G.S., Murthi, A.M.: Humeral head replacement: techniques and soft-tissue preparation. *Instr Course Lect* 51: 11–20, 2002.
2. Brems, J.J.: Complications of shoulder arthroplasty: infections, instability, and loosening. *Instr Course Lect* 51: 29–39, 2002.
3. Brems, J.J., Wilde, A.H., Borden, L.S., et al.: Glenoid lucent lines. *Orthop Trans* 10: 231, 1986.
4. Cameron, B., Galatz, L., Williams, G.R.: Factors affecting the outcome of total shoulder arthroplasty. *Am J Orthop* 30: 613–623, 2001.
5. Cofield, R.H.: Total shoulder arthroplasty with the Neer prosthesis. *J Bone Joint Surg Am* 66: 899–906, 1984.
6. Craig, E.V.: Total shoulder arthroplasty. In: Chapman, M., ed.: *Operative orthopaedics*, 2nd ed. Philadelphia: JB Lippincott Co., 1721–1752, 1993.
7. Dutta, A.K., Matthys, G., Burkhead, W.Z.: Glenoid resurfacing in shoulder arthroplasty. *Instr Course Lect* 51: 21–27, 2002.
8. Iannotti, J.P., Norris, T.R.: Influence of preoperative factors on outcome of shoulder arthroplasty for glenohumeral osteoarthritis. *J Bone Joint Surg Am* 85: 251–258, 2003.
9. Ibarra, C., Craig, E.V.: Soft-tissue balancing in total shoulder arthroplasty. *Orthop Clin North Am* 29: 415–422, 1998.
10. Ibarra, C., Dines, D.M., McLaughlin, J.A.: Glenoid replacement in total shoulder arthroplasty. *Orthop Clin North Am* 29: 403–413, 1998.
11. Neer, C.S.: Neer hemiarthroplasty and Neer total shoulder arthroplasty in patients fifty years old or less: long-term results. *J Bone Joint Surg Am* 81: 295–296, 1999.
12. Neer, C.S. II, Morrison, D.S.: Glenoid bone-grafting in total shoulder arthroplasty. *J Bone Joint Surg Am* 70: 1154–1162, 1988.
13. Neer, C.S. II, Watson, K.C., Stanton, F.J.: Recent experience in total shoulder replacement. *J Bone Joint Surg Am* 64: 319–337, 1982.
14. Norris, T.R., Iannotti, J.P.: Functional outcome after shoulder arthroplasty for primary osteoarthritis: a multicenter study. *J Shoulder Elbow Surg* 11: 130–135, 2002.
15. Smith, K.L., Matsen, F.A.: Total shoulder arthroplasty versus hemiarthroplasty: current trends. *Orthop Clin North Am* 29: 491–506, 1998.
16. Waldman, B.J., Figgie, M.P.: Indications, technique, and results of total-shoulder arthroplasty in rheumatoid arthritis. *Orthop Clin North Am* 29: 435–444, 1998.

sive tear can be present. Typically, it is thinned superiorly and may have a medium to large tear that is superior in location rather than anterosuperior. In old trauma, bony deformities predominate with associated rotator cuff stretching, tearing, or contracture, dictated by the position of the tuberosity. In osteonecrosis, the rotator cuff is almost always intact but may be involved with an inflammatory process that renders the tissues somewhat tighter and stiffer than usual. In rotator cuff tear arthropathy, there is always a massive tear involving the supraspinatus, the infraspinatus, and often a portion of the subscapularis. In surgery for revision of a previously placed prosthesis, in addition to bone, rotator cuff, and capsule deficiencies and possible neurologic impairment, the surgeon must address scar tissue that infiltrates the remaining tissues.

An issue in preoperative planning is glenohumeral stability. When the glenohumeral joint is stable, a small amount of bone deficiency can often be tolerated and accepted as a part of the reconstructive process. When instability is present, the bone deficiency will need to be more fully corrected to ensure postoperative stability of the artificial joint. This situation most commonly arises in osteoarthritis, because the posterior glenoid wear may be associated with substantial posterior humeral subluxation, requiring the bony deficiency to be more fully corrected than if subluxation is not present.

Last, the degree of glenohumeral stiffness must be carefully evaluated. This may be related to incongruity of the joint surfaces, but often depends on the condition of the shoulder capsule and surrounding rotator cuff. To have a mobile joint after surgery, these joint contractures usually have to be released. When there is bone deficiency, more exposure is usually needed to correct it, and there is more extensive tissue release in the reconstructive procedure. The latter includes release of the inferior shoulder capsule, release or lengthening of the anterior structures, and perhaps release of the superior and posterior aspects of the shoulder capsule, depending on the preexisting structural abnormalities.

Thus, a thorough preoperative analysis of the pathologic anatomy is essential to the reconstructive procedure. Not only must one have adequate imaging to define the alterations in bone quality, quantity, and position, but one must also have a good understanding of the condition of the surrounding musculature and the shoulder capsule. In addition, it is important to consider the possibility of neurologic compromise and the various patient selection factors. If there has been previous surgery, one also must rule out the possibility of occult or low-grade infection with hematologic studies, aspiration arthrography, or bone and indium-labeled scans.

If a history of previous trauma or physical examination findings suggests deficiency of muscle groups such as the deltoid, more thorough evaluation of neurologic status by a preoperative electromyogram may be considered.

Some patients with a neuropathic glenohumeral joint have extensive humeral or glenoid bone loss and destruction. Fortunately, many of these patients do not have pain in the involved joint despite extensive bony destruction. Radiographic evidence of a neuropathic joint should prompt the clinician to do a careful peripheral neurologic examination and consider imaging studies of the cervical spine, because a cervical spine syrinx is a common pathologic entity leading to a neuropathic shoulder.

SURGERY

When doing additional work on the glenoid, five "pre-steps" should be considered: extended exposure and extended arthrotomy, ample humeral bone removal, capsule releases, and the availability of special retractors. The patient is placed in a beach-chair position, semisitting, with the head secured to the operating table. An interscalene block is given, but general anesthesia and endotracheal intubation are usually required, particularly with a lengthy operation as may occur if there is extensive bone loss. The arm is draped free. For implantation of the humeral component, hyperextension of the arm is often needed. In contrast, for glenoid exposure, resting the arm on a draped Mayo stand will help keep the proximal humerus retracted posteriorly, giving better access.

During total shoulder arthroplasty, one of the most difficult aspects is exposure of the

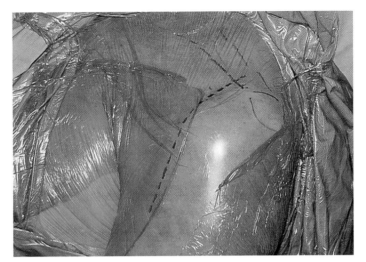

Figure 29-1. Skin incision for total shoulder arthroplasty.

glenoid. When bone deficiency exists in the glenoid, the exposure must be somewhat fuller, and when deficiency exists in the humerus, it may be necessary to extend the incision distally.

The exposure begins with the skin incision. I believe it is helpful to comment on certain aspects of exposure in the presence of glenoid and humeral bone deficiencies. The most useful incision is on the anterior aspect of the shoulder, extending from approximately 1 cm medial to the distal aspect of the clavicle, downward to the anterior aspect of the insertion of the deltoid muscle on the humerus (Fig. 29-1). This skin incision is directly over the tissues involved in most of the surgical procedure, preventing the need for retracting the skin incision further during the various surgical manipulations. It is necessary to raise a small medial flap (Fig. 29-2) to identify the deltopectoral interval and then to retract the deltoid laterally (Fig. 29-3). One must open the entire length of the deltopectoral interval from the clavicle to the insertion of the deltoid on the humerus, and, when the deltoid is somewhat stiff, it is helpful to elevate the anterior portion of the deltoid insertion in continuity with the distally extending periosteum. The fascia lateral to the conjoint tendon is then incised, and the conjoint tendon is retracted medially, affording the opportunity to free the subscapularis from contracted bursa or related scar. The subacromial and subdeltoid spaces are then fully freed of scar tissue to further facilitate the deeper exposure.

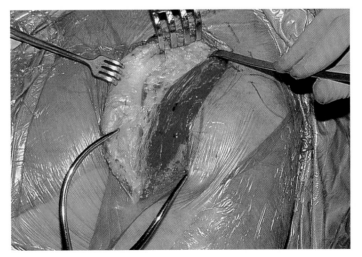

Figure 29-2. Small medial skin flap developed to expose the deltopectoral interval.

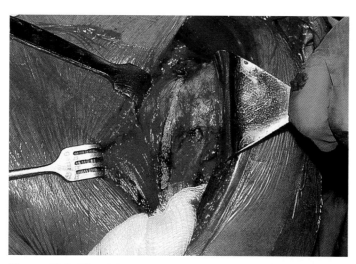

Figure 29-3. The deltoid is retracted laterally and held in position with a large retractor. The conjoined group is retracted medially. The long arthrotomy incision has been outlined with electrical cautery.

Ample exposure of the glenoid is likely to be desired, and it is useful to have a long arthrotomy incision extending from the supraglenoid tubercle (just anterior to the attachment of the long head of the biceps tendon), along the anterior aspect of the intraarticular portion of the long head of the biceps, and then curving distally at the capsular attachment on the humerus (Fig. 29-4). In the lower portion of the subscapularis, the branches of the anterior humeral circumflex vessels are coagulated, and the incision is directed onto the humeral neck. One can then, by externally rotating the humerus, release most of the inferior shoulder capsule from the humeral neck. One then has an arthrotomy (if this is a left shoulder) extending from the 11-o'clock position to the 6-o'clock or 5-o'clock position. Following removal of humeral osteophytes and excessive humeral metaphyseal bone, and

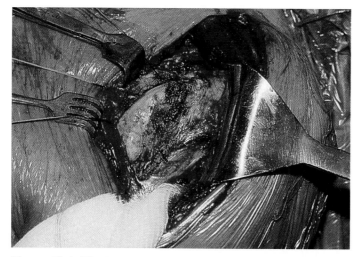

Figure 29-4. The long arthrotomy incision has been performed. It extends from the supraglenoid tubercle (anterior to the insertion of the intraarticular portion of the long head of the biceps tendon), along the interval, distally over the insertion of the shoulder capsule, and inferiorly along the glenoid neck proximal humeral shaft. By creating this long exposure, the entire anterior half of the shoulder joint will be exposed, and after humeral osteotomy, there will be ample exposure for dealing with glenoid or humeral bone deficiencies.

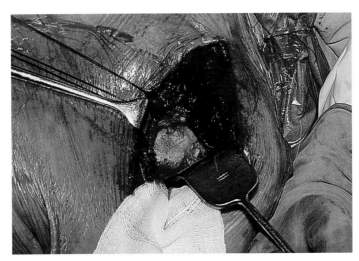

Figure 29-5. Glenoid exposure. A ring retractor holds the remaining humeral head posteriorly, and a knee retractor holds the subscapularis anteriorly. The entire glenoid face is exposed.

following osteotomy of the humeral head, there is ample exposure of the glenoid (Fig. 29-5). If the joint is still too tight, intraarticular scar can be excised, and a portion of the superior or posterior capsule can be incised at the glenoid rim. This exposure should allow one to easily address central glenoid wear and peripheral, asymmetric glenoid wear such as that typically seen in osteoarthritis. There are rare segmental glenoid deficiencies that may not be addressed by this approach. Exposure techniques for these unusual circumstances will be described later.

If there is a deficiency of the proximal humerus, it may be necessary to extend the skin incision distally along the anterolateral aspect of the arm (Fig. 29-6). The lateral portion of the brachialis muscle is incised, and the tissues are elevated medially and laterally to expose distal, uninvolved humeral bone (6). One must take great care to protect the radial nerve in the lateral aspect of the wound.

Glenoid Bone Deficiencies

It is very important to consider bone quality (Tables 29-1 and 29-2). Typically, there will be a glenoid subchondral plate that is 1 to 2 mm thick, and beneath this will be rather firm, cancellous bone surrounded by a thin, cortical shell. However, the bone quality varies considerably. The bone may be pockmarked with cysts, there may be severe osteopenia, or, perhaps more typically, the bone may be very sclerotic, extending throughout the glenoid neck, compromising fixation capabilities. Many surgeons consistently use methylmethacrylate bone cement as an adjunct to glenoid component fixation; others turn in some situations toward a tissue-ingrowth component. The ideal bone for methylmethacrylate fixation is also the ideal bone for placement of a tissue-ingrowth component. When the bone is very osteoporotic, one leans toward the use of bone cement as an adjunct to fixation, but

Table 29-1. *Classification of glenoid bone deficiencies*
Mild (any type)
Central
Resorption
Large cavity
Peripheral
Segmental

Table 29-2. *Reconstruction of glenoid deficiencies*
Focal bone graft
Focal bone cement
Extra reaming and a thicker component
Humeral head replacement (alone)
Asymmetric surface preparation and an "angled keel" component
Structural bone graft
Augmented component

the fixation will be less secure than if the bone was of typical density. When the bone is extremely sclerotic, fixation is impaired with the use of bone cement or with the use of a tissue-ingrowth component. Some surgeons might lean more toward the use of a tissue-ingrowth component in this setting, but that is not always better.

When assessing the remaining glenoid bone, it is important to consider the glenoid bone surface, its size, and its orientation. Often, variation in size can be addressed by using a

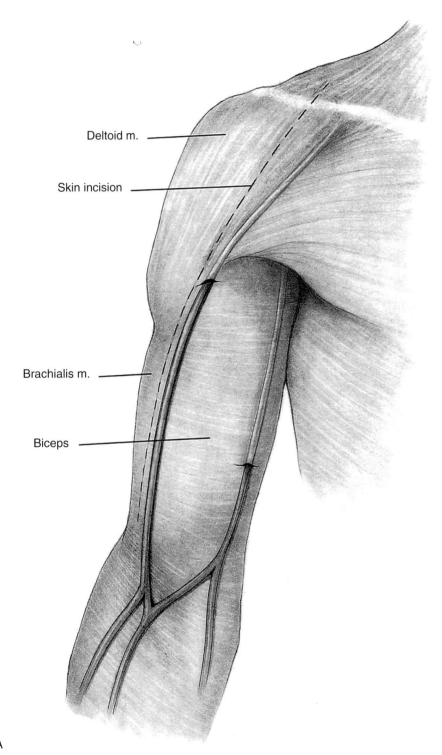

A

Figure 29-6. A: Line of skin incision for distal extension of total shoulder arthroplasty exposure. The length of the distal extension is modified according to the exposure needed. *(continued)*

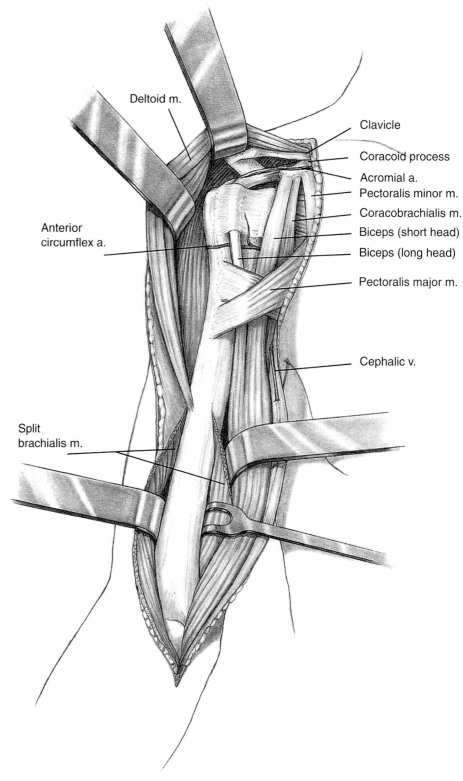

Deltoid m.

Clavicle

Coracoid process

Acromial a.

Pectoralis minor m.

Coracobrachialis m.

Biceps (short head)

Biceps (long head)

Anterior
circumflex a.

Pectoralis major m.

Cephalic v.

Split
brachialis m.

B

Figure 29-6. *Continued.* **B:** As can be appreciated from this dramatic illustration, an extensive amount of exposure is possible using this operative approach. Usually, only the upper half of the humerus will need to be exposed for even the most extensive humeral deficiencies encountered during total shoulder arthroplasty. *(continued)*

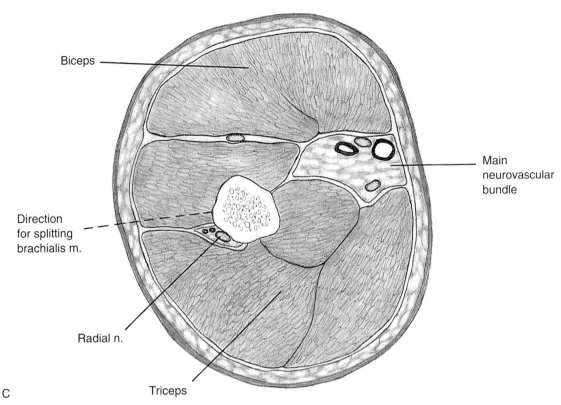

Biceps

Main
neurovascular
bundle

Direction
for splitting
brachialis m.

Radial n.

Triceps

C

Figure 29-6. *Continued.* **C:** As a part of the description of the exposure shown in **A** and **B,** it was suggested that the direction of brachialis splitting be rather anterior in the brachialis. From a practical standpoint, this splitting can be much closer to the radial nerve when the brachialis is stretched anteromedially over the humerus.

component of a corresponding size, that is, using a smaller component for a smaller glenoid and so forth. It is important to determine the length of the glenoid neck to ascertain whether there will be enough remaining bone to secure the keel or the columns of the various types of glenoid components. It is helpful to have 2 cm of depth to the glenoid neck. When it becomes less than this, compromise of fixation occurs. At a depth of approximately 1.5 cm, fixation will probably still be secure; at a depth of 1 cm, fixation will be significantly compromised. It is probably true that the depth of the glenoid neck can be slightly less when one uses a columned component than that for a component with a keel, because the columns can penetrate into the junction of the glenoid neck with the body of the scapula and gain some purchase. It is very difficult to accomplish this with the keellike component that requires methylmethacrylate bone cement for fixation.

Central Bone Loss. There are two types of central bone loss of the glenoid. The first and probably most significant occurs when the entire glenoid face resorbs medially (Fig. 29-7). The glenoid is shaped like a funnel, and, as the bone is worn medially, substantially less bone remains to allow secure fixation of the component. This situation most commonly arises in rheumatoid arthritis (Fig. 29-8). When it is identified on preoperative radiographs and intraoperatively, it may be prudent to place a centering hole to ascertain the depth of the glenoid neck (Fig. 29-9). If 1 cm or less of glenoid neck remains, one might consider recontouring the remaining glenoid surface with a burr or reamer and placing a humeral head component without a glenoid prosthesis (Fig. 29-10). In this situation, pain relief is more likely with a humeral head replacement alone than it would be with a total shoulder arthroplasty with an insecurely fixed glenoid component (2).

The second type of central wear involves a circumscribed defect (Fig. 29-11). Often this is present in conjunction with periarticular cysts. The cyst is removed, the glenoid surface and the cylinders for the columns or the slot for the keel are prepared, and the central defect is filled with bone graft from the humeral head; occasionally, methylmethacrylate bone

(text continues on page 561)

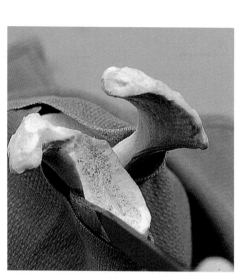

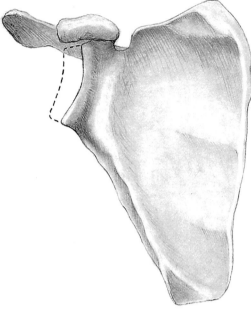

A

B

Figure 29-7. A: Bone model showing central resorption of the glenoid. The glenoid face is narrow and is positioned at or medial to the base of the coracoid process. **B:** Illustration depicting the central glenoid erosion. As the bone resorbs, the volume of bone remaining is much decreased as the glenoid is shaped not unlike a funnel.

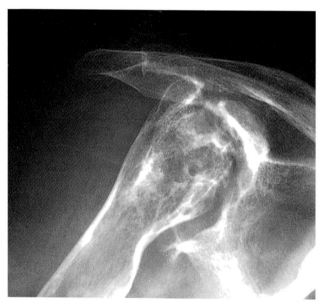

Figure 29-8. Radiograph of a patient with rheumatoid arthritis and severe central glenoid resorption.

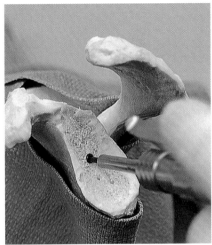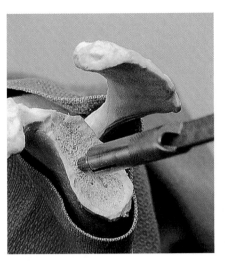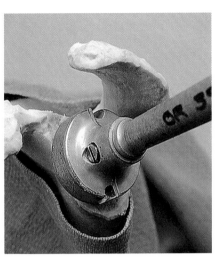

A, B   C

Figure 29-9. When central glenoid resorption is identified radiographically, it may be helpful to further image this using narrow-section computed tomography. During surgery, the
depth of the remaining glenoid neck is a critical determination in the decision as to whether
or not a glenoid component can be placed. **A:** Small central hole being developed to define
the depth of the remaining glenoid neck. **B:** Depth gauge inserted into pilot hole. If 1.5 cm
of depth is present, it should be possible to place a glenoid component. If less than 1 cm of
depth remains, fixation for a glenoid component may be inadequate. Between these two
measurements, bone remaining for glenoid fixation is marginal, and the decision to place a
glenoid component will depend on many factors. **C:** When there is insufficient bone to support a glenoid component, the remaining glenoid face can be recontoured with a pediatric
hip reamer, or a special "hemiarthroplasty" reamer.

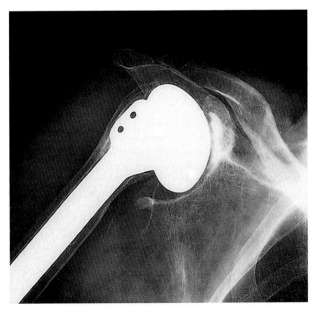

Figure 29-10. Postoperative radiograph of the shoulder of
the patient shown in Fig. 29-8. There was not enough
glenoid bone remaining to support a glenoid component, so
a humeral head component was placed against the recontoured glenoid surface.

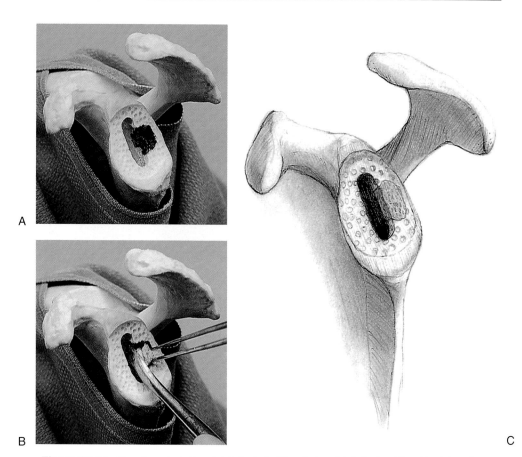

Figure 29-11. Focal central glenoid defect. **A:** Focal glenoid defect outlined by blue dye on a bone model. This often is present in patients with large periarticular cysts involving the glenoid. **B:** The focal central deficiency is being packed with bone graft material. If the deficiency is quite large, a structural bone graft may need to be fixed in position. **C:** Defect eliminated by bone graft material. The glenoid component may now be fixed in position with bone cement in the usual fashion.

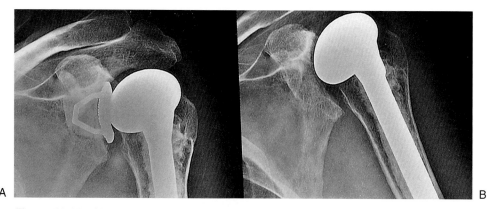

Figure 29-12. Glenoid with large central bone deficiency (cavity) following loosening of a previously placed glenoid component and glenoid bone resorption. **A:** Total shoulder arthroplasty with loosening of the glenoid component and periprosthetic glenoid bone resorption. **B:** Radiograph following removal of the loosened component and glenoid bone grafting. At surgery, only a shell of glenoid bone remained. Should pain relief not be adequate following this procedure, it may be possible at a later date to replace a glenoid component on the reconstituted glenoid bone.

cement is used instead. This minor defect does not usually represent a problem in a primary case, but in a revision case, the entire bone of the neck of the glenoid may be gone, with only the rims remaining and often even they have some perforations. With this extensive amount of central bone deficiency, one might consider bone grafting the deficiency and again placing a humeral head component without a glenoid prosthesis (Fig. 29-12).

Peripheral Deficiencies. Peripheral deficiencies are associated with asymmetric wear of the surface of the glenoid. In osteoarthritis, wear of the posterior aspect of the glenoid is common. After scar and any remaining cartilage are removed from the glenoid surface, one encounters two surfaces. The anterior surface represents the normal subchondral plate. The posterior surface represents the area of wear. Often, the two meet with a vertical crest not unlike a shallow, pitched roof. The ideal bone preparation would be such that the glenoid component would sit on the glenoid surface parallel to the normal subchondral plate. Posterior wear, however, may preclude this. Based on recent experience in total

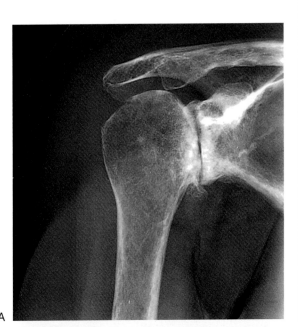

A

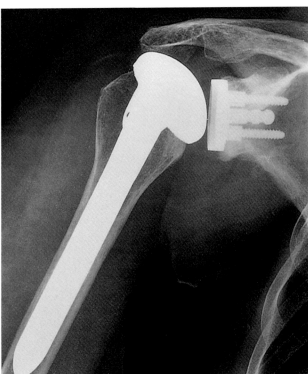

C

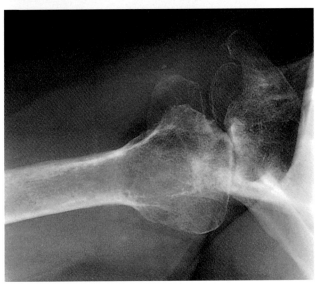

B

Figure 29-13. A: Shoulder radiograph of a patient with osteonecrosis following radiation therapy. There is a minor amount of central glenoid resorption. **B:** Axillary radiograph shows the resorption is not only central but also posterior. **C:** The glenoid deficiency was addressed by slight asymmetry to the reaming of the glenoid, with placement of a glenoid component thick enough to compensate for the bone loss and the cartilage destruction.

shoulder replacement, Neer et al. (9) outlined a number of options to be used in this circumstance. One can place the glenoid component on the remaining bone surface at a rather poor angle, often with excessive retroversion. One can build up the deficiency with bone cement. One can grind the normal subchondral plate to match the area of surface wear. One can use a special component augmented in thickness over the area of the deficiency. Finally, one can add a bone graft to the deficient area. Although a bone graft is seldom necessary, it may be the best choice when substantial wear is present (8).

The repair method chosen depends significantly on the amount of wear. If the amount of wear is minor (1 to 2 mm), the surface can be ground down so that the glenoid component is in a nearly normal position and the glenoid component can be seated on the remaining bone (Fig. 29-13). If the wear is slightly greater (3 to 5 mm), one might consider a compromise between the normal version for the component and the version created by asymmetric wear, that is, grinding the glenoid surface along the crest where the two surfaces meet (Fig. 29-14). This creates a glenoid component position that is not normal but is less

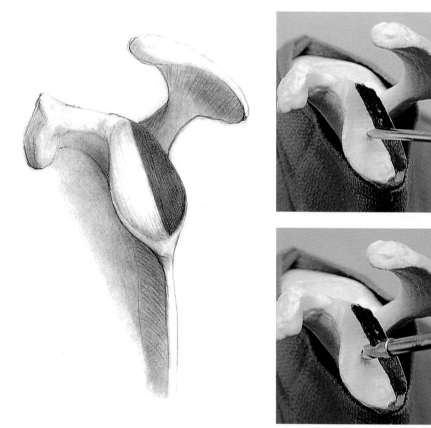

A

B

C

Figure 29-14. A–H: A minor amount of asymmetric wear (1 to 3 mm) of the posterior aspect of the glenoid. **A:** Bone model with blue area indicating an area of bone wear or deficiency on the posterior aspect of the glenoid. It is approximately 2 mm in depth at the glenoid rim relative to the normal position of the glenoid subchondral plate. **B:** An awl is used to identify the central point of the glenoid. **C:** A drill is placed in the identified central hole, and the hole is deepened in a direction that is a compromise between the direction of the normal subchondral plate and the area of bone wear. **D:** A reamer stabilized in the central hole has been used to grind the ridge between the two bone surfaces on the glenoid. This has, in effect, changed the direction of the glenoid face a few degrees, but it has also eliminated much of the bone deficiency, as illustrated by the reduction in the size of the blue-stained area. **E:** The template and drills are then used to further prepare the glenoid component. **F:** The margins of the keel slot have been identified by the three drill holes. **G:** The drill holes are then connected, and the holes are deepened in the axis of the glenoid neck. A polyethylene component with a slight angle between the face of the component and the keel is also shown. **H:** The component is now placed firmly on the recontoured glenoid surface and in the normal axis of the glenoid neck. This type of preparation can be done for a minor degree of asymmetric bone wear and in the presence of little or no humeral subluxation. *(continued)*

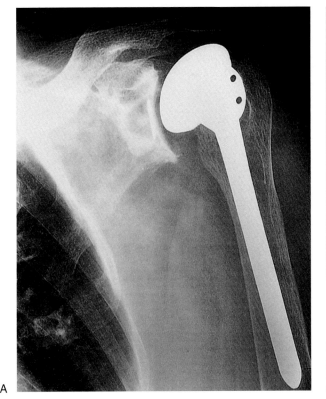

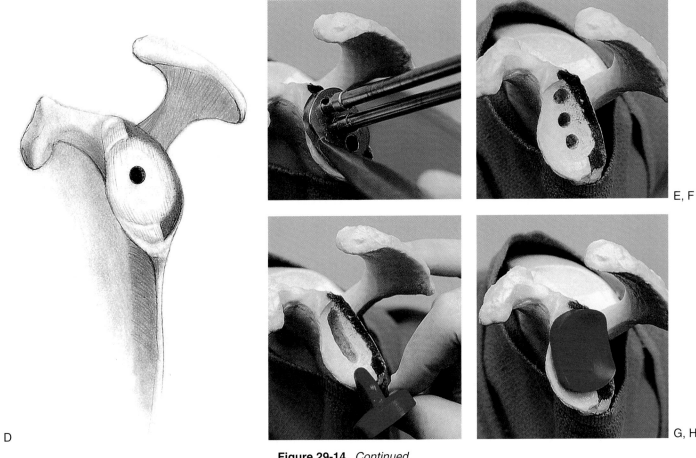

E, F

G, H

D

Figure 29-14. *Continued.*

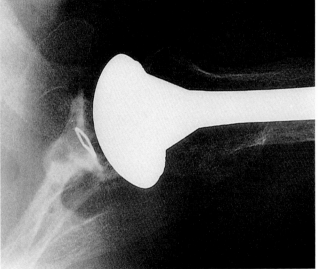

A

B

Figure 29-15. A: Total shoulder arthroplasty with a cemented glenoid component using the angled keel. **B:** Axillary view illustrates the asymmetric glenoid surface preparation and the absence of humeral subluxation.

abnormal than that which existed prior to the reconstruction. If there is no preexisting humeral subluxation in the direction of wear or the subluxation is only minor, this is an appropriate reconstructive technique. After preparation of the joint surface in this manner, the keel slot can be prepared as usual, and a component with an angle between the keel and the face can be cemented in position (Fig. 29-15). If one uses a component with columns, the component can be offset in the direction of the wear 2 to 3 mm, and the columns can be prepared perpendicular to the new position of the glenoid surface.

When using one of these two options, one cannot recontour and remove more than a few millimeters of the glenoid without compromising the size of the remaining glenoid face and the support obtained from the firm subchondral bone. Below the subchondral plate, the cancellous bone will be soft and inadequate to support the component.

If the asymmetric deficiency is 5 mm or greater, one has to adopt more complex measures. Building up the deficiency with extra bone cement does not seem realistic. Deficiency can be addressed occasionally by use of a special component (Fig. 29-16) but, perhaps more typically and most effectively, by placing a bone graft over the deficient area (Fig. 29-17). This bone graft is often prepared from a segment of the partially resected humeral head. The shape of the remaining glenoid surface is prepared. The column holes or the keel slots are placed, and then the bone graft is secured in position. This is often done most effectively with small screws, such as 3.5-mm cortical screws for a larger patient or slightly smaller screws for the smaller glenoid (Fig. 29-18).

Segmental Deficiencies. A few individuals have a defect that involves a segment of the glenoid. This most commonly occurs in old trauma, such as a fracture of the glenoid rim, that is enlarged by subsequent wear (Fig. 29-19). It may be necessary to bone graft this deficient region and place fixation perpendicular to the glenoid surface. This is usually accomplished with screws but on rare occasions may require a buttress plate. Such deficiencies on the anteroinferior aspect of the glenoid can be reconstructed through the typical surgical exposure with further incision of the anterior capsule. When there is a posterior deficiency, the remaining bed can be prepared, and the bone graft can be positioned,

(text continues on page 568)

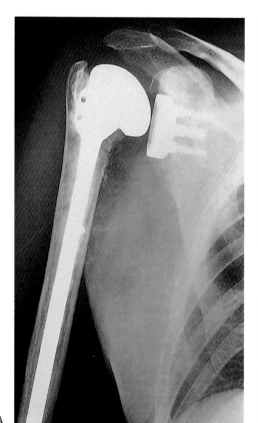

A

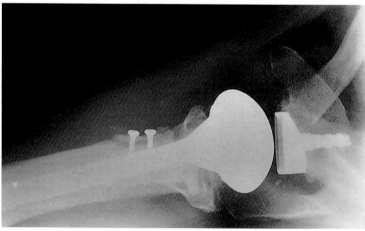

B

Figure 29-16. Active, middle-aged man with posterior shoulder instability and glenoid loosening following total shoulder arthroplasty. There were both central and posterior glenoid deficiencies. The central deficiency was addressed with bone grafting, and the posterior aspect of the deficiency with an augmented glenoid component. **A:** Anteroposterior radiograph. **B:** Axillary radiograph illustrating the posteriorly augmented glenoid component allowing secure fixation to the remaining glenoid bone and eliminating the posterior angle that had been present on the glenoid face. Note also that humeral component retrotorsion has been decreased somewhat, and no humeral subluxation exists.

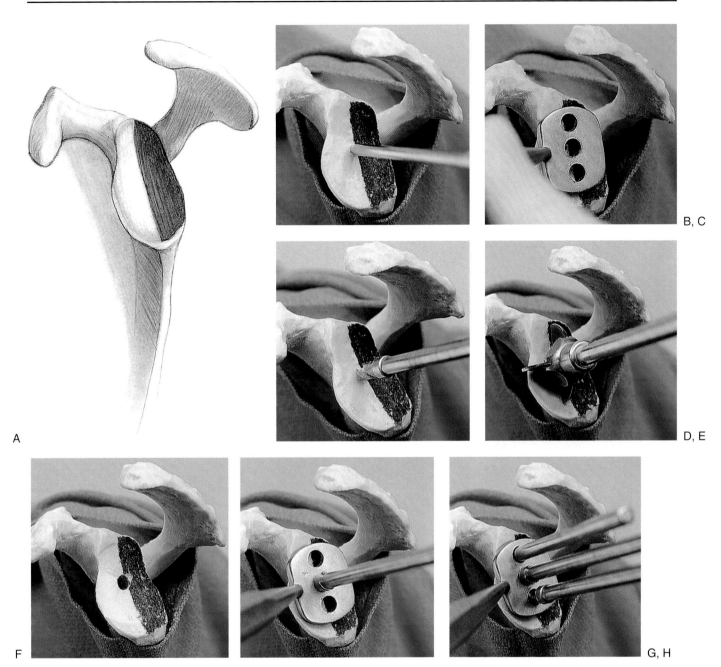

Figure 29-17. A–T: Asymmetric glenoid wear with posterior glenoid deficiency of 3 to 5 mm or greater. Reconstruction with structural bone grafting. **A:** Bone model illustrates in blue the area of glenoid wear on the posterior aspect of the glenoid surface and glenoid neck. The depth of the wear is to 5 mm. **B:** The central point of the normal glenoid is defined. **C:** A template is positioned to confirm the correct location of the central point. **D:** A drill is placed in the central hole and oriented perpendicular to the normal remaining anterior portion of the glenoid subchondral plate. **E:** A facing reamer is used to reshape the remaining anterior portion of the subchondral plate. **F:** This illustration shows the reshaped anterior portion of the subchondral plate. This shape now matches the undersurface of the glenoid component. Note that the blue area of bone deficiency has not been altered by use of the reamer. **G:** Glenoid template is reapplied, and the centering hole is deepened. **H:** Peripheral columns for the glenoid component are reconstructed in the central aspect of the glenoid neck. *(continued)*

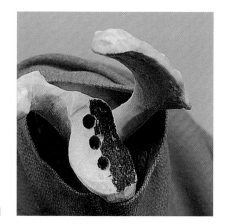

I

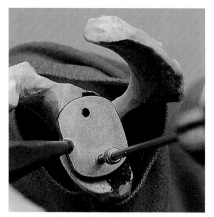

J

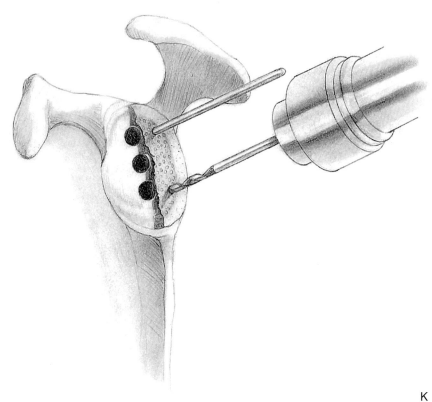

K

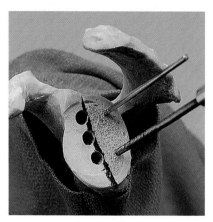

L

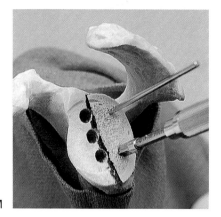

M

Figure 29-17. *Continued.* **I:** The three column holes have been prepared. **J:** The second template is applied to deepen the peripheral columns to allow subsequent seating of the cortical screws. **K:** The area of glenoid deficiency has been freshened to healthy, bleeding bone, and a bone graft contoured from the osteotomized portion of the humeral head has been placed in the defect. It is held in position with drills. In this situation, the drills for the 3.5-mm cortical screws have been used. **L:** The lower drill has been removed. A depth gauge has been inserted to determine the length of the screw. A tap is used to prepare the screw hole. **M:** A countersink may be used carefully to insert the screw heads. *(continued)*

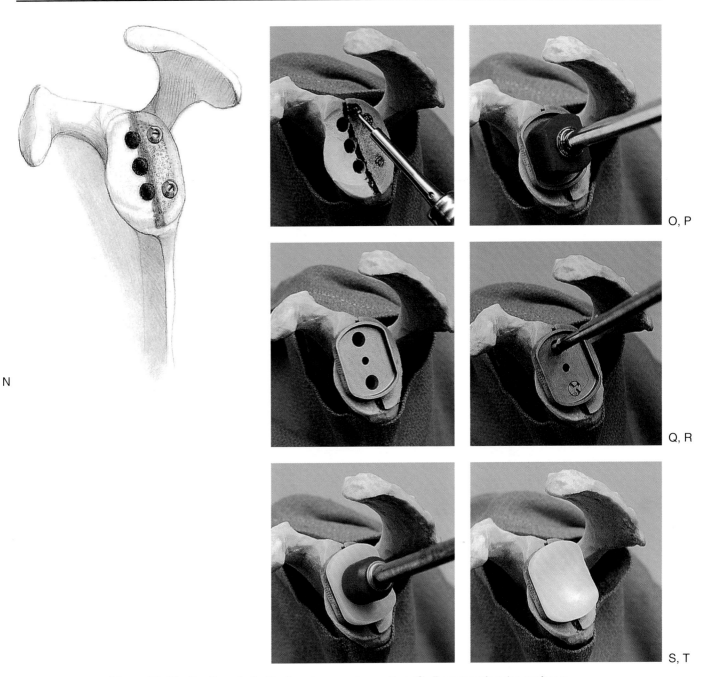

N

O, P

Q, R

S, T

Figure 29-17. *Continued.* **N:** Graft and screws in position. **O:** Recontouring the graft surface to match the previously prepared anterior portion of the glenoid. It may be necessary to grind the screw heads slightly so that they fit accurately into the contour. **P:** The tissue-ingrowth component is impacted into position. **Q:** The component is now in position and faces in the normal direction of the glenoid articular surface. **R:** The cortical screws are placed to hold the component firmly against the prepared glenoid surface and the bone graft. **S:** The polyethylene is impacted into position. **T:** The component in place. This sequence illustrates the use of a tissue-ingrowth glenoid component. It is also possible, in a similar fashion, to place a cemented glenoid component.

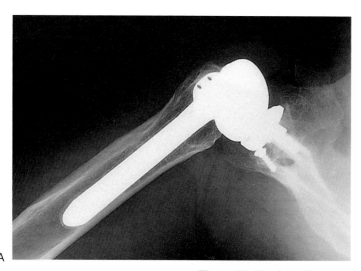

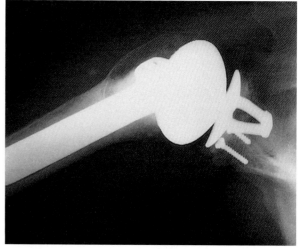

Figure 29-18. **A:** Axillary view of a tissue-ingrowth component that has been positioned as illustrated in Fig. 29-17. **B:** Axillary view of a cemented glenoid component positioned on a bone graft prepared as illustrated in Fig. 29-17.

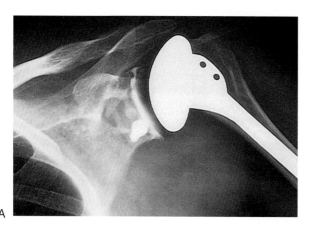

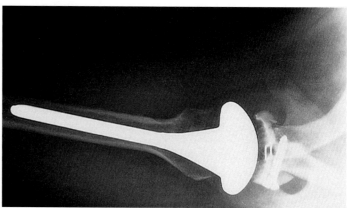

Figure 29-19. Total shoulder arthroplasty for a patient with posterior glenoid rim fracture, posterior shoulder subluxation, and subsequent development of traumatic arthritis. Approximately one third of the glenoid surface had been involved by the fracture and the subsequent glenoid wear. This was constructed with an anterior iliac crest bone graft at the time of total shoulder arthroplasty. The humeral head graft was too soft to use in this fashion. **A:** Anteroposterior view of the total shoulder arthroplasty. **B:** Axillary view showing the iliac crest bone graft screwed in position and the total shoulder arthroplasty cemented in place. Note that there is no tendency for posterior shoulder subluxation.

through the usual incision, but fixation will need to be accomplished through a second posterior incision. If the posterior defect is large, one may, in fact, have to do two fully separate approaches. As in the sequence performed for a bone graft placed on the face of the glenoid surface, this author prefers to prepare the glenoid surface and the keel or columns first and then add the bone graft to the prepared glenoid. By doing this, one can be more accurate in placing the fixation devices so that they will not inadvertently prevent seating of the glenoid component.

Humeral Bone Deficiencies

The most typical humeral deficiency involves the metaphyseal area (Table 29-3). Often, the bone below the resected portion of the humeral head is very osteopenic and may crush during surgical preparation, or there may be large cysts in the humeral head that create the defects. These crushed areas or cysts can be grafted (Fig. 29-20), or they can be filled with

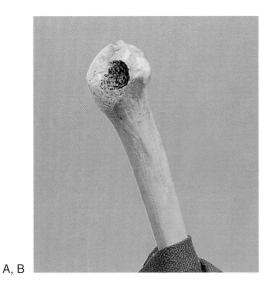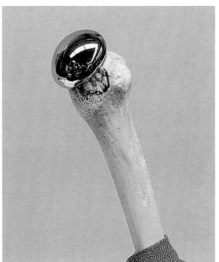

A, B

Figure 29-20. Reconstruction of humeral metaphyseal deficiency with bone graft. **A:** A humeral metaphyseal deficiency is outlined in blue. This may be the result of soft bone that crushes during the procedure or it may be present because of a large periarticular bone cyst. **B:** The deficiency has been corrected by packing bone graft in the deficiency and then seating the humeral component on top of the bone graft, further impacting it into position.

Table 29-3. *Reconstruction of humeral deficiencies*

Focal bone graft
Focal bone cement
Nonaxial component placement
Tuberosity osteotomy, repositioning, bone grafting
Long-stem implant with bone grafting
Long-stem implant with segmental allograft
Custom implant

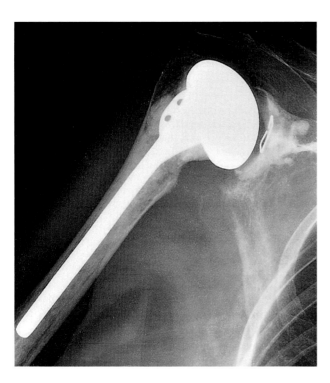

Figure 29-21. Previous resection arthroplasty of the humeral head for treatment of a malunited proximal humeral fracture. This has been reconstructed with a total shoulder arthroplasty. There was a large medial humeral metaphyseal defect that was eliminated with the use of bone cement.

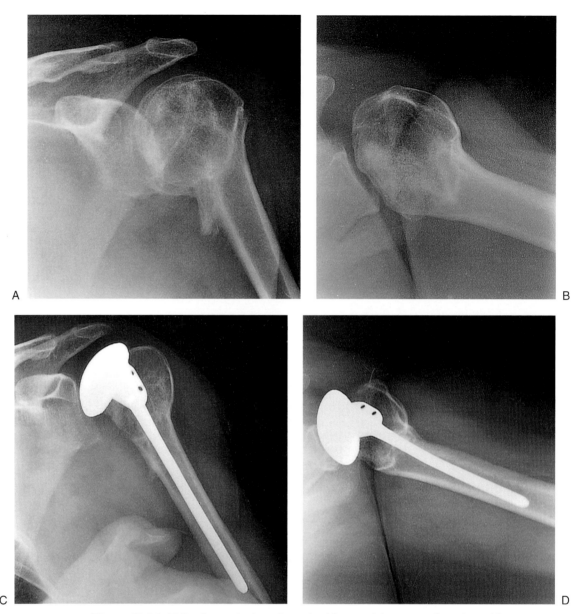

Figure 29-22. Following malunion of proximal humeral fractures, the tuberosities may remain in reasonable position relative to the head but may be malunited relative to the shaft. Reconstruction can be accomplished in a number of ways. One option is nonlinear placement of the humeral implant. **A,B:** Radiographs of a malunited humeral fracture with traumatic arthritis. The tuberosities are in near-normal position relative to the humeral head, but the head and tuberosities are malpositioned relative to the humeral shaft. **C,D:** Radiographs following prosthetic arthroplasty show nonaxial alignment of the humeral prosthesis. A three-point fit is illustrated with the prosthesis seated in normal anatomic position relative to the remaining humeral head and the tuberosities, but angulated relative to the humeral shaft. If fixation is not absolutely secure, it should be supplemented with bone cement.

cement. Both methods are appropriate. When stability can be achieved with local cancellous bone grafting, this is preferable; when it cannot, the addition of cement to the defect is quite reasonable (Fig. 29-21).

Special situations arise in the presence of old proximal humeral fractures. A fracture between the humeral head and the shaft of the humerus may have healed in such a way that the humeral head no longer sits on top of the humeral shaft but is offset. If this offset is minor, it might be addressable by asymmetric positioning of the humeral component (Fig. 29-22); if security is not obtained with press-fitting, fixation of the humeral component is supplemented with methylmethacrylate. If the degree of offset is more than can be tolerated with offsetting the humeral component, an osteotomy between the humeral head and the shaft may be necessary to reposition the humeral head on the shaft. The two fragments are then secured with the humeral prosthesis and additional tension-band suturing with heavy suture material, wire, or cable.

Tuberosity malposition is best addressed by adjusting the position of the humeral head and stem to match the malunion—if at all possible (Fig. 29-22). If tuberosity osteotomy is required, the osteotomy is often uniplanar if it involves the lesser tuberosity and bi- or triplanar if it involves the greater tuberosity. The tuberosities are fixed behind the implant and to the shaft of the humerus in the usual fashion. Additional bone graft should be used to

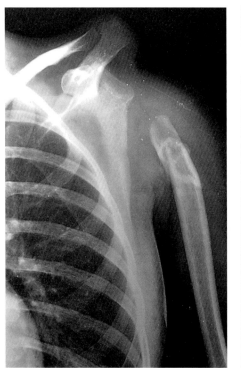

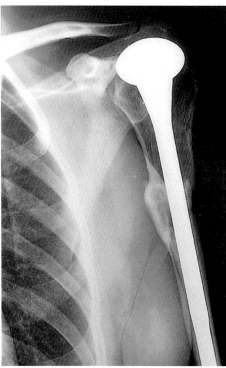

A   B

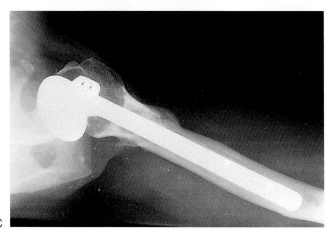

C

Figure 29-23. A: Substantial proximal humeral bone deficiency following shotgun wound and débridement. No neural injury was present. **B,C:** Radiographs following reconstruction using the long-stem humeral head prosthesis over which was placed a segmental allograft with rotator cuff attachments. These attachments were then sutured to the remaining rotator cuff. Bone healing has occurred at the allograft-humerus junction; only minor shoulder subluxation is present.

promote tuberosity-to-shaft healing. Also, if there is a bone deficiency of the tuberosity, it is best to add autogenous bone graft to the deficient area and secure the rotator cuff and any remaining tuberosity to the bone graft and to the prosthesis.

When there is a large deficiency of the proximal humerus, such as after a shotgun wound or resection for neoplasm, one must adopt the techniques used by oncology surgeons. Some orthopaedic oncologists would prefer to use only allografts for reconstruction of these deficiencies (5). Many others would consider allografts placed over long-stem humeral head prostheses (Fig. 29-23). Others would consider the use of a long-stem humeral head prosthesis surrounded by autogenous and allograft bone with the rotator cuff sutured to these bone grafts and to the prosthesis (Fig. 29-24). Finally, in extensive deficiencies, one might consider the use of a custom prosthesis. Some of these have included a fiber-metal covering to allow adherence of the soft tissues and bone to the implant (Fig. 29-25). When an implant such as this is used, a massive amount of autogenous and allograft bone is added around the implant. In almost all cases, the long-stem implant is fixed to the lower end of the humerus with methylmethacrylate bone cement.

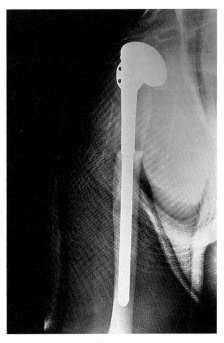

Figure 29-24. Reconstruction of a humeral deficiency, similar to that illustrated in Fig. 29-23, using a long-stem humeral head prosthesis. In this circumstance, autogenous iliac crest graft was utilized. This is best seen medially but is also present circumferentially around the implant. The rotator cuff is sutured to the bone graft and to the prosthesis. Here, the reconstruction was supported with a shoulder spica cast.

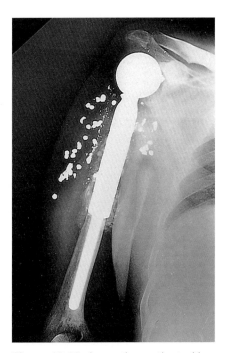

Figure 29-25. In another patient with a shotgun injury, the proximal humerus was destroyed and largely removed in sequential débridements. As was the case in the patient illustrated in Fig. 29-23, the neural structures were intact. Reconstruction in this situation was accomplished by the use of a custom prosthesis. The distal aspect of the prosthesis was cemented into the remaining humerus. The central portion of the prosthesis has a fiber-metal coating and was surrounded with bone graft material. The proximal portion of the prosthesis has a bipolar attachment for tensioning the scar surrounding the glenoid.

POSTOPERATIVE MANAGEMENT

In many situations involving glenoid bone deficiency, the postoperative management is the same as that for total joint shoulder arthroplasty in the absence of glenoid bone deficiencies. Early passive motion minimizes the likelihood of adhesions, and maximizes the chance that motion will be restored. The patient begins on passive forward flexion, external rotation, and internal rotation within 24 hours after surgery. Whether the patient can progress to an assistive program of rehabilitation with use of an overhead pulley depends largely on the patient's ability to safely perform these exercises, the security of the soft-tissue repair, and the stability of the implant itself.

Rehabilitation might be altered in those patients who have significant posterior glenoid erosion. In some instances, posterior glenoid erosion leads to a subluxation of the humeral head posteriorly with attendant stretching of the posterior capsular structures. In this situation there may be a tendency for the prosthesis to have an element of posterior instability when tested intraoperatively. Many intraoperative techniques can be utilized to augment the stability of the implant. However, if there is an element of posterior instability, avoiding those exercises that place strain on the posterior structures in the early postoperative period is probably wise. For instance, a patient may be instructed to use the overhead pulley in the plane of the scapula rather than in a straight anteroposterior plane, and the therapist providing passive forward elevation will perform this movement in the plane of the scapula rather than in the frontal plane. The proper early postoperative exercises should be determined by the surgeon on the basis of the position of implant stability and the adequacy of bony and soft-tissue reconstruction. After placement of a substantial glenoid bone graft, it might be prudent not to progress past the active-assisted motion routine until bone-graft healing is apparent radiographically. This may require a passive motion program for 4 to 6 weeks and then an active-assisted program without strengthening for another 2 to 4 months.

Postoperative management is significantly different in the presence of humeral bone deficiencies that involve the tuberosities or the proximal humeral shaft. In these cases, rotator cuff healing must occur to autogenous bone graft or allograft and will be quite prolonged. The active-assisted motion program might be maintained for 3 to 4 months or longer before considering active motion and certainly before considering muscle strengthening.

RESULTS

In a general sense, there are four situations to consider. The first is when the glenoid deficiency is too large to consider placing the glenoid component. This may be seen in primary cases, particularly rheumatoid arthritis where there is substantial central erosion. It is also seen in revision surgery when a loosened glenoid component and cement is removed along with the underlying histiocytic tissue. There is usually a large central cavity sometimes with peripheral wall deficiencies. In this latter situation allograft bone chips are packed into the deficiency to correct it and in both these situations, a hemiarthroplasty is then used. The results are parallel those of hemiarthroplasty in general for arthritic conditions. Approximately eight of ten people have satisfactory pain relief, and average active movement approximates two-thirds normal.

The second situation is when there is a segmental glenoid deficiency and a bone graft is placed usually along the posterior margin of the glenoid and a glenoid component is then applied over the graft and fixed to host bone. When glenoid fixation is secure, one can expect a result nearly equivalent to the result attained for those individuals without glenoid deficiencies. One might anticipate that the frequency of glenoid loosening would be slightly greater. This is not yet well defined in my patients or in the literature. The third situation, which is becoming all too common, is when there is humeral greater tuberosity deficiency. This often occurs following a complex proximal humeral fracture and use of a humeral head component. The tuberosities then resorb and do not heal, thus creating essentially a large rotator cuff tear. If revision surgery is necessary, I use autogenous posterior iliac crest bone graft to replace tuberosity deficiencies that have rerepaired the rotator cuff to the proximal humerus, the added bone graft, and the humeral prosthesis. In this setting, pain relief is anticipated to occur in better than nine of ten patients but active motion is seldom greater than one half of normal. In the fourth situation, there is a large amount of segmental proximal humeral bone loss. This can occur from shotgun wounds, neoplasia, or extensive osteolysis often associated with metallic synovitis related to titanium implants. This situation is clearly one of limited goals, trying to attain stability of the upper humerus and perhaps one third of active shoulder movement. It has been my experience that stability in nonneoplastic cases can be obtained in about two of three or three of four patients.

Several series are beginning to appear in the literature detailing the outcome for bone grafting for glenoid deficiency in total shoulder arthroplasty. Neer and Morrison (8) reported on 19 shoulders with an average follow-up of 53 months. When applying a rating system, there were 16 excellent results and one satisfactory result. Two shoulders were placed in a limited-goals category. The grafts were believed to have healed. No revision surgery was necessary. Incomplete lucent lines less than 1 mm wide were present in six cases. Hill and Norris (7) evaluated 17 shoulders with similar surgical treatment. The results were somewhat different. The authors reported detailed ratings of three excellent results, six satisfactory results, and eight unsatisfactory results. They report that the graft failed to maintain original correction in three shoulders. Five shoulders required revision surgery for persistent instability in two, rotator cuff tearing in one, improper component placement in one, and loss of graft fixation in one.

Steinmann and Cofield (10) reported on 28 shoulders having glenoid bone grafting for segmental glenoid wear as a part of total shoulder replacement. The average follow-up evaluation was slightly longer than 5 years. Autogenous humeral head grafts were used in 27 and 3.5-mm screws were generally used for fixation. Twenty-five patients had no or only slight pain. Postoperative active motion approximated two thirds of normal. When applying the same rating as Neer and Morrison (8) and Hill and Norris (7), 13 shoulders were excellent, ten were satisfactory, and five were unsatisfactory. The unsatisfactory shoulders were the result of symptomatic glenoid loosening in two, instability in two, and persistent unexplained pain in one. Three shoulders had complete lucencies at least 1.5 mm wide. These glenoids were considered loose and two, as mentioned above, were symptomatic. Thus, considering these three studies, if one can avoid other complications, bone grafting for the glenoid is usually effective but there is concern about the durability of the reconstruction given some of these radiographic changes.

In a related paper published by Antuna et al. (1) on glenoid revision surgery after total shoulder arthroplasty, 30 shoulders could undergo reimplantation of a new glenoid component but in 18, there was substantial glenoid bone deficiency. These patients underwent component removal and bone grafting for these bone deficiencies. In both groups, there was significant pain relief, improvement in active elevation and external rotation, and satisfaction with revision surgery. However, satisfactory pain relief was achieved in 86% of patients with a new glenoid and in 66% of patients who underwent glenoid component removal and bone grafting. As might be expected, the patients with the large glenoid deficiencies and bone grafting were less satisfied with the procedure than those patients who could have reimplantation of a new glenoid component. At an average 5 years of follow-up, revision surgery was necessary in two shoulders with a new glenoid component because of glenoid loosening and in three shoulders with bone grafting alone for the treatment of painful glenoid arthritis. Thus, the data from this study suggest that at the time of revision surgery if one can securely place the new glenoid component, the outcome will be somewhat better, but bone grafting these large deficiencies is also a satisfactory treatment option.

COMPLICATIONS

The complications that develop following total shoulder arthroplasty in the presence of bone deficiency are similar to those that occur in patients without bone deficiency, but some are slightly more common. The most notable complication is instability. If the bony deficiency is not appropriately addressed, instability can occur posteriorly, inferiorly, or in any other direction. This is often associated with stretching or partial disruption of the rotator cuff repair, because the repair is not adequately supported by a balanced placement of the components.

The frequency of glenoid component loosening when there was bone deficiency is undoubtedly somewhat greater than when components are placed in bone of ample quantity and quality. When a glenoid bone graft is placed, we can anticipate early healing to the host bone, and we can anticipate that the bone graft will probably remain in position for a period of years. Whether the bone graft becomes incorporated without collapsing or collapses at a later date is not yet understood. The frequency of problems following glenoid bone grafting is unknown, but at this point, it is assumed to be rather low.

When humeral bone deficiency involves the metaphyseal area, usually one would not anticipate any significant complication. If the bone of the humerus is distorted or deficient, the landmarks that allow accurate positioning of the component might not be available. Therefore, some component subluxation associated with stretching of the rotator cuff or capsule repair might occur. The largest problem occurs when the humeral deficiencies involve the tuberosities or a large segment of the proximal humerus. In this case, the rotator cuff attachments are compromised, and their healing is often delayed and weaker than usual. Subsequent stretching of the tissues may occur, resulting in less ample active movement or delayed joint subluxation.

RECOMMENDED READING

1. Antuna, S.A., Sperling, J.W., Cofield, R.H., et al.: Glenoid revision surgery after total shoulder arthroplasty. *J Shoulder Elbow Surg* 10(3): 217–224, 2001.
2. Boyd, A.D. Jr., Thomas, W.H., Scott, R.D., et al.: Total shoulder arthroplasty versus hemiarthroplasty: indications for glenoid resurfacing. *J Arthroplasty* 5(4): 329–336, 1990.
3. Cofield, R.H.: Degenerative and arthritic problems of the glenohumeral joint. In: Rockwood, C.A., Matsen, F.A. III, eds.: *The shoulder.* Philadelphia: WB Saunders, 678–749, 1990.
4. Cofield, R.H.: Integral surgical maneuvers in prosthetic shoulder arthroplasty. *Semin. Arthroplasty* 1(2): 112–123, 1990.
5. Gebhardt, M.C., Roth, Y.F., Mankin, H.J.: Osteoarticular allografts for reconstruction in the proximal part of the humerus after excision of a musculoskeletal tumor. *J Bone Joint Surg* 72(3): 334–345, 1990.
6. Henry, A.K.: *Extensile exposure,* 2nd ed. London: Churchill Livingstone, 25–37, 1970.
7. Hill, J.M., Norris, T.R.: Long-term results of total shoulder arthroplasty following bone-grafting of the glenoid. *J Bone Joint Surg Am* 73A: 877–883, 2001.
8. Neer, C.S. III, Morrison, D.S.: Glenoid bone grafting in total shoulder arthroplasty. *J Bone Joint Surg* 70(3): 1154–1162, 1988.
9. Neer, C.S. III, Watson, K.C., Stanton, F.J.: Recent experience in total shoulder replacement. *J Bone Joint Surg* 68: 319–337, 1982.
10. Steinmann, S.P., Cofield, R.H.: Bone grafting for glenoid deficiency in total shoulder replacement. *J Shoulder Elbow Surg* 9(5): 361–367, 2000.

30

Total Shoulder Replacement: Managing Soft-tissue Deficiencies

Robert J. Nowinski and Wayne Z. Burkhead, Jr.

INDICATIONS/CONTRAINDICATIONS

Management of the soft-tissue–deficient arthritic shoulder can present a formidable challenge to the operating surgeon. While preoperative planning is important, oftentimes the surgeon must rely on intraoperative decision making. Soft-tissue deficiencies encountered during shoulder arthroplasty can involve the capsule and the supraspinatus, infraspinatus, teres minor, and subscapularis tendons, or the deltoid muscle. The surgeon must therefore be equipped with an armamentarium of reconstructive options before embarking on surgery on these complex disorders. Because soft-tissue reconstruction can make the procedure more difficult, indications for total shoulder arthroplasty must be precise to prevent an unsatisfactory surgical outcome. Otherwise, other surgical options, such as hemiarthroplasty, may provide more reliable outcomes.

The most common soft-tissue defect likely to be encountered during shoulder arthroplasty is rotator cuff deficiency. Because the rotator cuff is responsible for a number of important tasks, including dynamic glenohumeral stability, humeral head depression, and secondary power for moving the arm, all reparable full-thickness rotator cuff tears encountered at the time of shoulder arthroplasty should be repaired. The cuff-deficient shoulder can be encountered with several arthritic conditions of the glenohumeral joint, including rotator cuff-tear arthropathy, rheumatoid arthritis, and degenerative osteoarthritis. Assigning them to one of these three diagnostic categories can facilitate surgical management of a rotator cuff–deficient arthritic shoulder.

The main indication for surgical management is unremitting pain that has proved resistant to a trial of nonoperative measures. These include rest, oral analgesics, nonsteroidal an-

R. J. Nowinski, D.O.: Ohio University College of Osteopathic Medicine, Athens; and Orthopaedic Specialists & Sports Medicine, Inc., Newark, Ohio.

W. Z. Burkhead, Jr., M.D.: Department of Orthopaedics, University of Texas Southwestern Medical School, W.B. Carrell Memorial Clinic; and Baylor University Medical Center, Dallas, Texas.

tiinflammatory medications, corticosteroid injections, fluid aspirations, and gentle range-of-motion exercises. Additional considerations, such as patient age, activity level, job requirements, and general health, are extremely important in individualizing a treatment plan. The integrity of the contralateral rotator cuff should also be assessed, as this may be important in planning postoperative rehabilitation. Patients who use canes or who are confined to wheelchairs may, during the first few postoperative months, apply increased stresses to the contralateral shoulder. A course of preoperative stretching before prosthetic arthroplasty may improve postoperative function (12).

Multiple surgical options exist for the arthritic, rotator cuff–deficient shoulder, including arthrodesis, resection arthroplasty, constrained arthroplasty, bipolar arthroplasty, nonconstrained total shoulder arthroplasty, humeral hemiarthroplasty, and more recently, reverse ball-and-socket designs. The decision to proceed with nonconstrained total shoulder arthroplasty for rotator cuff deficiency is based on several factors. First and foremost, the rotator cuff defect must be a repairable lesion. An intact, functional rotator cuff has been shown to reduce eccentric glenoid loading by centering the humeral head on the glenoid during dynamic shoulder motion. This is a mandatory requirement for glenoid resurfacing because the amount of superior migration of the humeral component directly correlates with the degree of glenoid loosening. Therefore, every attempt should be made to repair the rotator cuff.

Next, the glenoid must demonstrate significant degenerative changes to indicate polyethylene resurfacing. Total shoulder arthroplasty has been shown to provide superior pain relief compared with hemiarthroplasty for patients with glenohumeral osteoarthritis; however, absolute indications for glenoid replacement are still evolving. Severe glenoid bone loss in osteopenic patients may contraindicate the use of a cemented glenoid component (Fig. 30-1). This may be particularly pronounced in the rheumatoid patient with severe disease and extensive erosion of the glenoid. Biologic resurfacing of the glenoid may provide a better option for these patients and for young patients with severe degenerative changes of the glenoid.

Specific contraindications to surgery also include neurologic conditions resulting in severe weakness of the deltoid and rotator cuff, motion disorders that would preclude rotator cuff healing, and an irreparable detachment or denervation of the anterior deltoid. Even if the cuff defect is repairable or reconstructable, attempts at restoring motion and balancing forces coupled with prosthetic replacement and soft-tissue reconstruction are fruitless if the anterior deltoid is nonfunctional.

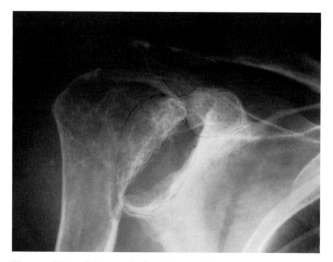

Figure 30-1. Advanced glenohumeral arthritis with soft-tissue deficiency, as seen in this radiograph of a rheumatoid shoulder, demonstrates extensive glenoid erosion. Total shoulder arthroplasty is contraindicated under this circumstance due to loss of glenoid bone stock.

PREOPERATIVE PLANNING

The preoperative planning stage begins with a detailed history and physical examination. Patients with cuff-deficient arthritic shoulders are typically elderly (seventh decade or older) and female. Most commonly, it is the dominant extremity that is involved. Patients usually present with a long history of progressively increasing pain that is worse at night and is intensified by glenohumeral motion. They will also report loss of active shoulder motion.

Rotator cuff–deficient arthritic shoulders can be diagnostically categorized into those with rotator cuff-tear arthropathy, degenerative arthritis (osteoarthritis) with cuff deficiency, or rheumatoid arthritis with cuff deficiency. Categorization is based on specific clinical, radiographic, and laboratory findings. These designations help the surgeon anticipate the quality of the tissues, the natural history of the disease, and the ultimate surgical outcome.

Patients with osteoarthritis and rotator cuff tears often relate a history of progressive pain and stiffness. It is not uncommon for these patients to relate an acute traumatic event followed by increased shoulder weakness and symptoms. Patients with rotator cuff tears and rheumatoid arthritis generally have a long history of polyarthritis and medical treatment for their systemic disease. They may have pain in other joints of the hands, wrists, elbows, hips, or knees. Patients with either rheumatoid arthritis or osteoarthritis can have mild swelling, but this is usually synovial-tissue thickening rather than fluid that can be aspirated. These patients may also have physical findings involving other joints, such as deformity, contractures, or instability.

In patients with rotator cuff-tear arthropathy, atrophy of the supraspinatus and infraspinatus muscles and weakness of external rotation and abduction are typical physical examination findings. Active and passive attempts to move the shoulder through a functional range of motion are limited by weakness, pain, and stiffness. This is most apparent in external rotation and abduction. A rupture of the biceps tendon may be detected. A large shoulder swelling, or "fluid sign," which results from chronic, excessive fluid pressure in the subacromial bursa, may also be present (Fig. 30-2). This excessive subacromial pressure can lead to concomitant perforation of the acromioclavicular joint (Fig. 30-3). Aspiration of the fluid, which may be bloody or blood-streaked, followed by cortisone injection,

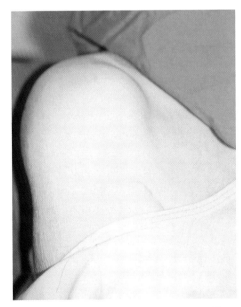

Figure 30-2. A subacromial hygroma, illustrating the fluid sign of communication between the glenohumeral joint and subacromial and subdeltoid bursa in an elderly patient with cuff-tear arthropathy.

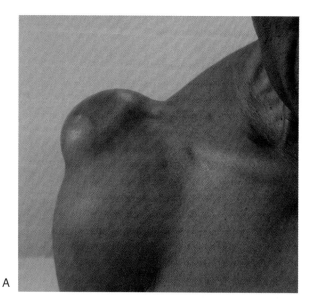
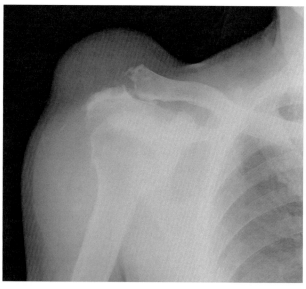

A   B

Figure 30-3. A: Excessive subacromial fluid pressure in severe cuff-tear arthropathy can create a one-way valve in a degenerative acromioclavicular joint, thereby leading to overlying cyst formation. **B:** Radiograph demonstrates the radiographic appearance of this patient with severe cuff-tear arthropathy and degenerative acromioclavicular joint pathology.

is an excellent temporizing measure that can be attempted to avoid surgery. Recurrence after aspiration, however, is common.

The preoperative integrity of the subscapularis muscle is very important because the tendon can be transferred superiorly to close supraspinatus defects. Physical examination, including the subscapularis lift-off test and belly-press test, provides assessment of subscapularis muscle function. An increased amount of passive external rotation compared to a normal contralateral side can also indicate deficiency of this tendon. Insufficiency of this tendon may indicate the need for direct repair versus pectoralis major transfer during arthroplasty.

Our standard radiographic evaluation of the arthritic shoulder is a three-view series, including anteroposterior (AP) views in internal and external rotation and an axillary view. For patients with a prior surgical procedure, we add an AP view in neutral rotation and a scapular Y-view. Radiographs of osteoarthritic shoulders typically show subchondral sclerosis and cyst formation, humeral head and glenoid osteophytes, and posterior erosion of the glenoid. In contrast to rheumatoid arthritis and cuff-tear arthropathy, osteopenia is not characteristic of conventional osteoarthritis. Relatively symmetric juxtaarticular erosion and minimal subchondral sclerosis and osteophyte formation characterize rheumatoid shoulders. Rotator cuff-tear arthropathy findings include humeral head collapse, periarticular osteopenia, reduced acromiohumeral distance, and erosions of the glenoid, acromion, and acromioclavicular joints (Fig. 30-4). Erosion of the proximal humerus may be so extensive that the humeral head is worn beyond the surgical neck. Axillary lateral views can reveal a fixed anterior or posterior glenohumeral dislocation.

The differential diagnosis must always be considered in the evaluation of an arthritic shoulder with suspected cuff deficiency. The radiographic appearance of the glenohumeral joint with metabolic arthritis, such as gout, pseudogout, or hemochromatosis, can resemble that of osteoarthritis. The rotator cuff, however, is typically intact with metabolic arthritis. In some advanced cases, the radiographic findings can be similar to those seen with advanced rotator cuff arthropathy. Blood and joint-fluid chemistries and synovial biopsy can help confirm a diagnosis of gout, pseudogout, hemochromatosis, and other types of metabolic arthritis. Patients with Charcot (neuropathic) joints and osteonecrosis usually have intact rotator cuffs. Clinical workup typically reveals the underlying cause, such as corticosteroid use, alcohol abuse, tabes dorsalis, or syringomyelia. Radiographs of the shoulders of patients with advanced hemophilic arthropathy may also resemble those of patients with rheumatoid arthritis or, less commonly, osteoarthritis. Finally, patients with septic arthritis are often debilitated due to a generalized disease process such as rheumatoid arthritis.

Although magnetic resonance imaging (MRI) is not necessary for the routine workup of patients with straightforward osteoarthritis and obvious clinical and radiologic findings indicative of a full-thickness rotator cuff tear, it is helpful in patients with physical findings that are difficult to interpret. These include those patients who cannot do a lift-off or belly-press test because of pain and motion loss and for whom preoperative determination of the subscapularis tendon integrity is required. Because cuff tears may have unexpected configuration and sizes and the cuff tissue may be of poor quality, the surgeon must be prepared to use alternative methods in reconstruction or repair. These can include autografts, allografts, or tendon transfers. These intraoperative decisions are facilitated by preoperative knowledge gained with MRI.

Although not routinely obtained, a preoperative computed tomography (CT) scan of both shoulders can be useful for comparing glenoid version in some patients. This may be particularly helpful for the evaluation of posterior glenoid erosion and subluxation of the humeral head that can occur with severe end-stage osteoarthritis. In severe rheumatoid arthritis and cuff-tear arthropathy with extensive glenoid erosion, CT scanning is used for

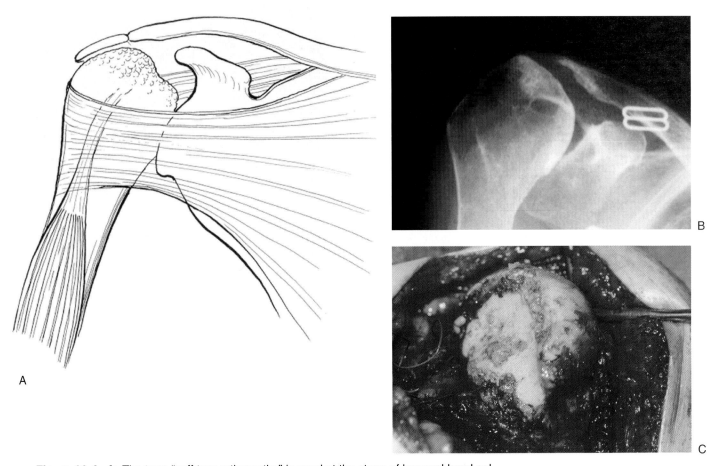

Figure 30-4. A: The term "cuff tear arthropathy" is used at the stage of humeral head collapse. The glenohumeral joint becomes eroded by the incongruous and unstable humeral head, and eventually the coracoid is eroded. Advanced changes in subacromial impingement, which include erosion of the acromioclavicular joint within the anterior part of the acromion and outer aspect of the clavicle are shown. Radiographic **(B)** and intraoperative **(C)** appearance of advanced rotator cuff tear arthropathy. (Figure 4A from Cantrell, J.S., Itamura, J.M., Burkhead, W.Z.: Rotator cuff tear arthropathy. In: Warner, J.P., Iannotti, J.P., Gerber, C., eds.: *Complex and revision problems in shoulder surgery.* Philadelphia: Lippincott–Raven, 303–318, 1997.)

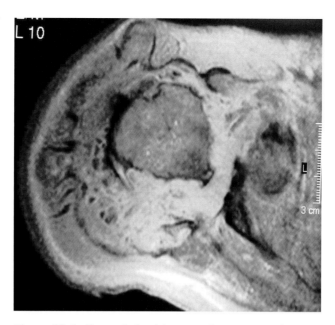

Figure 30-5. Computerized tomography or magnetic resonance imaging with certain sequencing can be extremely valuable for the evaluation of remaining glenoid bone stock as demonstrated by this scan of a rheumatoid shoulder.

evaluation of remaining glenoid bone stock (Fig. 30-5). Superior glenoid wear and cystic changes in the glenoid and humeral head can also be identified with CT scanning. The information gained helps the surgeon to anticipate both the location and the amount of bone augmentation or removal that may be needed.

CT arthrography is used for those patients who cannot undergo an MRI examination because of medical reasons. CT arthrography is also used for the evaluation of revision cases where previously placed metal suture anchors in the humeral head would produce too much scatter on MRI. In addition, this test is valuable during the assessment of the failed shoulder arthroplasty. Bundled software packages on most high-end CT scanners include programs that can digitally subtract the scatter produced by metal implants for better visualization of the soft tissues and for evaluation of humeral component retroversion. An aspiration of the glenohumeral synovial fluid is obtained prior to the arthrogram to rule out occult or low-grade infection.

Additional testing is occasionally required for those patients with a history of previous trauma or surgery with physical examination suggestive of muscle deficiency, such as the deltoid. Preoperative electromyography and nerve conduction testing are used to evaluate for deltoid muscle activity and axillary nerve function. Significant atrophy in the supraspinatus or infraspinatus fossa should also be evaluated, especially if plain film evaluation does not suggest rotator cuff-tear arthropathy. Such atrophy can be related to chronic rotator cuff tears, dysfunction of the suprascapular nerve, or possibly chronic disuse.

Before arthroplasty, preoperative radiographs are used for templating the humerus and glenoid. If severe deformity is present and the patient has unilateral disease, the noninvolved humerus should be used for templating. The AP view is used to check for depth of the glenoid vault and for superior/inferior glenoid bone stock. The axillary radiograph is reviewed for AP bone stock. In the osteoarthritic patient, careful note of posterior erosion must be made. If marked posterior erosion is present, alternatives include bone grafting, posteriorly versus removing bone selectively from the anterior surface.

SURGERY

The arthritic shoulder with soft-tissue deficiencies presents a formidable challenge for surgical reconstruction. Fortunately, only an estimated 4% of full-thickness rotator cuff tears

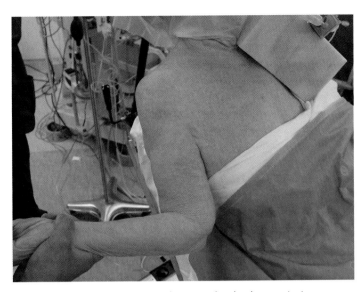

Figure 30-6. Examination under anesthesia demonstrates excessive external rotation consistent with subscapularis deficiency in this patient with arthritis and rotator cuff deficiency.

progress to cuff-tear arthropathy (9). Neer et al. (9) recognized three factors that need to be addressed by the treatment approach: (a) pain caused by incongruity of the glenohumeral joint, (b) subacromial impingement, and (c) massive rotator cuff tearing. Several options have been presented in the literature, including total shoulder replacement, humeral replacement alone (with various sizes of heads, with or without rotator cuff repair), reverse ball-and-socket arthroplasty, bipolar arthroplasty, arthrodesis, and superior reconstruction. This chapter will specifically focus on the techniques of soft-tissue management with hemiarthroplasty versus total shoulder arthroplasty.

Our standard technique for shoulder arthroplasty begins with endotracheal intubation. The patient is positioned in the beach-chair position, which involves flexion of the operating table, elevation of the back, and lowering of the legs. The patient is placed on a beanbag, which is inflated under the affected scapula to increase glenoid exposure. A Mayfield headrest is used for stabilization of the head and neck during surgery. The head is secured with a surgical towel and heavy tape around the forehead. The patient's body is brought as far laterally as possible on the operating table toward the side of the operated extremity. This allows extension of the shoulder and facilitates humeral shaft exposure and reaming. A 10-minute iodine prep with sterile orthopaedic draping technique is utilized. Unless contraindicated, a first-generation cephalosporin (Ancef, 1 g) is used as a preoperative prophylactic antibiotic.

Preoperative examination of range of motion under anesthesia is needed to determine the amount of fixed capsular and subscapular contracture. Frequently, external rotation is significantly improved while the patient is anesthetized, indicating no fixed contracture. Excessive external rotation, especially compared to the contra lateral side, typically indicated either partial or complete absence of the subscapularis tendon attachment (Fig. 30-6).

The standard deltopectoral approach is used for almost all arthroplasty cases (the Kessel approach and indications will be described later). The bony landmarks are palpated and the skin incision is drawn. The incision runs from the distal clavicle to the deltoid insertion centered over the coracoid process. The skin incision is then infiltrated with 0.125% bupivicaine with epinephrine for early hemostasis and postoperative pain relief. Once the skin incision is made, the fascia over the deltopectoral interval is identified. The areolar tissue obliquely between the muscle planes identifies the deltopectoral groove where the cephalic vein is located in most shoulders. Because of the need for proximal dissection, it is most often easier to take the cephalic vein medially with the pectoralis. Vascular clips are used for smaller lateral feeding vessels into the cephalic vein. Occasionally, the cephalic vein requires ligation, but this is not routinely recommended due to a noted increased incidence of postoperative swelling, pain, and phlebitis when the vein has to be ligated. Care must be exercised, especially with patients with rheumatoid arthritis, because the cephalic vein is quite fragile and can be lacerated by overzealous retraction.

Once deep to the deltopectoral interval, the upper 1 cm of the pectoralis major tendon can be incised to aid in the exposure. It is best to incise the pectoralis major tendon with cautery to avoid bleeding within the tendon. The clavipectoral fascia is incised and the conjoined tendon is visualized. After dissection on the lateral border of the conjoined tendon, the axillary nerve can be palpated in the quadrilateral space and the musculocutaneous nerve palpated on the undersurface of the coracobrachialis. Proximally, the coracoacromial ligament is preserved to prevent postoperative superior migration of the humeral head in patients with a massive cuff tear. If the ligament must be divided for visualization purposes, it is repaired at the completion of the case. Gentle retraction on the conjoined tendon is frequently enough to facilitate exposure of both the proximal humerus and glenoid. However, in patients with marked medial glenoid erosion, a portion of the conjoined tendon may be incised or the coracoid osteotomized. If the coracoid is osteotomized, the assistant holding retractors must be careful to avoid pulling too hard on the conjoined tendon and injuring the brachial plexus.

Frequently, especially in old trauma and severe arthritis, the anatomy is quite distorted. The biceps tendon is frequently dislocated or ruptured in the arthritic cuff–deficient shoulder. However, when the biceps tendon is present in its groove, it serves as an excellent landmark. It can then be traced toward the proximal humerus, where dissection of the biceps tendon is carried up through the rotator interval, defining the soft spot between the supraspinatus and subscapularis. Opening the rotator interval is critical all the way to the glenoid rim.

The role of the biceps tendon in the shoulder, not only as a stabilizer to prevent superior humeral migration but also as a potential source of pain, remains controversial. In our practice, a biceps tenotomy is routinely performed at its attachment to the superior glenoid rim. The tendon is then tagged for tenodesis to surrounding soft tissue at the completion of the case. In the severely arthritic shoulder, the biceps tendon, when present, is often diseased. It will commonly lose any function as a head depressor prior to rupture and can act as a significant source of pain. Walch and associates (4) recently presented the results of a series of 259 total shoulder arthroplasties done for osteoarthritis in which tenodesis of the long head of the biceps tendon was performed in 30% of patients. The patients who underwent a tenodesis reported significantly better pain relief than did those in whom the biceps was left intact. No complications were associated with the tenodesis. Moreover, Murthi et al. (7) showed histologically that glenohumeral arthroses are associated with biceps disease.

Intact Subscapularis with Deficient Supraspinatus/Infraspinatus

Although many patients with an intact subscapularis have a negative lift-off test, they may have marked weakness with active forward flexion and external rotation. For these patients, a standard deltopectoral approach is appropriate. Once the bicipital groove has been identified, the subscapularis tendon is dissected sharply from the lesser tuberosity, beginning at the bicipital groove and taken medially. Subperiosteal dissection with the arm in maximum external rotation will protect the axillary nerve behind the elevated soft-tissue envelope. The proximal neck is exposed and cautery, ligatures, or vascular clamps are used to ligate the circumflex vessels as required. Careful subperiosteal dissection is required in this area to avoid injury to the axillary nerve. Tag sutures are placed in the subscapularis tendon at this point to assist with mobilization and prevent retraction. As an assistant externally rotates the humerus, the capsule is further incised and the humeral head is dislocated.

Lateral detachment of the subscapularis tendon will effectively maximize the tendon length for medial attachment to the osteotomy site. This technique of medialization can increase external rotation by 20 to 30 degrees, even in shoulders with severe internal rotation contractures. A Z-plasty lengthening of the subscapularis tendon and anterior capsule, although an option, is typically not required.

The humeral osteotomy is perhaps the most critical step in shoulder replacement. The average retroversion of the humeral head ranges from 28 degrees to 45 degrees, and therefore, version of the humeral component requires individualization to best restore the natural anatomy. Certain pathology requires additional alteration. In patients with posterior subluxation from osteoarthritis, less retroversion (< 35 degrees) may be appropriate to prevent postoperative posterior instability or dislocation. Conditions such as rheumatoid arthritis with a thin, functionless cuff or rotator cuff-tear arthropathy may require more retroversion (> 35 degrees) to center the humeral head under the acromion and to avoid postoperative anterosuperior instability.

An aggressive humeral osteotomy is performed for patients with an intact subscapularis and deficient supraspinatus/infraspinatus superior complex (Fig. 30-7). This will remove more bone than usual. The osteotomy follows a line extending laterally from approximately 1 cm above the lateral flare of the greater tuberosity to a point medially where, with firm manual downward traction on the arm, the humeral neck meets the inferior aspect of the glenoid. This satisfies three objectives: (a) it leaves an osseous margin to which the distal ends of the supraspinatus, infraspinatus, and subscapularis can be repaired; (b) it shortens the distance that the mobilized tendons must traverse; and (c) it centers the humeral head on the glenoid. Despite aggressive capsular releases inferiorly, the humeral head cannot be centered without this more aggressive bone resection.

At this point, the amount and quality of repairable rotator cuff tissue are assessed. In cases with retracted, inelastic musculotendinous units, extensive intraarticular and extraarticular releases are required to lateralize the tendon for repair into the greater tuberosity.

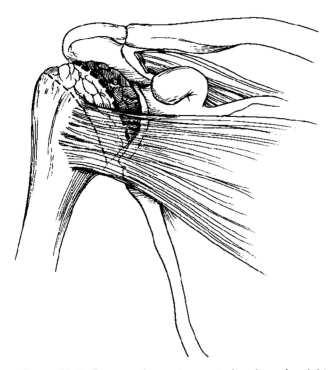

Figure 30-7. Preoperative anteroposterior view of a right shoulder with a cuff tear and severe glenohumeral arthrosis. The broken line drawn obliquely across the proximal humeral head represents the direction of an osteotomy performed when there is an intact rotator cuff. The dotted line drawn obliquely across the more distal humeral head represents the more aggressive osteotomy used when performing an arthroplasty in shoulders with large, retracted rotator cuff tears. (From Zeman, C.A., Arcand, M.A., Cantrell, J.S., et al.: The rotator cuff-deficient arthritic shoulder: diagnosis and surgical management. *J Am Acad Ortho Surg* 6(6): 337–348, 1998, with permission.)

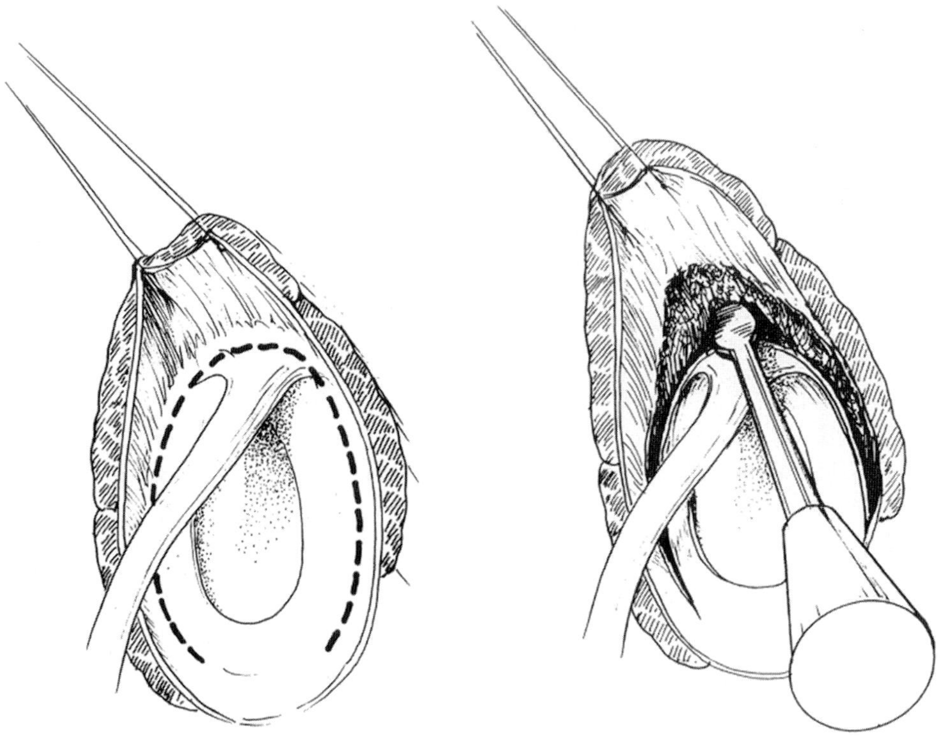

Figure 30-8. A: The technique of mobilization and repair of a retracted, chronic supraspinatus tendon tear begins with division of the coracohumeral ligament. The intraarticular release of the tendon is performed by dividing the labrum and the capsule, so that the labrum is left on the glenoid. **B:** Intraarticular mobilization of the rotator cuff is performed with a Cobb elevator or Darrach retractor, followed by release of the rotator interval tissue. (From Warner, J.J.P., Gerber, C.: Massive tears of the postero-superior rotator cuff. In: Warner, J.P., Iannotti, J.P., Gerber, C., eds.: *Complex and revision problems in shoulder surgery.* Philadelphia: Lippincott–Raven, 177–201.)

These mobilization techniques are similar to those used for repair of massive rotator cuff-tears without arthritis. All visualized bursal tissue is removed in order to release any adhesions and to define the true margins of the cuff tissue. The coracoacromial ligament is left intact to avoid progressive postoperative anterosuperior instability. If it must be divided for visualization, it is then repaired at the completion of the case. Tag sutures are next placed into the supraspinatus and infraspinatus tendons to assist with mobilization. The coraco-humeral ligament is then divided by pulling on the supraspinatus tendon sutures and cutting soft-tissue extensions to the base of the coracoid. If sufficient length is not obtained, the interval between the superior labrum and rotator cuff is sharply divided, thereby creating an intraarticular release of the tendon. Intraarticular mobilization of the cuff tendons can then be performed with a Cobb elevator carefully over the glenoid rim (Fig. 30-8).

At this junction, it must be determined whether to resurface the glenoid with a polyethylene component. This decision is made by several factors, including the degree of arthritic wear on the glenoid cartilage, but more important, by an assessment of the reparability of the superior supraspinatus tendon complex. The tag sutures in the supraspinatus tendon are pulled to the greater tuberosity, thereby distracting the tendon to its bony insertion. If an adequate supraspinatus repair with good quality tissue is achievable under little or no tension, then polyethylene glenoid resurfacing is indicated. If a tension-free repair is possible with the arm in slight abduction (< 45 degrees), an abduction pillow can be used postoperatively to protect the repair. Hemiarthroplasty is indicated when an adequate supraspinatus repair is impossible; therefore, preparation of the glenoid surface is required.

Adequate exposure of the glenoid is critical for proper glenoid preparation. It is important that a capsular-type retractor (Bankart) be used so that there is not a direct pull on the plexus, but merely a levering back on the conjoined tendon. Careful palpation along the rim of the glenoid and into the subscapularis recess will provide a feel for how much bone is left on the glenoid, as well as an idea of orientation. A glenoid retractor is inserted posterior to the glenoid rim, positioning the humerus posteriorly. A capsulotomy opening the subscapularis recess is performed (Fig. 30-9). The labrum is maintained if normal, otherwise it is removed.

When there is marked superior erosion of the glenoid, a burr is used to selectively remove bone from the inferior aspect of the glenoid until a superior shelf is created, thereby constructing a more concave surface for articulation with the humeral head. The combination of using a smaller humeral head combined with medialization of the joint line, lowering the instant center of rotation, and mobilization of the cuff increases the effective length of the subscapularis. These factors facilitate the superior transposition of the subscapularis for covering large defects in the retracted supraspinatus tendon at the completion of the case.

The humeral shaft is prepared by extending and externally rotating the shoulder, thereby bringing the cut surface of the humeral head into the wound for preparation of the medullary canal. A small Hohmann retractor is frequently helpful in retracting the remaining posterior rotator cuff tissue and levering the humerus out away from the deltopectoral incision. The canal can then be sounded with a curette or drill. Medullary reamers are utilized by hand to prepare the humeral shaft. Hand reaming is especially important in patients with rheumatoid arthritis and in patients with osteopenia to avoid distal perforation of the humeral shaft. A stepwise approach with the reamers is used, beginning with the smallest reamer and advancing in increments. Because most humeral stems in this patient population are cemented, aggressive reaming to achieve the tightest canal fit is not recommended.

After the humeral canal is reamed, the proximal portion of the humerus is prepared with the broach. Appropriate retroversion of humeral stem is individualized to the patient's pathology in order to assure stability. When the posterior glenoid is not eroded, the pros-

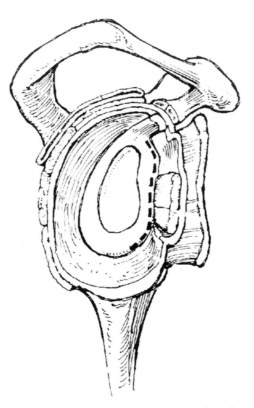

Figure 30-9. A capsulotomy opening the subscapularis recess is performed to allow placement of an anterior capsular-type retractor, as well as to assist with mobilization of the subscapularis tendon.

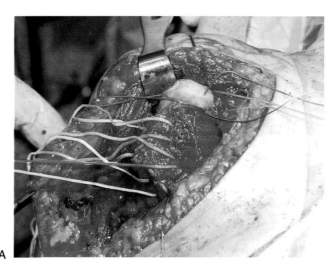
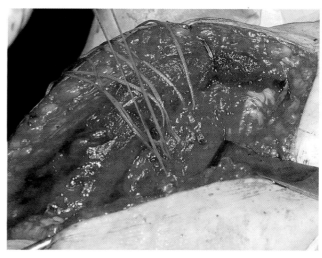

A   B

Figure 30-10. Preparation for rotator cuff closure begins with drill holes off the greater tuberosity for supraspinatus closure and off the lesser tuberosity for subscapularis closure **(A)**. The holes for subscapularis closure are placed as superiorly as possible. This will effectively allow superior transposition of the subscapularis tendon for closure of any superior defects and to allow easier approximation to the supraspinatus tendon **(B)**.

thesis should generally be retroverted more than usual (45 to 60 degrees), placing the greater part of the prosthetic head under the acromion. This maneuver ensures that at the very least, the shoulder has captured-fulcrum mechanics. This will also assist in avoiding postoperative anterosuperior instability of the proximal humerus.

At this point, a trial reduction is performed. If the broach appears stable in all planes, the flat proximal surface of the broach can be used as an intramedullary saw guide to remove more bone if necessary. Once the broach is fully seated, a metal trial head is inserted in a snap-fit manner onto the broach and the trial reduction is performed. When choosing the correct humeral head size for soft-tissue balance, there are several considerations. A large humeral head size will increase tension in the soft tissues, as lateralization of the center of rotation takes place. Greater stability is afforded and increased power may be generated. The trade-off is a head that is too large and may put too much tension on the soft tissues so that translation is not possible, and a tight painful result may lead to eccentric loading of the glenoid component. A smaller head, alternatively, creates less soft-tissue tension and permits easier rotator cuff closure, increased translation, and more motion. The repaired rotator can therefore provide static and dynamic stability for the smaller head.

Preparation is made for rotator cuff closure prior to implanting the final humeral component. Drill holes with a 2-mm bit are made in the proximal humerus, approximately 1-cm from the humeral cut, to facilitate rotator cuff closure. Holes are drilled off the greater tuberosity for supraspinatus closure and off the lesser tuberosity for subscapularis closure. The holes for subscapularis closure are placed as superiorly as possible. This will effectively allow superior transposition of the subscapularis tendon for closure of any superior defects and to allow easier approximation to the supraspinatus tendon. We use 1-mm Cottony Dacron suture through the drill holes at this point, and apply hemostats to keep the individual sutures separated (Fig. 30-10).

Because most of these patients present with significant osteopenia of the proximal humerus, cementing of the humeral stem is recommended in almost all cases. The canal is prepared first with pulsatile lavage for cleaning, followed by thorough drying with sponges. A cement plug is inserted to prevent distal extravasation of the cement. Pressurized cement is inserted into the canal via a hand held cement gun to assure a complete canal fill. The humeral component, usually at least one diameter size smaller than the trial broach, is then inserted into the canal at the appropriate height and version. The humeral component we use is a cobalt–chrome collarless stem, which allows subtle adjustments of height and version during final cementing.

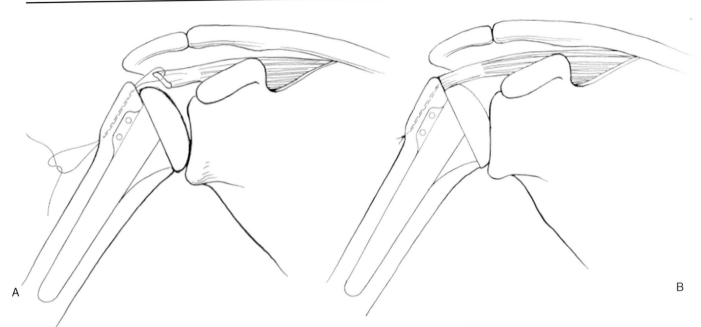

Figure 30-11. After an aggressive humeral osteotomy and adequate soft-tissue mobilization, the supraspinatus tendon **(A)** can more easily be repaired to the proximal humerus **(B)**. (From Cantrell, J.S., Itamura, J.M., Burkhead, W.Z.: Rotator cuff tear arthropathy. In: Warner, J.P., Iannotti, J.P., Gerber, C., eds.: *Complex and revision problems in shoulder surgery.* Philadelphia: Lippincott–Raven, 303–318, 1997.)

Once the cement has hardened and excess cement has been removed, a final trial reduction is performed. Again, a head size slightly smaller than the osteotomized head is chosen to facilitate supraspinatus closure. The male taper of the humeral stem is dried completely and any remaining soft tissue or cement is removed. The final selected humeral head is then impacted onto the humeral stem.

Rotator cuff closure begins posteriorly. The infraspinatus and supraspinatus are reapproximated first, if necessary, using a 1-mm Cottony Dacron suture in a side-to-side fashion with a running baseball stitch, similar to the McLaughlin technique. This will effectively bring the supraspinatus closer to the greater tuberosity attachment. The previously placed Cottony Dacron sutures in the greater tuberosity are then passed through the supraspinatus tendon and tied (Fig. 30-11). The arm may require slight abduction for a tensionless repair, which can be treated postoperatively with an abduction pillow for protection and support. The Cottony Dacron sutures in the proximal portion of the lesser tuberosity are then passed through the subscapularis tendon and tied. The holes in the superior portion of the lesser tuberosity effectively transpose the tendon superiorly for coverage of any superior defects and to allow closure of the rotator interval (Fig. 30-12). Finally, the rotator interval is reapproximated with a running baseball stitch using no. 2 Ethibond suture (Ethicon, Inc., Somerville, NJ). Final steps include closure of the deltopectoral interval with a running no. 2 Vicryl suture (Ethicon) (Fig. 30-13). A drain is typically used under the deltopectoral interval.

Formal transposition of the proximal half to two thirds of the subscapularis tendon is an alternative method for reconstruction of larger tears of the rotator cuff, especially those associated with widespread scarring in the surrounding tissue, retraction of the supraspinatus, or loss of available tissue for repair (Fig. 30-14). The technique begins at the lesser tuberosity, where the proximal half of the subscapularis tendon is dissected free from the underlying capsule. At its musculotendinous junction, the muscle is incised along the source of its fibers, obliquely downward and medially, with attention paid to the proximity of the musculocutaneous and axillary nerves. Any subcoracoid or subconjoined adhesions of the tendon are released. The proximal half of the subscapularis is mobilized sufficiently to facilitate superior and lateral advancement. The inferior border of the transferred tendon is then secured along the medial aspect of the greater tuberosity. The lateral free edge and superior border of the transferred tendon are then sutured to the edges of the infraspinatus and supraspinatus tendons to close the superior defect.

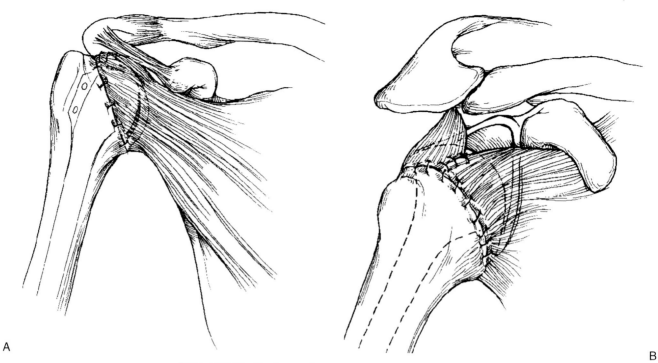

A   B

Figure 30-12. Postoperative anteroposterior **(A)** and oblique (superior-to-inferior) **(B)** views show use of a superiorly transposed subscapularis tendon to cover a large cuff defect. The prosthetic humeral head has been recentered using this technique. (From Zeman CA, Arcand MA, Cantrell JS, et al. The rotator cuff deficient arthritic shoulder: diagnosis and management. *J Am Acad Orthop Surg* 6(6): 337–348, 1998, with permission.)

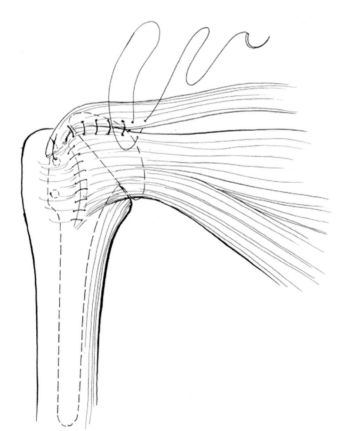

Figure 30-13. The rotator interval tissue is reapproximated with a running baseball stitch to close the defect between the supraspinatus and subscapularis tendons. (From Cantrell, J.S., Itamura, J.M., Burkhead, W.Z.: Rotator cuff tear arthropathy. In: Warner, J.P., Iannotti, J.P., Gerber, C., eds.: *Complex and revision problems in shoulder surgery.* Philadelphia: Lippincott–Raven, 303–318, 1997.)

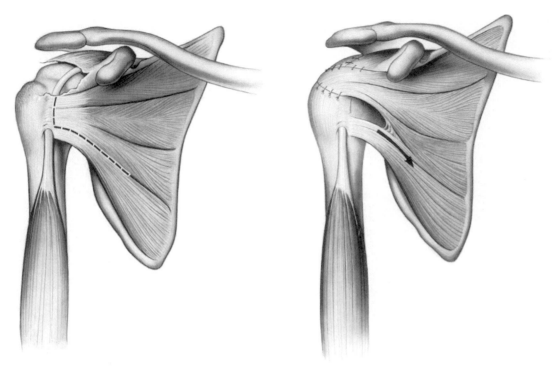

Figure 30-14. Subscapularis transfer is considered for large irreparable defects of the supraspinatus and infraspinatus. Detachment of the longest possible flap of subscapularis from the underlying capsule is performed, avoiding injury to the axillary nerve. The inferior border of the flap is sutured to the greater tuberosity lateral to the anatomic neck, beginning immediately posterior to the bicipital groove. The leading edge of the subscapularis and its superior border are then approximated to the free edges of the supraspinatus and infraspinatus tendons to close the defect. (From Neer, C.S. II: *Shoulder reconstruction.* Philadelphia: WB Saunders, 1991, with permission.)

Deficient Subscapularis

If the patient has positive lift-off and belly-press tests, the subscapularis is involved in the massive tear, and the patient will have marked weakness with almost all active motions of the shoulder. A complete preoperative examination with comparison to the contralateral side should be completed in all cases to plan for subscapularis pathology. Although a deltopectoral approach is commonly used for most shoulder arthroplasties, including those with a known deficient subscapularis, the surgeon must be prepared to deal with the unexpected subscapularis deficiency. The deltopectoral approach is useful for two circumstances: primary repair of the subscapularis and transfer of the pectoralis major tendon.

Primary repair of the subscapularis is indicated when sufficient tissue is available for a substantial repair. Mobilization techniques are used in a fashion similar to those previously described. All bursal and soft-tissue adhesions are released from both sides of the tendon to the base of the coracoid. Any remaining tissue in the rotator interval area is also released. Suture tags are placed through the tendon to aid immobilization. Assessment of the ability to primarily close the subscapularis is made after the humeral osteotomy. Drill holes are inserted through the proximal humerus along the osteotomy line as previously described. The drill holes are made more inferior on the humeral neck cut if the tendon cannot be mobilized to the superior portion of the osteotomy. This will effectively allow partial repair of the subscapularis by decreasing the required distance to transverse the glenohumeral joint.

A transfer of the pectoralis major muscle is commonly used for augmentation of a weak subscapularis repair or for irreparable rupture of the tendon. The tendon of the pectoralis major is exposed over its full length at the humerus by extending the deltopectoral incision distally. The size of the subscapularis defect determines the amount of tendon to transfer. For smaller defects, one half of the superior portion of the tendon is detached from the

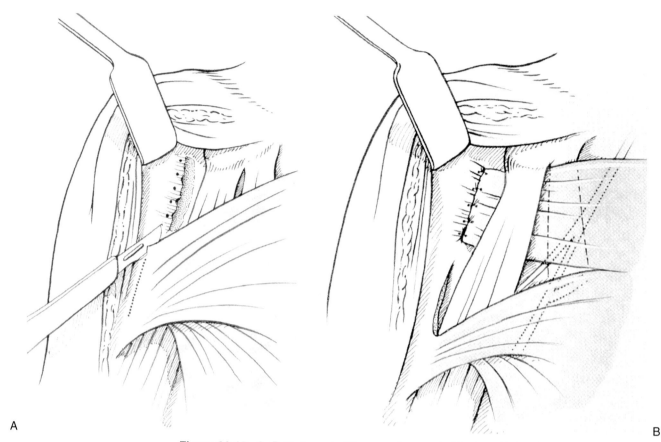

Figure 30-15. A: Detachment of the superior one half to two thirds of the pectoralis major tendon from the humerus. **B:** View of the course of the newly transferred pectoralis major tendon under the conjoined tendon. (From Resch, H., Povacz, P., Ritter, E., et al.: Transfer of the pectoralis major muscle for the treatment of irreparable rupture of the subscapularis tendon. *J Bone Joint Surg Am* 82(3): 372–382, 2000, with permission.)

humerus (Fig. 30-15). For larger defects, the entire tendon is harvested (Fig. 30-16). When only a portion of the tendon is transferred, the muscle fibers corresponding to the detached section of the tendon are split by blunt dissection over a length of approximately 10 cm between the clavicular and sternal portions to take only the clavicular part for transfer, working from the insertion medially. The muscle fibers of the sternal portion that radiate from dorsal into the proximal part of the tendon are transected. This leaves the clavicular portion of the pectoralis major muscle attached to the tendon with the exception of the transected muscle fibers just mentioned. The sternal portion is left intact unless the entire tendon needs to be transferred.

The space between the pectoralis minor and the conjoined tendon is entered, and the area behind the conjoined tendon is exposed with finger dissection. The musculocutaneous nerve is palpated at its entrance into the muscle. This is very important for assessment of the space for the transferred muscle when it passes between the nerve and the conjoined tendon. Stay sutures attached to the tendon of the pectoralis major are then grasped with curved forceps and the muscle is advanced behind the conjoined tendon but in front of the musculocutaneous nerve. The tendon is then attached through drill holes at the osteotomy site with 1-mm cottony Dacron suture. For irreparable superior defects, the tendon is attached not only to the lesser tuberosity area but also transferred superiorly to the anterior part of the greater tuberosity.

Deficient Deltoid

Even if the cuff defect is reparable or reconstructable, attempts at restoring or balancing force coupled with prosthetic replacement and soft-tissue reconstruction are fruitless if the

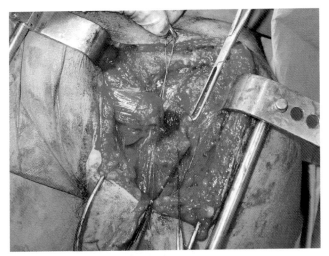
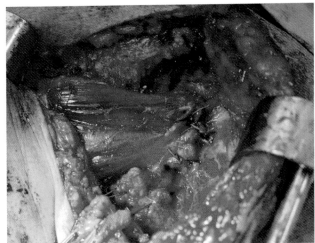
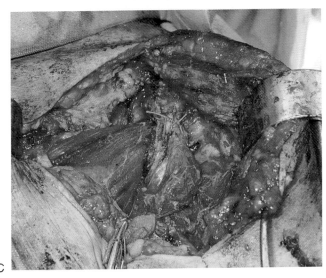

Figure 30-16. For larger subscapularis defects, the entire pectoralis major tendon can be transferred. **A:** The pectoralis major tendon is released from its insertion site on the humerus and mobilized to release all adhesions. The conjoined tendon was released for this particular case to avoid nerve injury. **B:** The pectoralis tendon is attached to the lesser tuberosity through drill holes with nonabsorbable suture. **C:** Completion of the transfer with repair of the conjoined tendon to the coracoid process.

anterior deltoid is deficient due to large areas of detachment or denervation. A thorough preoperative evaluation of axillary nerve function must be made for any questionable cases. In the event of permanent axillary nerve injury, glenohumeral fusion with the use of pelvic reconstruction plates, autogenous and/or allogenic bone graft, and postoperative management of medical problems or metabolic bone disease make this an attractive alternative even for those patients in their late 70s or 80s.

Areas of deltoid avulsion from the anterior portion of the acromion are occasionally encountered during arthroplasty cases for failed rotator cuff repairs. Factors related to the success of deltoid repair after dehiscence has occurred include the size of the defect, the duration of detachment, the osseous integrity of the acromion, the quality of the soft tissues, and the degree of soft-tissue deficiency. Overall, factors associated with a satisfactory outcome include isolated disruptions of the anterior deltoid, an intact acromion, preservation of rotator cuff function, and evidence of a healed deltoid reconstruction. Conversely, poor results are associated with a prior lateral acromionectomy, involvement of the middle deltoid, a concomitant and poorly compensated massive rotator cuff tear, and duration of symptoms longer than 12 months.

In selected cases, repair of long-standing deltoid dehiscence may be indicated (Fig. 30-17). However, patient education about the likely events of prolonged postoperative immobilization and rehabilitation and about the unpredictability of outcome should be emphasized. The surgical method requires accurate identification of the detached muscular segment, adequate mobilization, and secure transosseous repair. Division of scar and tendon approximately 1 cm proximal to the muscular margin provides a sufficient cuff of tis-

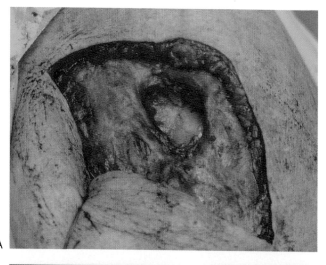

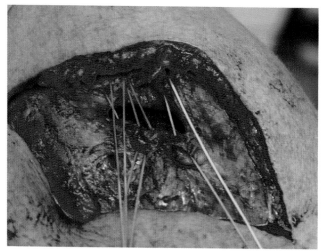

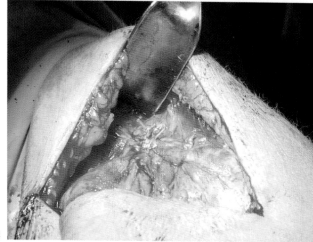

Figure 30-17. A: In certain cases, direct repair of deltoid avulsion injuries can be attempted, as demonstrated by this small dehiscence after previous rotator cuff repair. **B:** The avulsion is secured to the acromion with nonabsorbable suture. **C:** Final closure of the defect reapproximates the muscle edges and allows a functional recovery.

sue for repair to the remaining acromion. In cases with a small area of detachment (< 4 cm) and with minimal retraction (< 4 cm), a side-to-side closure of the deltoid may be considered, or a direct repair to the acromion may be accomplished with heavy nonabsorbable suture. Most commonly, it is the lateral deltoid that detaches before it heals. When this occurs, the deltoid retracts to the upper brachium, but usually maintains a thin layer of scar that is connected to the lateral acromion. This scar can be folded back on the deltoid to create a thick fascial insertion (Fig. 30-18). A running suture is placed along the tissue to create a tendinous structure. With mobilization and abduction of the arm, the deltoid origin is approximated to the residual acromion. Then sutures can be placed behind this permanent suture so that the sutures are pulling against the suture and not the muscle or newly created tendon. Postoperatively, shoulder immobilization is recommended with an abduction pillow. The period of immobilization depends in part on the quality of tissue, the size and tension of the repaired defect, and any concomitant repair of the rotator cuff.

Rarely, deltoid transfer from lateral to anterior or posterior to lateral is required to allow closure of the defect. For patients in whom lateral acromionectomy has resulted in deltoid dehiscence, Neer (8) has recommended a sliding osteotomy of the spine of the scapula to recreate, as best can be done, an acromion (Fig. 30-19). Even less common, although occasionally useful in certain situations, is the latissimus dorsi transfer through the axilla. This technique, described for replacement of a paralyzed anterior deltoid, frees and rotates the latissimus dorsi with its neurovascular pedicle and then places it over the anterior part of the paralyzed muscle. The lever arm of the transposed muscle is as long as that of the deltoid, and the muscle volume is enough to restore the natural contour of the shoulder.

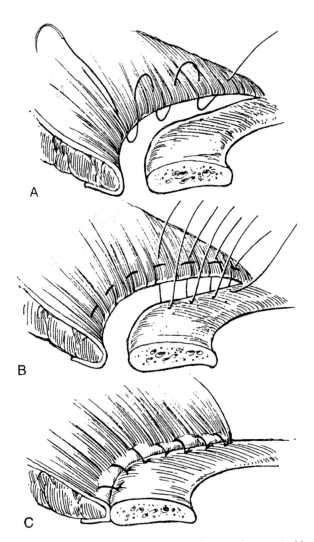

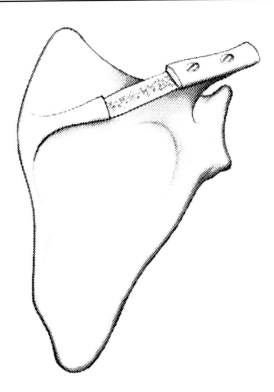

Figure 30-19. Sliding osteotomy of the spine of the scapula to recreate an acromion, as recommended by Neer. (From Neer, C.S. II: *Shoulder reconstruction.* Philadelphia: WB Saunders, 1990, with permission.)

Figure 30-18. A: A thick fascial insertion can be created by folding the residual scar back onto the deltoid, then placing a running suture to hold it in place. The length of the new tendon can be altered based on the degree to which the underlying deltoid can be mobilized. **B:** With mobilization and abduction of the arm, the deltoid origin is approximated to the residual acromion. Note the sutures can be placed behind the permanent suture so that the pull is against the suture and not the muscle. **C:** Tying down the sutures via drill holes in the acromion. (From Burkhead, W.Z., Cantrell, J.S.: Management of failed rotator cuff repairs. In: Burkhead, W.Z., ed.: *Rotator cuff disorders.* Baltimore: Williams & Wilkins, 399–407, 1995.)

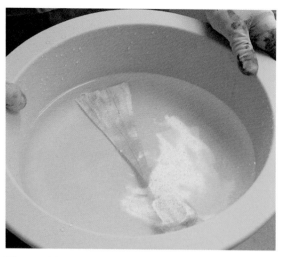

Figure 30-20. The cadaveric Achilles tendon allograft is soaked in lukewarm water for thawing.

Biologic Glenoid Resurfacing

An interesting alternative for the management of glenoid pathology in patients with arthritis and soft-tissue deficiency is biologic resurfacing. The senior author (W.Z.B.) has described this technique, initially using the anterior glenohumeral joint capsule or an autologous fascia lata graft (2). Our current graft of choice for biologic glenoid resurfacing is a cadaver Achilles tendon, which provides a much thicker graft material compared with that of anterior capsule or fascia lata. The tendoachilles graft also provides other advantages over the anterior capsule technique. Because the capsule-resurfacing technique involves leaving a medial soft-tissue attachment, persistent sympathetic nerve fibers in the capsule can act as a potential source of pain. This potential problem can therefore be avoided with the use of allograft tissue.

The tendoachilles resurfacing technique begins with thawing of the graft in lukewarm water (Fig. 30-20). Hot water is avoided due to potential destabilization of the graft. Next, a 15-blade scalpel is used to resect the tendon from the bony calcaneal attachment, attempting to preserve as much tendon as possible (Fig. 30-21). Alternatively, a portion of the bony insertion can be left attached to the tendon and used as bone graft in areas of glenoid insufficiency.

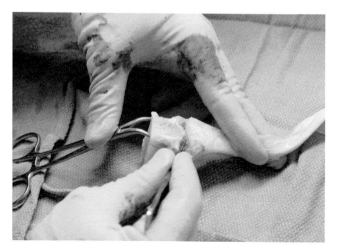

Figure 30-21. The calcaneal bone is sharply removed from the graft, thereby maximizing length on the tendon.

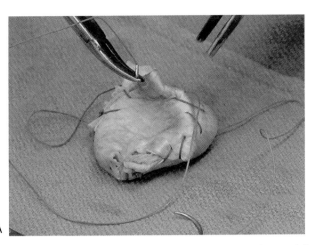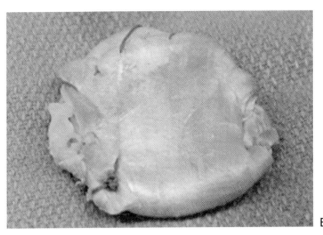

A   B

Figure 30-22. The tendon is contoured into the shape of the glenoid **(A)** and held together with suture **(B)**.

The graft is then contoured by folding the tendon back onto itself several times to create a glenoid shape of appropriate size (Fig. 30-22). Number 2 Ethibond or Panacryl suture (Mitek Worldwide, Norwood, MA) is used to secure the shape of the graft. The glenoid surface is then decorticated with a burr to create a bleeding surface. Currently, we are using four or five Mitek Panalok anchors (Mitek Worldwide) with Panacryl suture for graft fixation to the glenoid. Metal anchors are avoided due to potential loosening in the soft bone and erosion through the graft into the joint. Four anchors are inserted into the glenoid in a diamond-shaped pattern, and additional anchors are used if necessary. The sutures are then individually passed through the contoured tendon graft in a mattress fashion. The graft is pushed down the sutures and abutted against the glenoid, at which point the sutures are tied (Fig. 30-23).

The tendoachilles graft also has the advantage of being used to resurface the undersurface of the acromion and for coracoacromial ligament augmentation or reconstruction. In patients with cuff-tear arthropathy or rheumatoid arthritis with superior head migration and articulation to the undersurface of the acromion, the Achilles graft works well as an interposition. The graft is prepared by suturing the distal end back onto itself once for glenoid resurfacing, leaving a long strip of proximal tendon free (Fig. 30-24). The graft is anchored to the glenoid as previously described, positioning the free strip superiorly (Fig. 30-25). The strip of tendon is then positioned on the undersurface of the acromion and sutured in

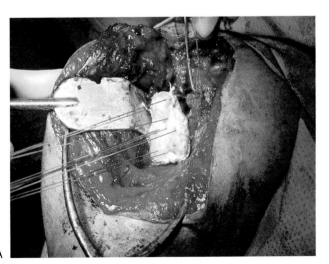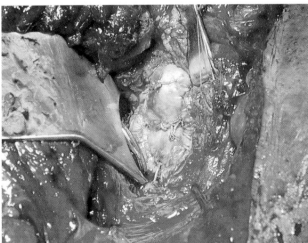

A   B

Figure 30-23. The sutures are passed through the graft **(A)** and tied to the glenoid **(B)**.

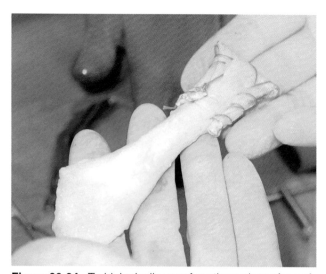

Figure 30-24. To biologically resurface the undersurface of the acromion, the Achilles graft is doubled-back onto itself only once, thereby creating a long strip of free tendon to place under the acromion.

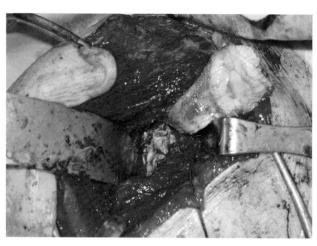

Figure 30-25. The graft is fixed to the glenoid with suture anchors, leaving the free strip of tendon at the superior portion of the glenoid fixation.

place (Fig. 30-26). Two mattress sutures are used for fixation through the graft. The first suture is secured through the soft tissue in the superior notch medial to the acromion. The second is secured through the soft tissue just lateral to the acromial edge. Subcutaneous tissue dissection will need to be performed to expose these two areas. Alternatively, the proximal aspect of the incision can be extended laterally in curved fashion to expose these areas. The two ends of each mattress suture are then tied over the trapezial and deltoid fascia respectively. Any free tendon can be removed with trimming or sutured back to itself on the undersurface of the acromion.

In cases of coracoacromial ligament insufficiency, the free end of the tendon graft can be used for augmentation or substitution of the ligament to prevent migration of the humeral head (Fig. 30-27). The free end of the tendon graft is first secured to the glenoid and undersurface of the acromion as previously described. The terminal free end is then brought back and sutured to the remaining coracoacromial ligament if present. This will act as an augmentation to anterosuperior migration of the head. When the ligament is absent,

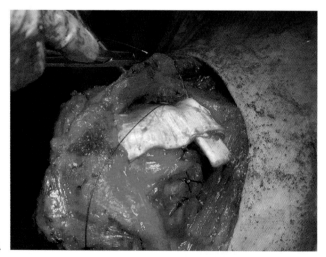

A

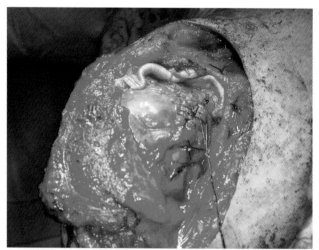

B

Figure 30-26. A: The free tendon edge is sutured to the soft tissue of the deltotrapezial fascia on both sides of the acromion. Alternatively, drill holes through the acromion may be used for suture fixation. **B:** Final resurfacing demonstrates complete coverage of the undersurface of the acromion.

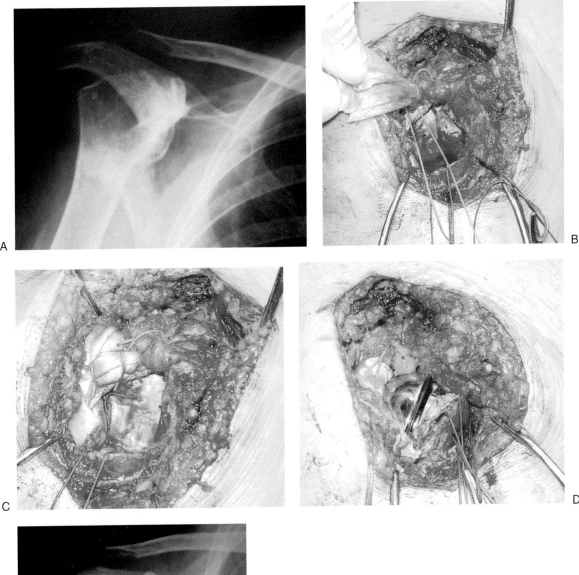

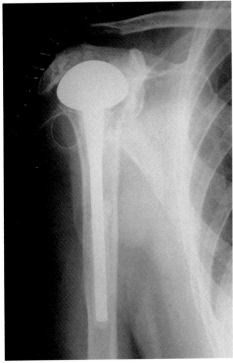

Figure 30-27. **A:** Preoperative radiograph of glenohumeral arthritis with rotator cuff deficiency and significant medial glenoid erosion. **B:** After humeral head osteotomy and canal preparation, the glenoid is resurfaced with an Achilles tendon allograft. **C:** The proximal free strip of tendon is first used to resurface the undersurface of the acromion. The remaining tendon is then diverted to the coracoid process to reconstruct the coracoacromial ligament. **D:** The humeral stem is placed in increased retroversion to center the humeral head under the acromion, thereby preventing anterosuperior instability. **E:** Postoperative radiograph demonstrating proper position of the humeral head under the acromion.

as commonly found in revision cases, the free end of the tendon graft is brought back from the acromion to the coracoid to recreate the ligament. The graft is secured to the coracoid by soft-tissue fixation to the superior portion of the conjoined tendon with heavy nonabsorbable suture. Alternatively, a suture anchor placed in the coracoid process may also be used for fixation. This will effectively substitute for the absent ligament and again act as a restraint to anterosuperior instability of the humeral head.

Reverse Total Shoulder Arthroplasty

Newer interest has been evolving regarding the use of reverse ball-and-socket shoulder arthroplasty for the rotator cuff–deficient arthritic shoulder (Fig. 30-28). The design rationale of this new category of shoulder replacement accommodates certain conditions. These involve the deficient rotator cuff in which functional outcomes of rotator cuff arthropathy or hemiarthroplasty with superior escape of the humeral head are severely limited, difficult to manage symptoms of glenoid erosive disease from osteoarthritis or failed hemiarthroplasty, or instability due to soft-tissue loss is that unmanageable by traditional arthroplasty techniques. The goal of this implant is to offer a constrained prosthetic option when the shoulder is functionally disabled and no other viable solution for providing functional rehabilitation is available. Although not intended to withstand normal activity loads of a healthy shoulder, it is a means of restoring mobility and reducing pain for many patients. Long-term results with this prosthetic design are unfortunately not yet available, but preliminary results are promising.

Reverse arthroplasty designs are indicated for several conditions. These include rotator cuff arthropathy or failed hemi- or total shoulder arthroplasty (Fig. 30-29), incompetent rotator cuff or erosive glenoid disease, evidence of upward displacement of the humeral head with respect to the glenoid, and loss of the glenohumeral joint space. Most important, indications for this implant rely on a functional deltoid muscle, which is necessary for the biomechanical fulcrum created by this component. The contraction force of the deltoid muscle forces the arm into the glenoid ball, thereby regaining elevation function through the fulcrum mechanism.

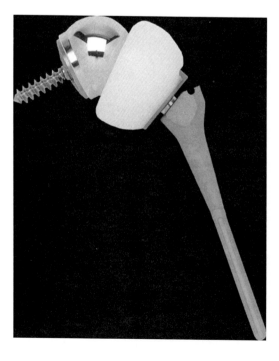

Figure 30-28. The reverse shoulder prosthesis. (From Encore Medical Corporation, Austin, TX, with permission.)

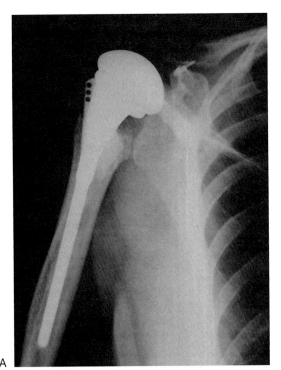
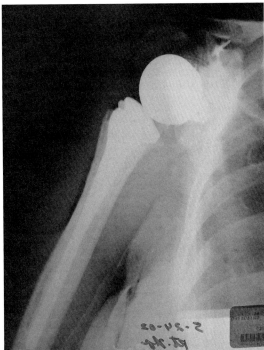

A   B

Figure 30-29. A: Loss of tuberosity fixation led to failure of this hemiarthroplasty treated for an initially four-part proximal humerus fracture. Note the absence of the tuberosities and superior migration of the implant, indicating absence of the rotator cuff. **B:** Revision of this case to a reverse ball-and-socket design restored deltoid tension to provide better functional elevation of the arm.

POSTOPERATIVE MANAGEMENT

Postoperative management begins with preoperative education of the patient and his or her family, emphasizing that pain relief is the primary goal of surgery, and realistic expectations for range of motion and strength are typically limited (9). On the first or second postoperative day, patients are taught passive exercises, which are continued alone for at least 8 weeks. These initially include gentle Codman pendulum exercises, forward elevation with a pulley, external rotation with a stick, gentle elbow flexion/extension, and isometric hand range-of-motion exercises. The limits of passive motion are determined by the integrity of the soft-tissue repair. Typically, forward elevation to 90 degrees and external rotation to neutral are initially allowed. These exercises may be delayed for 3 weeks if additional protection of the rotator cuff repair is required. When the rotator cuff repair is tenuous, an abduction pillow can be used for the first 4 to 6 weeks. If an abduction pillow is used, the passive exercises are performed above the level of the pillow.

Passive exercises are maintained exclusively for at least 8 weeks before subjecting the superior repair to the vertical shear force of the deltoid. Between 8 and 12 weeks, depending on the size of the cuff tear and tissue quality, full passive stretching is allowed. This includes full forward elevation and external rotation, with the addition of abduction and extension stretching with a stick and internal rotation stretching up the back. At this time, gentle active motion is allowed in all planes, beginning first with an active-assisted program. Resisted strengthening with Theraband exercise is begun between 8 and 12 weeks. Short-arc internal and external rotation Theraband exercises with the arm at the side are started first and continued every other day for 4 weeks. After 4 weeks, forward elevation, abduction, and extension Theraband exercises are added. Yellow Theraband (lowest resistance) is used almost exclusively for the duration of the strengthening program.

We rely primarily on a home-based, patient-performed therapy program, and rarely use formal physical therapy. Preoperatively, our nurses instruct patients on pendulum, pulley, and stick exercises in the office. These home exercises are started three times per day before surgery to maintain preoperative motion and to provide instruction for the postoperative period. On the first or second postoperative day, hospital physical therapists review exercises with the patient and instruct on any adjustments in the home program. Passive exercises are performed three times per day. Theraband instruction is performed by our nurses at the appropriate follow-up visit and performed by the patient every other day at home. Formal physical therapy is only used for those patients who require a more disciplined postoperative therapy program.

RESULTS

Over the years, one of us (W.Z.B.) has tried several methods to improve the results of shoulder arthroplasty for this difficult group of patients. In a small series compiled at our institution, four types of surgical management were previously used to improve results in this group of patients: (a) bipolar prosthesis without cuff repair, (b) large-head hemiarthroplasty without cuff repair, (c) small-head hemiarthroplasty with subscapularis transposition, and (d) nonconstrained total shoulder arthroplasty with cuff repair. Eighteen patients were initially followed up for at least 2 years. At the most recent follow-up evaluation, shoulders treated by replacement using a smaller humeral head with subscapularis transposition and an attempt at cuff repair gave superior results to any of the other three approaches (Fig. 30-30).

Sanchez-Sotelo et al. (11) have recently reviewed their results of 33 shoulders treated with hemiarthroplasty for glenohumeral arthritis associated with severe rotator cuff defi-

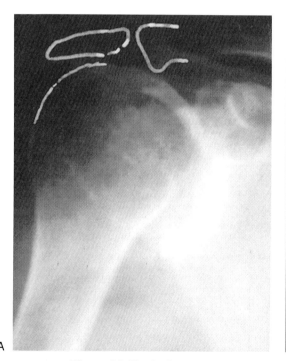
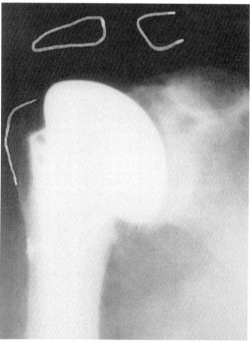

A

B

Figure 30-30. A: Preoperative radiograph of an 83-year-old woman with glenohumeral arthritis and soft-tissue deficiency. **B:** Postoperatively, the prosthesis is centered under the acromion in 45 to 60 degrees of retroversion. (From Cantrell, J.S., Itamura, J.M., Burkhead, W.Z.: Rotator cuff tear arthropathy. In: Warner, J.P., Iannotti, J.P., Gerber, C., eds.: *Complex and revision problems in shoulder surgery.* Philadelphia: Lippincott–Raven, 303–318, 1997.)

ciency. Partial repair of the subscapularis was possible in 23 shoulders, and partial repair of the infraspinatus was possible in three. The supraspinatus remnants were sutured to the subscapularis muscle in three shoulders. Improvements were demonstrated in mean pain score and active elevation. Overall, the result was graded as successful for 22 shoulders (67%).

The results of hemiarthroplasty with cuff repair versus total shoulder arthroplasty have been reported in the literature by other authors. Pollock et al. (10) reported 30 shoulders with severe rotator cuff deficiency that underwent arthroplasty. There were 19 hemiarthroplasties and 11 total shoulder arthroplasties performed. Meticulous attempts at reconstruction of the rotator cuff were made for all patients, and poor coverage was obtained in 15 of these shoulders. Total shoulder arthroplasty and hemiarthroplasty in their series were found to have similar results with respect to pain relief, functional improvement, and patient satisfaction. Cuff repair was facilitated in the hemiarthroplasty group because the joint line was not lateralized. These authors concluded that treatment of choice in rotator cuff–deficient shoulders associated with glenohumeral arthritis is a humeral arthroplasty with cuff repair, which is an important difference from the conclusions of Williams and Rockwood (12) and Arntz et al. (1), who did not advocate cuff repair for this group of patients.

Lohr et al. (6) studied 22 shoulder replacements in patients with rotator cuff tear arthropathy. They evaluated hemiarthroplasty, unconstrained arthroplasty, and semiconstrained total shoulder arthroplasty. There was a high degree of radiographic and clinical findings of loosening of the glenoid components in the unconstrained and semiconstrained total shoulder groups. However, patients with hemiarthroplasty had poor pain relief. They concluded that every attempt should be made to obtain rotator cuff repair and the unconstrained devices gave the best results in their series.

COMPLICATIONS

Complications that develop after shoulder arthroplasty with soft-tissue deficiency are similar to those that occur without soft-tissue deficiency. Unconstrained total shoulder arthroplasty has a high glenoid failure rate in patients with massive cuff deficiency because of continued instability. Positioning both components so that the loading of the glenoid is symmetric can be very difficult. With time, the humerus will continue to migrate superiorly with associated wear of the acromion, leading to eccentric glenoid loading and loosening. Hemiarthroplasty has been the most successful arthroplasty performed in patients with massive, irreparable cuff deficiency. The pain relief, although not as complete as in total shoulder arthroplasty, is still good.

Continued instability and weakness can be present after hemiarthroplasty, especially if the humeral head is small and the rotator cuff is unable to be closed. Overstuffing the glenohumeral joint with an oversized humeral head can cause potential stiffness and loss of function. Persistent instability due to humeral stem malrotation is also a common complication. Excessive retroversion in the osteoarthritic patient with posterior glenoid wear can lead to posterior dislocation of the humeral component. Conversely, excessive anteversion, especially in those patients with a deficient coracoacromial arch, can lead to anterosuperior instability or anterior dislocation. Anterior deltoid dysfunction may also lead to anterior instability. Constant awareness of axillary nerve position and awareness of its proximity during retraction and dissection are mandatory to avoid injury to this nerve.

Complications following arthroplasty in the cuff-deficient shoulder also include potential intraoperative fracture of the glenoid or humerus. The rate of fracture is higher in patients with rheumatoid arthritis, owing to increased osteopenia and fragility. Although not always considered as such, inadequate range of motion is a complication occurring after shoulder arthroplasty. The arthroplasty techniques designed for cuff deficiency have a primary goal of pain relief, and a secondary goal of increased motion. Appropriate soft-tissue techniques as described in this chapter will therefore serve to maximize outcomes of active motion.

RECOMMENDED READING

1. Arntz, C.T., Jackins, S., Matsen, F.A.: Prosthetic replacement of the shoulder for the treatment of defects in the rotator cuff and the surface of the glenohumeral joint. *J Bone Joint Surg Am* 75(4): 485–491, 1993.
2. Burkhead, W.Z., Hutton, K.S.: Biologic resurfacing of the glenoid with hemiarthroplasty of the shoulder. *J Shoulder Elbow Surg* 4(4): 263–270, 1995.
3. Cantrell, J.S., Itamura, J.M., Burkhead, W.Z.: Rotator cuff tear arthropathy. In: Warner, J.P., Iannotti, J.P., Gerber, C., eds.: *Complex and revision problems in shoulder surgery.* Philadelphia: Lippincott–Raven, 303–318, 1997.
4. Godenèche, A., Boileau, P., Favard, L., et al.: Prosthetic replacement in the treatment of osteoarthritis of the shoulder: early results of 268 cases. *J Shoulder Elbow Surg* 11(1): 11–18, 2002.
5. Grammont, P.M., Baulot, E.: Delta shoulder prosthesis for rotator cuff rupture. *Orthopedics* 16(1): 65–68, 1993.
6. Lohr, J.F., Cofield, R.H., Uhtoff, H.K.: Glenoid component loosening in cuff tear arthropathy. *J Bone Joint Surg Br* 83[Suppl 2]: 106, 1991.
7. Murthi, A.M., Vosburgh, C.L., Neviaser, T.J.: The incidence of pathologic changes of the long head of the biceps tendon. *J Shoulder Elbow Surg* 9: 382–385, 2000.
8. Neer, C.S. II: *Shoulder reconstruction.* Philadelphia: WB Saunders, 1991.
9. Neer, C.S. II, Craig, E.V., Fukuda, H.: Cuff-tear arthropathy. *J Bone Joint Surg Am* 65: 1232–1244, 1983.
10. Pollock, R.G., Deliz, E.D., McIlveen, S.J., et al.: Prosthetic replacement in rotator cuff-deficient shoulders. *J Shoulder Elbow Surg* 4(1): 173–185, 1992.
11. Sanchez-Sotelo, J., Cofield, R.H., Rowland, C.M.: Shoulder hemiarthroplasty for glenohumeral arthritis associated with severe rotator cuff deficiency. *J Bone Joint Surg Am* 83: 1814–1822, 2001.
12. Williams, G.R., Rockwood, C.R.: Hemiarthroplasty in rotator cuff-deficient shoulders. *J Shoulder Elbow Surg* 5(5): 362–367, 1996.
13. Williams, G.R., Rockwood, C.A.: Massive rotator cuff defects and glenohumeral arthritis. In: Freidman, R.J., ed.: *Arthroplasty of the shoulder.* New York: Thieme Medical Publishers, 204–214, 1994.

31

Surface-replacement Arthroplasty of the Shoulder

Stephen Copeland

INDICATIONS/CONTRAINDICATIONS

The fundamental premise of the Copeland surface implant is minimal removal of bone and cementless fixation. The initial development of this implant began in 1979, and the prosthesis was first used clinically in 1986. Since 1993, the entire surfaces of both glenoid and humeral components have been hydroxyapatite-coated for later biologic fixation after initial mechanical fixation. Instrumentation has emphasized simplicity while affording anatomic placement of the humeral head.

Advantages of Surface Replacement

1. Anatomic placement of the head to allow infinite variation of version, offset, and angulation.
2. No intramedullary canal reaming is required, affording less trauma in an elderly patient. There is no risk of fat embolus or hypotension and no cement is required.
3. May be used even if the intramedullary canal has already been previously violated with cement, stem of an elbow replacement from below, rods, or screws. If there is malunion at the proximal end of the humeral with secondary osteoarthritis, the malunion can be left undisturbed and just the humeral articular surface replaced.
4. Lack of stem extending down the humeral shaft produces no stress riser effect and no possibility of fracture at the tip of the prosthesis.
5. May be used in some congenital abnormalities of the humerus that do not allow the passage of standard intramedullary stem prostheses.

S. Copeland, M.D., F.R.C.S.: Shoulder Surgery Unit, Berkshire Independent Hospital, Coley Park, Reading-Berkshire, Reading, United Kingdom.

6. Humeral head bone is preserved, making revision easier. Remaining bone can be used if grafting is necessary.

Primary and secondary arthritis of the shoulder are the common indications. The prosthesis has been used for osteoarthritis, rheumatoid arthritis, avascular necrosis, cuff arthropathy, instability arthropathy, posttrauma arthritis, postinfective arthritis, arthritis secondary to glenoid dysplasia, and epiphyseal dysplasia. It is not intended for use in fresh fractures.

The results of surface replacement, as in any other shoulder replacement, depend on the indications and diagnosis. The best results are achieved in osteoarthritis with an intact cuff and the worst results in cuff tear arthropathy and posttraumatic arthritis. It can be used in moderate to severe degrees of erosion of the humeral head as the humeral head is often bone grafted at the same time as the surface replacement. Once the humeral head shaper has been used, if there is more than 60% apposition between the undersurface of the trial prosthesis and bone, surface replacement is used. Up to 40% of the humeral head may be replaced by autograft. Bone for this can be taken from the drill holes, head-shaping reamings, osteophytes, and sometimes from the excision arthroplasty of acromioclavicular joint and acromioplasty.

Hemi or Total. There is no long-term randomized study concerning whether a total or hemiarthroplasty is the ideal procedure for arthritis, although in some studies, the pain relief in total shoulder replacement may be more complete than in hemiarthroplasty. However, the long-term failure rate of shoulder replacement relates to glenoid loosening failure and wear. Therefore, the comparison must always be made between the possibility of glenoid erosion pain by a humeral hemiarthroplasty related to the rate of late glenoid loosening because of high-density polyethylene wear debris. The trade-off is accepting not-quite-as-good short-term pain relief with the possible long-term failure of a glenoid and late revision surgery. This must be taken into account if the prosthesis is used in younger patients with higher expectations and increased longevity.

In our series, we found that there has been little clinical difference in the functional results of those with and those without a glenoid. We know that the long-term survival of any total joint replacement is directly related to the volume of high-density polyethylene wear debris, therefore our preference is to avoid the introduction of polyethylene. The only indication for a total replacement is nonconcentric erosion or a very elderly patient. However, when a hemiarthroplasty is done, the glenoid is not ignored. Multiple 2-mm drill holes are made in the osteochondral hard bone to encourage secondary fibrocartilage. The conversion rate from hemi- to total replacement between stemmed and surface replacement is statistically different (stemmed: average, 12%; surface, 1.3%). This is thought to be due to correct version and head size in the surface replacement. If a normal modular prosthesis is used as a hemiarthroplasty then the surgeon tends to err on the side of making the head diameter too small compared to the original anatomic size therefore the possibility of point

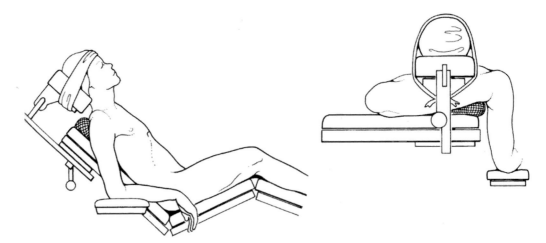

Figure 31-1. The patient is now placed in a beach-chair position, with the involved extremity draped free. An arm board adjacent to the patient permits support of the humerus, while permitting extension during humeral implantation.

erosion of the glenoid is high. With the surface-replacement system, the tendency if any is to err toward a larger head size and hence there may be rim erosion rather than point erosion. There is no doubt that if the humeral head is not being removed as part of the procedure, it is more difficult to actually replace the glenoid, as access is restricted and difficult. However, if it has been decided to insert a glenoid component, exposure can be achieved by more extensive capsular release which is always possible.

SURGERY

Patient Positioning

Apply an antiseptic pad to the shoulder 1 hour preoperatively to cover the axilla and operation site. Place the patient in a beach-chair position with a sandbag underneath the medial scapular border to thrust it forward (Fig. 31-1). Use a neurosurgical headpiece to allow the patient to be positioned on the edge of the table in the semi-reclining position with the head supported. Drape the arm free to allow full movement at the shoulder. An arm board is attached to the table at the level of the elbow, to allow the arm to be extended.

Technique

Approach. Until 1993, I used the standard anterior deltopectoral approach and since September 1993, by preference, the anterosuperior approach (Fig. 31-2) as described by

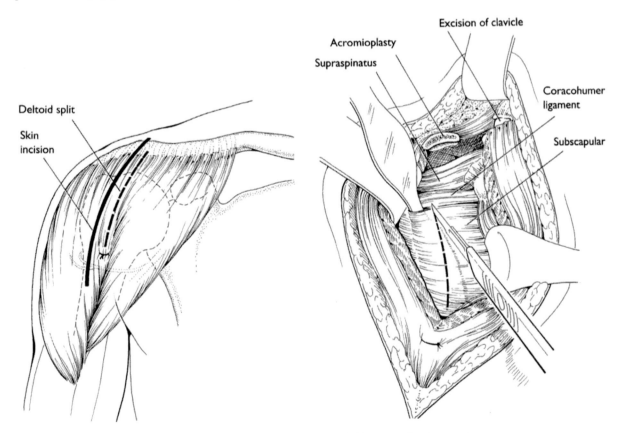

Figure 31-2. The anterosuperior surgical approach (deltoid split). Because the humeral head is not resected, a less extensile exposure is used. The split between the anterior one third of deltoid and the posterior two thirds is developed, the conjoint tendon is retracted immediately, and the rotator interval is identified. The subscapularis tendon is divided from superior to inferior, from the level of the rotator interval to the anterior humeral circumflex vessels. This division of the subscapularis permits anterior dislocation of the humeral head.

Mackenzie (5). The prosthesis is suitable for insertion via either technique. The advantages of the latter approach are a smaller and neater scar, shorter postoperative recovery, easier access via rotator interval to the glenoid, and better access to the posterior and superior rotator cuff for reconstruction. It also allows excision arthroplasty of the acromioclavicular joint and acromioplasty if these are indicated. The acromioclavicular joint excision could be a very useful source of bone graft for use later.

If the rotator cuff is intact or a repairable rotator cuff defect is seen, do an anterior acromioplasty with partial resection of the coracoacromial ligament. Leave the coracoacromial arch undisturbed if the rotator cuff is extensively torn or nonfunctional. If preoperative radiographs have shown arthritic changes of the acromioclavicular joint and symptoms suggest this is a site of pain, do an excision arthroplasty at this stage. This further improves the surgical exposure. I do an acromioclavicular excision almost as routine for patients with osteoarthritis because often preoperatively they do not have an adequate range of motion to determine problems arising here clinically. At least 80 degrees of forward flexion is required to induce pain at this site and this could be the source of pain after shoulder replacement has been done and a good range of motion has been achieved.

Identify the rotator interval and longitudinally incise along the line of the long head of the biceps to define the insertion of subscapularis. Detach the subscapularis and dislocate the humeral head anteriorly. If the long head of the biceps is intact, displace it posteriorly over the humeral head.

Humeral Component. The key landmark for determining anatomic positioning of the humeral component is the anatomic neck of humerus. Demonstrate this by removing osteophytes around the neck (Fig. 31-3) [Sizing is determined by radiograph template or direct visual comparison with the trial prostheses (five sizes are available).]

Place the humeral drill guide over the head with its free edge parallel to the anatomic neck (Fig. 31-4A). The guide jig should be central on the humeral head, parallel to the anatomic neck with an equal amount of humeral head anteriorly and posteriorly (Fig. 31-4B–D), this automatically adjusts for version, inclination, and offset. Drill a guidewire through the center of the head and on through into the lateral humeral cortex, using the drill guide (Fig. 31-5A). Remove the guide jig and check the position of the guidewire visually as being in the center of the head (see Fig. 31-5B). If you believe that the guidewire is not central at this point, reposition it now.

When you believe that the guidewire is placed exactly central in the humeral head, drill the pilot hole with the correctly sized spade cutting drill (Fig. 31-6). All the sizes are color-coded (e.g., if the standard size is being used, then use the black guide, drill, shaper and trial prosthesis).

Having made the central peg hole, remove the guidewire. Ream the head with the appropriately sized reamer (Fig. 31-7A). The centralizing peg on the reamer is a sloppy fit in the pilot hole. Ream the head until reamings are seen exiting from all the holes in the shaper (Fig. 31-7B). Ideally, all remnants of articular and fibrocartilage should be removed and the subchondral bone left intact as far as possible. Save all the morselized bone generated for later grafting and mix it with the patient's blood scavenged from the wound.

Insert the trial component (Fig. 31-8). If only a hemiarthroplasty is to be done, test the stability of the humeral component and the range of movement. Check the tension of the subscapularis with the shoulder reduced to ensure adequate external rotation.

Glenoid Preparation. Leave the trial humeral component *in situ* so that the prepared head is not damaged by subsequent retraction. Retract the humeral head posteroinferiorly with a Murphy skid or Fukuda retractor. An extensive capsulotomy must be performed, sparing only the origin of biceps to provide adequate exposure of the glenoid (Fig. 31-9).

The decision concerning glenoid replacement is now made. My present management is to only replace the glenoid if the glenoid surface is noncongruent and there is sufficient bone to hold a glenoid component. Preoperative imaging using an axillary view radiograph and computed tomography is also helpful in this regard.

If glenoid replacement is not intended, it is my routine practice to drill the bone with a 2-mm drill bit repeatedly just through the hard osteochondral surface of the glenoid to induce bleeding and some fibrocartilagenous regeneration.

(text continues on page 615)

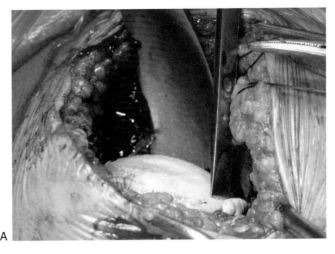

A

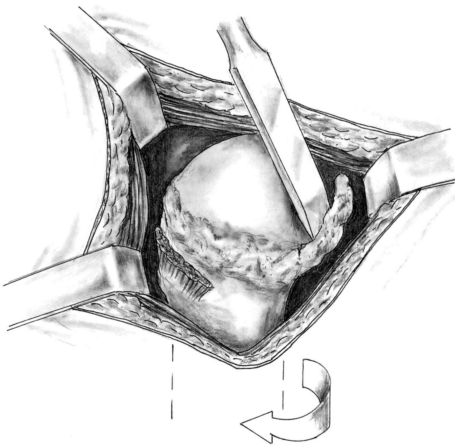

B

Figure 31-3. Copeland humeral component. **A:** The key for insertion of the humeral component is the anatomic neck of the humerus. This is more easily defined by removing all osteophytes. **B:** Removal of osteophytes may be made easier by rotation of the humeral head, thereby exposing the circumferential osteophytes. Osteophytes adjacent to the bicipital groove and tuberosities most clearly define the area of the anatomic neck.

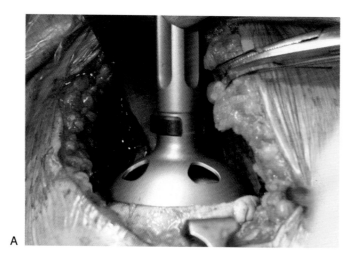

A

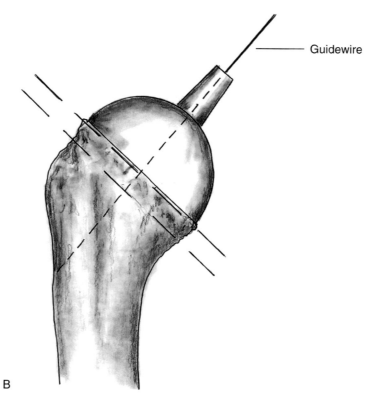

Guidewire

B

Figure 31-4. A: The humeral drill guide is placed over the humeral head, with its free edge parallel to the anatomic neck of the humerus. The guide position should be central on the humeral head and parallel to the anatomic neck, thus automatically adjusting for retroversion and inclination. **B:** In this position, a guidewire is drilled through the center of the head and into the lateral humeral cortex. *(continued)*

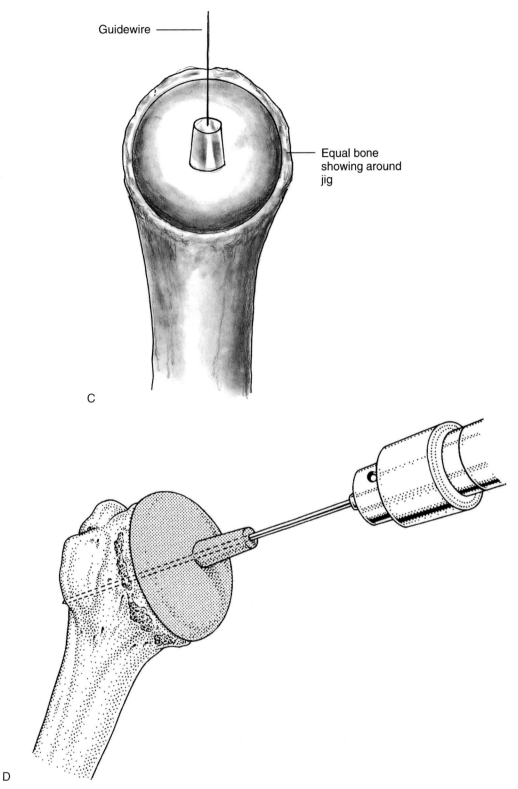

Figure 31-4. *Continued.* **C,D:** The guide jig should be central on the humeral head, with equal amounts of humeral head anteriorly and posteriorly.

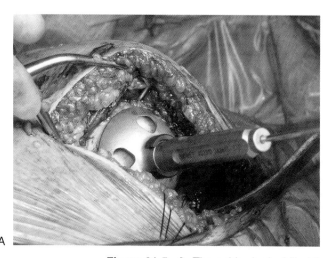
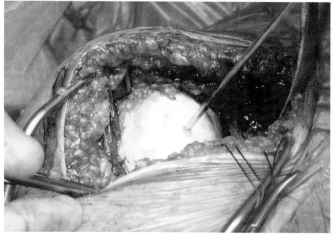

A

B

Figure 31-5. A: The guidewire is drilled through the center of the head and on into the lateral cortex. **B:** The guide is then removed and the position of the guidewire is visually confirmed. If the guidewire is not central, it is repositioned at this time.

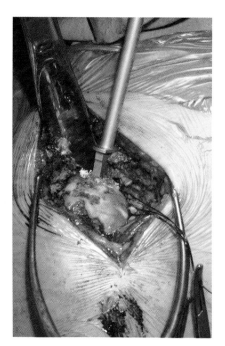

Figure 31-6. Once the position of the guidewire has been confirmed as being central in the humeral head, the pilot hole is drilled with the correctly sized spade cutting drill. All sizes are color-coded. For example, if a standard size is to be used, the surgeon will use the black guide, drill, shaper, and trial implant.

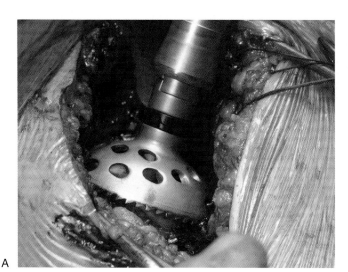

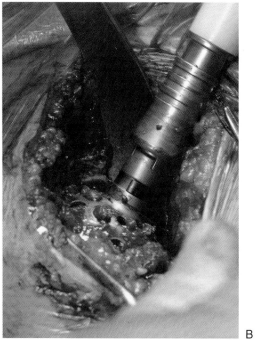

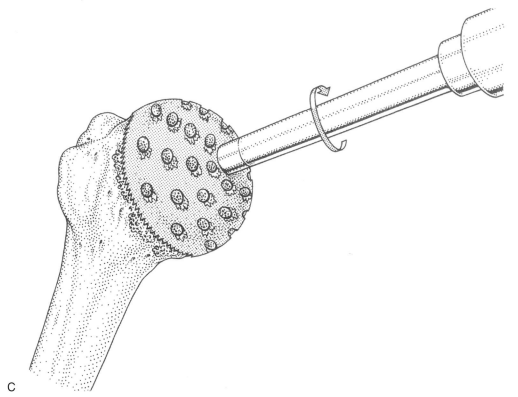

Figure 31-7. A: The humeral head. Once the central peg hole is made, the guidewire is removed, and the head is reamed with the appropriately sized reamer. The centralizing peg on the reamer is a "sloppy" fit in the pilot hole. **B:** Ream the head until reamings are seen exiting from all the holes in the shaper. This removes all remnants of articular and fibrocartilage, while leaving the subchondral bone intact. **C:** Bone can be seen extruding from the holes in the reamer.

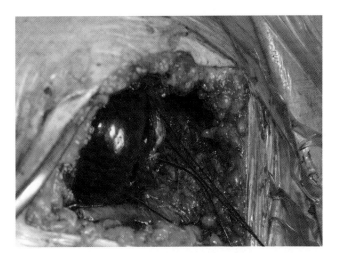

Figure 31-8. Trial humeral component is inserted. If a glenoid is not to be used, mobility and stability of the implant in all positions are recorded. With the humerus reduced in the glenoid, tension and ability to close the subscapularis tendon are checked; external rotation should be permitted with the subscapularis approximated to the point of its division.

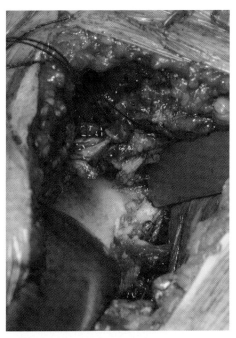

Figure 31-9. For adequate exposure of the glenoid, capsulotomy is usually performed. If inadequate exposure of the glenoid is present, more extensive capsulotomy is usually required. The humeral head may be retracted with a blunt retractor such as a Fukuda. The trial humeral component is left *in situ* so that the prepared head is not damaged by subsequent retraction during glenoid exposure.

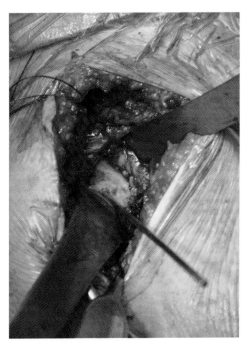

Figure 31-10. The glenoid drill guide is inserted to find the precise center of the glenoid. Osteophytes may confuse the surgeon as to the precise glenoid center.

Glenoid Replacement. Apply the glenoid drill guide (left or right) to determine the center of the glenoid. Palpate the base of the coracoid and drill the guidewire from the center of the glenoid face toward the base of the coracoid and just through the cortical bone (Fig. 31-10). If the guidewire passes through both cortices, this gives it stability for the pilot drill. Pass the appropriately sized cannulated spade drill over the guidewire and drill the pilot hole for the glenoid peg (Fig. 31-11). Save all bone reamings for grafting. Prepare the glenoid articular surface with the glenoid surface shaper placed in this pilot hole (Fig. 31-12). If glenoid erosion is asymmetric, anterior or posterior grafting may be required, but this is very rare. It is better to ream down the high side than graft the low side if this is possible.

In primary and secondary osteoarthritis, retain as much as possible of the hard subchondral surface of bone to provide a firm foundation for the prosthesis. If there is a large surface of hard sclerotic bone, this is made more reactive by drilling multiple holes with a 2-mm drill (Fig. 31-13). Once again, do a trial reduction and test for range and stability.

Mix the bone harvested from the drill holes and reaming with the scavenged blood. Apply the "paste" graft mix to the hydroxyapatite-coated surface of the glenoid component (Fig. 31-14) and impact it flush with the surface of the bone using the impactor (Fig. 31-15A) and two or three smart blows with the mallet. Irrigate away the excess bone paste to prevent new bone formation and ensure that the prosthesis is solidly fixed (Fig. 31-15B).

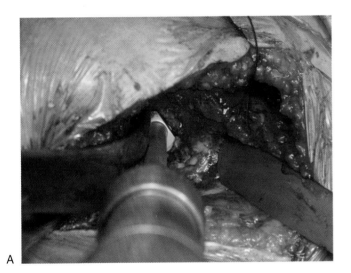

A

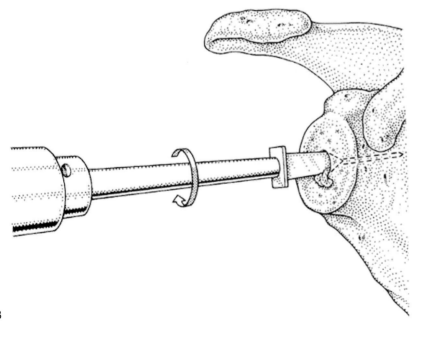

B

Figure 31-11. A: The cannulated spade drill has passed over the guidewire and the pilot hole for the pegged glenoid is made. **B:** All bone reamings are preserved for grafting and the glenoid face is contoured to accept the implant.

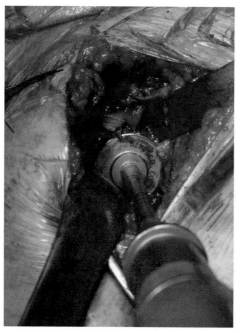

Figure 31-12. The glenoid articular surface is prepared, with the glenoid surface shaper placed in the original pilot hole. Assessment should be made as to asymmetric wear in the glenoid. If there is wear on the glenoid (such as occurs with osteoarthritis), symmetric reaming may be used to even the two sides so that the implant sits precisely on subchondral bone anteriorly and posteriorly. While glenoid bone grafting may be considered, it is usually not needed. Satisfactory subchondral seating of the implant can usually be achieved by asymmetric reaming of the glenoid face.

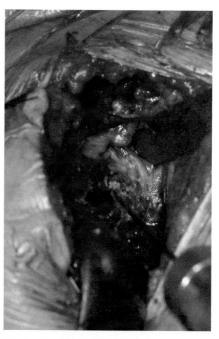

Figure 31-13. It is helpful to retain subchondral surface of the bone as much as possible to provide a firm foundation for the prosthesis. Drilling of multiple holes through the exposed surface may encourage growth into the implant.

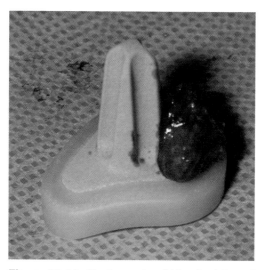

Figure 31-14. Paste made of blood, clot, and harvested bones is applied to the coated surface of the glenoid component.

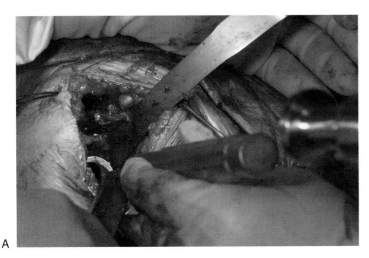

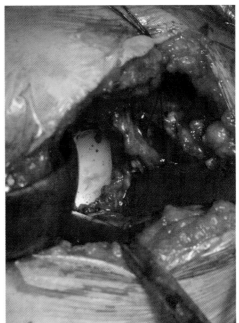

A

Figure 31-15. A: The glenoid component is inserted using the glenoid impactor. **B:** A prosthesis is then examined to make certain that it is solidly fixed, seating on subchondral bone, and excessive bone paste is irrigated and removed.

B

Now turn attention to the humerus again and do multiple 2-mm drill holes just through the sclerotic subchondral bone to make this more reactive (Fig. 31-16). Similarly, empty the bone-graft mix into the humeral cap component (Fig. 31-17) and finger press it into the pilot hole and again impact it with the mallet (Fig. 31-18). Irrigate excess bone away. Reduce the joint and test for stability again.

Closure. As the center of rotation may have been lateralized, make an attempt to gain relative length in subscapularis either with a stepwise cut in the tendon or by medialization of the insertion of subscapularis to the free edge of the prosthesis. Close only the lateral part of the rotator interval. If there is any rotator cuff deficiency, and this is repairable, repair it at this stage. Capsulotomy or sutures may be required at this stage to balance the reduction.

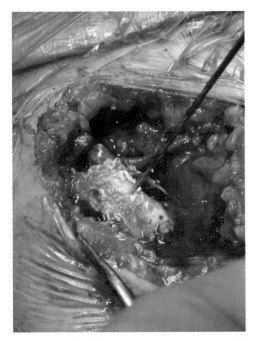

Figure 31-16. Subchondral humeral bone is drilled with a spaced, 2-mm drill.

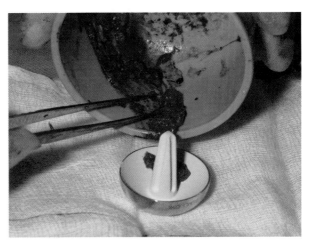

Figure 31-17. The bone graft/clot/blood mix is packed into the coated surface of the humeral implant.

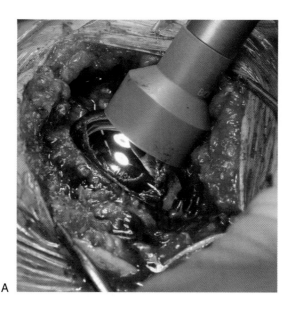

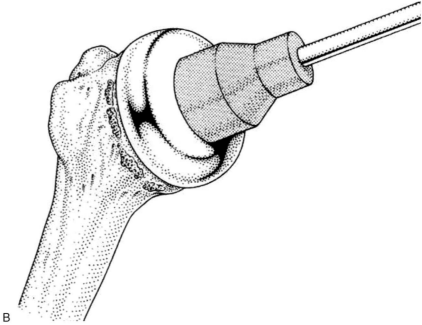

Figure 31-18. A: The humeral component is "finger pressed" into the pilot hole and held in place with the inserter. **B:** Using the humeral head impactor, a solid seating of the humeral component is ensured.

POSTOPERATIVE MANAGEMENT

Only allow passive movement for the first 48 hours and passive assisted for five days. Begin active movements at one week if pain allows and discard the sling at 3 weeks. Encourage the patient to stretch and strengthen for many months as improvement will continue up to 1 year postoperatively.

COMPLICATIONS

In a personal series, complications included the following:

- Myositis ossificans—0.7%
- Aseptic loosening—5.1% (before hydroxyapatite coating, 0% since hydroxyapatite coating)

- Periprosthetic fracture—0.7% (at anatomic neck)
- Deep infection—0.7%

RESULTS

More than 400 surface-replacement arthroplasties have been implanted in our unit.

The results of the Mark 2 design (before hydroxyapatite coating) were published in 2001 (4). One hundred three shoulders were implanted into 94 patients (nine bilateral). There were 73 women and 21 men. The mean age at the time of surgery was 64.3 years (range, 22 to 88 years). Total shoulder replacement was used in 68 cases and hemiarthroplasty in 35. The average length of follow-up was 6.8 years (range, 5 to 10 years).

Constant Scores

The preoperative average Constant Score (functional score as a percentage) was 15.4 points or 24% after adjustments for age and gender. Best results were achieved in cases of primary osteoarthritis with Constant scores of 93.7% for total shoulder replacement and 76% for rheumatoid. The poorest results were encountered in patients with cuff arthropathy, instability arthropathy, and other causes (arthropathy, post septic arthritis) with adjusted Constant Scores of 61.3%, 62.7%, and 58.7%, respectively. Active elevation improved by an average of 69 degrees to an average of 133 degrees for osteoarthritis and avascular necrosis and to an average of 105 degrees for rheumatoid arthritis. For instability arthropathy and cuff arthropathy, this increased to an average of 97 degrees and 73 degrees, respectively. Preoperative and postoperative differences were statistically significant for all the disease groups ($p<0.001$).

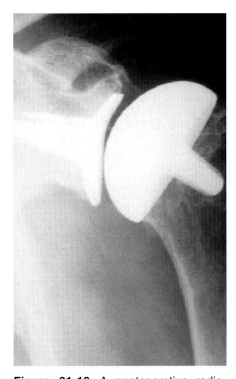

Figure 31-19. A postoperative radiograph of a surface-replacement humerus and glenoid. Note the absence of radiolucent lines and the apparent apposition of bone to the implant surface, and the excellent remaining bone stock.

Radiographic Results

There was a 5.1% incidence of progressive lucent lines of more than 2 mm, with signs of definite loosening in three glenoids. The relevance of the radiolucent line is uncertain, but seems unrelated to the clinical outcome and is obviously of long-term concern. In five shoulders, some degree of mild humeral prosthesis subsidence was found. There seemed to be no effect of the mild subsidence on the clinical result (Fig. 31-19).

Since using the hydroxyapatite-coated implants, no lucent lines have been observed and no loosening has occurred.

The revision rate at 5 to 10 years of using the Mark 2 design has been 5.9%. The indications have included the following:

1. Instability
2. One case of periprosthetic fracture
3. One case of disassociation of the polyethylene glenoid from the metal part of the glenoid component (obviated by immediate design change)
4. One case of glenoid fracture/loosening following a fall
5. Two cases of aseptic loosening

Revision surgery was greatly simplified because of initial bone preservation. At the time of revision of a surface-replacement arthroplasty, the only bone lost was the bone that would have been removed had a stemmed prosthesis been used at the first operation.

RECOMMENDED READING

1. Antuna, S.A., Sperling, J.W., Cofield, R.H., et al.: Glenoid revision surgery after total shoulder arthroplasty. *J Shoulder Elbow Surg* 10(3): 217–224, 2001.
2. Cofield, R.H., Edgerton, B.C.: Total shoulder arthroplasty: complications and revision surgery. *Instr Course Lect* 39: 449–462, 1990.
3. Copeland S.A. Cementless surface replacement arthroplasty. In: Copeland, S.A., ed.: *Operative shoulder surgery*. Churchill Livingstone, 1995.
4. Levy, O., Copeland, S.A.: Cementless surface replacement arthroplasty of the shoulder. 5- to 10-year results with the Copeland Mark-2 prosthesis. *J Bone Joint Surg Br* 83(2): 213–221, 2001.
5. Mackenzie, D.B.: The anterosuperior exposure of a total shoulder replacement. *Orthop Traumatol* 2: 71–77, 1993.
6. Roberts, S.N.J., Swallow, H.M., Wallace, W.A., et al.: The geometry of the humeral head and the design of prostheses. *J Bone Joint Surg Br* 73: 647–650, 1991.
7. Rydholm, U, Sjögren, J.: Surface replacement of the humeral head in the rheumatoid shoulder. *J Shoulder Elbow Surg* 2: 286–295, 1993.
8. Walch, G., Boileau, P.: Prosthetic adaptability: a new concept for shoulder arthroplasty. *J Shoulder Elbow Surg* 8(5): 443–451, 1999.
9. Wirth, M.A., Rockwood, C.A. Jr.: Complications of shoulder arthroplasty. *Clin Orthop* 307: 47–69, 1994.

32

Revision Shoulder Arthroplasty

Tom R. Norris and Stephen B. Gunther

Approximately 25,000 shoulder arthroplasty surgeries are performed in the United States per year, with an increase annually. In 2002, 16,840 humeral head and 8,150 total shoulder arthroplasties were carried out. The 35% of total shoulder arthroplasties also are increasing annually. The most common indications for these procedures are osteoarthritis and fractures. As the numbers of arthroplasties increase each year, the numbers of complications that require revision surgery increase. There are four major causes for revisions. An increasing number of total shoulders have been in long enough for polyethylene wear to become a significant issue. Component materials and nonanatomic designs are two issues that were likely a step backward during the second-generation designs. Lastly, with 80% to 85% of surgeons performing only one to three shoulder revisions each year, many of the technical points of shoulder reconstructions are often not as well appreciated or executed as by those who perform a larger volume.

In assessing the multiple reasons for failure in a given case, one must consider issues from material wear to surgical errors in prosthetic size and position and in choices when patient tissues are compromised. For example, stiffness may be from an oversized or proud prosthesis or from inadequate rehabilitation. Cuff dehiscence may occur from a proud prosthesis with areas of contracture as the prosthesis is forced away from areas of tightness. Often, multiple reasons are identified for a given revision. The causes are not necessarily the same in each case; thus, classification and treatment recommendations are difficult. All of the failure mechanisms must be addressed to produce the most successful result.

T. R. Norris, M.D.: Department of Orthopaedics, University of California, San Francisco; and Department of Orthopaedic Surgery, California Pacific Medical Center, San Francisco, California.

S. B. Gunther, M.D.: Department of Orthopaedics, California Pacific Medical Center, San Francisco, California.

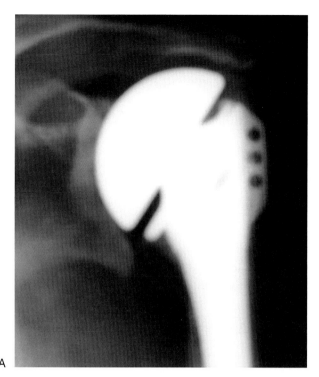

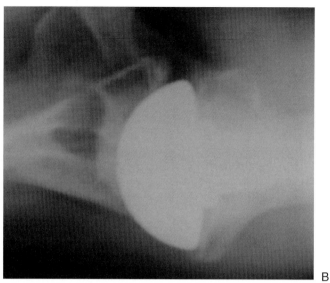

A

B

Figure 32-1. **A:** Glenoid arthritis rapidly developed following a humeral head replacement. **B:** An axillary view demonstrates the posterior glenoid erosion. These views are preoperative for a conversion to total shoulder replacement for glenoid arthritis.

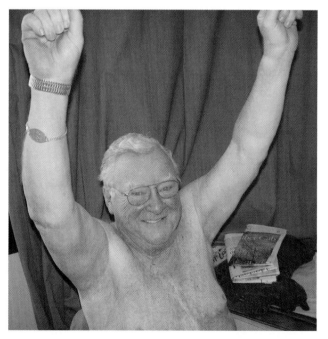

Figure 32-2. Elevation is successful after his conversion for bilateral glenoid arthritis from humeral head replacement to total shoulder replacement in a paraplegic poliomyelitis victim. His rehabilitation was complicated by the need to avoid use of the operated arm for transfers for up to 6 months after surgery to protect his repairs.

INDICATIONS/CONTRAINDICATIONS

The decision to revise a previous shoulder arthroplasty is based primarily on pain, obvious pathology, and sometimes, on loss of function. Radiographic evidence of pending precipitous failure with extensive osteolysis most frequently precedes significant clinical symptoms. Does one proceed with a complicated revision maximizing the chance there is still enough bone for an exchange of the glenoid, or wait for pain with more glenoid bone loss, which may include the anterior or posterior wall? Patients need to have as clear an understanding as possible as to the consequences of proceeding with revision surgery. In addition, they should understand whether the condition will worsen in the absence of any intervention. The most common cause for revision of a humeral head replacement (HHR) is glenoid arthrosis (Fig. 32-1). Levine et al.(7) at Columbia have shown that HHRs alone, with uneven posterior glenoid erosion, fare poorly. The HHRs as a group show progressive deterioration with midterm 3- to 5-year follow-up in their subsequent report. In these patients, conversion to a total shoulder replacement (TSR) is the treatment that has the best chance of relieving pain, but the results are not as stellar as the total shoulder as an incident procedure (Fig. 32-2).

The most common early cause for the revision of a TSR and the third most common cause for revision of a humeral head is instability (Fig. 32-3). Later, stiffness, rotator cuff tears, glenoid loosening, humeral loosening, and complications related to polyethylene wear with osteolysis lead to revision surgery and become more critical (Fig. 32-4).

In prosthetic fracture reconstruction, dehiscence of the greater tuberosity is the most frequent cause for failure (Fig. 32-5). Sutures placed through the unpolished holes in a prosthetic keel may easily break, leading to early loss of tuberosity fixation (Fig. 32-6). Sutures placed around the polished calcar provide more secure fixation for fracture healing without the stress riser rupturing the sutures (Fig. 32-7). Other indications for revision surgery include prosthetic malposition, periprosthetic fracture, and infection. Each of these complications requires a stepwise approach during preoperative planning, operative execution, and postoperative rehabilitation.

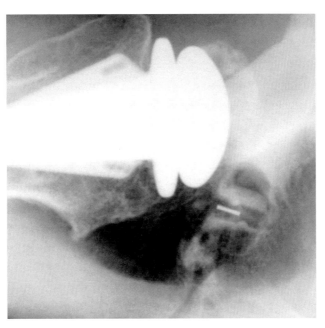

Figure 32-3. Anterior dislocation, subscapularis dehiscence, and glenoid loosening are a terrible triad following a total shoulder arthroplasty.

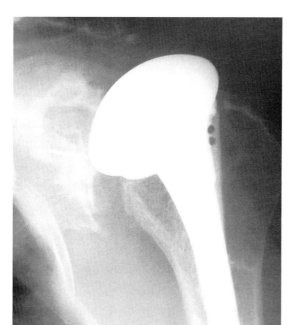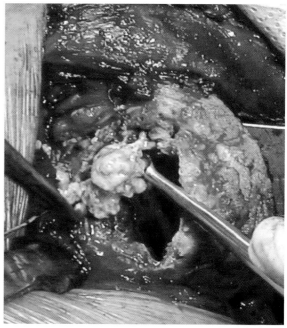

A   B

Figure 32-4. A: Osteolysis is secondary to hylamer polyethylene wear. The proud humeral prosthesis is associated with stiffness and is a second cause for more rapid wear. **B:** Humeral osteolysis requires exchange of the component and removal of the reactive tissue from the humeral metaphysis and the glenoid cavity.

Relative contraindications include the following:

Infection. One will consider a primary or delayed exchange, but rarely would one consider an irrigation and débridement while leaving the prosthesis *in situ*. A simple incision and drainage might be considered only for an acute infection with a low-virulence organism. Chronic infections usually require revision surgery with implant removal with or without an antibiotic spacer followed by a secondary exchange 12 weeks later (Fig. 32-8).

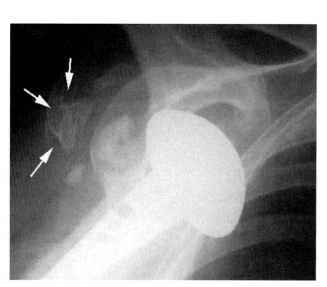

Figure 32-5. The greater tuberosity dehiscence with anterior dislocation of humeral head replacement for fracture reconstruction occurred from use of suture fixation through the unpolished holes in the humeral component.

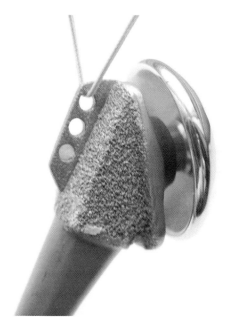

Figure 32-6. Sutures through the stress riser (unpolished holes in the humeral fin) lead to early tuberosity dehiscence.

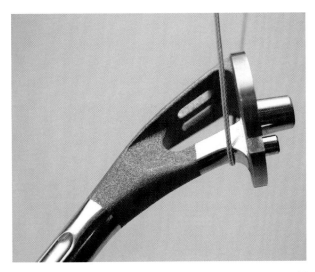

Figure 32-7. Sutures placed around smooth calcar avoid the stress riser of the fin holes and avoid early breakage.

Rotator Cuff Deficiency. With irreparable cuff deficiency, a revision to a standard TSR is contraindicated. Because the cuff cannot center the humeral head in the glenoid, a rocking-horse phenomenon occurs with subsequent glenoid loosening followed by pain. Other options are conversion to an HHR if the glenoid is loose or a reverse prosthesis if adequate bone is or can be made available to hold the base plate for the glenoid sphere.

Deficient Glenoid Bone Stock. Insufficient bone stock to resurface the glenoid is another contraindication for glenoid resurfacing. Alternatively, one may choose to bone graft the glenoid deficit and convert to a humeral head or TSR.

Medical Comorbidities. Severe medical conditions should be considered. Advanced cardiac disease may preclude revision surgery in a patient that otherwise would qualify for

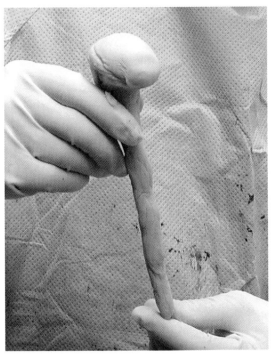
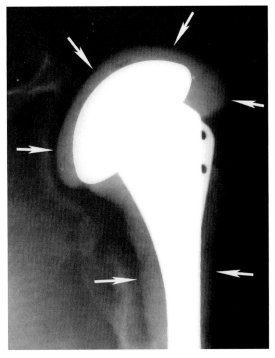

A   B

Figure 32-8. A: An antibiotic methylmethycrylate spacer is created over an undersized humeral prosthesis. **B:** The temporary antibiotic spacer permits placing the greater tuberosity out to length for 3 months while awaiting clearing of the infection. *(continued)*

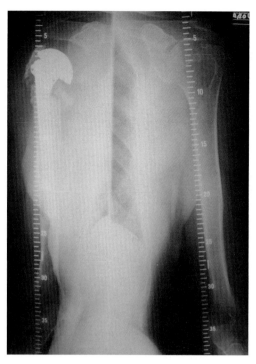

C

Figure 32-8. *Continued.* **C:** Scanograms allow comparison of the height of the humeral prosthesis with the opposite side. In this case, there is low placement of the humeral head replacement in a four-part fracture reconstruction complicated by a greater tuberosity dehiscence and sepsis.

the procedure. Uncontrollable alcoholism or other personality disorders may preclude the cooperation needed for the complicated rehabilitation postoperatively.

PREOPERATIVE PLANNING

In all revision cases, the type of prosthesis to be removed should be identified if possible by radiographs and/or previous operative reports. Bone stock should be assessed with the plain films or a computed tomography (CT) scan. If there appears to be an abnormality in the height of the prosthesis, bilateral humeral scanograms assist in differentiating prosthetic malposition or subsidence from muscular atony figure (Fig. 32-8C). A preoperative CT scan also can facilitate in determining glenoid bone version as well as depth of bone that might hold a glenoid component.

Preoperative assessment with electromyography and nerve conduction studies not only permits the surgeon to be aware of the prerevision nerve status, it also may protect the surgeon after the revision surgery from complex medicolegal issues that might later arise in the event the changes predate the revision. Lynch et al. (8) reviewed 417 TSRs and found a 4% incidence of neurologic complications. The long deltopectoral approach, use of methotrexate, and shorter operations were found to be significant risk factors. Neurologic recovery was rated "good" in most (11 of 16) patients.

A cell saver is routinely used for return of the patient's own blood if there is sufficient intraoperative loss. This has proven superior to having the patient predonate blood and then start the procedure with the patient having a depleted hematocrit.

Special gouges and punches should be available. The most effective leverage point for prosthetic removal is an upward disimpaction blow on the calcar area of the prosthesis (Fig.

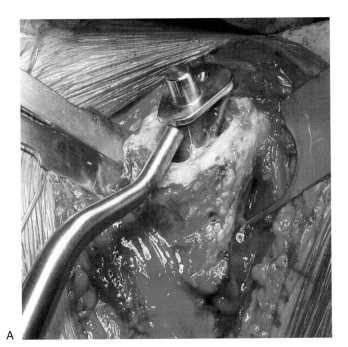
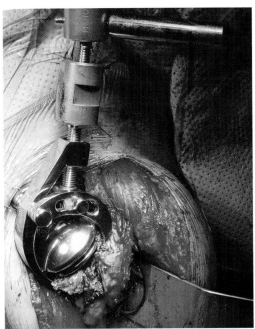

A   B

Figure 32-9. A: The calcar provides the best purchase for prosthesis extraction with a punch. **B:** A universal head and collar grasper attached to a slap hammer is useful when one wishes to avoid potential bone loss at the calcar.

32-9A). Alternatively, devices that grasp the head or stem attached to a slap hammer provide a longitudinal extraction force but without as much power as the calcar-placed punch (Fig. 32-9B). Long- and extralong-stem humeral implants, cerclage cables, and allograft bone struts are available for revision cases to create a stable shaft.

SURGERY

Most failed arthroplasties have stiffness as a significant component. If this is the only identifiable reason and if the patient has been unable to make any headway with physical therapy, a release without violating the cuff attachments would permit therapy to be restarted the day following surgery. Having scratched the pristine humeral head with the metal arthroscopic sheath in a tight shoulder, I would caution against this or any other technique that might damage the surfaces of the polyethylene or humeral components. For stiffness alone, if the disability is significant enough to require additional surgery, the deltopectoral approach permits lysis of any extraarticular adhesions with a wide opening of the rotator interval with preservation of the cuff attachments for intraarticular releases. The subacromial space is freed with blunt and sharp dissection back to the scapular spine. The coracoid base is freed of the coracohumeral ligament. The superficial subscapularis tendon is separated from the undersurface of the coracoid muscles. The coracoacromial ligament is initially left in place early in the exposure in the event that there is a cuff-deficient shoulder to prevent anterosuperior humeral head escape.

The axillary nerve is dissected free of the subscapularis and gently retracted when the entire inferior capsule is released from the humerus. The long head of the biceps is identified as an anatomic landmark between the greater and lesser tuberosities. As loose bodies, spurs in the biceps groove, and fraying of the tendon can contribute to postoperative pain, release or tenodesis avoids an additional cause of postoperative pain.

Through the rotator interval opening, all capsular attachments around the glenoid can be elevated. Exposure is provided with inferior traction on the humerus with the arm placed in the McConnell arm holder. This accomplishes what can be done with the cuff attachments intact and release of all intraarticular adhesions (Fig. 32-10A). Assuming the glenoid is intact, closure with plans for early motion is in order.

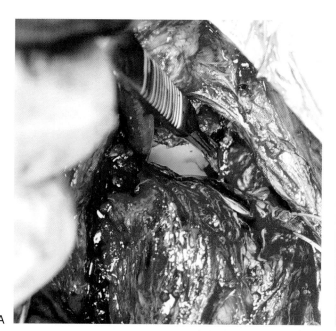
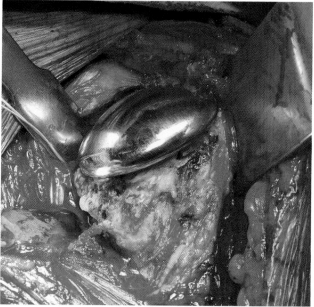

A

B

Figure 32-10. A: Through the deltopectoral and rotator intervals, all capsular attachments are released without any muscle detachments. If necessary, the subscapularis can be elevated from the scapular neck and the posterior structures are elevated short of the suprascapular nerve to restore the anteroposterior glide. This permits the head to be centered again by overcoming the obligate translations that occur when one side remains too tight. **B:** Elevate the entire inferior humeral capsule in the calcar area. This assists in releases for the humerus and is the first step in an adequate glenoid exposure. Avoiding injury to the axillary nerve is crucial because it is the midway between the humeral and glenoid insertions of the capsule.

For additional procedures, the subscapularis is elevated while leaving 1 cm of distal attachment on the lesser tuberosity. Removal of the entire tendon from bone with the recession of the insertion at closure only serves to weaken the internal rotators and provides less tissue to heal the subscapularis. If possible, subscapularis dehiscence is to be avoided. This begins with the operative approach. The inferior capsule and both the upper portions of the pectoralis and latissimus dorsi are released (Fig. 32-10B).

In revisions, a humeral component may need extraction because of an overly large collar, improper head size, or malposition. Once the subscapularis is open and retracted, the

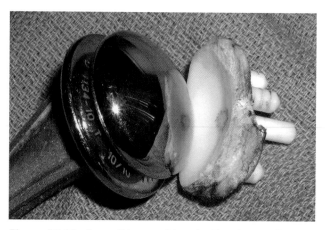

Figure 32-11. A small humeral head with a larger diameter humeral collar impinges on the glenoid. This results in erosion and rapid destruction of the polyethylene component.

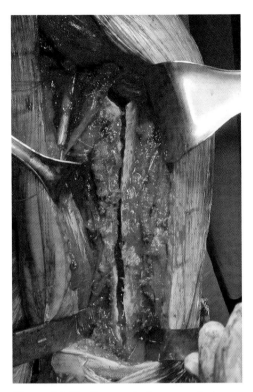

Figure 32-12. Removal of a cemented prosthesis may be difficult. An episiotomy or controlled longitudinal split of the shaft with a side-cutting burr avoids unnecessary fragmentation of the shaft. Reconstruction is possible around a new prosthesis with cables with or without bone grafts.

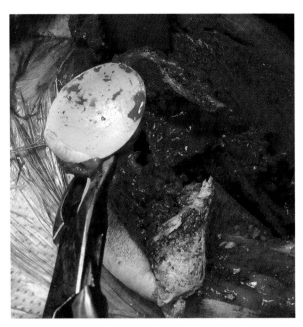

Figure 32-13. Removal of loose glenoid component and débridement of any soft tissue underneath prepare the remaining glenoid cavity for glenoid bone grafting and conversion of a total shoulder replacement to a humeral head replacement.

humeral prosthesis can be approached with an extraction device if the manufacturer has one available. An overlarge collar on the humeral stem compared to the head size will destroy the glenoid (Fig. 32-11). The advantages of modularity are lost if the prosthesis is too high, too low, or malrotated. The entire stem needs to be removed. Extraction of the humeral implant is facilitated by loosening the proximal fixation with flexible and rigid osteotomes and the Ultradrive (Biomet, Inc., Warsaw, IN) ultrasonic cement removal system. If the component is extremely well fixed distally, an extended episiotomy of the humeral shaft facilitates removal while avoiding uncontrolled comminuted humeral shaft fractures (Fig. 32-12). In case of sepsis, this may facilitate removal of all the foreign-body cement and scar in preparation for antibiotic treatment. A high-speed burr such as the Midas Rex (Medtronic, Fort Worth, TX) should be available to split the humerus from the lateral aspect of the biceps groove, down the humerus, and past the tip of the prosthesis. Ideally, the pectoralis insertion is left with the medial fragment. This spares the bone infinitely more than the piecemeal comminution with repetitive impacts in removal of stem that is well fixed with bone ingrowth or cement. Long humeral stems should be available to bypass the tip of the prosthesis by two to three humeral diameters. Cerclage cables securely close the osteotomy. Cortical allograft bone struts give the option for additional fixation while dispersing the force on any specific point of fixation.

If the humeral component is well aligned and well fixed, it is advisable to change only the modular humeral head. This avoids the problem of humeral shaft fracture. Many current prostheses allow adaptations of humeral head coverage and translation through more anatomic eccentric humeral head placement.

The glenoid component should be carefully examined for loosening and for signs of wear. Loose glenoid components should be removed (Fig. 32-13). There are also some ex-

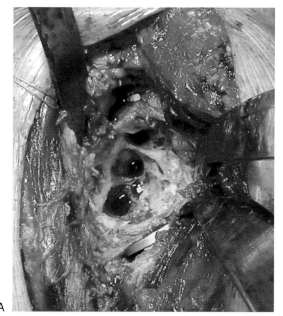

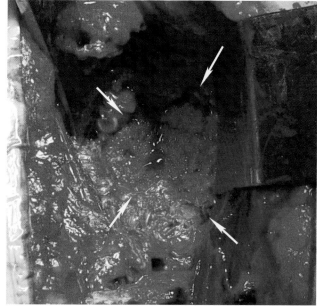

A

B

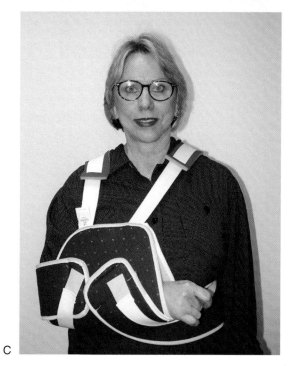

C

Figure 32-14. A: A cavernous defect is left in the glenoid from hylamer osteolysis once all the reactive tissue is removed. **B:** Autogenous or allograft bone graft is tightly impacted into the glenoid cavity. **C:** A Zimmer sling provides upward support in the early postoperative period.

amples of well-fixed glenoid implants with significant wear that continue to shed particulate debris, causing osteolysis. These implants may need to be removed as well. In general, better results with pain relief and motion can be obtained if the glenoid can be reimplanted. However, the entire glenoid vault may be absent with more advanced loosening and severe osteolysis. As this worsens, the anteroposterior scapular cortical wall deficiencies may progressively develop. (Fig. 32-14). If there is not enough good bone for glenoid exchange with recementing, meticulously clean out all the fibrous tissue and cement and then impact firmly the glenoid vault with autograft or allograft bone chips, preferably with one's favorite bone morphogenic protein (Fig. 32-14B). This permits bone incorporation and glenohumeral stability to be restored. There is recent work on containing the bone graft with impaction and acellular jackets. The glenoid can be resurfaced with a new component 6 months to a year later in the infrequent cases in which patients complain of ongoing pain.

In cases of glenohumeral instability, one should ensure that anatomic humeral version and height have been restored. It is not desirable to overstuff the shoulder joint with a large humeral head or increase the lateral offset due to the additional gap added when there is a space between the head and the stem that was present in some of the second-generation prostheses. Instead, it is preferable to balance the soft tissue anteriorly and posteriorly. Anterior instability is often addressed with a repair of the subscapularis. In my experience, a shoulder is rarely unstable anteriorly without dehiscence of a portion or the entire subscapularis tendon. Fixation of the subscapularis should be performed through drill holes in bone and to any remaining laterally based tendon. In more extreme situations, subscapularis deficiencies require a pectoralis transfer, a hamstring tendon graft, or an Achilles-calcaneal allograft fixed to the scapular neck and humerus (Figs. 32-15 and 32-16). Fixation of tissue to the prosthesis alone is not a viable method for healing.

The most common cause for a posterior instability is a stretched out posterior capsule with or without alterations of glenoid version (Fig. 32-17). Neither may have been addressed with the primary surgery. If there is no glenoid resurfacing to be done, sutures in the mid-posterior capsule to the labrum or posterior glenoid will tighten the posterior capsule to restore stability (Fig. 32-18). This is anticipated at the incident procedure in osteoarthritis with posterior glenoid wear in which the posterior capsule has been stretched out and the anterior capsule is too tight. The anterior capsule needs to be released from the anterior scapular neck to prevent this tight anterior structure from pushing the head backward, and the posterior capsule needs to be tightened to balance the humeral component over the glenoid. One can readily understand that using an oversized component to achieve posterior stability will only make the tight anterior structures more difficult to close. Instead, the posterior capsule can also be shifted superiorly through drill holes in the posterior glenoid rim if necessary. At the same time, the correct version is restored. A glenoid is added if the cuff is repairable and there is adequate scapular bone remaining to seat a component. The depth of the scapular neck often can be determined with preoperative CT scans.

For inferior instability, the usual cause is a low-set prosthesis. Scanograms can be used to compare ipsilateral and contralateral humeral lengths. Correction of the deformity would

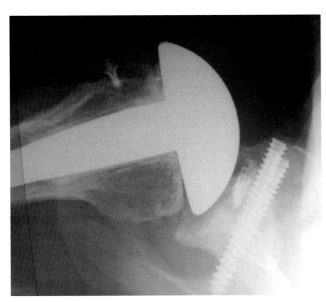

Figure 32-15. A calcaneal-Achilles allograft and a pectoralis subcoracoid transfer are substituted for an irretrievable subscapularis for anterior stability.

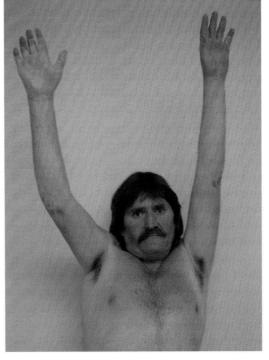

Figure 32-16. Elevation following pectoralis transfer and calcaneal-Achilles allograft is functional but not complete.

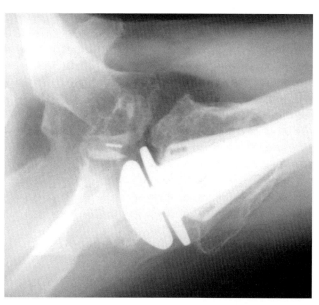

Figure 32-17. Posterior subluxation and glenoid loosening occur if the glenoid version is not restored and the capsular laxity is not corrected at the incident replacement.

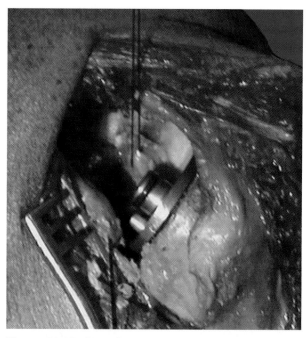

Figure 32-18. Posterior capsular plication from the deltopectoral approach permits reduction of the stretched out capsule with a series of sutures from the mid capsule to the labrum.

then require a humeral revision. Rarely, an inferior capsular shift is required. Consider and evaluate the axillary nerve function as another cause for inferior subluxation with a humeral component out to length. For a humeral prosthesis of proper height with early postoperative inferior subluxation, upward support with a special sling is usually sufficient.

Revision for rotator cuff tears requires an appreciation of the size or number of tendons and chronicity of the tear as well as the possibility of coexisting lesions in the shoulder. If it is clear that no other problem exists other than rotator cuff tear, one might consider using an anterosuperior rotator cuff approach. I personally have been less happy with the mini-open deltoid split approach because of damage to an overly retracted deltoid that may occur when exposure is suboptimal. A 3-cm deltoid elevation off the anterolateral acromion requires no additional time for healing than does the cuff repair. For an isolated supraspinatus tear, repair with standard rotator cuff techniques would be appropriate. However, if there is a problem with the humeral component or glenoid component, return to the deltopectoral approach, remove the humeral head, and repair the rotator cuff repair through the larger opening from below. This permits more options for transfers without endangering the axillary nerve.

Of increasing concern has been the vertically fixed position with subsequent rotator cuff ruptures seen in the bipolar prostheses (Fig. 32-19). These have no easy Food and Drug Administration (FDA)–approved treatment, but the custom reverse prosthesis holds promise, and has been the practice in Europe for the past 15 years (Figs. 32-20 and 32-21). In my experience as well as that of Walch, in revising similar cases with both a deficient glenoid from prior osteolysis or hypoplasia and a deficient rotator cuff, glenoid bone grafting and supplemental acromial support with an extra bar and screws for the glenoid sphere has proven satisfactory in four custom cases (Fig. 32-22). Mechanical loosening has been implicated as the primary cause of glenoid implant failure. However, recent reports have also documented polyethylene wear mechanisms, particulate debris, and osteolysis in the shoulder. Clinically, these patients usually present with months of gradually increasing pain, loss of motion, and radiographic findings that are suspicious for glenoid loosening. Micronsized polyethylene particles can be seen microscopically using polarized light. Grossly, slivers to fragmented portions may be seen (Fig. 32-23). This process, a particulate-induced

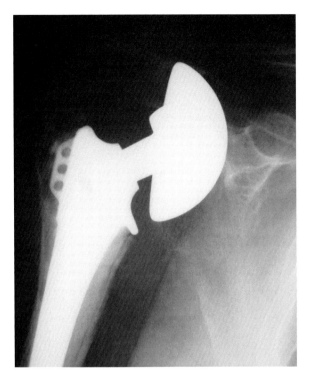

Figure 32-19. The nonanatomic bipolar prosthesis assumes a vertically fixed position and proceeds to rupture the superior cuff.

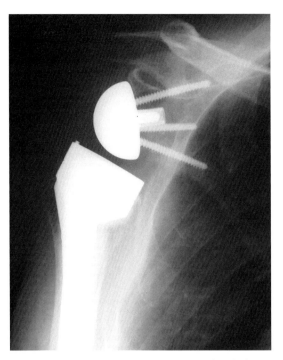

Figure 32-20. A custom reverse prosthesis is an option for revision of a bipolar prosthesis with a cuff that is not reconstructable.

foreign-body reaction mediated by giant cells, produces an inflammatory reaction that weakens soft tissues and progressively destroys bone. The hylamer glenoid implants are especially susceptible to this destructive process. It is not currently known whether this wear pattern is a result of the hylamer material, oxidation resulting from the sterilization process, or, more likely, from a combination of the two. In retrieval studies at U.C. Berkeley by

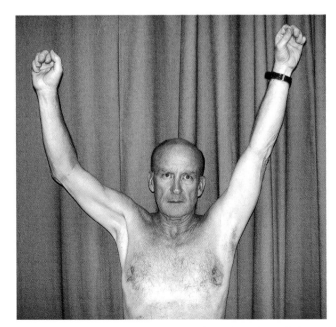

Figure 32-21. Elevation restored and pain relief are achieved at 1-year follow-up with the custom prosthesis for an irreparable cuff.

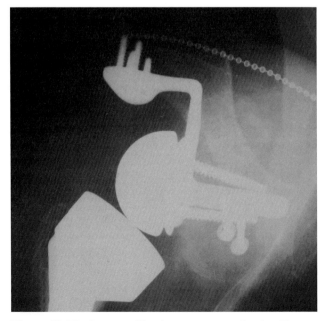

Figure 32-22. A custom Tornier reverse prosthesis with supplemental acromial support is used when there is significant glenoid deficiency.

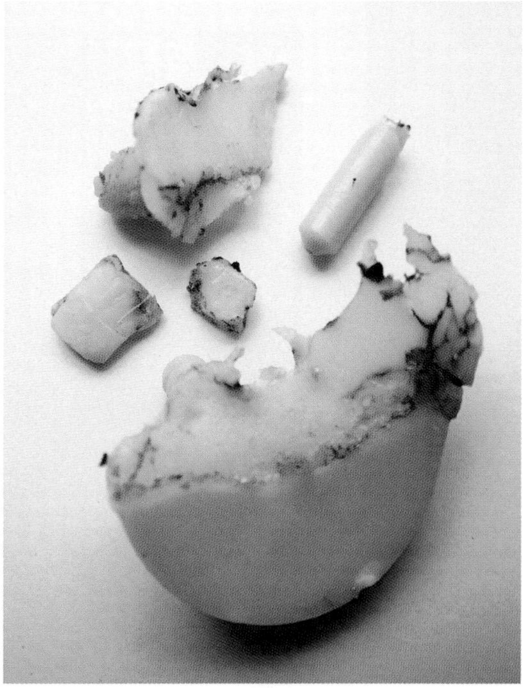

Figure 32-23. The hylamer glenoid has fragmented after 5 years in place.

Gunther et al. (5), hylamer with any forms of sterilization has lasted only half the time of other polyethylenes. The surgeon must beware that plain radiographs usually underestimate the amount of bone destruction. This has important implications in the timing for revisions. Removal of the failed glenoid component is necessary. Removal of the humeral component may also be necessary because of humeral osteolysis and subsequent implant loosening. One does not wish to leave this reactive tissue behind to continue its destructive

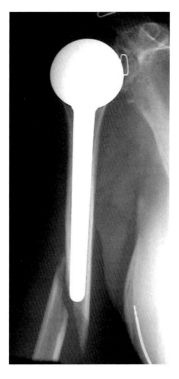

Figure 32-24. Periprosthetic fracture at the tip of the prosthesis is unstable.

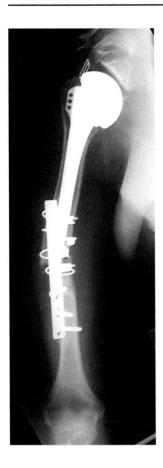

Figure 32-25. Plates with cables or screws above and screws below may not provide adequate fixation for healing.

process with the newly implanted components. Bone grafts and revision implants should be available for these cases.

Periprosthetic fractures can occur during the primary procedure. Intraoperative fractures are usually caused by overzealous reaming of the humeral canal, torque on the humerus during glenoid preparation, or hoop stresses during forceful impaction of a humeral prosthesis (Fig. 32-24). These fractures should be addressed at the time of the primary procedure. Immediate exchange with a longer-stem prosthesis and multiple cables restores enough stability to allow normal postoperative rehabilitation. This is preferred to using a plate that overlaps the humeral stem but has poor purchase on the proximal fragment (Fig. 32-25).

For postoperative fractures, the surgeon must determine the stability of the prosthesis and the site of the fracture relative to the prosthesis. Many fractures associated with a well-fixed prosthesis proximal to the tip can be treated nonoperatively. A fracture associated with a loose prosthesis requires revision surgery, usually to a long-stemmed prosthesis. This requires the additional operative approach proximally through the subscapularis. Fractures at or distal to the tip usually occur at 45 degrees. Closed treatment of these fractures has been shown to have a higher rate of nonunion or malunion than operative fixation. Stiffness becomes a prominent feature with delays in motion while the fracture attempts to heal with the nonoperative approach. Therefore, my preferred technique is internal fixation using allograft strut supports prepared from a tibia or femur (Fig. 32-26). The struts are placed well proximal and distal to the fracture site and are secured with cables (Figs. 32-27 and 32-28). When the fracture site is exposed for this additional extramedullary fixation, the radial nerve falls posteriorly with the soft tissue (Fig. 32-29). It is protected by elevating all soft tissue about the fracture subperiosteally, beginning with the anterior aspect of the fracture site. This is a vital point in avoiding a serious complication for experienced as well as occasional surgeons operating in this difficult area. With this extended deltopectoral

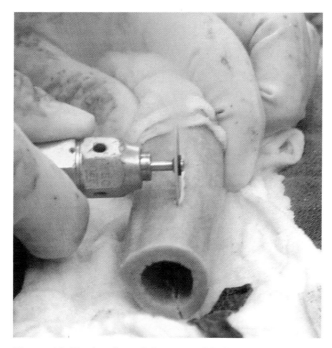

Figure 32-26. An allograft femur or tibia is split into longitudinal struts for secure fixation of a periprosthetic fracture with or without exchanging the humeral component.

approach, the fracture site always is approached on the anterior aspect of the humerus away from the path of the radial nerve. Beginning at the fracture or nonunion site, subperiosteal elevation of the muscles and/or scar will permit adequate exposure without endangering the radial nerve. This also will ensure that the radial nerve is not incorporated into the cable or allograft fixation, because all fixations can be safely applied to bone without soft-tissue interposition. Motion may begin as soft-tissue swelling decreases. One may advance stretch-

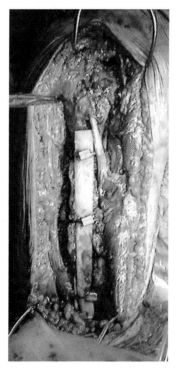

Figure 32-27. The allograft struts are secured with Dall-Miles cables. Supplemental allograft with bone morphogenic protein is packed in the gaps and at the ends of the struts.

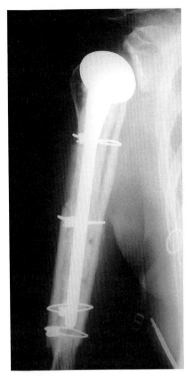

Figure 32-28. The cable–strut support for the fractures provides excellent fracture fixation for healing and permits early motion for better function.

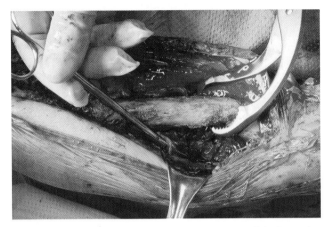

Figure 32-29. The radial nerve is exposed safely from the periprosthetic fracture site when the muscles are elevated from the deltopectoral approach.

ing when the fracture site is thought to have sufficient healing. This is usually by 3 to 4 months (Figs. 32-30 and 32-31).

The three situations that may require humeral revision of a well-fixed component include a periprosthetic fracture in a patient with advanced glenohumeral arthritis, humeral malposition (Fig. 32-32), or glenoid component loosening. In these cases, it is often advisable to

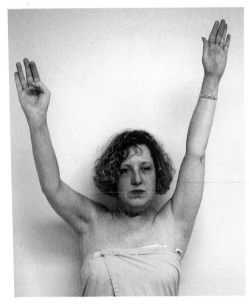

Figure 32-30. Elevation progresses at 4 months after the periprosthetic fracture reconstruction.

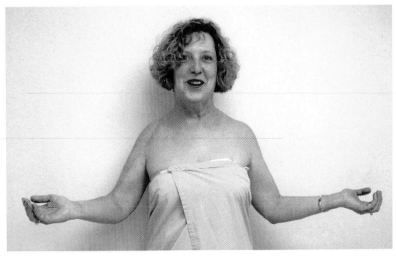

Figure 32-31. External rotation is regained with the early exercises permitted by the periprosthetic fracture reconstruction.

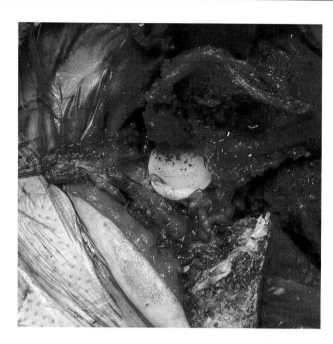

Figure 32-32. Revising a malpositioned humeral stem for glenoid wear and loosening resulted in fractures of the tuberosities.

revise the humeral component to a longer stem with cables. The glenoid is replaced at the same time for glenoid arthritis and replaced or bone-grafted for glenoid loosening.

COMPLICATIONS

The treatment of infection, as with other joint replacements, depends on the chronicity of the infection, the virulence of the organism, and medical condition of the patient. Some acute infections with low-virulence organisms can be treated with a simple incision and

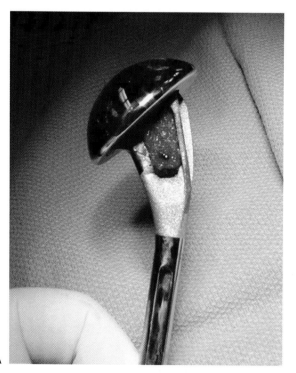

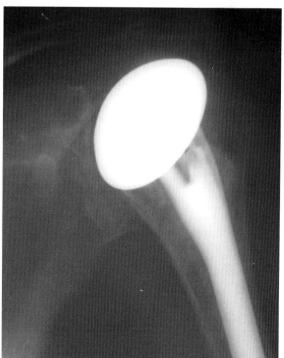

Figure 32-33. **A:** A fracture prosthesis with bone graft facilitates tuberosity healing. Its low-profile design facilitates placement in revisions when the greater tuberosity can be left intact and facilitates tuberosity repair when necessary. **B:** The fracture prosthesis is used as a revision prosthesis for its low profile with allograft bone in the opening.

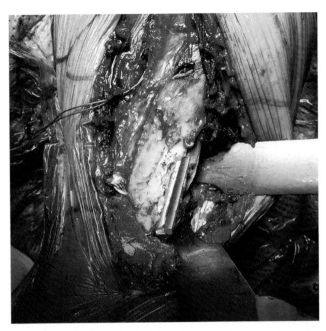

Figure 32-34. An undesirable option was chosen in the prior revision surgery in which the prosthetic stem was malpositioned in varus to avoid prior cement and the greater tuberosity. The stem protruded through shaft, was cut off, but was still painful.

drainage. Most infections, however, are chronic and thus require implant removal, extensive débridement, and selective antibiotic treatment. It is important to remove all foreign material, including all cement, from the primary procedure and to obtain good cultures before giving the antibiotics. The preferred treatment for most chronic infections is a secondary exchange 12 weeks after placing an antibiotic-impregnated cement spacer. Some authors have advocated using a primary-exchange technique using antibiotic-impregnated cement for low-virulence organisms.

Intraoperative complications during humeral stem removal may include a greater tuberosity fracture (Fig. 32-27). Although it is preferable to avoid this if possible, when it occurs, take advantage of the increased exposure to the glenoid for revision, bone grafting, and capsular releases, and proceed as if reconstructing a fracture case. Allograft bone with bone morphogenic protein is added to the construct (Fig. 32-28). The low profile of this prosthesis without the posterior keel now makes it my ideal choice for revision cases to get under the tuberosities that have not fractured (Fig. 32-33). When fractured, the greater tuberosity is fixed around the prosthetic stem. Meticulous care is taken to cement the humeral stem distally and out to length. Any cement at the fracture site is avoided or removed. With this method, one can avoid placing the prosthesis in varus, which could then perforate more distally through the humeral shaft (Fig. 32-34). The occurrences that I have seen of this were most uncomfortable.

POSTOPERATIVE MANAGEMENT

Postoperative care for most revisions consists of early passive motion as well as active-assisted motion if possible. Active motion must be delayed for most fractures and cases requiring rotator cuff repair. In addition, the subscapularis must be treated gently by delaying active exercises after multiple operations to avoid dehiscence. Although rehabilitation is dictated by the individual case, our most common protocol for revisions is to permit protected passive motion for 6 weeks, advance to active assisted motion for an additional 6 weeks, and begin gentle active motion at 3 months. In these cases, nothing is gained by in-

stituting early active exercises. Where tuberosity fractures are involved, the trend has been to protect the shoulder for 3 to 4 weeks with a sling before starting any passive motion. Since tuberosity dehiscence is the greatest problem in the fracture reconstruction, this additional protection has proved beneficial in lowering the rate of this complication by 50%.

RESULTS

The results of the most common revision, namely converting a humeral head arthroplasty to a TSR for glenoid arthritis, have generally shown improvement. Unfortunately, the procedures are not without risks and complications. The motion is seldom as good as a primary total shoulder, and the risks of nerve injury and infection increase with each revision. Sperling and Cofield's (14) report dispels the common misconception that one can easily convert a failed HHR to a TSR; hence, their good advice is to do the best operation the first time. Presently, the total shoulder revision rates are much lower than those for HHRs.

One of the best advances in prosthetic fracture treatment has been the avoidance of unpolished holes in the humeral fin for tuberosity fixation. This was advocated early on by Neer and Kirby (9) and was recently reinforced by Boileau et al. (1) when it reduced the tuberosity dehiscence by 50%. Traditionally, more than 50% of the fracture complications are attributable to complications of the greater tuberosity. This one technical point dramatically reduces the complications responsible for many poor results in prosthetic fracture reconstruction.

The results after revisions for glenoid loosening favor replacing the glenoid for pain relief and motion. Unfortunately, because osteolysis and early loosening are often silent before extensive bone destruction, adequate bone is not present for glenoid replacement in most cases. Less predictable pain relief occurs when the glenoid requires grafting. In the first 80 cases for conversion, four have been revised back to a total shoulder at 6 to 12 months for inadequate pain relief.

Results of revisions for instability fare well for posterior instability with few recurrences. Anterior instability results diminish when the subscapularis cannot be retrieved and more extensive transfers or allografts are required. Anterosuperior escape or instability denotes a massive cuff deficiency. Rerepair of the cuff is seldom effective. The reverse prosthesis holds great promise and has 17 years' experience in Europe with many international peer-review articles to support its emerging role as it awaits FDA approval in the United States. Until then, it is performed on a more limited basis as a custom procedure or with an investigational device exemption study sanctioned by the FDA.

RECOMMENDED READING

1. Boileau, P., Coste, J.S., Ahrens, P.M., et al.: Prosthetic shoulder replacement for fracture: results of the multicenter study. In: *2000 shoulder prostheses . . . 2 to 10 year follow-up.* Montellier, France: Sauramps Medical, 561–578, 2001.
2. Campbell, J.T., Iannotti, J.P., Norris, T.R., et al.: Periprosthetic humeral fractures: mechanisms of fracture and treatment options. *J Shoulder Elbow Surg* 7: 406–413, 1998.
3. Cofield, R.H., Edgerton, B.C.: Total shoulder arthroplasty: complications and revision surgery. *Inst Course Lect* 39: 449–462, 1990.
4. Gartsman, G.M., Roddey, T.S., Hammerman, S.M.: Shoulder arthroplasty with and without glenoid resurfacing for patients with osteoarthritis. *J Bone Joint Surg Am* 82(1): 26–34, 2000.
5. Gunther, S.B., Graham, M.S., Norris, T.R., et al.: Retrieved glenoid components: a classification system for surface damage. *Arthroplasty* 17(1): 95–100, 2002.
6. Klimkiewicz, J.J., Iannotti, J.P., Rubash, H.E., et al.: Aseptic loosening of the humeral component in total shoulder arthroplasty. *J Shoulder Elbow Surg* 7(4): 422–426, 1998.
7. Levine, W.N., Djurasovic, M., Glasson, J.M., et al.: Hemiarthroplasty for glenohumeral osteoarthritis: results correlated to degree of glenoid wear. *J Shoulder Elbow Surg* 6(5): 449–454, 1997.
8. Lynch, N.M., Cofield, R.H., Silbert, P.L., et al.: Neurologic complications after total shoulder arthroplasty. *J Shoulder Elbow Surg* 5(1): 53–61, 1996.
9. Neer, C.S. II, Kirby, R.M.: Revision of humeral head and total shoulder arthroplasties. *Clin Orthop* 170: 189–195, 1982.
10. Norris, T.R.: Complications of proximal humerus fractures: diagnosis and management. In: Iannotti, J.P., Williams, G.R. Jr., eds.: *Disorders of the shoulder: diagnosis and management.* Philadelphia: Lippincott, Williams & Wilkins, 687–708, 1999.

11. Norris, T.R., ed.: *Orthopaedic knowledge update: shoulder and elbow,* 2nd ed. Rosemont, IL: American Shoulder and Elbow Surgeons, American Academy of Orthopaedic Surgeons , 2003.
12. Norris, T.R., Lipson, S.R.: Management of the unstable prosthetic shoulder arthroplasty. In: *Instructional course lectures.* Rosemont, IL: American Academy of Orthopaedic Surgeons, 47: 141–148, 1998.
13. Petersen, S.A., Hawkins, R.J.: Revision of failed total shoulder arthroplasty. *Orthop Clin North Am* 29(3): 519–533, 1998.
14. Sperling, J.W., Cofield, R.H.: Revision total shoulder arthroplasty for the treatment of glenoid arthrosis. *J Bone Joint Surg Am* 80(6): 860–867, 1998.
15. Walch, G., Boileau, P., eds.: *Shoulder arthroplasty.* Berlin: Springer-Verlag, 1999.
16. Wirth, M.A., Rockwood, C.A. Jr.: Complications of total shoulder replacement arthroplasty. *J Bone Joint Surg Am* 78: 603–616, 1996.

33

Shoulder Arthrodesis

Robin R. Richards

INDICATIONS/CONTRAINDICATIONS

Shoulder arthrodesis can effectively restore function to patients with specific shoulder disorders. Patient selection is important in determining whether the procedure will be beneficial. Where a choice is possible, shoulder arthroplasty is preferable to shoulder arthrodesis, because arthrodesis results in the sacrifice of all glenohumeral rotation through the glenohumeral joint. Shoulders can be fused if an arthroplasty fails, although fusion in this situation is a technical challenge.

Paralysis of Both Deltoid and Rotator Cuff Muscles

Experts agree that the presence of a flail shoulder is an indication for shoulder arthrodesis. Patients with anterior poliomyelitis, those with irreparable proximal root and upper trunk brachial plexus lesions, and some with isolated axillary nerve paralysis are candidates for shoulder arthrodesis. These patients often prefer to keep the arm in a sling to relieve discomfort and avoid injuring it. In a patient with the prerequisite good function in the periscapular musculature, particularly the trapezius, levator scapula, and serratus anterior, glenohumeral arthrodesis successfully stabilizes the extremity and allows effective hand function. A flail shoulder can also result in painful subluxation or instability that can be improved by arthrodesis (Fig. 33-1).

Doi et al. (5) reported on restoration of prehension with the double free-muscle technique following completion avulsion of the brachial plexus and noted that secondary reconstructive procedures, such as arthrodesis of the carpometacarpal joint of the thumb, shoulder

R. R. Richards, M.D., F.R.C.S.C.: Department of Surgery, University of Toronto; and Sunnybrook and Women's College Health Sciences Centre, Toronto, Ontario, Canada.

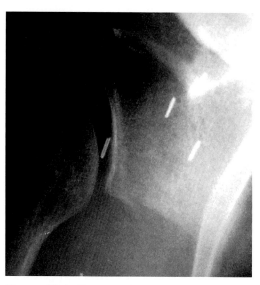

Figure 33-1. Preoperative radiograph demonstrates periarticular osteopenia and inferior subluxation of the humeral head.

arthrodesis, and tenolysis of the transferred muscle and the distal tendons were sometimes required to improve the functional outcome.

Axillary Nerve Paralysis

There is wide variability in the disability caused by axillary nerve paralysis. While muscle transfers may be available in carefully selected patients, and other patients may function quite well without any deltoid function, if there is significant limitation of shoulder function due to paralysis of the axillary nerve, arthrodesis should be considered.

Reconstruction after Tumor Resection

En bloc resection of periarticular malignant tumors often requires sacrifice of the rotator cuff, the deltoid, or both. In such a shoulder reconstruction, arthroplasty may be difficult. In some instances, arthroplasty with bone or soft-tissue allograft may be considered. However, arthrodesis is often a good solution for tumor reconstruction.

Infection of the Glenohumeral Joint with Painful Incongruity

Although total shoulder replacement may be considered if the history of infection is remote, active or recent infection is better handled with a shoulder arthrodesis.

Failed Total Shoulder Replacement

Although resection arthroplasty or revision may be considered if the patient is young, if there is history of infection or if the bone stock is adequate, arthrodesis should be considered as a salvage procedure.

Failure of Previous Repairs for Shoulder Instability, Particularly Multidirectional Instability

Occasionally, after multiple repairs, a patient will present with uncontrollable shoulder instability, particularly global laxity and multidirectional instability. If attempts at soft-tissue stabilization were satisfactory but there is still symptomatic uncontrollable instability, shoulder arthrodesis should be considered as a means to stabilize the shoulder, particularly when secondary osteoarthritic changes have begun to develop. These patients, however, may continue to experience problems and may not function at as high a level as other patients undergoing arthrodesis.

Failed Rotator Cuff Surgery, Especially if Accompanied by Deltoid Inadequacy or Excessive Acromial Excision

The combination of a massive rotator cuff deficiency, deltoid insufficiency, and an acromial excision is virtually insolvable with repeated rotator cuff surgery and is often associated with the development of secondary osteoarthritic change in the glenohumeral joint. Glenohumeral arthrodesis may provide these patients with a comfortable arm and glenohumeral stability, particularly if the patient is sufficiently symptomatic to exchange the loss of glenohumeral motion for the relief of pain.

Contraindications

Shoulder arthrodesis should be reserved for those situations that are not amenable to reconstruction by any other means. Many patients are amenable to arthroplastic reconstruction that preserves glenohumeral motion and has greater potential to restore function (4). The primary contraindications to shoulder arthrodesis include a progressive neurologic disorder with paralysis of the trapezius, levator scapula, and serratus and a contralateral shoulder arthrodesis. In addition, because shoulder arthrodesis requires a major effort by the patient to rehabilitate the shoulder, this procedure is contraindicated in a patient who cannot cooperate with such a program. I have not performed shoulder arthrodesis on elderly patients for this reason.

Alternative Techniques

The author's practice is limited to the treatment of adults. In pediatric patients, where it is desirable to preserve growth, alternative surgical techniques to that described in this chapter may be considered. For instance, Mohammed (11) reported on the use of a Rush pin introduced from the spine of the scapula through the glenoid into the medullary canal of the humerus to perform shoulder arthrodesis. Mohammed supplemented this fixation with tension-band wiring from the acromion to the neck of the humerus and a muscle pedicle graft attached to the acromion. Furthermore, a shoulder spica was applied for 4 to 6 weeks. Mohammed used this method on four patients with upper brachial plexus injuries and found that it did not affect bone growth in young patients, was effective in patients with osteoporosis, and gave a high rate of union. Kocialkowski and Wallace (8) reported on the use of an external fixator to obtain shoulder arthrodesis.

PREOPERATIVE PLANNING

The typical patient requiring shoulder arthrodesis complains of flail shoulder, symptomatic instability, and inability to use the elbow or hand because the shoulder cannot be stabilized. Unless there is a severe brachial plexus injury involving paralysis more distally, the functioning of the elbow and hand is often remarkably good. Examination of the shoulder may reveal atrophy of the deltoid or of the infraspinous or supraspinous fossae. The humeral head may be subluxated inferiorly at rest. Often there is excessive mobility of the humeral head in the glenoid. In the absence of glenohumeral arthritis, the range of passive motion is often normal, especially in those patients undergoing arthrodesis for paralysis. Muscle testing reveals weakness of internal and external rotators of the shoulder, and weakness or paralysis of the deltoid muscle. In those patients who present for tumor reconstruction, failure of prior rotator cuff or instability surgery, failed arthroplasty, or distant glenohumeral joint infection, the physical examination is usually specific for those conditions. Standard radiographs ordered are anteroposterior, lateral, and axillary views of the glenohumeral joint, giving the surgeon information about the presence or absence of arthritis, any developmental abnormalities of the shoulder, and the adequacy of bone stock if internal fixation is to be used in the surgical arthrodesis. Occasionally, if the neurologic condition of the shoulder girdle muscles is in doubt, an electromyogram of the deltoid, rotator cuff, or scapular muscles may be indicated.

Before shoulder arthrodesis, preparations by the patient, the operating room staff, and the hospital's rehabilitation personnel are necessary. Patients require some understanding of the operative technique and some insight into how glenohumeral arthrodesis can improve function and increase motion in the presence of a flail shoulder. The concept of the procedure is difficult for many patients. The most practical way to help them understand is to have them speak to a patient who has undergone the procedure. I attempt to provide the patient with the name of a former patient of the same sex, a similar age, and a similar diagnosis.

Shoulder arthrodesis requires a full set of the usual shoulder surgery instruments. In addition, pelvic reconstruction plates are used together with fully threaded cancellous screws. Plate-bending devices are required to contour the plate to the specific local anatomy of the individual patient. Curved osteotomes are used for decorticating the surfaces of the glenoid and humeral head and the undersurface of the acromion. Decortication of both the acromial humeral and the glenohumeral surfaces to increase the surface area available for arthrodesis is helpful in achieving solid arthrodesis. The operating room table must be adjustable so that the patient may be placed in a semisitting position intraoperatively. Although there are numerous methods for stabilization of a shoulder arthrodesis, the most popular method today is probably the AO technique with either a single plate or double plate.

Postoperative management requires the use of a thermoplastic orthosis appliance suspended from the opposite shoulder, although Riggins (17) has reported, from a small series of patients, that external immobilization is not needed after shoulder arthrodesis with plate fixation. In our institution, these appliances are custom-made for each patient and this can be a time-consuming task. Accordingly, the rehabilitation personnel must be aware of the anticipated postoperative requirements of the patient in advance. It is sometimes expeditious to construct the thermoplastic orthosis appliance on the afternoon before or on the morning of surgery so that only minor adjustments are needed in the immediate postoperative period. This can be helpful in reducing patient discomfort.

SURGERY

Patients are anesthetized in the supine position in the operating room (Fig. 33-2). The skin is shaved from the midline posteriorly to the midline anteriorly down to the elbow laterally. It is not necessary to shave the axilla. The patient is pulled proximally on the operating room table and shifted to the edge of the table on the affected side. A folded sheet is placed medial to the scapula to elevate it from the table. The head is placed on a donut. A footrest is secured to the bottom of the table. The table is adjusted to the semisitting position. The arm and shoulder are prepped to the midline.

The drapes are applied so that there is unrestricted access to the area of the scapula and anterior chest wall. The arm is draped free (Fig. 33-3). The skin incision is marked out and the dermis incised (Fig. 33-4). The subdermal plexus is infiltrated throughout the length of the incision with 1:500,000 adrenaline in saline (subject to approval by the anesthesiologist) to reduce bleeding from the skin.

The skin and subcutaneous tissue are incised down to the fascia throughout the length of the incision (Fig. 33-5). The spine of the scapula is exposed first by cautery and then by subperiosteal dissection (Fig. 33-6). The incision extends from the angle of the acromion to the anterior acromion. The deltoid is reflected from the acromion both medially and laterally so that wide exposure of the proximal humerus is obtained.

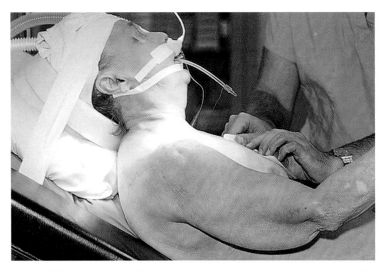

Figure 33-2. The patient is semisitting on the operating room table. The head is supported by a donut, and a folded sheet has been placed medial to the scapula to elevate it from the surface of the table. The distal portion of the incision is visible as it extends along the lateral aspect of the humerus. The incision travels distally in the deltopectoral groove. The deltoid can be split, if paralyzed, to facilitate exposure.

Distally, the deltopectoral interval is developed and the coracobrachial fascia incised. The biceps tendon is tenodesed in the biceps groove with a Bunnell-type suture of no. 1 braided polyester material. The rotator cuff is resected from the level of the subscapularis anteriorly to the level of the teres minor posteriorly. The muscle–tendon units are divided using cautery. Homan retractors are placed posterior to the glenoid, and the humeral head is retracted posteriorly. A ³⁄₈-in. curved osteotome or burr is used to resect or decorticate the glenoid joint surface, and the glenoid labrum is removed (Fig. 33-7).

The retractors are removed and the humeral head is brought anteriorly (Fig. 33-8). A ¹⁄₂-in. curved osteotome or burr is used to resect the articular surface of the humerus in its entirety (Fig. 33-9). It is often possible to remove the cartilage of the humeral head en bloc using this technique. The undersurface of the acromion is resected with a ³⁄₄-in. curved osteotome. Care is taken not to fracture the base of the acromion. The arm is flexed 30 degrees, abducted 30 degrees, and internally rotated 30 degrees so that, with elbow flexion,

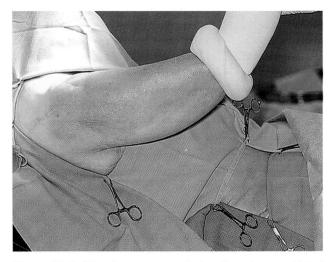

Figure 33-3. The drapes are applied so there is unrestricted access to the scapula, upper arm, and anterior chest wall. The arm is free draped.

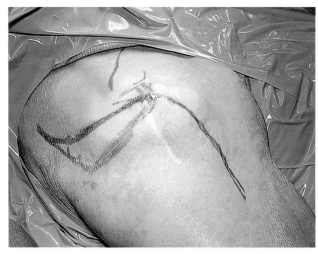

Figure 33-4. Superior view showing incision site extending from the spine of the scapula, over the acromion, and laterally along the humerus.

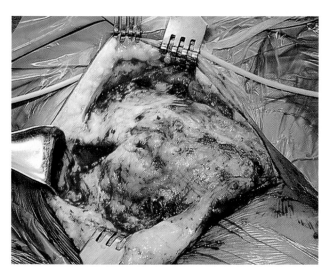

Figure 33-5. The skin and subcutaneous tissue are incised down to fascia throughout the length of the incision.

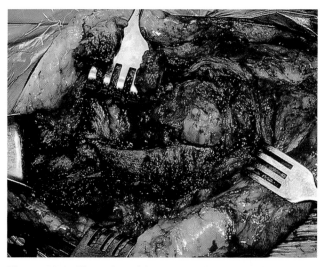

Figure 33-6. The spine of the scapula is exposed first by cutting cautery and then by subperiosteal dissection.

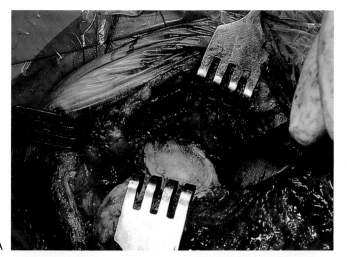

A

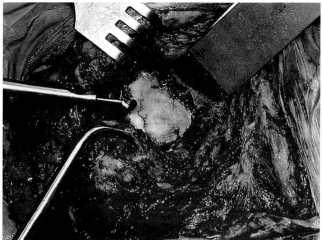

B

C

Figure 33-7. A: The humeral head is retracted posteriorly, exposing the glenoid. **B:** For glenoid cartilage resection, a ³⁄₈-in. curved osteotome or burr is used to resect or decorticate the glenoid joint surface. **C:** Labrum is removed and the glenoid joint surface completely decorticated.

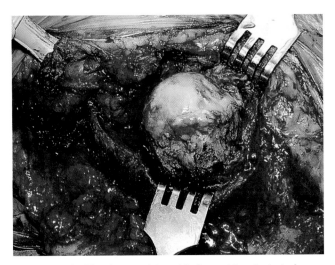

Figure 33-8. The humeral head is brought anteriorly in anticipation of cartilage resection.

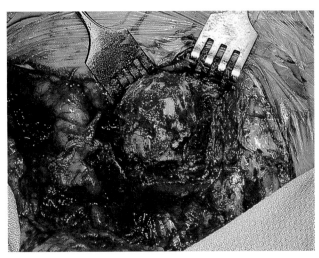

Figure 33-9. A burr or curved osteotome is used to remove articular surface of the humerus in its entirety.

the hand reaches the mouth (Fig. 33-10). The humerus is brought proximally to appose the decorticated undersurface of the acromion (Fig. 33-11). Folded sheets are placed between the thorax and the extremity, and an assistant standing on the opposite side of the table maintains this position throughout the application of internal fixation to the shoulder. A ten-hole, 4.5-mm pelvic reconstruction plate is contoured to run along the spine of the scapula, over the acromion down onto the shaft of the humerus (Fig. 33-12). It is necessary to bend the plate between the third and fourth holes and to contour it so that it lies comfortably along the zenith of the greater tuberosity, and then to contour it so that it is closely applied to the humeral shaft (Fig. 33-13).

With the arm held in the proper position and the plate held against the scapula and the humerus, a hole is drilled through the plate, through the humerus, and into the glenoid, using a 3.2-mm drill bit. The screw length is measured and is usually between 65 and 75 mm. The humeral cortex is tapped with a 6.5-mm tap. A short-thread cancellous screw is then inserted as a lag screw into the glenoid to apply compression to the arthrodesis site (2). Two more holes are drilled in a similar fashion. It is important that these screws be inserted first to obtain initial stability and to provide compression at the arthrodesis site (Fig. 33-14). At this point, the position of the arm is checked once again.

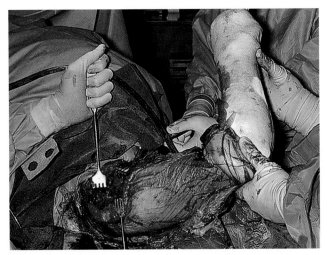

Figure 33-10. With the arm draped free, the position for arthrodesis can be determined. The arm is flexed 30 degrees, abducted 30 degrees, and internally rotated 30 degrees, so that with elbow flexion, the hand reaches the mouth.

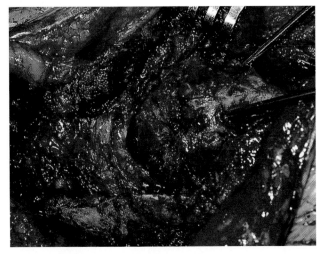

Figure 33-11. The humerus is brought proximally to appose the decorticated undersurface of acromion and medially to appose the decorticated surface of the glenoid.

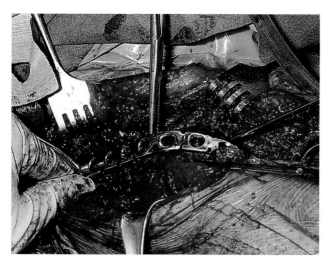

Figure 33-12. A pelvic reconstruction plate (ten-hole, 4.5-mm) is contoured to run along the spine of the scapula, over the acromion, and down onto the shaft of the humerus.

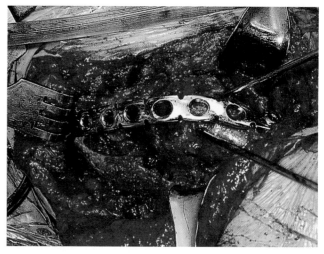

Figure 33-13. It is usually necessary to bend the plate between the third and fourth holes to increase the precision of the contour.

The remaining holes are then filled. Proximally, along the spine of the scapula, it is usually possible to place two or three screws. These screws can be fully threaded, cancellous screws if the scapula is osteoporotic. It is usually necessary to leave one screw hole empty as the plate crosses the acromion and extends down onto the shaft of the humerus. The distal screws are usually cortical screws.

After insertion of all the screws, they are individually tightened to obtain maximal purchases. At this point, the wound is thoroughly irrigated. Hemostasis is checked and closure begins. Two ⅛-in. suction drains are placed beneath the deltoid. The deltoid is carefully reattached, and an effort is made to cover as much of the plate as possible with the deltoid. Although most patients undergoing shoulder arthrodesis have extensive deltoid atrophy, coverage of the plate with the atrophic deltoid tissue is important from both a cosmetic and a functional perspective (Fig. 33-15). Skin closure is routine.

In the operating room, a pillow is placed between the arm and the chest. The arm is then wrapped to the chest with a swathe. The patients are allowed to ambulate on the evening of surgery. A thermoplastic orthosis is applied on the day after surgery and is adjusted as nec-

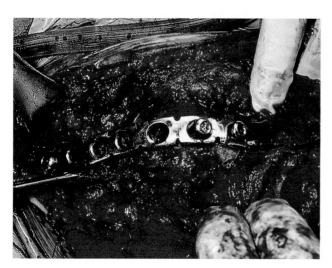

Figure 33-14. The lag screws from the plate into the glenoid are inserted first to apply compression to the arthrodesis site. Following this, the position of the arm is checked once again.

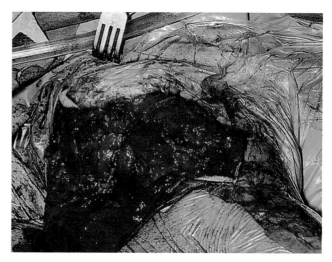

Figure 33-15. Despite the usual amount of atrophy, the deltoid is carefully reattached and an effort made to cover as much of the plate as possible.

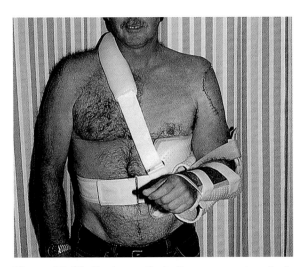

Figure 33-16. Postoperatively the upper extremity is supported by a thermoplastic orthosis. The orthosis may be constructed the day prior to surgery and the final adjustments made the day after surgery. The patient can remove the orthosis to bathe. This is typically worn for 6 weeks postoperatively.

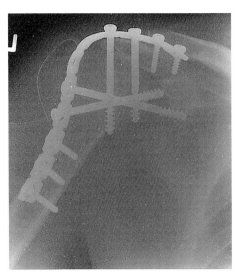

Figure 33-17. Radiograph 8 months postoperatively reveals a successful glenohumeral joint arthrodesis.

essary (Fig. 33-16). Patients are usually discharged from the hospital on the second or third postoperative day. Blood loss can be brisk during surgery at the time of joint surface resection, although bleeding usually decreases significantly once the first few screws have been placed and the arthrodesis becomes more stable. Most patients do not require a blood transfusion.

The patients are housed on the orthopaedic floor. Intensive care is not necessary. A radiograph is obtained in the recovery room to ensure that screw placement is satisfactory. Better radiographs are obtained within the first 24 to 48 hours, depending on the patient's condition. The patients are reviewed 10 to 14 days after surgery, at which time their staples or sutures are removed. A radiograph is not taken at this time. The next review is at 6 weeks when a radiograph is taken without the use of a splint. At this point, particular attention is paid to the internal fixation. The use of the brace is discontinued if there is no sign of loosening of the internal fixation. It is usually impossible to determine radiographically at 6 weeks whether or not union has occurred. Usually at this point, trabeculae are not seen crossing the arthrodesis site and the fixation is sufficiently rigid that external callus is not seen. Three months postoperatively, another radiograph is obtained. If the internal fixation remains intact, active range-of-motion exercises are initiated, concentrating, for obvious reasons, on thoracoscapular mobilization. Radiographs are taken periodically until union is sound (Fig. 33-17).

POSTOPERATIVE MANAGEMENT

The surgeon should carefully explain to the patient preoperatively the intent of the operation, and the limitations and gains in function that are likely to result from a successful glenohumeral arthrodesis. The successful surgery eliminates glenohumeral joint motion and thus all internal and external rotation. All movement of the shoulder comes from the thoracoscapular motion and is usually about one third of normal. After successful arthrodesis, the patient can usually reach the mouth, opposite axilla, belt buckle, and side pocket. The patient cannot reach or work overhead, cannot reach the back pocket or a bra strap, and rarely chooses to sleep on the fused side. Perineal care is often very difficult using the fused shoulder. The patient should also be told about the possible development of scapula fatiguing or pain and postoperative aching, and that the scapula may be prominent when the arm hangs by the side. The surgeon should also inform the patient about the possibility of pseudarthrosis, which reportedly occurs in up to 10% of patients, and that reoperation may be necessary to remove prominent hardware or internal fixation.

Rehabilitation

Patients are instructed to perform exercises to remobilize the hand, wrist, and elbow, until review at 3 months following surgery when further radiographs are taken. If there is no sign of loosening, physical therapy is prescribed with specific, shoulder-elevation exercises that maximize thoracoscapular motion. Once improvement in thoracoscapular motion plateaus, resistive exercises are added. If an elbow flexorplasty was performed at the same time as shoulder arthrodesis, rehabilitation is directed toward restoration of this function as well.

The rehabilitation process is slow following shoulder arthrodesis. The stress placed on the thoracoscapular musculature is significant, and patients require a great deal of adaptation to compensate for the loss of shoulder rotation. In many patients, a recovery period from 6 to 12 months is to be expected.

COMPLICATIONS

Groh et al. (7) reported that the most common complication of shoulder arthrodesis is malposition followed by nonunion, wound problems, and fractures occurring in relation to internal fixation devices. I have also observed thoracic outlet syndrome and pain after achievement of shoulder arthrodesis.

Malunion

Malunion can be avoided by the careful application of rigid internal fixation, the use of a splint postoperatively, and careful attention to positioning the patient intraoperatively. Thirty degrees of forward flexion brings the greater tuberosity directly beneath the acromion and this position must be maintained during the application of internal fixation. The most common error is to allow the arm to drift into too much internal rotation so that, with elbow flexion, the hand does not reach the mouth. The assistant maintaining the position of the extremity must do so with vigilance and must recognize the importance of this assignment.

When internal fixation is used, the position maintained in the operating room is, in general, the position maintained as union proceeds. We have not observed breakage, bending, or pullout of the internal fixation device, although this theoretically could occur. Furthermore, if internal fixation is not used, the extremity is free to change position and drift during the time required for solid arthrodesis to occur. Pruitt et al. (14) reported that excessive abduction or forward flexion should be avoided following arthrodesis and that the position of arthrodesis is not as important as the stability gained following the procedure.

Nonunion

Nonunion is rare following shoulder arthrodesis. Of 69 patients who have undergone the procedure, we have had three with nonunion. The low nonunion rate is probably a result of the mobility of the scapula, the use of internal fixation, the excellent vascularity of the periscapular tissues, and the use of a protective orthosis postoperatively. Stark et al. (21) performed 15 shoulder arthrodeses using plate fixation and only used abduction pillow immobilization following the surgery. Thirteen of 15 patients went on to unite without additional intervention.

We do not routinely perform bone grafting. If delayed union or nonunion does occur, the internal fixation should be revised and an iliac crest bone graft used. We have successfully obtained union in the three patients who did not unite, primarily by the use of bone grafting. When arthrodesis is performed in the presence of significant bone loss, as seen following failed total shoulder arthroplasty, bone grafting should be used primarily. It is not necessary, in my opinion, to use bone graft routinely.

Infection

Infection is rare following shoulder arthrodesis. We have had one postoperative infection, which required local drainage. The infection did persist, however, and did not resolve until the internal fixation device was removed after union was assured. If infection does occur following shoulder arthrodesis, the fixation should be left in place as long as it is holding firmly, and the infection should be treated by a drainage procedure.

Humeral Fracture

The presence of internal fixation does place the patient at risk for incurring a fracture of the distal humerus. We have observed two such fractures. Both fractures occurred at the distal end of the plate used for internal fixation. In one patient, the fracture occurred when he was arrested, in an inebriated state. His fracture was treated by open reduction and internal fixation. The same patient subsequently refractured his humerus while running from the police. The second patient sustained a fracture of the humerus at the end of the plate when he fell, in an inebriated state, directly onto his arm. This fracture was treated by application of a spica cast. In retrospect, these two complications were due to poor patient selection. Nevertheless, fracture of the humerus at the end of the plate remains one of the complications for the procedure.

Thoracic Outlet Syndrome

Shoulder arthrodesis places significant stress on the thoracoscapular musculature. If patients do not participate in a vigorous program of trapezius-strengthening exercises, the shoulder can droop and a thoracic outlet syndrome can develop. Two of our patients have undergone first rib resections at other institutions for thoracic outlet syndrome following shoulder arthrodesis. They remain symptomatic, and it is my belief and experience that most patients will respond positively to a physiotherapy program aimed at increasing the muscular reserve of their shoulder elevators. Accordingly, surgical treatment would be reserved for the most recalcitrant cases of thoracic outlet syndrome.

Pain

Most patients who undergo shoulder arthrodesis do so as part of a program of surgical rehabilitation following irreparable brachial plexus injury. All patients with brachial plexus injuries have a combination of sensory disturbance, motor dysfunction, and pain. Shoulder arthrodesis does not relieve neurogenic pain, although it can relieve the pain associated with glenohumeral subluxation due to paralysis. Patients should not undergo a shoulder arthrodesis with the expectation of total pain relief if neurogenic pain is present preoperatively. Our experience has demonstrated that pain is very much related to the preoperative diagnosis. Patients with osteoarthritic problems and pain due to glenohumeral instability secondary to neuromuscular weakness experience good pain relief following the surgery, although Vastamaki (22) reported that rotation of the shoulder is limited following arthrodesis and that some pain can persist following the procedure, if it is performed for arthrosis.

Patients with diagnoses such as refractory multidirectional instability who have pain of obscure origin do not experience complete pain relief following the procedure. Our approach to patients with pain has been to attempt to maximize the function in their extremity and to avoid the use of analgesic medication, transcutaneous electrical nerve stimulation units, and surgical modalities aimed purely at decreasing pain. It is our experience that most patients will tolerate their discomfort much better if they can effectively use their upper extremity.

RESULTS

Ruhmann et al. (20) compared function following transfer of the trapezius muscle to shoulder arthrodesis. Mean abduction was 36.4 degrees (range, 20 to 80 degrees) and forward flexion was 31.9 degrees (range, 10 to 90 degrees) following trapezius transfer. Following shoulder arthrodesis, mean abduction was 59.3 degrees (range, 40 to 90 degrees) and forward elevation was 50.7 degrees (range, 30 to 90 degrees). The authors concluded that shoulder fusion was more suitable for those patients who required the best possible function and strength in the shoulder.

Despite the advent of total shoulder arthroplasty, a role remains for shoulder arthrodesis that is heavily dependent on the preoperative diagnosis. The procedure is indicated only for specific diagnoses. The technique described offers a high fusion rate and a relatively low complication rate. The use of a thermoplastic orthosis postoperatively decreases morbidity and, together with plate fixation, probably reduces the nonunion rate. Shoulder arthrodesis deserves a role in the armamentarium of every shoulder surgeon.

RECOMMENDED READING

1. Beaton, D.E., Dumont, A., Mackay, M.B., et al.: Steindler and pectoralis major flexorplasty: a comparative analysis. *J Hand Surg* 20: 747–756, 1995.
2. Charnley, J., Houston, J.K.: Compression arthrodesis of the shoulder. *J Bone Joint Surg Br* 46: 614–620, 1964.
3. Clare, D.J., Wirth, M.A., Groh, G.I., et al.: Shoulder arthrodesis. *J Bone Joint Surg Am* 83: 593–600, 2001.
4. Cofield, R.H., Briggs, B.T.: Glenohumeral arthrodesis. *J Bone Joint Surg Am* 61: 668–677, 1979.
5. Doi, K., Muramatsu, K., Hattori, Y., et al.: Restoration of prehension with the double free muscle technique following complete avulsion of the brachial plexus: indications and long-term results. *J Bone Joint Surg Am* 82: 652–666, 2000.
6. Freidman, R.J., Ewald, F.C.: Arthroplasty of the ipsilateral shoulder and elbow in patients who have rheumatoid arthritis. *J Bone Joint Surg Am* 69: 661–666, 1987.
7. Groh, G.I., Williams, G.R., Jarman, R.N., et al.: Treatment of complications of shoulder arthrodesis. *J Bone Joint Surg Am* 79: 881–887, 1997.
8. Kocialkowski, A., Wallace, W.A.: Shoulder arthrodesis using an external fixator. *J Bone Joint Surg Br* 73: 180–181, 1991.
9. Macdonald, W., Thrum, C.B., Hamilton, S.G.: Designing an implant by CT scanning and solid modelling: arthrodesis of the shoulder after excision of the upper humerus. *J Bone Joint Surg Br* 68: 208–212, 1986.
10. Makin, M.: Early arthrodesis for a flail shoulder in young children. *J Bone Joint Surg Am* 59: 317–321, 1977.
11. Mohammed, N.S.: A simple method of shoulder arthrodesis. *J Bone Joint Surg* 80: 620–623, 1998.
12. Neer, C.S. II, Craig, E.V., Fukuda, H.: Cuff tear arthropathy. *J Bone Joint Surg Am* 65: 416–419, 1983.
13. Neer, C.S. II, Watson, K.C., Stanton, F.J.: Recent experience in total shoulder replacement. *J Bone Joint Surg Am* 64: 319–337, 1982.
14. Pruitt, D.L., Hulsey, R.E., Fink, B., et al.: Shoulder arthrodesis in pediatric patients. *J Pediatr Orthop* 12: 640–645, 1992.
15. Richards, R., Sherman, R.M., Hudson, A.R., et al.: Shoulder arthrodesis using a modified pelvic reconstruction plate: a review of eleven cases. *J Bone Joint Surg Am* 70: 416–421, 1988.
16. Richards, R.R., Waddell, J.P., Hudson, A.R.: Shoulder arthrodesis for the treatment of brachial plexus palsy. *Clin Orthop* 198: 250–258, 1985.
17. Riggins, R.S.: Shoulder fusion without external fixation. *J Bone Joint Surg Am* 58: 1007–1008, 1976.
18. Rockwood, C.A., Burkhead, W.Z.: The management of patients with massive rotator cuff defects by acromioplasty and radical cuff debridement. Presented at: The Orthopaedic Associations of the English-Speaking World. Washington, D.C., May 8, 1987.
19. Rowe, C.R., Pierce, D.S., Clark, J.G.: Voluntary dislocation of the shoulder: a preliminary report on a clinical, electromyographic and psychiatric study of twenty-six patients. *J Bone Joint Surg Am* 55: 445–460, 1973.
20. Ruhmann, O., Gosse, F., Wirth, C. J., et al.: Reconstructive operations for the paralyzed shoulder in brachial plexus palsy: concept of treatment. *Injury* 30: 609–618, 1999.
21. Stark, D.M., Bennett, J.B., Tullos, H.S.: Rigid internal fixation for shoulder arthrodesis. *Orthopaedics* 14: 849–855, 1991.
22. Vastamaki, M.: Shoulder arthrodesis for paralysis and arthrosis. *Acta Orthop Scand* 58: 549–555, 1987.

Subject Index

Page numbers followed by an "f" indicate figures; those followed by a "t" indicate tables.